Guide to
NURSING MANAGEMENT AND LEADERSHIP

The Latest *Evolution* in Learning.

Evolve provides online access to free learning resources and activities designed specifically for the textbook you are using in your class. The resources will provide you with information that enhances the material covered in the book and much more.

Visit the Web address listed below to start your learning evolution today!

▶ **LOGIN:** *http://evolve.elsevier.com/Marriner/guide/*

Evolve Learning Resources for Guide to Nursing Management and Leadership, 7th Edition, offers the following features:

- **Case Studies**
  Chapter-specific case studies demonstrate the practical application of the content presented.

- **Critical Thinking Activities**
  These activities and worksheets not only provide a practical application of content but strengthen comprehension and retention as well as serve as a valuable study tool.

- **WebLinks**
  An exciting resource that lets you link to hundreds of websites carefully chosen to supplement the content of the textbook. The WebLinks are regularly updated, with new ones added as they develop.

Think outside the book...*evolve*.

Guide to
NURSING MANAGEMENT AND LEADERSHIP

Seventh Edition

Ann Marriner Tomey, RN, PhD, FAAN
Professor
Indiana State University School of Nursing
Leadership and Management Consultant
Terre Haute, Indiana

Mosby
An Affiliate of Elsevier

An Affiliate of Elsevier

11830 Westline Industrial Drive
St. Louis, Missouri 63146

NOTICE

Nursing is an ever-changing field. Standard safety precautions must be followed, but as new research and clinical experience broaden our knowledge, changes in treatment and drug therapy may become necessary or appropriate. Readers are advised to check the most current product information provided by the manufacturer of each drug to be administered to verify the recommended dose, the method and duration of administration, and contraindications. It is the responsibility of the licensed prescriber, relying on experience and knowledge of the patient, to determine dosages and the best treatment for each individual patient. Neither the publisher nor the author assumes any liability for any injury and/or damage to persons or property arising from this publication.

Previous editions copyrighted 2000, 1996, 1992, 1988, 1984, 1980.

Library of Congress Cataloging-in-Publication Data

Marriner Tomey, Ann, 1943-
    Guide to nursing management and leadership/Ann Marriner-Tomey—7th ed.
        p.; cm.
    Includes bibliographical references and index.
    ISBN 0-323-02864-0
    1. Nursing services–Administration. 2. Leadership. I. Title: Nursing management and leadership. II Title.
    [DNLM: 1. Nursing, Supervisory. 2. Decision Making. 3. Leadership. 4. Personnel Management–methods. WY 105 M359g 2004]
    RT89.3.M37 2004
    362.17'3'068–dc22   2003065699

Senior Editor: Tom Wilhelm
Associate Developmental Editor: Jennifer Anderson
Publishing Services Manager: Catherine Jackson
Project Manager: Anne Gassett Konopka
Design Manager: Bill Drone

Printed in the United States of America.

Last digit is the print number: 9   8   7   6   5   4   3   2   1

To
H. Keith Tomey

Reviewers

Janice Boundy, PhD, MSN, RN
Professor, Director Graduate Program
Saint Francis College of Nursing
Peoria, Illinois

Deborah Kumer Coltrane, MSN, RN
Faculty Leadership and Management
Waynesburg College
Waynesburg, Pennsylvania
Director of Marketing
Pocket Nurse
Pittsburgh, Pennsylvania

Mary Ann Henriquez, PhD, RN
Instructor of Nursing
Mississippi College School of Nursing
Clinton, Mississippi

Merry McBryde-Foster, PhD, RN, CCM
Assistant Professor
Louis Herrington School of Nursing
Baylor University
Dallas, Texas

Larry Purnell, PhD, RN, FAAN
Professor
Department of Nursing
College of Health and Nursing Sciences
University of Delaware
Newark, Delaware

Charlotte Stephenson, DSN, MSN, MRE, BS, RN
Professor, Academic Coordinator
Mississippi College School of Nursing
Clinton, Mississippi

Christine Wynd, PhD, RN, CNAA
Professor of Nursing and Director of the PhD in Nursing Program
The University of Akron College of Nursing
Akron, Ohio

Preface

Guide to Nursing Management and Leadership is designed to teach nursing students about the management process and leadership and to supply the practicing nurse with practical information about nursing administration. The first edition was written during the 1970s, when nursing education emphasized clinical skills at the expense of managerial expertise and nurses who were interested in leadership and management had to turn to other disciplines. Now there are many books and journals about nursing leadership and management. The first edition was *Guide to Nursing Management*. It was organized around the management process—plan, organize, staff, direct, and control as the conceptual framework.

The rapid changes during the 1980s, with the increase in better-educated personnel and increased technology to handle management functions, brought about a focus on leadership, which was reflected in *Guide to Nursing Management and Leadership* in 1996. Continuous quality improvement, cost containment, free market competition, managed care, technology, increasing diversity, more focus on ethical issues, and the need for teams and transformational leadership were dominant during the 1990s, requiring a major transformation of the book for 2000. The book was then divided into two major sections: leadership and management. The content was refocused.

For the seventh edition, ethics, diversity, technology, and legal issues have been integrated into several chapters. Protection from workplace violence, bioterrorism, sources and categories of law, continuum of multiorganizational arrangements, disease management, demand management, private management companies, cultural imposition and imperialism, generational differences, character development, the Health Insurance Portability and Accountability Act (HIPAA), employment-at-will, COBRA, and liability issues have been added. Age, culture, and gender diversity; delegation; decision-making models; creativity techniques; ethics; emotional intelligence; politics; negotiation; mediation; arbitration; leadership; budgeting; variance reporting; recruitment and retention; staffing; and continuum of care have been expanded. I have added a new feature—Research Perspective boxes—to illustrate the findings of current research in the leadership and management field.

Also new to this edition is the Evolve website, providing course management software, weblinks keyed to each chapter, and student-generated frequently asked questions with answers from the author. The website provides students and faculty with continually updated information, numerous resources for additional study through the Internet, and interaction with the authors. Critical thinking activities, case studies, work sheets and bibliographies are also included on the website.

I have used literally hundreds of articles and books for the transformation of this edition. The assistance provided by numerous individuals in the University Library has been most helpful. Faculty at the Information Desk readily answered my questions and guided me to appropriate resources. Staff in the Interlibrary Loan unit did an outstanding job of retrieving numerous requested materials within my timelines. Also supportive and attentive to my needs was the staff at the Check-Out, Reserves, and Periodicals Desks. I cannot forget the behind-the-scenes staff who classify materials and maintain the collections, making it possible for all patrons to find the sources they need. I would like to express my appreciation to the following library staff: Information Desk: Melody Allison, Renee Englund, Ralph Gabbard, Steve Hardin, David Kaunelis, Christopher Mehrens, Judy Tribble, and Wilma Turetzky; Periodicals Desk: Tasha Hayne, John Lunceford, and Lee Walls; Check-Out/ Reserves/Interlibrary Loan Desks: Michael Boswell, Alberta Comer, JoAnn Hayden, Shirley Risley, Rebecca Stinnett, and Nancy Watkins; and Cataloging: Sally Baker, Cheryl Bealmear, Brian Clark, Debbie Considine, Valentine Muyumba, Karen Passen, Chris Robinson, Debra Taylor, and Carol Vanatti. I thank Betsy Hine for her leadership in information and library services and others such as student assistants who are too numerous to mention. I also want to thank my loving husband, H. Keith Tomey, for enriching my private life while supporting my professional activities and for helping me maintain balance.

Ann Marriner Tomey

Contents

Guide to

NURSING MANAGEMENT AND LEADERSHIP

PART ONE

LEADERSHIP

1

Communications

*"He who influences the thought of his times
influences the times that follow."* —Elbert Hubbard

Chapter Overview

Chapter 1 describes the communication process, communication
systems, barriers to communications, ways to improve communications,
communicating with difficult people, assertiveness, transactional analysis,
and life positions.

Chapter Objectives

- List the six steps in the communication process.
- List at least six barriers to communication.
- Formulate ways to improve communication.
- Describe how to deal with hostile-aggressive people.
- Plan strategies for dealing with a sniper.
- Describe how to handle complainers.
- List barriers to assertiveness.
- Diagram complementary transactions.
- Analyze crossed transactions.
- Describe three games people play.
- Compare the four life positions.
- Identify and stipulate at least three assertive techniques, and discuss how to
  use them.

Major Concepts and Definitions

Communication giving and receiving information via talk, gestures, writing, and so forth
Ideation decision to share an idea
Encoding putting meaning into symbols
Transmission sending the message
Receiving seeing and hearing a transmitted message
Decoding defining words and interpreting gestures
Feedback an evaluative response
Grapevine informal communication system
Informal communications casual, not according to prescribed ways
Formal communications according to prescribed rules
Verbal spoken
Nonverbal not spoken; body language, tone of voice, facial expressions, posture, gestures, pauses
Assertiveness the quality of being confident in stating one's opinions or needs
Transactional analysis a technique for analyzing discussions
Life positions an individual's assumptions about self in relation to others
Passive inactive, acted on
Aggressive active, bold, pushy
Broken record a technique involving repeating what one wants
Fogging agreeing with the truth
Negative assertion accepting negative aspects about oneself
Negative inquiry asking for more information about oneself

COMMUNICATION PROCESS

All the manager's functions involve communication. The communication process involves six steps:

$$\text{Ideation} \rightarrow \text{Encoding} \rightarrow \text{Transmission}$$
$$\text{Response} \leftarrow \text{Decoding} \leftarrow \text{Receiving} \leftarrow$$
$$\rightarrow \text{Encoding} \rightarrow \text{Transmission} \rightarrow \text{Receiving}$$
$$\text{Response} \leftarrow \text{Decoding} \leftarrow$$

The first step, ideation, begins when the sender decides to share the content of a message with someone, senses a need to communicate, develops an idea, or selects information to share. The purpose of communication may be to inform, persuade, command, inquire, or entertain. Whatever the reason, the sender needs to have a goal and think clearly or the message may be garbled and meaningless.

Encoding, the second step, involves putting meaning into symbolic forms: speaking, writing, or nonverbal behavior. One's personal, cultural, and professional biases affect the goals and encoding process. Use of clearly understood symbols and communication of all the information that the receiver needs to know are important.

The third step, transmission of the message, must overcome interference such as garbled speech; unintelligible use of words; long, complex sentences; distortion from recording devices; noise; and illegible handwriting.

Receiving is next. The receiver's senses of seeing and hearing are activated as the transmitted message is received. People tend to have selective attention (hear the messages of interest to them but not others) and selective perception (hear the parts of the message that conform to what they want to hear), which cause incomplete and distorted interpretation of the communication. Sometimes people tune out the message because they anticipate the content and think they know what is going to be said or are so busy formulating their response that they do not hear the message. The receiver may be preoccupied with other activities and consequently not be ready to listen. Poor listening is one of the biggest barriers in the communication process.

Decoding of the message by the receiver is the critical fifth step. The receiver defines words and interprets gestures during the transmission of speech. Written messages allow more time for decoding while receivers assess the explicit meaning and implications of the message based on what the symbols mean to them. The symbols are subject to interpretation based on one's personal, cultural, and professional biases and may not have the same meaning to the receiver as to the sender. The communication process depends on the receiver's understanding of the information.

Response, or feedback, is the final step. It is important for the manager or sender to know that the message has been received and accurately interpreted.

BASIC COMMUNICATION SKILLS

"The real art of communication is not only to say the right thing at the right place but to leave unsaid the wrong thing at the tempting moment."
—Dorothy Nevill

One can *ensure understanding* by *assuming value, clarifying,* and *confirming* and can then *enhance the value* by *identifying the merits, building* on the expressed ideas, and *balancing* the merits and concerns. One should *support* by expressing appreciation and being specific (*Advanced Executive Leadership Skills,* 1981).

Ensuring understanding is facilitated by *assuming value, clarifying,* and *confirming. Assuming value* is an attitude that the person is worth listening to that opens lines of communication so one can understand what the other person thinks

and feels. It helps one understand what the other person is saying and why and increases the chances that the other person will listen in return. *Clarification* is used when one is not sure what the other person is saying by asking a specific question such as "What do you mean when you say…," by making a statement such as "I don't understand what you mean," or by expressing open-ended interest by comments such as "and then?" *Confirmation* is used when one thinks there is understanding about what was said and why by checking for understanding and confirmation from the other person that one's understanding is accurate. Repeating what was said indicates one heard what was said but does not necessarily mean one understands. Saying "I understand what you said" indicates one thinks she understands what the other person said, but her understanding may not be the same as the speaker's. Stating one's understanding of what the speaker said and why is a more accurate way of confirming.

Enhancing value differs from criticism by *identifying the merits, building,* and *balancing* instead of rejecting the other's ideas and actions. We often criticize by telling others what we do not like about their ideas, what is wrong, and what will not work. That leads to demoralization, defensiveness, and oppressed innovation. We may be more effective if we do not criticize.

To *enhance value, identify the merits* mentally and ask yourself if you can improve on the idea or action without mentioning concerns. If yes, *build* by specifying the merits verbally and adding value. A merit is anything you like about what the other person said or did or what you want the person to keep doing despite the need for change. A merit may be a part of an idea, a good intention, an important issue that was addressed, or part of an action. If you have difficulty identifying merit, you can ensure understanding by asking people the value to their idea or act. Most people have good intentions. You can often enhance value by specifying the merits and suggesting slight refinement or changes by suggesting another way to reach the goal without mentioning your concerns. If a merit you have identified can be used as an example of what you want, the change you suggest is an alternative to reaching the goal, or if the person is not strongly committed to the previous idea or act, you can build by suggesting a minor change or refinement. Specify the merits verbally, add value by suggesting a refinement, and check back to confirm that the other person thinks that action is acceptable.

However, if the person asks you for an evaluation or needs to know what is wrong to be able to make necessary changes or if the situation requires a major change, you need to *balance.* You specify the merits and concerns, ask for suggestions or reaction, and check back. Invite suggestions after you identify the merits and your concerns to get the person involved in finding a solution, to get commitment to one's own ideas, and to get the other person's ideas instead of a confirmation of your ideas. Do not invite suggestions unless you do consider them or you think the person needs to know your ideas for the discussion. After you have invited and received suggestions, give your reaction, confirm or clarify, give another itemized response, and ask for the other person's response.

Supporting promotes cooperation by giving timely and specific feedback about the positive aspects of another's ideas or efforts and by acknowledging the value of the other's contributions to you and others. Most people need recognition for their efforts and accomplishments. There is a direct relationship between support given and cooperation. Less time is wasted if others know what is important to you. However, there are several reasons people are reluctant to support others. Some fear being perceived as weak or insecure, do not see a connection between giving and receiving, or fear generalization for a specific accomplishment to other situations. It is appropriate when someone shows the first signs of improvement or meets minimum requirements not usually met, meets the basic requirements, or exceeds minimum requirements. Give support by expressing appreciation. Be specific to provide recognition, prevent others from misunderstanding your intent, prevent others from thinking you like everything, make your support believable, and let others know you pay attention to what they are doing. By mentioning personal qualities, you reinforce those qualities and earn goodwill and support. By mentioning how others' accomplishments are important to you, you help them know that their efforts make a difference and are valued, make them feel more important, and increase their desire to continue contributing.

COMMUNICATION PRINCIPLES

De Ann Gillies (1994, p. 187) identifies some communication principles. The effectiveness of various media differs with educational level, with less educated people relying more on aural and pictorial media and more educated people relying more on print. People with low self-esteem are more easily influenced by persuasive communications than are people with high self-esteem. People are more likely to hear messages that are compatible with their expectations and are more likely to listen to messages on topics about which they have read. The more trustworthy the speaker, the less manipulative she is perceived to be. Majority opinion is more effective in changing attitudes than expert opinion.

METHODS OF COMMUNICATION

David Whetten and Kim Cameron (1998) present a five *s*'s approach to effective oral and written presentations: *strategy, structure, support, style,* and *supplement.* The strategy develops the purpose for the specific audience and occasion. The structure translates the strategy into specific content. Examples and illustrations are used to support or reinforce ideas. Style, or the way ideas are presented, is as important as the ideas expressed. Supplement means to give informed responses to challenges and questions related to the presentation.

Strategy involves identifying the general and specific purposes, understanding the needs and attitudes of the audience, and designing the message for the audience. The speech should be audience centered. More formal situations call for more formal presentations, whereas informal situations allow for slang. Both sides of issues should be presented if the audience is uncommitted or hostile.

Structure begins with a forecast of the main ideas to capture audience members' attention and give them a reason to listen or read. It gives the audience an outline of the message, making it easier for audience members to follow the presentation. Simple to complex, familiar to unfamiliar, and old to new are some ways to structure a presentation. Only a few main points should be made, transitions should be made among main points, and the presentation should end on a high note, calling for action or creating a good feeling.

Support from evidence and visual aids helps establish credibility. It is advisable to use a variety of supports and to keep visual aids simple and effective to aid comprehension and retention.

Style for oral communications involves preparing notes; practicing the presentation with the visual aids; and planning to engage the audience through use of eye contact, physical space, and body movement. Style for written communications involves mechanical and factual precision. Tone is related to word choice and should be adjusted to the formality of the situation. The proper format for the business letter, memo, proposal, or paper should be used.

Supplement the presentation by responding to challenges and questions by being prepared to answer questions in a specific format. First restate the objection. Then state your position. Offer support for your position, and speak to the impact of adopting your position.

USE OF COMPUTERS FOR COMMUNICATION

Word processing is commonly used and allows electronic writing, revising, storing, and printing of documents. *Spreadsheet software* allows manipulation of information in columns and rows as in accounting and allows writing, editing, graphing, storing, and printing of the data. *Database software* collects and catalogs information so that lots of well-organized data can be located and displayed. *Graphic software* allows use of clip art, icons, silhouettes, and line drawings to enhance written communications, whereas *presentation software* creates visual aids such as overheads and slides for oral presentations. *Electronic mail (e-mail)* allows users to send messages instantaneously using one-on-one interchanges, or e-mail can connect staff throughout an organization at one or many sites. It can get information, including graphics and sound, to listservs and newsgroups. *Voice mail* answers the telephone automatically, plays a message, and accepts and stores voice messages. *Calendar and scheduling software* in conjunction with e-mail allows networked users to access each other's schedules. The software can identify common free time and immediately book a meeting. *Chat rooms* can be used for exchange of written messages in real time without having to find a physical location for a meeting. Much committee work can be done asynchronously through e-mail. The *World Wide Web* links computers around the world and is a major source of information (Kreider and Haselton, 1997).

Health care providers have a professional, legal, and ethical obligation to protect patient information. Confidentiality, by disseminating information only to authorized individuals or organizations that have a need to know, is a major issue. Most confidentiality violations involve fired workers or other insiders motivated by blackmail, curiosity, humiliation, or revenge. Breaches of confidentiality may also be unintentional disclosures, uncontrolled secondary usage such as for marketing, and unauthorized access such as use of another's password (Saba and McCormick, 2001). Telehealth also raises issues of confidentiality and reimbursement of health services across state lines and quality of care. Major challenges are keeping

RESEARCH Perspective 1-1

Data from Alexander JW, Kroposki M: Using a management perspective to define and measure changes in nursing technology. *Journal of Advanced Nursing* 35(5), 776-783.

Purpose: The purpose of this study was to discuss the uses of the concept of technology from the management and medical science perspectives; to prepare a definition of nursing technology; and to present a study applying the use of the concept of nursing technology on nursing units.

Methods: A longitudinal study was done to measure the dimensions of nursing technology on nursing units 10 years apart. The 1980 and 1990 means scores on the technology dimensions for all the units were compared using *t*-tests. Of the 14 units used in both tests, four had significant changes in one or more of the technology dimensions. The four were a medical unit, two surgical units, and a labor and delivery unit.

Results/conclusions: The findings suggest that the dimensions of nursing technology change over time and support the need for nurse managers to assess nursing technology periodically before making changes on the unit.

costs down while maintaining quality of care and privacy and confidentiality of data (Ball, Hannah, Newbold, et al, 2000).

COMMUNICATION SYSTEMS

Study of small-group process has revealed various communication networks (Figure 1-1). The chain system is fast and accurate for simple problems. The middle person in the chain emerges as the leader, and the leadership position is stable. Unfortunately, morale is low, and so is the flexibility for problem solving.

The leader emerges at the location of highest centrality, which is the fork of the Y and the hub of the wheel. Both provide fast, accurate problem solving. The coordinator, who is centrally located, is generally satisfied, but the peripheral

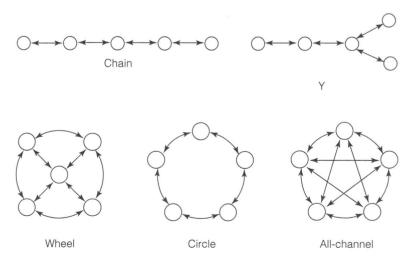

Figure 1-1 Communication systems: chain, Y, wheel, circle, all-channel.

members are less satisfied than members in less efficient systems. The wheel is an efficient, effective communication structure for simple problems.

The circular structure is slow and inaccurate. The structure does not influence the emergence of a leader. Because no one can communicate with everyone, there is no coordinator. However, morale is high, and there is considerable flexibility for problem solving.

When free to do so, groups tend to evolve to the all-channel network as problems become complex and shift back to a wheel structure as problems become simple. Greater amounts of information must be processed as task uncertainty and complexity increase. Consequently, an adaptive structure such as the all-channel system is best for completing complicated and unpredictable tasks. Essentially the right network is the structure that facilitates the communication necessary to accomplish the task.

DOWNWARD COMMUNICATION

The traditional line of communication is from the manager down through the levels of management (Figure 1-2). This downward communication is primarily directive and helps coordinate the activities of different levels of the hierarchy by telling staff associates what to do and by providing the information needed by staff associates to relate their efforts to the organization's goals. It includes oral and written indoctrination, education, and other information to influence the attitudes and behaviors of staff associates. Common forms of downward communications are employee handbooks, operating manuals, job description sheets, performance appraisal

interviews, employee counseling, a loudspeaker system, letters, memos, messages circulated with paychecks, posters, bulletin boards, information racks, company newspapers, annual reports, the chain of command, the grapevine, and unions. Downward communication contributes to greater staff associate dissatisfaction than upward communication, regardless of the quality of the message (Sullivan and Decker, 2001).

UPWARD COMMUNICATION

Newer management techniques encourage delegation of authority and more personal involvement in decision making, thus creating a need for accurate upward communication (Figure 1-3). Upward communication provides a means for motivating and satisfying personnel by allowing employee input. The manager summarizes information and passes it upward to the next level for use in decision making. That level then summarizes its action and transmits information to the next level. Because each level tends to bias the report by embellishing it with information that puts that level in the best light, there is a natural filtering process as information moves upward. By the time it reaches top management, it is highly refined.

In spite of this bias, staff associates are often in a position to assess the situation more accurately than are their managers. An employee may have a better solution to a problem than the first-line manager, who may know more about a situation than a middle manager, and so on. Consequently, accurate upward communication is important for effective problem solving. Staff associates must feel free to communicate both

Figure 1-2 Downward communication.

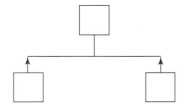

Figure 1-3 Upward communication.

solicited and unsolicited information upwardly and must have opportunity to do so, or management will lack needed information and both managers and staff associates will become frustrated. Common means for upward communication include face-to-face discussions; open-door policies; staff meetings; task forces; written reports; performance appraisals; grievance procedures; exit interviews; attitude surveys; suggestion boxes; counseling; the chain of command; ombudsmen; informers; the grapevine; unions; and participative, consultative, and democratic management in general.

LATERAL COMMUNICATION

Lateral, or horizontal, communication is between departments or personnel on the same level of the hierarchy and is most frequently used to coordinate activities (Figure 1-4). The need for lateral communication increases as interdependence increases. For instance, it becomes more important when one worker starts a job and someone else finishes it. It is also used by staff to transmit technical information to line authorities, and it may contain subjective and emotional aspects. Committees, conferences, and meetings are often used to facilitate horizontal communication.

DIAGONAL COMMUNICATION

Diagonal communication occurs between individuals or departments that are not on the same level of the hierarchy (Figure 1-5). Informal in nature

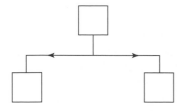

Figure 1-4 Lateral communication.

and frequently used between staff groups and line functions and in project types of organizations, it is another facet of multidirectional communication that is common when communications often flow in all directions at the same time.

THE GRAPEVINE

Informal methods of communication coexist with formal channels and are referred to as the grapevine. Informal communication is often rapid and subject to considerable distortion. The grapevine transmits information much faster than the formal channels because it uses cluster chain pathways involving three or four individuals at a time instead of going from one person to another as in manager-staff associate relationships. Communication passes at an increasing rate as individuals from clusters inform other small groups of people who work near each other or have contact with each other. Information spreads most quickly through the grapevine when it is recent, affects personnel's work (for example, pay increases or changes in policies),

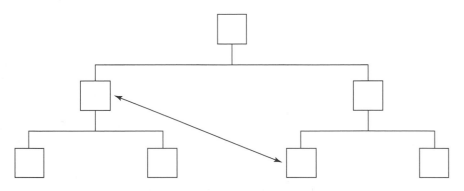

Figure 1-5 Diagonal communication.

and involves people they know. People who work near each other or come in contact with each other are likely to be on the same grapevine.

Information becomes distorted for a number of reasons. Grapevine information is often fragmentary and incomplete. Consequently, there is a tendency to supply the missing pieces. Some people seize this opportunity to express feelings of self-importance, thus compensating for feelings of insecurity but also distorting the message. Because the grapevine is informal, with no formal lines of accountability, individuals do not have to answer to their manager for misinforming others.

Managers can learn much by listening to the grapevine and can remedy distortions by using the informal channels to pass on correct information.

BARRIERS TO COMMUNICATION

"No man has a good enough memory to be a successful liar." —Abraham Lincoln

Thomas Gilovich (1991) indicates that misperception and misinterpretation of random data, misinterpretation of incomplete and unrepresentative data, biased evaluation of ambiguous and inconsistent data, seeing what we want to see, believing what we are told, and imagined agreement of others are *How We Know What Isn't So*.

Faulty reasoning and poorly expressed messages are major barriers to communication. Lack of clarity and precision resulting from inadequate vocabulary, poorly chosen words, platitudes, jargon, awkward sentence structures, poor organization of ideas, and lack of coherence are common. Talking too quickly or too slowly, slurring words, and not emphasizing important points lead to the faulty transmission of ideas. Memos that are poorly organized, ramble, and lack summaries also complicate the communication process. Words mean different things to different people. Communication is complicated when the sender uses words with which the

receiver is not familiar, does not communicate on the receiver's level, or makes the message long and complicated.

If senders lack information or omit facts they do know, they will pass on a distorted or filtered message. Filtering, whether intentional or unintentional, involves a biased choice of what is communicated. For instance, distortion is more likely when subordinates desire promotion, since they may pass on information about their merits and suppress less successful aspects of their work. Fear of the consequences of full disclosure contributes to such omissions. At other times individuals may not communicate some information because they do not believe it is important enough to do so. The receiver becomes confused when nonverbal cues such as facial expressions and posture conflict with the verbal communication or when the sender does not admit to the intent of, or to the emotions underlying, the message.

People use selective perception to hear what they want to hear in terms of their biases. Values, attitudes, and assumptions affect one's perception of the message. Making a value judgment about the worth of a message based on one's opinion of the sender or the expected meaning of the message allows the receiver to hear what she wants to hear. An attitude is a feeling toward someone or something that is based on experience or the lack thereof, and it is a common barrier to communication because of its screening effect.

Uncommunicated assumptions are common and can make a considerable difference between the message sent and the one received. For instance, when program evaluation is mandated, personnel may fear that the results will be used to terminate workers, whereas management's actual intention is to use the results for recruiting purposes. Trust or distrust of the sender also influences how the message is received.

The sender is judged along with the message because the receiver has difficulty separating what she hears from how she feels about the sender. In fact, nonexistent motives can be attributed to the sender. Messages from higher echelons are often considered authoritative, even when they are not intended to be. The higher in the hierarchy a message originates, the greater are its chances of being accepted because of the status of the sender. If the sender has status with the listener, the message is usually considered credible. If the sender does not, the message may be discounted.

Staff associates tend to pay attention to communications from managers, thus facilitating downward communication. Unfortunately, managers may give verbal and nonverbal cues about how busy and unapproachable they are. They probably value communications from higher-level managers more than those from staff associates and may not reward associates for communications. In fact, staff associates are sometimes punished for communicating. Staff associates will be reluctant to report problems or potential problems when they believe these will be viewed as a weakness in their performance appraisal. Similarly, middle managers may not report problems that would reflect unfavorably on their managerial skills.

Status symbols magnify role and status barriers by increasing the psychological distance and the perceived organizational distance. Time pressures also become barriers that prevent communication. Managers do not have time to see all their staff associates as much as desired, and staff associates may not take the time to report to the manager. Time pressures are also used as an excuse for not listening. Premature evaluation of what is going to be said, preoccupation with oneself, lack of readiness to hear, lack of receptivity to new ideas, and resistance to change interfere with listening. Physical distance, organizational complexity, temperature, noise, physical facilities (such as offices, meeting rooms, and an informal coffee shop), and technical facilities (such as telephones, loudspeakers, and duplicating equipment) also affect communications.

GENDER DIFFERENCES

Deborah Tannen (2001) indicates that women talk about their problems at length, whereas men want to find a solution or laugh them off. Women do rapport-talk, whereas men do report-talk. Women tend to be more talkative than men, initiate turn taking, make more frequent interruptions of others' comments, ask most of the questions, keep the conversations going, and use a larger vocabulary (Douglas, 1996). In *Men Are from Mars, Women Are from Venus,* John Gray (1992) indicates that men want to reason, whereas women want to be heard and validated. When stressed, men become focused and withdrawn, whereas women become emotionally involved and overwhelmed. Women have difficulty supporting a man who is not talking, whereas men have difficulty listening to women without giving advice.

Four stylistic modes of verbal communication between genders have been identified as follows (DeYoung, 2003):

1. Direct versus indirect style with males characterized as relatively direct, open, straightforward, and honest and females characterized as relatively indirect, ambiguous, tactful, and face saving
2. Succinct versus elaborative style with males characterized as succinct and using elliptical sentences ("great movie") whereas females are more elaborative and use metaphors, similes, and flowery expressions
3. Personal versus contextual style with males using the role-centered contextual style and females using the personal style stressing equality
4. Instrumental versus affective style with males using instrumental style with reference to quality and females using affective style focusing on people's emotions

CULTURAL DIFFERENCES

Culture is a learned pattern of beliefs, customs, language, norms, and values that is shared by a group of people. How that learned pattern of behavior is expressed distinguishes cultures from each other. Cross-cultural communication involves having respect for, tolerance of, and nonjudgmental attitudes toward people with different attitudes, behaviors, and values; obtaining knowledge of other cultures; and being sensitive to cultural differences. One should assume differences until similarity is indicated, emphasize description rather than evaluation and interpretations, and treat interpretations as working hypotheses to be tested.

Cross-cultural communication occurs when someone from one culture correctly understands a message sent by someone from another culture. Cross-cultural miscommunication occurs when someone from the second culture misinterprets the sender's message. No two people have exactly the same cultural background, so every communication is somewhat intercultural. The greater the cultural differences, the greater the communication challenges and probability that the message sent will not be the message received. As attitudes, behaviors, and values are shared, people change and the cultural process continues (Douglas, 1996; Hein, 1998).

Stereotypes form expectations regarding how strangers will act and influence the way we process information. We tend to remember more favorable information about in-groups and less favorable information about out-groups. Then our processing of information is biased in the direction of maintaining our preexisting belief systems. That produces cognitive confirmation of our stereotypes. Our stereotypes are automatically activated when we contact strangers, and we unconsciously try to confirm our expectations when we communicate with them. Rigidly held inaccurate or negative stereotypes can lead to misunderstandings and inaccurate predictors of others' behaviors. Although our stereotypes of in-groups are more accurate than our stereotypes of out-groups, we tend to assume that people in a group are more alike than they really are. Consequently even valid stereotypes can cause misinterpretations of the behaviors of atypical group members. Our stereotypes of others can influence their views of themselves. The more traits included in our stereotype of a group that group members have of themselves, the more accurate our predictions of their behavior (Gudykunst, 1998).

To form supportive environments in order to work better with others, we should be descriptive rather than judgmental, define mutual problems and express a willingness to find a solution collaboratively, be spontaneous instead of strategic, express empathy to show concern for others' welfare, treat others as equals, be open to different viewpoints, and be willing to experiment with other behaviors (Gudykunst, 1998). Through conversations, we can celebrate a togetherness by building something that is "ours" (Casmir, 1997).

IMPROVING COMMUNICATION

Ideas should be clear before one speaks. What is the purpose of the message? Is it to seek information, inform, persuade, or initiate action? To formulate a message, one must gather the information needed and seek consultation from others as appropriate. Considering the goals and attitudes of the receivers helps the sender convey something of help or value to the receivers. One must also determine the mode of communication—by written or oral messages or through gestures. Face-to-face contact involves nonverbal behavior that further clarifies intent and allows for feedback to validate understanding of the message. Feedback through mutual exchange decreases the chance for misunderstanding. A climate that allows people to say what they think facilitates feedback.

One must also consider the setting in which one communicates and time one's messages for maximal impact. Should the communication be made in public or private? What is the social climate, and what effect will that have on the tone of the communication? What are the customs and practices of the audience, and how does one's message conform to its expectations? It is helpful for the message to refer to something the person has experienced and for it to be timed for immediate use by the receiver. For example, a building evacuation plan will be better received during fire prevention week, when personnel are expecting a fire drill, than at most other times.

Communications should be well organized and expressed in simple words, a clear style, and the shortest sentences possible. Redundancy— the repetition of the message verbatim or its presentation in several different ways—ensures that the message is understood. The amount of redundancy depends on the content of the message and the experience and background of the receiver. Repetition is especially important when the information is important and the directions are complicated. However, redundancy can become a barrier to communication if the message is simple and personnel are familiar with it. Employees are likely to stop listening because they know what is going to be said.

Because actions speak louder than words, the message is more forceful if the sender acts congruously. Communications should be followed up to make sure they were understood, and one should seek to understand as well as to be understood.

Listening, an active process that requires conscious attention, is critical to good communication. Trust is a prerequisite, because nurses will not share feelings with people they do not trust. The speaker must be convinced that disclosures will be kept confidential, that feelings will be respected and not judged, and that the information will be used appropriately and not used against the speaker.

Once trust is established, empathetic listening is needed. We think faster than we talk. Consequently, when listening to another person talk, we have time left over for thinking, time that is frequently misused. There is less time for irrelevant thoughts when one concentrates on what is being said. One can think ahead of the speaker, try to guess the points that will be made next, consider what the conclusion will be, listen between the lines, try to understand the speaker's point of reference, review, and summarize the points made.

Active listening involves refraining from talking while trying to understand the speaker's attitude and feelings. One should listen to the whole story, talking as little as possible and avoiding leading questions, arguing, or giving advice. Silent pauses encourage the speaker to continue. Attentiveness is indicated by comments such as "yes," "uh huh," "go on"; restatement (repeating what was said); paraphrasing (saying what was said in different words); clarifying (asking the speaker what was meant); reflecting (responding to the feelings communicated); and summarizing (reviewing the major points made). By saying little, receivers can concentrate on listening instead of on what they are going to say in return (Ellis and Hartley, 2000; Swansburg and Swansburg, 2002).

Written communications usually have the advantage of being more carefully formulated than oral communications. They also may save time and money and can be retained as legal records and reference sources. Written communications are sent downward, upward, or horizontally. Policies, procedures, handbooks, annual reports, bulletin boards, and house newspapers are usually directed downward. Attitude and morale surveys, suggestion systems, and written grievances are directed upward. Letters, memos, and reports may be upward, downward, or horizontal communication. Among department heads they are horizontal.

Before writing, one must first consider the purpose of the communication. For a planned and organized message, the writer develops thoughts logically, gives evidence to back up statements, and carefully selects words. Writers must ask themselves whether the communication answers who, what, when, where, and why questions and should appraise the tone of the document. Because writing is not easy, one should expect to edit original drafts.

Dictation is a valuable communication skill. Dictating probably requires more effort at first, but it can soon become easier than writing in longhand. In dictation one must again consider the purpose of the communication and plan and organize one's remarks. One starts dictation by indicating who is dictating what (letter or memo), the subject, type of paper needed (letterhead stationery, memo pad), and the number of copies needed. One should state the format (headings, double space, tabular outline, new paragraph), punctuation (capitalization, hyphen, period, commas, question marks, italics), and spell out unusual or unfamiliar words. Conversational instructions are given as one dictates. For example, "Mary, list the following statements and precede each with a dash." One should not smoke, eat, or chew gum while dictating. Background noises should be reduced as much as possible. Closing the office door during dictation can eliminate interference. Dictation should be given at a normal talking speed, with the words pronounced clearly and correctly. The sender can conclude dictation by saying "end of memo." If one cannot complete the dictation, instructions for the incomplete correspondence should be dictated. The dictator may want to keep a list of what is dictated and mark the items off as they are processed.

Telephone etiquette takes into account the needs of the sender and the receiver. One should answer the telephone promptly and speak clearly and distinctly to identify the agency, unit, and self. One should establish the purpose of the telephone call, determine the appropriate respondent, and ask questions to verify the message. One should answer questions with discretion, describe options appropriately, and identify actions for follow-up. Then the message is documented if indicated. To send a telephone message, one should gather the information needed and anticipate questions, call the number, identify the sender and receiver of the message, state the purpose of the call, exchange information, identify the follow-up, and document the call if indicated (Wywialowski, 2004).

Communications are critical for the functioning of an organization. Nurses need to be familiar with the communication process, communication systems, and directions communications can take. There are numerous barriers to communication. Managers need to know them and ways to overcome them.

JAHARI WINDOW

The process of giving and receiving feedback is illustrated by the Jahari Window (Figure 1-6). Two columns represent the self, and two rows represent the group. The left column represents

Figure 1-6 Jahari Window. (From Jones JE, Pfeiffer JW, editors: *The 1973 annual handbook for group facilitators*, La Jolla, Calif, 1973, University Associates.)

things one knows about oneself. The right column represents things one does not know about oneself. As one solicits more feedback from the group, the pane moves to the right, enlarging the arena area, where what one knows about oneself and others also know is represented. The pane varies as the level of mutual trust and feedback in the group changes. The arena is characterized by free and open exchange of information between self and others.

The second pane, the blind spot, contains information one does not know about oneself but members of the group may know. One communicates to group members in verbal and nonverbal ways of which one may not be aware. The person with the large blind spot interacts primarily by giving feedback but solicits very little. The person may be a poor listener or may be insensitive to the feedback, or she may respond to feedback with undesirable responses, such as anger, crying, or leaving, which makes others reluctant to give feedback. Soliciting feedback can decrease this pane.

In the third pane, the façade, one knows something that the group does not know. The person with the large facade asks questions of the group but does not give information or feedback. The information may be hidden from the group because of fear of rejection, attack, or other hurtful behavior. When one perceives supportive elements in the group and does self-disclosure, the pane can decrease. One needs to disclose some information to test one's assumptions about the supportiveness of the group. Keeping information to oneself may be used to control and manipulate others.

In the fourth pane, unknown, neither the person nor the group knows. The person neither solicits nor gives feedback. As the arena gets larger through feedback and self-disclosure, the other panes get smaller. However, there will probably always be some unknown information, such as intrapersonal dynamics, early childhood memories, and latent potentialities that are unconscious. A receptive attitude to feedback and self-disclosure increases the arena and reduces the blind spot, the facade, and the unknown. The goal is to solicit self-disclosure and feedback to move information from the facade and the blind spot into the arena, making the information available to everyone.

COMMUNICATING WITH DIFFICULT PEOPLE

"It is easier to swallow angry words than to have to eat them." —Anonymous

One requires special communication skills to deal with some personalities, including hostile-aggressive, complaining, negative, unrespon-sive, and overly nice. Some hostile-aggressive types seem to attack in an abrupt, abusive, intim-idating manner that pushes others to acquiesce against their better judgment. These people tend to know what others should do, need to prove themselves right, and lack trust and caring. One must stand up to a hostile-aggressive person or feel overrun and frustrated. It is important to do this without fighting, or the conflict will escalate. It can be advantageous to give the hostile-aggressive person time to run down for a while and then interrupt to stand up for oneself. There may be no opportunity to speak between sen-tences, thus making it necessary to interrupt before the other person has finished speaking. It is also likely that the other person may interrupt. Then one must state firmly, "You interrupted me," and start again, preferably with a smile. One needs to get the other person's attention to do problem solving. Calling the person by name

may help get the person's attention. Deliberately dropping a book is a more dramatic way to get attention. By standing up, one may also get attention. In addition, the other person may be less aggressive when sitting down. Then one needs to state ideas forcefully in a friendly manner that does not belittle the other person. It is important to avoid fighting with the hostile-aggressive person because such a battle will likely be lost. Even if the battle is won, the hos-tile-aggressive person's righteous anger will likely increase, and the war may be lost. When one stands up to a bully, one may become a friend. When dealing with hostile-aggressive people, it is important to stand up for oneself without fighting.

Exploders are another type of hostile-aggres-sive personality. Adult tantrums are the grown-up version of childhood tantrums that are a defense mechanism to cope with fear, helpless-ness, and frustration. Adult tantrums are sudden, almost automatic responses to feeling threatened. The exploder typically feels angry first and then blaming or suspicious. People act on their perceptions, but people are likely to perceive the same situation differently. Consequently, the other person may be unaware that the exploder has been threatened and be surprised by the outburst. The exploder should be given time to finish the tantrum and regain self-control. If the exploder does not finish, a neutral statement such as "stop" may interrupt the tantrum. Then one can show that the person is taken seriously by a comment such as "I can see this is important to you. I want to discuss this with you but not like this." Possibly one should change the pace by getting a cup of coffee and seeking a private place for a problem-solving session.

Sniping is an aggressive response to an unre-solved problem. It causes distress rather than positive actions. Unfortunately, the unsolved problems become worse, and the resulting stress causes more difficult behavior such as innuen-does, not-too-subtle remarks, and nonplayful teasing.

First of all, it is important to expose the attack by comments such as "That sounded like a putdown; did you mean it that way?" Usually snipers will deny any attack. Sniping is not possible without a camouflage that works. Standing up to the attack without escalating it will help one proceed with problem solving. It gives the sniper an alternative to a direct contest. It is appropriate to get other points of view that confirm or deny the sniper's criticism and then try to solve any problems that have surfaced. Sniping can be prevented by establishing regular problem-solving meetings.

Complainers may dump on you directly or may complain about other "awful" people. Complaining helps people appear blameless and innocent, at least to themselves. One should listen attentively to the complaints, paraphrase an acknowledgment of what was heard, and confirm one's perception of how the complainer feels. One should not agree with or apologize for the allegations and should avoid the accusation-defense-reaccusation pattern. It is preferable to simply state and acknowledge the facts without comment and then proceed with problem solving.

Negatively thinking people believe that any task that is out of their hands will fail and that others do not care and are self-serving. One should beware of being dragged down by their despair. One can make optimistic but realistic comments about past successes in similar situations but should not try to argue negativists out of their pessimism. It is better not to offer solutions or alternatives until the problem has been thoroughly discussed or to ask people to act before they feel ready. During the problem-solving session, the negative events that could occur if the option is implemented should be explored. One should be ready to take independent action if the group refuses to do so and announce these plans without equivocation.

Unresponsive people cannot or will not speak when input is needed from them. It is difficult to know what their silence means. The most important strategy is to get the silent person to speak by asking open-ended questions, waiting calmly for a response, and not talking to fill the silence. If an open-ended question gets no response, one should comment on what is happening, for example, "I'm not getting any feedback from you," and end the observation with another open-ended question such as "What are you thinking?" Attention should be given when the person does speak. If the person never speaks, one should terminate the meeting by stating what will be done because no discussion occurred.

Superagreeable people are equally difficult because they lead one to believe that they are in agreement but let one down when it comes to taking action. They have strong needs to be liked and accepted and help others feel approved to get approval themselves. They run into trouble when their need for approval conflicts with negative aspects of reality. They commit themselves to actions that they do not complete. Once again, problem solving is important. One must try to learn what prevents people from taking action and let them know that they are valued by telling them so and by asking questions about their interests, hobbies, and family to get to know them better. One should ask them what is not as good as they would like it to be and what could interfere with good relationships. Listening to their humor for hidden messages in teasing remarks and being prepared to do problem solving are also important (Bramson, 1997).

ASSERTIVENESS

BARRIERS TO ASSERTIVENESS

Communication styles are passive, aggressive, or assertive. Assertiveness is the best style for nurse managers and the one they should foster in their personnel. However, there are barriers that nurses must overcome to become assertive. The most pervasive barrier is female gender role socialization. Whereas men are characterized as aggressive, competitive, independent, objective, analytical, task oriented, confident, self-disciplined, and emotionally controlled, women are expected to be passive, dependent, subjective, intuitive, empathetic, sensitive, interpersonally oriented, weak, inconsistent, and emotionally unstable.

The nursing socialization process and the nature of nursing are additional barriers. Both nursing schools and health care agencies usually have organizational hierarchies with authority and power concentrated at the top. This arrangement usually promotes compliance and conformity. Nurses are taught to value sacrifice, humility, and service to others. They have been taught not to state their thoughts or feelings. Although they give intimate physical nurturing, they are not to become emotionally involved with patients. Nurses have been socialized into a subservient role. They are expected to follow physicians' orders and to be professional but not to anticipate equal financial reimbursement for their education and responsibilities. They are expected to be a part of the health care team but not to make decisions or policies. They tend to keep so busy that they ignore their own rights.

In addition to these male-female role competition problems, nurses face female-female relationship problems. Men are more competitive with women than with other men, and women are more competitive with women than with men. Consequently, attempts to develop support systems for nurses are not usually successful. Instead, the queen bee and the trashing syndrome emerge.

The queen bee identifies with men, enjoys being told that she is different from most women, and feels superior to other women. The queen bee usually has to work very hard to become a success in a male-dominated society. She is likely to need to be cooperative and non-threatening to achieve and maintain her successful position. She probably feels little animosity toward the system and the men who allowed her to become successful. Consequently, she is likely to identify with her male colleagues instead of with other women. However, protective of her own position and aware of the high price she

paid for it, she makes it no easier for other women to succeed.

Trashing is a form of character assassination that divides women against one another. It is self-destructive and leads to impotent rage. Rather than exposing disagreements to resolve differences, trashing is done to destroy. It can be done to one's face or behind one's back, in public or in private. It questions one's motives, stresses one's worthlessness, and breaches one's integrity. The victim may be ignored, or anything she says or does may be interpreted in the most negative manner. Others' unrealistic expectations about her ensure failure. The trasher may give misinformation to others about what the victim does and thinks or tell her lies about what others think of her. Whatever method is used, it is manipulative, dishonest, and destructive. Women in general and nurses specifically need to become aware of what they are doing to each other, commit themselves to supportive instead of destructive behavior, learn to analyze interpersonal communication, and learn assertive behavior.

TRANSACTIONAL ANALYSIS

Transactional analysis is a technique that can be used by nurses for analyzing and understanding behavior. It was developed by Eric Berne (1964, 1996) and popularized by Thomas Harris (1964, 1969) and Muriel James and Dorothy Jongeward (1996). Transactional analysis is an outgrowth of the freudian concepts of id, ego, and superego—elements of the psyche that stimulate, monitor, and control behavior. Berne calls these ego states parent, child, and adult.

Ego States

The *parent* ego state controls and is the source of values, opinions, rules, regulations, and social conscience. The two major types of parent ego states are nurturing parent and critical parent. The nurturing parent guides, teaches, advises, and supplies "how to" information. The critical parent prohibits and supplies "should" and "should not" information. The parent ego state is a result of cultural traditions, social programming, and responsibilities. Parental judgments are drawn heavily from natural parents, older siblings, teachers, and other parent figures.

The *child* ego state is dominated by emotions and is the feeling state. It is the id ego state in which strong feelings are triggered by immediate experiences. People are in the child state when they are experiencing childlike natural impulses, such as joy, delight, and gaiety or anger, hostility, and rage. The child ego state may be happy or destructive. The natural child is spontaneous, trusting, joyful, living, creative, and adventurous. The adapted child is suppressed and may express anger, rebellion, fear, or conformity.

The *adult* is the ego state that monitors one's behavior. It is the unemotional, thinking, problem-solving state. The adult ego state collects information, sets goals, compares alternatives, makes decisions and plans, and tests reality. The adult ego state is an unemotional state in which rational decision making takes place.

Every individual exhibits behavior from the three ego states at different times. A healthy individual maintains a balance among them. Unfortunately, some people are dominated by one or two of the ego states and are likely to create problems for managers. Parent-dominated individuals may not participate in problem solving because they think they already have the answer and know what is right and wrong. Child-dominated individuals do not engage in rational problem solving either. Screaming and being emotional have helped them get what they wanted before. It is likely to be difficult to reason with someone dominated by the child ego state. Working with adult-dominated individuals may be boring

because they work so hard. A balance among the three ego states produces the healthiest worker.

Transactions

When people interact, they participate as parent, child, or adult. A transaction or an observation unit is an exchange between people that consists of at least one stimulus and one response. Transactional analysis is done to identify the participant's ego state and consists of complementary or crossed types (Figure 1-7). The basic principle of the complementary type is that the response to the stimulus is predictable and expected.

Adult-to-adult transactions are the manner in which much business is conducted (Figure 1-8). For instance, a supervisor says, "Would you please give Mr. Jones his prn medication before you give Mrs. Smith her 8 AM medications?" A staff nurse replies, "Yes, I understand that Mr. Jones is complaining of surgical pain."

Parent-to-parent interaction is often a short-term sharing of opinions (Figure 1-9). One staff nurse says to another, "Those new graduate nurses certainly don't know how to function." The other nurse replies, "That's for sure."

Child-to-child interactions usually involve an emotional exchange (Figure 1-10). As long as both parties are in a child ego state, they are unable to think rationally and solve problems. The first staff nurse says, "I just gave Mrs. Smith her 8 AM medications, and when I went to chart them, you had signed for giving them. Why don't you sign right after you give medications so they won't be repeated!" The second nurse answers, "Why don't you give me a chance to sign before you go and give them again!"

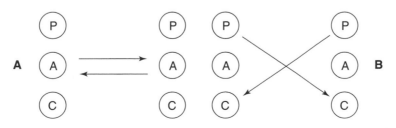

Figure 1-7 Transactions. **A,** Complementary. **B,** Crossed.

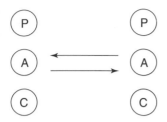

Figure 1-8 Adult-to-adult complementary transaction.

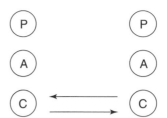

Figure 1-10 Child-to-child complementary transaction.

In *parent-to-child* interactions one person takes a psychologically superior position over the other (Figure 1-11). A manager says, "I want to see you in my office." A staff nurse answers, "Yes, ma'am."

Crossed transactions result in closing communications at least temporarily (Figure 1-12). The response may be inappropriate or unexpected and may confuse or threaten the sender of the stimulus. A supervisor says, "Miss Jones, could I see you about this in my office right away?" Miss Jones replies, "No! Can't you see I'm busy? You'll have to wait."

Transactions usually proceed in a programmed series with rituals and procedures being the simplest kinds. Rituals are a series of simple complementary transactions that provide mutual stroking with no real commitment. Most rituals have been used so often that the form has become more important than the content, but they provide structure for greeting people and expressing religious beliefs. Greeting rituals such as "Hi," "How are you?" and "I am fine" are not intended to supply information. The person who goes from office to office participating in rituals may get promoted because she is "a

good guy." Rituals work for the person who can still get the job done. People who work hard to develop themselves may become apathetic when they realize socializing is more effective for obtaining promotions than hard work. Rituals may have started as a series of complementary adult transactions intended to manipulate reality, but they have lost their procedural validity over time.

Pastimes are pleasant ways to pass time with others to learn if you have enough in common to warrant further interaction. Common small talk includes topics such as cooking, fashions, costs, sports, recreation, and mutual acquaintances. There is no goal or emotional closeness involved. People who spend too much time participating in pastimes may sense that their lives are happy but empty, whereas the person who spends too little time making small talk may not have much fun and may feel harassed. Pastimes become a problem for the organization when they are an alternative to work.

GAME PLAYING

In *Games People Play* Eric Berne (1996) writes: "A game is an ongoing series of complementary ulterior transactions progressing to a well-defined,

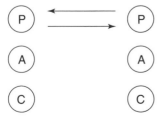

Figure 1-9 Parent-to-parent complementary transaction.

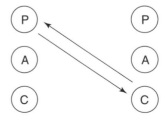

Figure 1-11 Parent-to-child complementary transaction.

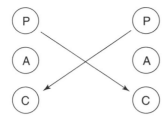

Figure 1-12 Crossed transaction.

predictable outcome." Games have a high stroke or recognition potential, but the payoff is usually negative. Games have hidden agendas that prevent both people and organizations from becoming winners. While playing games, people dwell on their own sorrows and inadequacies, make mistakes, catch others making mistakes, pass the buck, and fail to meet their obligations. People receive negative strokes and get hurt while real problems go unsolved. Productivity is limited because people use their energies to play games instead of to get the job done. Attention is given to past events rather than to the present. While realities of the current situation go unperceived, problems go unsolved.

People need strokes, and negative strokes are better than no strokes. Consequently, in work environments that do not provide positive strokes, people have a need to play games. People who are bored with their jobs are also likely to play games. Games discourage openness, honesty, and intimacy. They take many forms. Games that blame others include "If it weren't for you" and "See what you made me do." Games that attack others include "Blemish," "Now I've got you, you SOB," "Bear trapper," "Corner," "Rapo," "Uproar," and "Let's you and him fight." Self-pity is reinforced by games such as "Poor me," "Kick me," "Stupid," "Wooden leg," "Harried," and "Lunch bag."

"If it weren't for you" is a blaming game in which people who feel inadequate blame others for their inability to achieve. People who blame their inability to be innovative on rigid policies may fear their own creative abilities. "If it weren't for . . ." is a clue that the game is being

played. When managers hear an employee say this, they should suspect that the complainer would not function better under different circumstances but would likely become frustrated and request a transfer or quit. Changes may be made on a trial basis to test suspicions.

"See what you made me do" and *"You got me into this"* are closely related blaming games. The player avoids responsibility by being vindictive. It is common for workers to blame managers for problems and for democratic managers to blame workers for mistakes or poor decisions. The manager decides whether or not to use the input from the workers and needs to accept that responsibility.

Many games attack others. The *"Blemish"* player looks for inconsequential, unimportant flaws. Instead of looking at purposes, the player concentrates on minutiae and zeroes in on trivial mistakes. Any positive stroke is discounted with a blemish. Blemish players also play "I was only trying to help you." The victims become resentful and may become the persecutor by playing *"Now I've got you, you SOB."* In this game the persecutor waits for the victim to make a mistake or sets the victim up for failure. The manager may be indulging in this game by setting standards too high to achieve, assigning people to work for which they are not qualified, creating impossible working conditions, or giving incomplete or unclear instructions. The worker may use grievance procedures or lawsuits against managers playing this game.

The *"Bear trapper"* often baits someone with false promises and then lets the trap fall. Organizations play this game in hiring practices when glamorous job descriptions are presented. This tends to result in high turnover. Workers learn the shortcomings of the job and become disillusioned. Presenting both the advantages and disadvantages of jobs is a more realistic approach.

The *"Corner"* player's victim is in a lose-lose situation. No matter what the victim does, it is wrong. A woman manager is damned if she is aggressive because that is not considered feminine and damned if she is not because aggressiveness is a desired managerial quality. A manager can corner someone into not completing work on time by not accepting the work that is done.

"Corner" can lead to *"Uproar."* Uproar often starts with a critical remark and results in an attack-defense dialogue that is often loud.

"Rapo" is a sexual game. A woman may wear revealing clothing and move in provocative ways. When a man responds, she rejects him. This game is problematic when men and women work together. Organizations require concentrating on equality and using human resources regardless of gender.

In *"Let's you and him fight,"* one person gets a second and a third person into a fight. When one person tells a second person the "bad" things a third person said about the second, the first person is fostering a fight.

There are several versions of self-pity games. *"Kick me"* players provoke putdowns and make comments such as "I could kick myself for that." *"Stupid"* players collect putdowns about their intelligence. Managers need to give immediate feedback and take corrective actions to prevent the Stupid game. The *"Wooden leg"* player uses a physical or social handicap to avoid work. A deprived background may be used as an excuse to underachieve. The manager needs to set and maintain standards to minimize this game.

Managers play *"Poor me"* games also. *"Harried"* executives work hard to maintain the sense of being OK. They are likely to work nights and weekends to appear competent and confident. "I'm not OK" feelings are hidden by appearing super OK.

The Harried executive may also participate in the *"Lunch bag game."* Managers carry leftovers in a used paper bag and eat at their desk instead of going out to lunch with peers. This technique can be used to make other people feel guilty.

Games always involve putting someone down. To decrease games in organizations, one must stop putting oneself and others down. One should not play the complementary role but should give and receive positive strokes and invest time in activities and intimacy.

Managers should integrate the goals of the workers and the organization and decrease boredom through job enrichment and personnel development. With good organization and management, positive strokes can become an intrinsic part of the job. Managers should foster an "I'm OK, you're OK" atmosphere.

Activities such as working and learning are goal directed and have a high stroke potential. They are a highly rewarding way to spend time. Workers must be careful not to take on so many activities that they neglect rituals and pastimes, and managers should not overload themselves with activities and leave the workers with idle time.

Intimacy is an open sharing of experience with others, usually by people with close relationships but sometimes by strangers. It is the most rewarding way to spend time. It is also the most risky. Although intimacy is without ulterior motives or exploitation, one needs high self-esteem to risk the openness of intimacy. It requires and fosters the "I'm OK, you're OK" atmosphere.

LIFE POSITIONS

Life positions are more permanent than ego states. As individuals mature, they make assumptions about themselves and others. They consider themselves as OK or not OK and see others as OK or not OK. Four positions result: *"I'm OK, you're OK," "I'm OK, you're not OK," "I'm not OK, you're OK,"* and *"I'm not OK, you're not OK."* OK feelings are associated with a sense of power, personal worth, well-being, capability, and lovableness. Not-OK feelings result from a sense of inability, weakness, helplessness, worthlessness, anxiety, and a feeling of being insignificant and unlovable. Most people develop a basic life position early in childhood that tends to be reinforced by the person's selective perceptions and reactions to experiences.

In the I'm OK, you're OK position, individuals feel interdependent with others and the environment. They are happy, active people with a positive outlook on life who like reinforcement for being OK but are not dependent on it.

They use the happy child and nurturing parent ego states. Because they feel OK about themselves, they have little difficulty feeling others are OK.

People in the I'm OK, you're not OK position do not believe they can rely on anyone but themselves. They think people are worthless and are likely to be enemies and consequently tend to blame others. The critical parent ego state is dominant. A manager in this position possesses a Theory X philosophy, implements a Likert type I system, and supervises people closely because they cannot be trusted.

People in the I'm not OK, you're OK position are burdened with self-defeating attitudes and a lack of confidence. They take a psychologically inferior stand to others and assume that they are less competent and less influential than others.

Individuals in the I'm not OK, you're not OK position are maladjusted. They think they are worthless and so are others. Lacking confidence in themselves and trust in others, they are suspicious and anxious, disconnected from others, alienated from the environment, and miserable, and they tend to give up.

During infancy individuals have a mixture of OK and not-OK feelings, with the not-OK feelings predominating. The infant feels OK when physical needs are met and positive strokes are received. Most of an infant's experiences provide negative strokes and not-OK feelings. Because adults can satisfy the infant's needs, they are viewed as OK. Consequently, for most people the I'm not OK, you're OK position is established early and continues into adulthood. Socialization of women and nurses particularly reinforces the position that they are not OK. Therefore they need a lot of positive reinforcement to move to an I'm OK, you're OK position. Assertiveness can help one achieve and maintain that position. Once it is learned, there will be less passive-aggressive behavior.

ASSERTIVENESS TECHNIQUES

"If one tells the truth, one is sure sooner or later to be found out." —Oscar Wilde

Communication styles are commonly passive, aggressive, or assertive. Passive persons are often self-denying and inhibited and allow others to choose for them. Consequently, their goals are not achieved and they feel hurt, anxious, and frustrated. Aggressive persons are self-enhancing at others' expense. They are expressive, choose for others, deprecate others, and achieve their goals by using others. Aggressive behavior generates hatred and sometimes revenge. Assertive persons are self-enhancing. They are expressive, choose for themselves, and can achieve their goals. Consequently, they are likely to feel good about themselves.

Passive persons tend to be at a loss for words, do not say what they really mean, use many apologetic words, and hope people will understand what they want without telling them. They tend to have a weak, hesitant voice; downcast eyes; and fidgety hands; and they nod frequently.

The aggressive person is loud; uses loaded, subjective words; makes accusations; and sends "you" messages that blame others. A flippant, sarcastic style with an air of superiority and rudeness is common. The person is likely to stand with hands on hips, feet apart, narrowed eyes, pointing a finger and talking in a superior, demanding, authoritarian manner.

Assertive persons say what they want in direct statements that say what they mean. They use objective words, send "I" messages, and make honest statements about their feelings. They are attentive listeners who give the impression of caring. They use eye contact and spontaneous verbal expressions with appropriate gestures and facial expressions while speaking in a well-modulated voice.

The style used governs how situations will be handled. Suppose, for instance, that a manager has noted that a staff nurse has been arriving at work late for the past 3 days. The passive manager may not mention the problem at all. The aggressive manager might say, "How about getting here on time or looking for a new job? What do you think we pay you for anyway?" The assertive manager would be likely to speak to the staff nurse in private and might say, "I've noticed you have been late the past 3 days. Why haven't you been getting to work on time?" The last approach gives an impression of caring and facilitates problem solving.

Assertiveness is the most desirable style for a nurse manager. To achieve assertiveness, one must substitute verbal persistence for silent passivity or verbal abuse. Broken record is a technique managers can use to reach a compromise by indicating what they want and by keeping other people from talking them into what the others want to do. With the broken-record technique managers keep repeating what they want:

Manager: I expect you to get to work on time.

Staff nurse: But I'm a night person. I stay up late, and it's difficult to get up so early to come to work. I'm so tired that I shut off my alarm and go back to sleep. Then when I do get up, I stumble around in the dark to find my clothes so I won't wake my husband.

Manager: You are scheduled to work the day shift this rotation, and I expect you to be at work on time. If you are a night person, would you like to be assigned to the night shift permanently?

Staff nurse: No. I wouldn't be able to see my husband then. He works 9 AM to 9 PM and gets home about 9:30 PM. I would have to come to work at 10:30, and I could see him for only about an hour. I would get home just in time for him to go to work.

Manager: You are scheduled to work the day shift this rotation, and I expect you to get to work on time. However, we could assign you to the evening shift permanently. Would you want that?

Staff nurse: Working the evening shift would allow me to see my husband after work and to sleep in. Yes, I would prefer the evening shift.

Manager: I will see how quickly we can get your schedule changed to permanent evenings. I do expect you to be here by 7 AM until we get your schedule changed.

Fogging, negative assertion, and negative inquiry are techniques for dealing with criticism, whether it is self-directed or from another source, real or imagined. They help minimize the negative emotional response of anxiety to criticism that manipulates one into defending what one wants to do instead of doing it. Consequently, one feels less at conflict with oneself and more comfortable with both the negative and positive aspects of one's personality.

Fogging is agreeing with the truth, agreeing in principle, or agreeing with the odds rather than denying the criticism, getting defensive, or counterattacking with criticism. It helps desensitize one to criticism and leads to a reduction in the frequency of criticism from others. It sets up psychological distance, is a passive skill, and does not encourage the other person to be assertive. It also encourages a person to listen to what the critic says, to respond only to what the critic says rather than to what is implied, and to consider probabilities. For example:

Staff nurse: You scheduled me to double back from evenings to days twice in a 2-week time schedule.

Manager: I see that I scheduled you to double back the first Wednesday and the second Friday (agreeing with the truth).

Staff nurse: When I double back, I have less than 7 hours of sleep. I get tired, have trouble functioning, and fear making mistakes.

Manager: I understand that you get tired when you double back and fear making mistakes. It seems logical that one would make more mistakes when tired than when alert (agreeing with the odds).

Staff nurse: We need a policy to prevent having just one shift off between shifts.

Manager: I agree. We do need staffing policies that would provide for adequate rest periods between shifts (agreeing in principle).

With negative assertion people assertively accept negative aspects about themselves. This reduces the need to seek forgiveness for one's mistakes or the need to counterattack with criticism.

Staff nurse: Your new uniform really reveals how fat you are.

Manager: I'm overweight because I eat too much. I eat just about everything in sight except the kitchen sink. I've even seen the cat get worried (negative assertion).

Staff nurse: Well, that new uniform sure makes you look like a blimp.

Manager: These new styles don't complement my figure (negative assertion).

Negative assertion is not appropriate for physical or legal conflicts or for relating to people on a close interpersonal basis. The persistence of the critic will determine if one needs to use other assertive techniques.

Negative inquiry fosters assertiveness in the critic. In an unemotional manner, the criticized person asks for more information that may be negative. This provides a basis for problem solving and consequently reduces repetitive criticism.

Staff nurse: You don't look good today.
Manager: Is it me or what I'm wearing?
Staff nurse: It's your face. You look so tired.

Manager: I don't feel tired. What about my face makes me look tired?

Staff nurse: Your eyes look so tired. They're so dark. There are bags under them.

Manager: What can I do to make them look less tired?

Staff nurse: If the problem isn't fatigue, I guess you could use a creme cosmetic over the bags and use light instead of dark-colored eye shadow.

Assertive behavior is more than demanding your rights from others and keeping others from manipulating. In a social sense assertiveness is the ability to communicate with others about who you are, how you live, what you do, and what you want and the ability to make them feel comfortable talking about themselves. Free information—information offered without being asked for—gives you something to talk about and reduces awkward silences. Self-disclosure reveals how you think, feel, and react to others' free information. This social conversation allows you to discover mutually rewarding relationships or to identify people with whom you have few common interests.

RESEARCH Perspective 1-2

Data from Sa TL, Cohen J, Marculescu G: Nurse practitioners' attitudes and knowledge toward current procedural terminology (CPT) coding. *Nursing Economic$* V19(3):100-106, 2001.

Purpose: The purpose of this study was to describe nurse practitioners' attitudes and knowledge about current procedural terminology.

Methods: This research was an exploratory, descriptive nonexperimental study. Data were collected using a mailed survey that was sent to the nurse practitioners in California who were members of a state nurse practitioner organization. The instrument used was a self-administered questionnaire developed by the researchers. All items in the attitudinal survey were placed on a continuum from positive to negative responses. Descriptive statistics using frequencies, percentages, and means were used.

Results/conclusions: Nurse practitioners lacked the required knowledge about coding and did not perceive the significance of this reimbursement strategy. Nurse practitioners need to be taught the coding and the importance of using it to get reimbursement.

Chapter Summary

Chapter 1 covered the following:
Communication Process
Basic Communication Skills
Communication Principles
Methods of Communication
Use of Computers for Communication
Communication Systems
    Downward Communication
    Upward Communication
    Lateral Communication
    Diagonal Communication
    The Grapevine
Barriers to Communication
    Gender Differences
    Cultural Differences
Improving Communication
    Jahari Window
Communicating With Difficult People
Assertiveness
    Barriers to Assertiveness
    Transactional Analysis
        Ego states
        Transactions
    Game Playing
    Life Positions
    Assertive Techniques

On-line Resources

evolve   Additional critical thinking activities, worksheets, and case studies are available on-line at http://evolve.elsevier.com/Marriner/guide/

References

Advanced executive leadership skills, Stamford, Conn, 1981, Xerox Learning Systems.

Ball MJ, Hannah KJ, Newbold SK, et al: *Nursing informatics: Where caring and technology meet*, New York, 2000, Springer.

Berne E: *Games people play,* New York, 1964, Grove Press, Inc.

Berne E: *Games people play,* New York, 1996, Ballantine.

Bramson RM: *Coping with difficult people,* New York, 1997, Doubleday.

Casmir FL: *Ethics in intercultural and international communication*, Mahway, NJ, 1997, Lawrence Erlbaum Associates, Publishers.

DeYoung S: *Teaching strategies for nurse educator*, Upper Saddle River, NJ, 2003, Prentice Hall.

Douglas LM: *The effective nurse,* St Louis, 1996, Mosby.

Ellis JR, Hartley CL: *Managing and coordinating nursing care,* ed 3, Philadelphia, 2000, Lippincott.

Gillies DA: *Nursing management: A systems approach,* Philadelphia, 1994, WB Saunders.

Gilovich T: *How we know what isn't so,* New York, 1991, Free Press.

Gray J: *Men are from Mars, women are from Venus,* New York, 1992, HarperCollins.

Gudykunst WB: *Bridging differences: Effective intergroup communication,* ed 3, Thousand Oaks, Calif, 1998, Sage.

Harris TA: *I'm OK—you're OK: A practical guide to transactional analysis*, New York, 1969, Harper & Row.

Hein EC: *Contemporary leadership behavior: Selected readings,* Philadelphia, 1998, Lippincott.

James M, Jongeward D: *Born to win,* Oxford, 1996, Perseus Press.

Jones JE, Pfeiffer JW, editors: *The 1973 annual handbook for group facilitators,* La Jolla, Calif, 1973, University Associates.

Kreider NA, Haselton BJ: *The systems challenge,* Chicago, 1997, American Hospital.

Saba VK, McCormick KA: *Essentials of computers for nurses: Informatics for the new millennium*, New York, 2001, McGraw-Hill.

Sullivan EJ, Decker PJ: *Effective leadership and management in nursing,* ed 5, Upper Saddle River, NJ, 2001, Prentice Hall.

Swansburg RC, Swansburg RJ: *Introduction to management and leadership for nurse managers,* ed 3, Boston, 2002, Jones and Bartlett.

Tannen D: *You just don't understand: Women and men in conversation,* New York, 2001, Quill.

Whetten DA, Cameron KS: *Developing management skills,* Reading, Mass, 1998, Addison-Wesley.

Wywialowski EF: *Managing client care,* ed 3, St Louis, 2004, Mosby.

2

Stress Management

*"There is little difference in people, but that little
difference makes a big difference. The little
difference is attitude. The big difference is whether
it is positive or negative."* —*W. Clement Stone*

Chapter Overview

Chapter 2 presents sources of stress, stress response, symptoms of
stress, stress control, relaxation, time management, delegation,
procrastination, and ways to maximize organization time.

Chapter Objectives

- Identify at least six sources of stress.
- List at least 12 symptoms of stress.
- Identify and discuss at least 12 stress management techniques.
- Predict how planning relates to time management effects.
- Delineate at least five ways to streamline paperwork.
- Formulate at least five ways to make telephone communication efficient.
- Select at least five ways managers can help meetings be effective and efficient.
- Assess responsibility, authority, and accountability as they relate to delegation.

STRESS MANAGEMENT

SOURCES OF STRESS

Adjustment to change is stressful. Many events in life produce individual stress reactions. Death of a spouse or close family member, divorce, marital separation, marriage or remarriage, and personal injury or illness are highly stressful events. Change in the health of a family member, pregnancy, gain of a new family member, marital reconciliation, increased arguing with spouse, sexual difficulties, changes in financial state, mortgages, trouble with in-laws, a son or daughter leaving home, and the death of a close friend are stressful. Changes in living conditions and personal habits, such as changes in work, residence, school, recreation, church activities, social activities, sleeping habits, and eating habits, cause stress. Even personal achievements, vacations, and holidays are stressful. These personal stressors can affect one's job performance.

In addition to personal stressors, there are many sources of stress at work. Dismissal and retirement are highly stressful. Business readjustments such as changing jobs or responsibilities, changes in working hours or conditions, and problems with the boss are stressful. Even outstanding achievement is stressful. Poor physical working conditions; physical danger; work overload; time pressures; responsibility for people; role ambiguity and conflict; conflicts with superiors, peers, and subordinates; restrictions; little participation in decision making; overpromotion or underpromotion; and lack of job security are stressors common to jobs.

Nurses face stress with life-and-death situations; heavy workloads involving physical and mental strain; knowledge of how to use numerous pieces of equipment and the consequences of equipment failure; reporting to numerous bosses; communication problems among staff members, physicians, families, and other departments; and awareness of the serious consequences of mistakes. A hospital is one of the most stressful work environments.

People often needlessly increase their own stress. The difference between demands people place on themselves or perceive from others and the resources they perceive as available to meet the demands is a threat or stress. Individuals are typed by the demands they place on themselves. Type A people set high standards, are competitive, and put themselves under constant time pressure. They are very demanding of themselves even in leisure and recreation activities. Type B people are more easygoing and relaxed. They are less competitive and more likely to accept situations than fight them.

STRESS RESPONSE

Stress is impossible to avoid. It is a nonspecific response of the body to any demand. There are two types of stress: (1) eustress, a positive force that adds excitement and challenge to life and provides a sense of well-being, and (2) distress, a negative force caused by unrelieved tension that threatens effectiveness. Whether one will experience eustress or distress largely depends on the person's perceptions, physical activity or inactivity, mental activity or inactivity, sound nutrition, and meaningful relationships.

A stressor is anything an individual perceives as a threat. Stressors produce a state of stress by disrupting homeostasis. There are three stages in the stress response (Box 2-1). First, the alarm reaction is the mobilization of resources to confront the threat. Second, in the resistance stage, there is a large increase in energy consumption. Once the reserve energy has been used, the body needs time to recover and to replenish the supply. When stress continues for long periods of time, the energy is used but not replaced and the third stage, exhaustion, results.

Consequently, unrelieved stress interferes with one's physical and mental well-being. After the stress event the body returns to a state of equilibrium. Stable periods for bodies to restore adaptive energy allow one to meet new stressful situations.

SYMPTOMS OF STRESS

Numerous symptoms indicate that stress is becoming distress. These include but are not limited to those shown in Box 2-2.

High stress levels accumulated over several months are likely to result in physical and psychological reactions. The amount of stress necessary before one manifests symptoms varies, depending on factors such as heredity, habits, personality, past illnesses, and previous crises and coping mechanisms. Well-educated, intelligent, creative people in management are at high risk for burnout. They may become workaholics but get little accomplished, experience chronic fatigue, feel they do not want to go to work,

---

BOX 2-1 Three Stages in Stress Response

Alarm reaction—mobilization of resources to confront threat
Resistance stage—increase in energy consumption
Exhaustion—depletion of the body's energy reserves

BOX 2-2 Symptoms of Stress

Fatigue
Depression
Tearfulness
Restlessness
Nervousness
Withdrawal or sudden gregariousness
Irritability
Anger
Feeling of being unloved
Insecurity
Feeling of vague anxiety
Pessimism
Self-criticism
Frequent frustration
Loss of interest in going out
Loss of interest in people and things
Decrease in self-care
Disorganization
Inability to relax or rest
Accidents
Arthritis
Asthma
Colds
Colitis attacks
Nightmares
Early morning waking
Feeling of not being able to get anything done
Feeling that everything is too much
Forgetfulness
Lack of concentration
Tendency to be demanding
Loss of appetite or overeating
Indigestion
Constipation or diarrhea
Nausea
Coughing
Headaches
High blood pressure
Rapid pulse
Heart palpitation
Perspiration
Aching neck and shoulder muscles
Low back pain
Allergy problems
Dermatitis
Influenza
Hives
Menstrual distress
Ulcers

take increasing amounts of sick time, become negative, blame and criticize others, engage in backbiting, and talk behind others' backs.

STRESS CONTROL

"The secret of happiness is to count your blessings while others are adding up their troubles."
—Anonymous

Nurse managers can prevent and control burnout by setting personal and professional goals, establishing priorities, practicing good health habits and relaxation techniques, improving their self-esteem by obtaining the skills they need, and using support systems.

Values Clarification

Values clarification is a useful activity. Values should be chosen freely from alternatives with thoughtful consideration to the consequences of each alternative. They should be cherished and shared with others. The value should be integrated into one's lifestyle, and actions should be consistent with the values. To help clarify one's values, one may assign priorities to a list of values such as the following:

Affection	Pleasure
Duty	Power
Expertise	Prestige
Family	Security
Health	Self-realization
Independence	Service
Leadership	Spirituality
Parenthood	Wealth

One can also list in order of priority characteristics such as the following:

Ambitiousness	Honesty
Broadmindedness	Imagination
Cheerfulness	Independence
Cleanliness	Logic
Courage	Lovingness
Forgiveness	Responsibility
Helpfulness	

Goal Setting

Goals should be consistent with one's values, and one should consider goal alternatives. To do this, one considers why a goal is desired. One may want a promotion for recognition or for economic reasons. If the promotion is not forthcoming, one may receive recognition through community service. Money might be generated through wise investments or fees for community services. The achievement of desired outcomes through different approaches increases flexibility and decreases stress caused by unmet goals.

Stress Avoidance and Regulation

When reappraising situations, one should avoid troublesome transactions. The frequency of stress-inducing situations should be minimized. Every change takes energy. Therefore during periods of high stress, routines and habits should be maintained as much as possible. One should be cautious about moving and starting a new job at the same time one is getting a divorce. That also would be a particularly poor time to try to stop smoking or lose weight. Unnecessary changes should be prevented during periods of high stress. Deliberately postponing some changes helps one deal with unavoidable change constructively and reduces the need for multiple adjustments at one time. However, increasing positive sources of tension that foster growth, such as learning a sport, can help offset the deleterious effect of negative tension.

Time Blocking

Time blocking is the setting aside of specific time for adaptation to a stressor. To reduce the stress from having been promoted to a management position, you can set aside time for reading about management or for observing a manager. This helps ensure that concerns are addressed and tasks accomplished. It decreases anxiety, time urgency, and feelings of frustration. Define off-limit times, and set aside time when you will not be interrupted by phone calls or individuals except for emergencies. Schedule free time and exercise time, and put social events on the calendar like you would a business appointment.

Time Management

Time management helps control stress. Much time can be conserved when one knows one's value system and acts consistently with it, sets goals, and plans strategies for accomplishment of those goals. One can also use organizers such as to-do lists and calendars to plan good use of one's time.

Assertiveness

When one asserts oneself, one increases self-esteem and reduces anxiety, thus reducing stress. As with time management, assertiveness involves thinking through goals and acting consistently with one's values through the use of effective work habits and by setting limits on others' attempts to block one's goals. It involves stating what one wants and how one feels, making requests, taking compliments, handling putdowns, and setting limits. An assertive person makes eye contact with others; stands straight; sits in an open, listening posture; and speaks in a clear voice. Assertive people choose for themselves and achieve desired goals through self-enhancing behavior that reduces stress.

Feeling Pauses

Feeling pauses are useful. One should take time to identify a feeling, label it, distinguish between thinking and feeling, and accept the feeling for what it is rather than talking oneself into what it should be. One should be aware if one is feeling the following:

Amusement	Hope
Calmness	Joy
Care	Love
Compassion	Passion
Elation	Relaxation
Excitement	Satisfaction
Forgiveness	Thrill
Happiness	

One should also acknowledge negative feelings, such as the following:

Anger	Fear
Anxiousness	Frustration
Confusion	Hurt
Depression	Jealousy
Embarrassment	Restlessness
Envy	Terror

Then one should determine whether the feeling is appropriate for the situation and decide how to express the feeling in a safe and appropriate way. Feelings can be expressed in "I feel" messages rather than "you" messages that blame or attack others. Feelings can be talked about with an uninvolved person. One can fantasize about how one would like to handle the situation better the next time. Negative feelings may be acted out symbolically by punching a pillow, drawing a picture, or writing a poem. One may set aside negative feelings by getting involved in something pleasant, such as exercise, hobbies, music, television, or talking to a friend. Feelings can also be experienced vicariously by getting involved in another's experience through reading a book, watching a movie, or listening to someone.

Inner Shouting

Inner shouting is the process of shouting "I feel …" inside one's head; the person blurts the feeling out spontaneously rather than saying it quietly. Anger should be viewed as a symptom. Pains should be focused on to help one take responsibility for feelings of hurt and humiliation.

Anchoring

Anchors are associated feelings that are initiated either by an event or by the memory of that event. Anchors may be sounds, sights, smells, tastes, or touches that stimulate positive or negative feelings. Birds chirping may remind one of happy, lazy mornings with the family. One may recall an awful accident at the sight of blood. One might remember fall walks through the woods with a lover at the smell of dry leaves. A taste may revive memories of Grandma's home cooking. A light touch to the face may remind one of earlier loving moments and cause one to experience a sense of well-being. Our lives are filled with anchors that cause associations. We can use anchoring in a useful way to experience desired feelings. Because touch can be inconspicuous and easy to replicate, one can associate a positive feeling with a familiar touch to the body. This may be as simple as clasping one's hands and being reminded of soft music, beautiful colored glass, and the peaceful sanctuary of church. Exact pressure at a very specific spot makes the anchor work most accurately and should be done when one desires to bring back a pleasurable feeling.

Sorting

Sorting is choosing the interpretation of an event. One can have an optimistic or pessimistic interpretation of events. Is the glass half full or half empty? We become what we think and therefore can make ourselves happy or miserable. To be happier and more fun loving, one should focus on the positive aspects of situations.

Thought Stopping

Thought stopping helps get rid of negative thinking. Excessive rehearsals in our minds of negative past events are unhelpful thoughts that waste time, reduce our self-esteem, and encourage maladaptive behavior patterns. To prepare for thought stopping, one should think of beautiful, pleasant experiences: a sunrise, a waterfall, a flower, a pet, favorite music, baking bread, holding hands. One should also identify not-so-helpful thoughts: I'm stupid; I'm fat; nobody likes me. One should identify the negative thoughts that are most bothersome. In private one can think about a negative thought momentarily and suddenly yell, "Stop!" while clasping one's hands or hitting one's head or leg. One startles oneself, and the thought escapes. Immediately one should insert a pleasant thought. If the negative thought returns, the

procedure can be repeated. It is reinforced when the negative thoughts are stopped. Thoughts lead to feelings that can lead to behaviors, so by changing the way one thinks, one can change the way one behaves. Thought stopping should not be used, however, when physical or emotional safety and grieving are involved.

Compartmentalization

Compartmentalization of thought is the deliberate decision to think negative thoughts at specified times of the day. During the allotted time one thinks about worry, guilt, or jealousy. One does not allow oneself to think these thoughts at other times of the day.

Environmental Changes

Environmental changes can be designed to reduce stress. This may be as extreme as changing jobs or residence or as minor as painting a room a favorite color or adding a picture, candle, or basket. The short time inconvenience of remodeling may be worth the long-term stress reduction. Temporary changes in jobs can add variety and stimulation.

Humor

Humor related to an attitude toward life is most likely to reduce stress. There is a cluster of qualities that characterize this frame of mind, including flexibility, spontaneity, unconventionality, shrewdness, playfulness, humility, and irony. These are qualities that can be developed. Flexibility is the ability to examine all sides of the issues. One should try to look at a situation from several different viewpoints: the boss's, the subordinate's, the client's. Spontaneity is the ability to swing from one mood to another quickly. One might practice the body language of several emotions, including fear, anger, sadness, and love. One can free oneself from current values, places, and occupations through unconventionality and imagine living a day as a favorite animal, a famous historical person, an Eskimo, a Native American, or an astronaut. Shrewdness is refusal to believe that people or things are what they appear to be. One can think of a list of people and things and give an example of how each is not what it seems to be. Playfulness is the ability to see life as an amusing game. One can visualize life as a game and give the game a name. One should identify times of various emotions—fun, enjoyment, fear, anger, sadness—and chart wins and losses. Humility is a willingness to question the importance of one's values, ideas, achievements, and existence. One must consider the meaning of one's life and consider how difficult situations have brought happiness and how happy relationships have included suffering. Irony is the ability to see that situations are not black or white.

Centering

Centering helps reduce stress by bringing the mind and body back into balance. With left-sided dominance, intuitive, aesthetic, and creative functions are reduced under stress. To center oneself, one is to put one's tongue on the centering button, which is about one quarter of an inch behind the upper front teeth. This spot apparently stimulates the thymus gland, weakens the effect of stress, and balances the cerebral hemispheres. Other activities that seem to balance the two hemispheres of the brain include reading a poem in a rhythmic fashion; listening to a person with a soothing voice; listening to classical music; listening to natural sounds such as cats purring, birds chirping, or brooks or waterfalls babbling; looking at pictures of pleasant landscapes or smiling people making caring gestures; swinging one's arms during a vigorous walk; and taking a shower. Good posture is also beneficial.

Nutrition

Good nutrition helps maintain the body for full functioning. Eating a balanced diet, taking vitamin supplements, and drinking plenty of water are important. In general, people in the United States need to reduce fat and cholesterol, sugar, salt, and food additive consumption. Their diets contain high levels of fat and cholesterol, which

are abundant in red meats, eggs, cheese, and prepared foods. Excessive consumption of fat is associated with cardiovascular diseases. They are obtaining an increasing proportion of their calories from sugar, which is associated with obesity, tooth decay, diabetes, and heart disease. There is a growing concern that additives and pollutants are related to cancer. These food additives include preservatives, coloring, flavoring, and stabilizers that extend shelf life and make processed food taste better. In addition, pesticides and other chemical pollutants are health hazards.

The increasing consumption of saturated fats and sugar, coupled with a decrease in activity levels, contributes to a widespread occurrence of obesity. In general, people in the United States need to increase exercise while decreasing caloric intake, particularly from fats and sugars. At the same time, the percentage of calories from foods containing fiber, such as fresh fruits, vegetables, and whole grains, should be increased. Canned, frozen, and prepared foods are usually devoid of their original fiber content and often have sugar and salt added. The grains we eat have often been refined to white flour and rice, thereby losing much of the roughage. Although improving eating habits may not prevent stress, it is one way to maintain the level of fitness needed to fight stress.

Exercise

Regular, vigorous exercise can also help one withstand chronic stress. Aerobic exercise elevates the heart rate during and for a period after the exercise. The range of elevation necessary to produce an aerobic effect is from 60% to 80% of the maximal heart rate the person can achieve, which is calculated at 220 minus the person's age in years. Jogging, cycling, and swimming are particularly good aerobic exercises. Dance allows one to stretch and strengthen muscles and to reduce tension.

Regular exercise develops greater capacities in several areas of function. It increases the strength of cardiac contractions, the size of the coronary arteries, the blood supply to the heart, the size of the heart muscle, and the blood volume per heartbeat. It decreases the heart rate at rest and with exertion and reduces vulnerability to cardiac dysrhythmias. It increases the blood oxygen content, blood volume, and efficiency of peripheral blood distribution and return. Exercise increases the blood supply to the lungs and the functional capacity during exercise. It increases lean muscle mass and functional capacity during exercise. Exercise also reduces strain and nervous tension resulting from psychological stress and reduces the tendency for depression.

Sleep

Sleep is also important for dealing with stress. Sleep needs decrease with age, and people may awaken several times during the night as they grow older. This should not be confused with insomnia, which is a prolonged inability to sleep. There are three types of insomnia: (1) initial, when it takes more than 15 minutes to fall asleep; (2) intermittent, with awakening during the night and difficulty returning to sleep; and (3) terminal, with early morning awakening and inability to go back to sleep.

Physical, emotional, and nutritional factors may contribute to insomnia. A lack of physical exercise, digestive problems, heart trouble, and high blood pressure interfere with sleep. Disturbing emotional states such as anger, fear, guilt, depression, and anxiety create tension that interferes with sleep. An unbalanced diet, alcohol, caffeine consumption, and a large meal shortly before bedtime can interfere with sleep.

To foster a good night's sleep, the day's activities should be tapered off before getting ready for bed. Regular exercise promotes deep sleep but should not be done for several hours before bedtime. Likewise, biofeedback and meditation have stress-reducing properties that foster sleep but should not be done before bedtime because they can boost energy and alertness. Chocolate, cola, coffee, tea, and other foods and beverages containing caffeine should be restricted, particularly in the evening. Overeating, particularly heavy foods, should also be avoided at night. The bed should be associated with sleep, and the room should be dark and quiet.

RELAXATION
Abdominal Breathing

Numerous techniques can be used to foster relaxation. Abdominal breathing is a quick method. When stressed, people tend to breathe in short, shallow breaths. Consequently, the lungs do not fill up completely. The remaining air is stale, and oxidation of tissues is incomplete. Muscle tension results. Without being conspicuous, one can take a few abdominal breaths almost anywhere at any time. It is best to do abdominal breathing for 5 to 10 minutes once or twice daily while sitting upright. It may be done during normally low times or to reverse the stress response when it has been triggered. To do abdominal breathing, one should inhale slowly through the nose while keeping the back straight. First the abdomen expands, then the chest, and finally the shoulders. Then one should exhale slowly and hold the breath for 1 or 2 seconds before starting another inhalation.

Massage

Massage can relieve tension, provide a passive form of exercise, and foster tactile communication. It stimulates relaxation and flexibility. Self-massage can be done from a chair. It can be done as a full-body massage or to a part of the body that is particularly tense. To do a full-body massage, one may start by placing both hands on the top of the head and moving them in slow circular motions down the back of the head, neck, and shoulder area. The neck and shoulder are common sites for tension. They may be most easily massaged by crossing hands over so that the right hand massages the left shoulder and the left hand massages the right shoulder. Then the hands are returned to the top of the head and moved forward in circular motions over the forehead, face, neck, and chest. To relax the right arm, one grasps the fingertips of the right hand with the left hand and moves up the hand and arm to the shoulder in circular motions with the fingers on top and the thumb on the underside. Then one massages down the right side of the chest. The procedure is repeated up the left arm and down the left side. Then hands are placed on the lower abdomen with fingertips touching. Circular motions are used up to the chest.

The low back is another area that is commonly tense, particularly from sedentary work. One places the hands on the lower back with fingertips touching at the coccyx. The fingertips then massage up as high as one can reach. A foot should be massaged with the massage continuing up the foot, over the ankle, and up the calf and thigh. Then the massage should be repeated on the other foot and leg. This full-body massage can be done after a warm bath at bedtime to foster sleep.

Progressive Relaxation

Progressive relaxation may also be used to foster sleep. It is the conscious contraction and relaxation of muscles. By deliberately tensing muscles, one can learn to identify what muscles are tight and learn to relax them. It can be used before, during, or after an anxious situation. If done routinely once or twice daily, it can help keep one's anxiety level down.

Progressive relaxation can be done in a standing, sitting, or lying position. There is greater likelihood of falling asleep in a lying position. In a sitting position, one should keep the head squarely on the shoulders, back against the chair, feet on the floor, legs uncrossed, and hands on the lap in a relaxed position. During progressive relaxation one tenses specific muscles to a maximal degree and notes how tight the muscles feel for about 5 seconds. Then the muscle is relaxed, and the pleasant feeling of relaxation is enjoyed for about 10 seconds. For a head-to-toe progression, one starts by wrinkling up the forehead and noting where it feels particularly tense. Then one relaxes that part slowly, identifies the muscles

that are relaxing, notes the difference between tension and relaxation, and enjoys the relaxed feeling. Box 2-3 contains abbreviated instructions for other body parts.

With experience in progressive relaxation, one can also learn to relax without tension. One first concentrates on relaxing each body part and then on generalized relaxation with deep breathing. One takes a deep breath, holds it, and then exhales slowly while relaxing the entire body from head to toe, saying "relax" so that the "x" is said as the focus reaches the toes.

Biofeedback

Biofeedback uses mechanical devices to gain self-regulation to control autonomic responses. The galvanic skin response uses electrodes attached to the fingertips to measure skin resistance, which is moisture of the skin that indicates nervousness. Arteries contract under stress and dilate with relaxation. A thermistor on the finger detects changes in peripheral skin temperature that are associated with activity of the

---

BOX 2-3 Progressive Muscle Relaxation

Close eyes tightly.
Wrinkle nose.
Place teeth together, and press lips against teeth into a forced smile.
Press tongue hard against the roof of the mouth.
Clench teeth.
Pucker lips.
Pull chin toward chest.
Put head back as far as it will go.
Press head to right shoulder.
Press head to left shoulder.
Hold arm out straight, make a fist, and tighten the whole arm or pull elbow tightly into side.
Repeat with the other arm.
Push shoulder blades toward each other.
Pull chest in.
Pull stomach in.
Tighten muscles in lower abdomen, buttocks, and thighs, and raise self in the chair.
Push foot against the floor; then point toes toward the head and repeat with the other leg and foot.

smooth muscles in peripheral arteries. This skin temperature is particularly useful for control of migraine headaches. The electroencephalograph uses electrodes attached to the scalp to detect electrical activity on the brain's cortex. Different brain wave patterns are associated with different states of mind. The electromyograph uses electrodes attached to the forehead or forearm to measure muscle tension from electrical impulses generated by muscles. People with migraine and tension headaches, hypertension, and gastrointestinal problems have responded well to biofeedback. Because the instruments convert skin resistance, skin temperature, brain waves, and muscle tension into readily observable signs, people can tell if they are controlling their body responses or not. They can also learn to read and interpret body signals without the use of instruments to modify their responses.

Autogenic Training: Self-Hypnosis

Autogenic training produces deep relaxation through self-hypnosis. These regular but brief sessions of passive concentration on physiologically adapted stimuli reduce other extraneous stimuli and have helped people with asthma, arthritis, constipation, hypertension, migraine headaches, and sleep disturbances.

To do self-hypnosis, one should lie down with eyes closed in a quiet room and take a few deep breaths. Each autogenic training session should last 2 to 20 minutes, preferably 20 minutes two or three times daily. There are six phrases. When learning autogenic training, only one phrase should be added at a time once per week.

The first phrase focuses on heaviness, the next on warmth, then on heartbeat, breath, the solar plexus, and the forehead. Supporting phrases such as "I am relaxing" or "I am at peace" are interspersed between induction phrases. For the heaviness induction, one systematically concentrates on thinking that each part of the body feels heavy: "My face is heavy. I am relaxing. My neck is heavy. I am at peace. My shoulders are heavy. I am resting. My chest is heavy. I am quiet."

For the warmth induction phrase, one substitutes "warm" for "heavy" in the previous phrases. The heart induction phrase is, "My heartbeat is calm and regular." Then one concentrates on "My breathing is relaxed and comfortable." Next one puts one's hands on one's abdomen to create warmth and repeats, "My solar plexus is warm." Finally, one thinks, "My forehead is cool." To return to an alert state, one takes a few deep breaths and thinks, "I will arise refreshed and alert," then moves one's arms and legs, opens one's eyes, and slowly gets up.

Meditation

Meditation focuses attention on an experience, helps one become aware of one's response, and facilitates the integration of the physical, mental, emotional, and spiritual aspects of one's life. There are many methods for meditating. One may focus on an object such as a candle, chant, listen to music, or meditate on one's own breath. To meditate on one's breath, one can count while breathing: one on inhalation, two on exhalation, three on inhalation, and four on exhalation. That process can be repeated until the allotted time for meditation is over. Usually people experience an inner calm and sense of well-being from meditation.

Visualization and Mental Imagery

Visualization and mental imagery can be used to relax. One starts in a relaxed position and visualizes pleasant thoughts. One can meditate on a visualized colored object such as a blue sky, white cloud, green tree, red apple, or pink flower. One can imagine being in a favorite place such as on a sandy beach, in the mountains, or in front of a fireplace in a favorite room listening to music. One can concentrate on the sights, sounds, smells, tastes, and feelings of the pleasant thoughts.

Poetry

Poetry reading or writing is useful for reducing tension, particularly if one is depressed and movement and verbalizing have not worked sufficiently. Poems are chosen for their rhythm, their mood, and the feelings expressed. Poems can be read in a one-to-one or group meeting. Discussions about the meaning can help verbalize feelings.

Music

Soft classical music can help release feelings and emotions and bring about relaxation.

Baths

Water is a relaxant. One should fill the bathtub with water that is body temperature and immerse oneself up to one's neck for about 15 minutes.

ENHANCING SELF-ESTEEM

"You yourself, as much as anybody in the entire universe, deserve your love and affection."
—Buddha

Positive affirmations can be used to enhance one's self-esteem. One can become more comfortable with positive thoughts about oneself and decrease the amount of self-devaluation. Several methods can be used. One might imagine positive scenes and see oneself as one wants to be. One can repeat positive affirmations such as "I am happy," "I am healthy," or "I am beautiful." One can also write positive affirmations on cards, put them in conspicuous places, and read them often. People may take turns making positive comments about each other.

SUPPORT GROUPS

Support systems are synergistic. One can accomplish more through support groups than alone. Support groups provide a feeling of being accepted, valued, loved, and esteemed and a sense of belonging. In addition to providing emotional support, support systems help provide a social identity and are a source of information, services, and material aid.

Wheatly (2002) says that many people feel isolated or invisible and want to talk about concerns and struggles. Telling our stories creates a relationship and helps us move closer to one another. It's difficult to hate someone whose story we know. Wheatly (2002) encourages the following principles: (1) acknowledging each other as equals, (2) staying curious about each other, (3) recognizing that we need each other's help to become better listeners, (4) slowing down to think and reflect, (5) understanding that conversations are a way to think together, and (6) expecting messiness.

There are several types of support systems. Usually the family is the natural support system that constitutes the primary support group. Peer support groups are also important. They are composed of people who have had similar experiences, have adjusted, and want to share their insight. A head nurse may receive support from other head nurses or a jogger from other joggers. Religious organizations provide a congregation that sets guidelines for living, shares values, and provides traditions. Voluntary service groups and self-help groups provide support for specific purposes such as to lose weight, to stop drinking alcohol, to quit smoking, or to adjust to a mastectomy or a stoma. Family, friends, and peers are usually sought out before professional support systems, but the helping professions are available when support from others is inadequate.

It is extremely important that managers take excellent care of their own well-being. They can function at their best if they are healthy. They need considerable energy to be supportive of others and will not have strength to share if they are hurting. Likewise, staff nurses need a sense of health and well-being to provide the best nursing care. Managers are responsible for providing care to the caregivers.

The manager should help protect personnel from undue stress. Personnel may be taught identification of stress symptoms and stress management. Annual physical examinations could be required. Vacations are provided and encouraged. Counseling and referral services can be provided as support systems. Nutrition, educational, and health promotional programs are presented, and nutritious food is served in the cafeteria. Exercise programs can be provided and encouraged. Managers should monitor stress levels and intervene when necessary.

PROTECTION FROM WORKPLACE VIOLENCE

Dysfunctional families, anger about illness and dying, disgruntled workers, and consequently workplace violence are too common. People may express their stress through violence. Sheehan (2000, p. 24) suggests asking the following questions to assess the risk of violence: "Does the patient have a history of aggressive behavior? Does the patient exhibit anger, irritation, or illogical thought processes? Does the patient exhibit confusion and agitation? Does the patient lack emotion or have a dull demeanor?" Then she recommends the following strategies to reduce the risk (Sheehan, 2000, p. 25):

Establish a zero-tolerance policy for violent behavior. Identify patients with a history of aggressive or violent behavior, and communicate this behavior to staff while maintaining confidentiality. Transfer violent patients to units with higher staffing ratios or with staff trained to deal with violent behavior. Enforce visiting hours and visitor passes.... Don't let employees work alone in isolated units or units with walk-in patients. Don't allow employees to be alone with patients during intimate physical examinations. Don't let employees enter seclusion rooms alone.

TIME MANAGEMENT

If productivity were a function of time only, one would expect all to produce equally. And yet, although everyone has the same number of hours in a day and the same number of days per week, some people accomplish more than others. Granted, some people work longer and harder than others to accomplish more, but some just make better use of their time. Because nurses work long hours, they should work smarter—not harder—to get more done in less time.

PERSONAL TIME MANAGEMENT

Stephen Covey (1989) speaks to *The 7 Habits of Highly Effective People: Powerful Lessons in Personal Change.* He says one needs to start by being proactive and accepting responsibility for one's actions and attitudes. The more one exercises freedom to choose responses, the more proactive one becomes. Then opportunities are fed and problems are starved.

Second, one should begin with the end in mind. One should begin with a clear understanding of the desired direction and destination. Things are created mentally before they are created physically. Quality is designed and built in. Ineffective people use old habits and environmental conditions. They may climb the ladder to success only to find once they get to the top that the ladder is against the wrong wall.

Third, put first things first. Personal management is organizing and managing according to personal priorities to get where you want to go. It is important to give less time to things that are urgent but not important, such as pressing matters and nonproductive meetings, and to spend more time on things that are important but not urgent, such as relationships, prevention, planning, preparation, taking opportunities, and recreation.

Fourth, think win-win. Effectiveness is often accomplished by cooperative efforts of two or more people. A win-win attitude explores options until a mutually satisfactory solution is reached. Desired results, guidelines, accountability, resources, and consequences are made explicit. It is an abundance mentality that builds on synergy rather than a scarcity mentality that leads to win-lose strategies.

Fifth, seek first to understand, then to be understood. Communications are important to building win-win relationships. Our perceptions come from our experiences. Credibility problems usually involve differences. Empathetic listening is therapeutic. Once people feel they are understood, they lower their defenses. Once one understands the other person's point of view, it is easier to problem solve a win-win solution.

Sixth, synergize. Synergy comes from teamwork or creative cooperation. Diversity can produce a synergy, where the whole is greater than the sum of its parts. Synergy results from bringing different perspectives together in a spirit of mutual respect to seek the best solution.

Seventh, sharpen the saw. The longer one saws, the duller the saw gets and the harder one works to get less and less accomplished. People need physical, spiritual, mental, social, and emotional self-renewal. One needs to give priority to a balanced program for self-renewal.

Habits involve knowledge, attitudes, and skills. Effective habits can be learned, and ineffective habits can be unlearned. As one practices the seven habits of highly effective people, one is changed from the inside out.

In *First Things First* Covey (1994) teaches the six steps to empowerment by putting first things first. Start by connecting to the mission. Write a personal mission statement. Identify up to seven roles. Second, review your roles. Third, identify your goals related to each role. Concentrate on relationships, prevention, preparation, planning, seizing opportunities, and recreation. Fourth, organize your week by prioritizing activities to reach your goals for each role. Schedule your priorities on your calendar. Fifth, exercise integrity toward the first things in your life. Start each day by previewing the day, prioritizing, and being sensitive to important commitments. Watch for opportunities to live your mission. Sixth, evaluate, learn, and live.

In *Fast Cycle Time* Christopher Meyer (1993) discusses how to align purpose, strategy, and structure for speed instead of working faster. He indicates that analyzing strategy and core processes enables management to detect and correct problems earlier and leverage knowledge toward improved innovations and increased value.

MAXIMIZE MANAGERIAL TIME

"From what we get, we make a living; what we give, however, makes a life." —Arthur Ashe

INVENTORY ACTIVITIES

Nurse managers may start a plan for maximizing use of their time by conducting an inventory of their activities. After recording what they did every 15 minutes for a typical week, they assess how they spent their time. How much time was spent in which activities? Was the way the time was spent determined by conscious decisions, habit, work demands, default, or spontaneity? What do they like to do? What activities do they want to increase? What do they want to decrease? How can they reduce the time wasters (Box 2-4)?

SET GOALS

Next, nurses determine their short-, medium-, and long-range goals. What do they want to accomplish? What do they want to do soon? Which goals must be completed before others? Which will take the longest to achieve? Setting priorities helps resolve goal conflicts and directs how they will spend their time.

PLAN STRATEGIES

Once they have determined and ranked their goals, they plan strategies for how to accomplish them. What activities must they do? What are low-priority activities that can be eliminated? Next the nurse manager schedules activities. A tickler box with divider cards for months and weeks can be used by filing task cards behind the appropriate month and week card. As they look at their major responsibilities for a whole year, they may have some flexibility in determining when certain jobs are done and can use those to help balance the workload around tasks that have to be done at certain times, such as preparing the budget. Various calendar systems can also be used: one may do major project planning

---

BOX 2-4 Time Wasters

Poor planning
Failure to establish goals
Failure to set objectives
Failure to plan strategies to accomplish goals
Unwillingness to say no
Ineffective use of transition times
Cumbersome paperwork
Poor filing system
Poor reading skills
Poor listening and memory techniques
Telephone interruptions
Unorganized office visits
Poorly planned meetings
Lack of delegation
Lack of information
Poor communication
Lack of feedback
Procrastination
Indecisiveness
Haste
Management by crisis

---

on a year-at-a-glance calendar; desk ink blotters that depict a month at a time can help regulate that month's work; a week-at-a-glance or a day-at-a-glance calendar is convenient for carrying in one's purse. Daily work sheets depicting what work should be done during which hour may also be useful. Commercial planning systems such as Filofax, Franklin Day Planner, Day Runner, and Day Timer are available. Computer software packages such as PalmPilot are also available for desktop or hand-held computers. Calendars can be on computer systems so that meetings can be scheduled when the most people are available. Computer files of correspondence, reports, or other documents can be stored on the computer in readily retrievable ways (Grohar-Murray and DiCroce, 2003; Marquis and Huston, 2000; Sullivan and Decker, 2001).

PLAN SCHEDULE

Nurse managers need to assess their peak and low times to plan a detailed schedule more effectively. Are they most alert and creative in the early morning or late at night? Are they slow starters in the morning? Do they reach a low energy point in the middle of the afternoon? The nurse's prime internal time—the most creative time for working alone—is a good time to schedule work that should not be interrupted. When is their prime external time, their best time to work with others? If they reach a low point in the afternoon, that may be a good time to schedule office visits. They may offer their guests a cup of coffee or tea, which tends to facilitate communication, sip on their own drinks, and listen.

Time should be set aside for certain activities each day. Scheduled activities are recorded. Scheduled and unscheduled times are noted, and contact and thinking times are identified. The secretary may be given available hours for scheduling office visits.

A few minutes at the beginning of each day should be allowed for planning. A running list of what the nurse manager needs to do in order of importance can be made each morning to plan what will be done that day. Desk-organizing files—which are merely folders with such labels as urgent, return calls, dictate, read, file, and low priority—can help determine what to do each day. Scheduled free time can be used to deal with these activities. A few minutes at the end of the day are used to evaluate what happened.

SAY NO

Learning how to say no graciously, especially regarding low-priority work, saves time. It is advisable for nurse managers to acknowledge the request, state and explain their position, check back for understanding with the other person, and avoid defensiveness. For example, when asked to speak at a meeting, they might respond, "I would love to discuss our institutional goals with your committee. However, I have another commitment at that time. Barbara Jones and Sue Smith are both very familiar with the institutional goals. Perhaps you could ask one of them to speak. Does that sound agreeable to you?"

USE TRANSITION TIMES

Managers can accomplish much during transition times. Incoming mail may be read while one is on hold when returning phone calls. Reports can be read while commuting to and from work, or audiotapes can be listened to while driving. Isometric exercises can be done at almost any time. Lunch and coffee breaks may be used for personal business. Because many people are watching their weight, lunch breaks may be better used for exercise such as walking and jogging or for meditation than for eating a large lunch.

ACCELERATE LEARNING

Leaders and managers need to be familiar with relevant information. An accelerated learning program includes *clear, realistic learning goals* that can be achieved in days. It is often better to quickly learn and act on the available information in a few days or weeks rather than to wait to retrieve all the information and wait for months or years to act. *Collect the information in one place.* Discard irrelevant and redundant materials, and rapidly skim the rest. Organize the materials into a logical sequence, and use speed-reading techniques to reread it. *Group the material into small study units.* Abstract the study unit information into a short paragraph. *Format the material* into a style you will study repeatedly. *Review the material,* preferably at least twice daily, to quickly comprehend and memorize it. Accelerated learning can help leaders learn a large volume of information without anxiety and overload (Bennis, Mason, and Mitroff, 1993).

IMPROVE READING

Learning speed-reading techniques, such as tapping, L pattern, S swirl, area reading, and reading for meaning, can help overcome common reading problems of single-word fixation, involuntary regression by rereading, subvocalization of words as one reads, and inability to concentrate.

IMPROVE MEMORY

Listening and memory techniques also save time. When listening for understanding, one should assume value in what the speaker is saying by being attentive, delaying judgment, maintaining eye contact, and using attentive body language. One then needs to assess the content of the information by focusing on central ideas, looking for relationships between ideas, and selecting an organizing structure such as main and supporting ideas, advantages and disadvantages, or putting information into chronological order. One should analyze the information by listening to what is being said, identifying how it is being said by inferring emotions from body language and tone of voice, and considering the speaker's motivation for saying it. Distractions may have to be reduced so the listener can concentrate.

Verbal, physical, and mental techniques can be used to stimulate memory (Box 2-5). Repeating, clarifying, and summarizing are effective verbal techniques. Physical techniques for stimulating memory are note taking, filing, and follow-up memos. Focusing, imaging, linking, locating, and chunking are mental techniques.

Focusing by putting attention on one thing at a time helps block out distractions.

Imaging creates a vivid mental image that helps one remember something. For example, when introduced to Leona Dean, the nurse might picture her leaning on a dean of a specific school to help remember her name.

Linking makes associations between things that make them easier to remember later. Associations may be cause and effect, parts of a whole, or things that are near each other, logically go together, contrast with each other, or happen concurrently. Creating an association

BOX **2-5** Memory Techniques		
VERBAL TECHNIQUES	**PHYSICAL TECHNIQUES**	**MENTAL TECHNIQUES**
Repeating	Note taking	Focusing
Clarifying	Filing	Imaging
Summarizing	Follow-up memos	Linking
		Locating
		Chunking

that leads from point one to point two to point three and creating an image of those associations will help one remember a speech.

Locating is a memory technique that uses a known structure, often one's home, to arrange and remember information by putting it in specific locations. One might progress through an orientation program by visualizing the hallway in the office and thinking of who is in each office as one walks through the hall and what service that person provides new staff.

Chunking helps one remember by dividing large amounts of information into smaller, more manageable pieces. One could chunk information needed into separate sections of a report, or the nurse could locate what items are needed in specific, separate offices.

CRITICAL THINKING

Critical thinking is needed to excel in the information age. It is a reflective problem-solving style of thinking. One should *focus on the right questions*, define terms, and list critical issues. *Analyze arguments* by identifying and examining assumptions, positions, reasons, and conclusions. *Question, challenge,* and *clarify* by asking who, what, when, where, and why questions. Distinguish between facts and inferences. Request more information as needed. *Judge the credibility of the sources.* Consider the reputation, expertise, and possible conflicts of interest of the source. *Use logic,* including inductive and deductive reasoning. Evaluate the related research. *Use high-level thinking strategies,* such as analyzing, clarifying, comparing, inferring, and problem solving.

Avoid faulty thinking such as overgeneralization, use of selected cases instead of a wide-based foundation of facts, and use of inadequate sources. Emotion-laden words that elicit strong emotions can camouflage weaknesses. Highly ambiguous language and poorly defined terms can lead to multiple interpretations. Unrelated and irrelevant points can cause distractions from the key points of an argument. Repetition in a variety of places by a number of people becomes

more believable regardless of its truthfulness. Acceptable statements make unacceptable conclusions more believable. Expert opinion is not necessarily the truth. Denigration of opponents is sometimes used to discredit another's arguments, so conclusions should be separated from the person presenting the issues.

STREAMLINE PAPERWORK

Much time can be saved by streamlining paperwork. Scheduling a block of time to answer mail prevents interruptions. If the situation warrants, a standard reply can be used. Some responses can be made on the query memo if no file copy is needed, and typing carbon responses to letters onto the back of the query letter saves filing time and space. Keeping as little as possible and only what is needed saves time. Color coding is useful, and recording of destruction dates on files reduces the need to review the materials later. Dictation usually takes less time than writing by hand, and calls can be used when a record is not necessary. Computerization and e-mail also save time. Invisible information (spoken word) can be recorded on a steno pad kept by the phone with each page dated sequentially. Unfortunately that information is difficult to move to priority areas. A spiral-bound message pad with no carbon required can be used to tear off the top sheet and send wherever needed while still keeping a chronological record. The disadvantage is that there is little space for writing on the form. Recycled paper by each phone can be used when a permanent record is not needed. Some calendar systems have forms for recording conversations and can be treated like phone message sheets. Selective reading by scanning tables of contents and reading summaries at the end of long responses and reports saves time. Managers should not concentrate on details unless necessary, because they are quickly forgotten. Scanning for major points is often adequate.

USE COMPUTERS FOR TIME MANAGEMENT

Computers can replace a hodgepodge of record-keeping procedures with a uniform system. With the use of a computer, printer, and accounting and payable software, information can be entered one time into a database and sent electronically anywhere that the technology is available. A graphic interface program can merge a computerized mailing list of names and addresses into letters, address envelopes and mailing labels, do mathematical calculations on the screen while the letter is being composed, spell check the entire document, identify more interesting words using the on-screen thesaurus, print out multiple copies, make global changes in all documents if the letter is revised, and preview the letter on the screen before printing it. It can also check a calendar for a date or schedule an appointment; set an alarm for the appointment; dial a phone number; send and receive faxes; calculate figures; address envelopes; create a macro of often-used addresses or phrases; create, save, and delete files; and locate a file and insert it into another document. Computer software can be used to organize projects and keep and track the progress relative to performance objectives. Files should be saved frequently and backed up on hard disk and floppy disk or tape. Computer files can duplicate the paper files. Clutter should be removed from both computer and paper files. Portable printers and fax machines or a phone jack and a fax-modem board inside a portable computer allow receiving and sending data anywhere the technology is available (Allen, 1995; Lively, 1996).

USE TELEPHONE CALLS

Telephone calls instead of office visits or correspondence save time. Secretaries can screen calls so that other activities are not interrupted and, in fact, may be able to handle much of the business. A call-back system can be used to complete the business the secretary cannot handle. If late morning and late afternoon are chosen for returning calls, calls are likely to be kept short, because people are eager to eat lunch or to go home.

Paging and beeping systems, call forwarding, call back, call waiting, speed dialing, three-way calling, voice mail, and conference calls make telephoning more efficient. A long cord or portable phone allows one to move around and work while using the telephone. Cell phones can be used at the patient's bedside or while walking between patients. Car phones can be used during transition times.

Forms for telephone messages are less likely to get lost than scraps of paper. It is helpful for phone messages to be collected in one place. A secured pen or pencil by the phone is convenient. One should keep a list of commonly called phone numbers handy. If major topics for conversation are outlined before making a call, it is less likely that one will forget something and need to call back. One can set the tone of the call. A businesslike call started by "What can I do for you?" will accomplish more in less time than a friendly call started with "How are you?" Conference calls also save time by focusing more on business than socializing. The purpose for the conversation helps determine whether a meeting or a conference call is necessary.

SCHEDULE OFFICE VISITS

Secretaries may also screen office visits. Again, they may be able to handle much of the business themselves. When managers schedule reception hours, secretaries can schedule appointments for the appropriate length of time and inform managers of the purpose of the meeting so that they can be adequately prepared. One may need to close the office door to complete a task without interruptions. Sitting with one's back to the door may decrease interruptions because people will note that the manager is busy.

CONTROL VISIT TIME

The length of a meeting can be better controlled if it is not in the manager's office. Managers may go to the staff associates' work area or meet visitors in a reception area, where they are free to leave whenever they desire. By standing up when someone drops into the office, managers prevent the visitor from sitting down, thus controlling the situation. They can assess the priority, make an appointment for another time, keep the visit short, or invite the visitor to sit down for a longer discussion. Many drop-in visits can be prevented by scheduling lunch with staff associates on a regular basis. This allows the manager opportunity to keep informed, discuss matters of common interest, and eat lunch at the same time. Staff can be informed through memos and routing slips.

USE MEETINGS EFFECTIVELY

Managers spend considerable time in meetings, much of which is wasted. Meetings are used for participative problem solving, decision making, coordination, information sharing, and morale building. Managers first consider the purpose of the meeting; if it is not necessary, they do not conduct it. Key participants are identified, and if they cannot attend, the meeting is not held. People who do not need to attend are not invited. Managers should consider alternatives to a meeting, such as a memo, telephone call, or conference. Staff associates can represent the manager at some meetings both to save managerial time and to develop the staff associates. Managers may limit their time in meetings by attending only that segment when they are to make a contribution. Scheduling meetings before lunch and quitting time facilitates ending meetings on time. A centrally located meeting place saves travel time. The purpose of the meeting should be clearly defined, and an agenda should be circulated before the meeting.

Meetings should start on time, because time is expensive. Starting a meeting 15 minutes late for 20 people who earn $10 an hour costs $50 in downtime. Stating the purpose of the meeting and following the agenda are the manager's responsibilities. The manager should start with high-priority items so that only low-priority items will be left over. The manager should control interruptions, restate conclusions, make assignments and deadlines clear, and end the meeting on time. If the business is completed early, the manager dismisses the meeting. Minutes are circulated preferably within 1 day after the meeting; this allows people to be informed without having to attend the meeting unless their input is specifically needed. Minutes also remind participants of their assigned tasks (Ellis and Hartley, 2000).

DELEGATION

The manager decides what task should be done, when, where, and by whom. Responsibility and authority should be assigned. The manager needs to evaluate the risk involved in delegating by assessing the criticality of the expected results and the confidence in resources. The planning strategy ascertains specifications, including the expected results, rationale, requirements, and constraints. The delegated authority should be specified, and support needed should be anticipated. When communicating the delegated assignment, the manager should ensure understanding, give and receive feedback, and address concerns. To monitor the delegated assignment, the manager should set up a milestone-tracking system, review scheduled status reports, and give feedback on the interim reports. Support is provided by responding to the delegatee's needs, acknowledging the status reports, and being available for guidance and problem solving. The manager should intervene only when the action seems warranted and, even then, by avoiding interference and explaining one's actions. Reverse delegation can be avoided by clarifying specifications, transferring authority, and expressing confidence in the delegatee. The results should be evaluated by examining the specifications, evaluating the monitoring results, and giving feedback on the final results.

Establishing routines improves learning curves, success, and productivity. Routines can reduce tension, errors, and wasted time. The manager decides what to delegate, selects the appropriate person, communicates the responsibilities to that person, grants authority with the responsibility, provides support, monitors the situation, and evaluates the results (Sullivan and Decker, 2001).

RESEARCH Perspective 2-1

Data from Anthony MK, Standing TS, Hertz JE: Nurses' beliefs about their abilities to delegate within changing models of care. *The Journal of Continuing Education in Nursing* V32(5):210-215, 2001.

Purpose: The purpose of this study was to describe the nurses' beliefs about their abilities to delegate and supervise direct nursing activities and studied differences on professional and job-related factors.

Methods: A mailed self-report survey was sent to 516 licensed nurses including 403 registered nurses and 113 licensed practical nurses/vocational nurses working in three practice settings. One hundred forty-eight questionnaires (30%) were usable. Descriptive statistics using frequency and means were used.

Results/conclusions: In general, nurses believed they were well prepared and competent to delegate. Differences were found in nurses' beliefs based on education, practice setting, and type of work responsibilities. They rated their educational preparation for delegation the lowest. Most of the nurses in the sample had over 15 years of experience. Continuing education classes or practical experience could lead to feelings about being well prepared and competent to delegate.

Reasons for Delegating

Delegation saves time and can help develop others. Delegation maximizes the use of the talents of staff associates. It uses latent abilities in personnel that contribute to their growth and development. Staff members learn by doing. Their involvement tends to increase their motivation and commitment to accomplish goals while freeing the manager to manage. This also reduces managerial costs.

The Four Rights of Delegation

The four rights of delegation are (1) task, (2) person, (3) communication, and (4) feedback. The right task should be within the scope of the person's practice and consistent with the job description. The right person should have the appropriate license or certificate, an appropriate job description, and demonstrated skill and is checked off on the skill checklist to delegate in the first place and to accept the delegated responsibility in the second place. The right communication should be clear, concise, complete, and correct. The right feedback should ask for input, get the person's recommended solution to

the problem, and recognize the person's efforts (Hansten, 1998).

Delegation Decision-Making Process

A National Council of State Boards of Nursing position paper (http://www.ncsbn.org/files/delegati.html) describes the assessment, planning, implementation, and evaluation of delegation. First, the Nurse Practice Act should permit the delegation, authorize the task or tasks to be delegated, and authorize the nurse to decide delegation. The delegator needs the appropriate education, skills, and experience; the appropriate scope of authority; and demonstrated and documented evidence of current competency. The delegatee needs appropriate education, skills, and experience and demonstrated and documented evidence of current competency. The delegator needs to assess the needs of the patient, the circumstances, and availability of adequate resources. Then the delegator needs to plan for the task or tasks to be delegated by specifying the knowledge and skills required to do the nature of each task, by requiring documented or demonstrated current competency to do each delegated task, and by determining the implications for the patient and others. To ensure appropriate accountability, the delegator accepts accountability for the performance of the delegated task or tasks and verifies that the delegatee accepts the delegation and accountability for the delegated task or tasks. Then the delegator supervises performance of the task by providing directions and clear expectations about how the task or tasks are to be performed; monitoring the performance to ensure compliance to established standards of practice, policies, and procedures; intervening as necessary; and ensuring documentation of the task or tasks. Finally, the delegator evaluates the delegation process, evaluates the patient and the performance of the task or tasks, and receives and gives feedback. The delegator adjusts the plan as necessary.

Conditions That Facilitate Delegation

Several conditions facilitate delegation. First, managers need to understand the concept of delegation and have a generally positive attitude toward people. They need to overcome feelings of loss of prestige through delegation and develop a positive atmosphere for their staff. They should help achieve results through effective communication instead of by doing the job themselves. Thus they concentrate on the accomplishment of overall goals and objectives rather than the day-to-day details.

Top management clarifies policies, goals, and objectives, and these are further developed by each succeeding lower level. For example, top management sets the overall budget, but each department then works with its own budget. Specifying goals and objectives directs personnel and determines priorities and the use of resources. Management by objectives promotes this.

Job descriptions provide a definition of the responsibility and authority involved with each position. Everything that must be done for the organization to meet its goals is part of someone's job. Consequently, job descriptions are based on the functional needs of the agency and clarify the responsibility of the individual's position and the objectives of the work.

Before writing job descriptions, management decides which assignments to delegate. To do so, managers should be aware of the capabilities and characteristics of their staff associates. Testing employees to learn what they can and cannot do and providing the necessary training help overcome many personnel failures. Staff members are often asked to perform skills for which they are not qualified or in which they are not interested. People tend to put off tasks they find unpleasant and then do them poorly. It is not necessary to delegate equally. By knowing individual capabilities, the manager can delegate according to the associate's interests and abilities.

Job descriptions are not always advantageous in small or rapidly changing organizations because those staffs often assume different roles at different times. Generalization is more common than the specialization required in larger, more stable organizations. Some employees outperform the requirements of their job descriptions, whereas others are not able to do some of the duties described. Job descriptions can be redefined according to the person's capability and organizational needs. If employees are unable to handle the required duties, they may be transferred to another area, given further training, supplied with an assistant to supplement their weak areas, or fired.

Controls based on goals, rather than means, are important. The manager checks on how well the delegated responsibilities are being performed, and the staff know whether or not they are meeting their responsibilities. Performance standards clarify how the manager measures achievement. These standards cover the quantity and quality of work expected and the time allowed for its accomplishment. The standards should be broad enough to allow individuality. If the standards are perceived as reasonable and fair by both manager and staff associates, they will both be happier with their jobs. Staff associates like their work to be noticed and appreciated. The manager meets their need for recognition and appreciation by having a general knowledge of what is happening, using an open door policy, expressing willingness to give assistance and support, and taking a personal interest in their problems. A "snoopervisor," however, is not appreciated.

It is the manager's responsibility to assess the results of delegation. One of the most satisfactory ways of being aware of what is happening is by being among the staff associates. Formal and informal meetings, systems of reporting, quality control, and statistical sampling are other means. Although inspection is perceived as unpleasant, most staff associates accept it as necessary. However, they do object to unnecessary inspections that disturb routines.

Even though people may receive satisfaction from knowing that they are doing a good job, having those efforts recognized by others is appreciated. Managers err if they do not give praise for work well done. People should also be rewarded for their continued contributions to the agency through raises and promotions. If staff associates err, they should be corrected as soon as possible. But when staff associates participate in goal setting, when the emphasis is on the goal rather than individual personalities, and when training is a continuous process, corrections that otherwise would have been made by the manager may be unnecessary. The system encourages self-correction.

Learning to live with differences may be difficult for managers, especially if they once performed their staff associates' tasks and now find that they are being done differently. It is even more threatening when the staff associate does a better job than the manager once did. It has to be recognized that there will be differences in quantity and quality of work accomplished and methods used between the manager and staff associate or between staff associates.

Responsibility, Authority, and Accountability

Assignment of responsibility, delegation of authority, and creation of accountability are the three concepts most often mentioned in relation to the delegation process (Box 2-6). Responsibility denotes obligation. It refers to what must be done to complete a task and the obligation created by the assignment. The manager and the staff associate must understand the activities for which the staff associate is responsible, what results are expected, and how performance is to be evaluated. Managers need a clear idea of what they want done before they can communicate that to others. To clarify ideas for themselves, the managers may put their ideas in writing. By so doing, they are then less likely to give incomplete directions. The assignment of responsibility is not complete, however, until the staff associate decides to accept the obligation.

Authority is the power to make final decisions and give commands. People to whom responsibility has been assigned need the authority to direct the performance of delegated duties. They need authority of sufficient scope to include all related activities without frequent consultation with their manager. The granting of too little authority is a common problem, because organizational policies and procedures are often limiting, and sometimes the person may have little control over the actions of others.

People with delegated authority perform for the manager. Although authority is delegated so that the staff associates can fulfill their responsibilities, the manager maintains control over the delegated authority and may recall it. Delegation of authority involves the staff associate's knowledge, abilities, skills, and potential contribution and the manager's guidance. During the initial phase of delegating authority, staff associates present their ideas and plans. The manager raises questions, explores alternatives, and helps identify potential problems and ways

BOX **2-6** Aspects of Delegation

Responsibility
Authority
Accountability

to prevent them. Then mutual agreement is reached. The manager offers continuing support by providing staff, resources, and information needed by the staff associate for the completion of the delegated responsibility. Good communications, sharing of information, and feedback are important.

Accountability refers to liability. Staff associates incur an obligation to complete work satisfactorily and to use authority appropriately when they accept delegated responsibility. They are accountable to their manager. Managers are accountable for the performance of the task, the selection of the person to complete it, and both the staff associate's and their own performance. Head nurses are responsible for delegation to team leaders, who are accountable for delegation to team members. Each remains accountable for the work delegated (Marrelli, 1997).

Cultural Considerations for Delegation

Communication is affected by culture. Context of speech, dialect, kinesics (stance, gestures, eye movement), use of touch, and volume have cultural variables and influence how one is perceived. Delegation given in a soft voice may not be considered as important as directions given in a louder tone. A quiet passive worker may be perceived as unable to do the work. Interpersonal space varies among cultures with most French and African Americans comfortable with closeness and middle class Caucasian Americans wanting 2 to 3 feet of personal space. Past, present, and future orientations vary among cultures. People with a past orientation may be particularly good for having elderly people reminisce, but a future-oriented person will be better adapted for strategic planning. Social organization differs among cultures. Some are more individualistic, and others more family oriented. People also differ in internal and external control, with some thinking they can control their environment and others leaving that to fate, luck, or God's will. There are also biopsychosocial differences, putting some people at more risk for some conditions than others.

These cultural differences affect the relationship between the delegator and delegatee (Marquis and Huston, 2000).

Reasons for Underdelegating

There are numerous reasons for underdelegating. Managers may think they can do the job more quickly themselves, resent interruptions to answer questions, or not want to take the time to check what has been done. They may get cooperation from other departments more easily than from staff associates or be unwilling to take risks for fear of being blamed for others' mistakes.

Some managers do not have confidence in their staff associates and are afraid that their staff associates will not keep them adequately informed. Or they may not trust their staff associates and complain that they lack training and sufficient experience. They may argue that their staff associates have little understanding of the organizational objectives and are specialists without the general knowledge needed for problem solving. In some cases, they may even be afraid that their staff associates will outperform them.

Therefore managers may like to do the work themselves and think that they can do it better. They receive personal recognition for and satisfaction from the work and prefer to do the real things instead of just plan with others. Such people often expect perfection, consider themselves indispensable, and desire to dominate. They are afraid of losing power and prestige and are aware that their poor operating procedures and practices may be exposed (Swansburg and Swansburg, 2002).

Reasons for Not Accepting Delegation

Staff associates have their reasons for not accepting delegation. Some depend on their manager and find it easier to ask the boss. Others lack self-confidence and fear failure and criticism. This fear is often related to how mistakes have been handled. Emphasis on the mistake itself is more threatening than using the situation as a learning experience.

Lack of guidelines, standards, and control are additional problems. Duties are not always clearly defined, authority not specified, or necessary information and resources not readily available. Some staff associates are already overworked. The incentives are inadequate, and they do not want to perform work if their manager receives the credit.

PROCRASTINATION

"What we see depends mainly on what we look for." —Sir John Lubbock

REASONS FOR PROCRASTINATION

Reasons for procrastination may be divided into two basic categories: emotional reasons and non-emotional reasons. Box 2-7 lists some of the most common reasons in each category.

Emotional Reasons

There are several emotional causes of procrastination. People may fill present moments with trivia to escape an overwhelming task or choose a pleasant task to escape an unpleasant one. Procrastination can be used as an excuse for poor work with comments such as "I just couldn't get to it until the last minute." Some play victims of circumstances to gain sympathy. Although it is preferable to delegate than to play "poor me,"

BOX **2-7** Reasons for Procrastination	
EMOTIONAL REASONS	**NONEMOTIONAL REASONS**
To escape an overwhelming task	Lack of goals
To escape an unpleasant task	Goals without deadlines
To excuse poor work	Unrealistic time estimates
To gain sympathy	Insufficient information
To get someone else to do the job	Inadequate follow-up
	Interruptions
	Overcommitment

---

there are those who try to get someone else to do the job through procrastination.

Nonemotional Reasons

Lack of goals, goals without deadlines, and unrealistic time estimates are some reasons for procrastination. Some people have insufficient information to do a job, do inadequate follow-up, or have so many interruptions they cannot get a job done. Others are just so overcommitted that they do not have time to do everything they have agreed to do.

TECHNIQUES TO STOP PROCRASTINATION

Dividing and conquering, or breaking a large job down into smaller, more manageable tasks, is a good way to overcome procrastination. Doing a start-up task to get in the mood and taking advantage of moods help. Starting with what one does not like to do and the highest priorities and giving oneself incentives are helpful. Considering the consequences of not doing the job can motivate some people into action (Yoder-Wise, 2003).

Consider using the money you earn by doing things you like to do to hire someone to do what you do not like to do. Consider switching jobs with someone, or divide up the job so you do what you like to do, such as the review of the literature, while someone else does what she likes to do, such as the statistical analysis of the data. Make a commitment to someone to help overcome procrastination.

It is appropriate to ask yourself, "What's the best use of my time now?" Then set goals, plan realistic time schedules, and gather the necessary information to do the job. Avoid overcommitment, and give yourself rewards for jobs well done. Box 2-8 summarizes techniques to help stop procrastination.

MAXIMIZE ORGANIZATION TIME

PLAN

Much time can be saved through appropriate organizational planning. The purpose for the existence of the agency should be determined, and

RESEARCH Perspective 2-2

Data from Payne N: Occupational stressors and coping as determinants of burnout in female hospice nurses. *Journal of Advanced Nursing* 33(3):396-405, 2001.

Purpose: The purpose of this study was to study the level of burnout among hospice nurses; to ascertain which aspects of nursing work were positively or negatively related to burnout; to examine the relative contributions made by those different variables; and to suggest individual and organizational interventions to reduce levels of burnout.

Methods: A battery of questionnaires consisting of the Maslach Burnout Inventory, Nursing Stress Scale, Ways of Coping Scale, and a demographic form was sent to eighty-nine nurses from nine hospices. Multiple regression analyses were used to analyze the data.

Results/conclusions: The level of burnout characterized by high emotional exhaustion, high depersonalization of patients, and low personal accomplishment was found to be low. Death and dying, conflict with staff, accepting responsibility, and higher nursing grade contributed to emotional exhaustion. Conflict with staff, inadequate preparation, escape, and reduced planful problem-solving contributed to depersonalization. Inadequate preparation, escape, reduced positive reappraisal, and fewer professional qualifications contributed to lower levels of personal accomplishment. Stressors made the greatest contribution to burnout, and demographic factors contributed the least.

---

the goals and objectives should be defined and ranked in order of importance. Nurse managers determine who is responsible for coordinating activities, who makes what decisions, and who needs to be informed about certain decisions. They also determine what decisions need to be

BOX 2-8 Techniques to Stop Procrastination

Break a large job into smaller tasks.
Do a start-up task.
Take advantage of your moods.
Consider the consequences of not doing the task.
Consider hiring someone to do the task.
Consider switching jobs with someone.
Make a commitment to someone or a wager with someone.
Ask yourself, "What's the best use of my time now?"
Set goals.
Set realistic time schedules.
Gather necessary information.
Avoid overcommitment.
Give yourself rewards.

made before others, what action needs to be taken first, and what deadlines must be set. The determining and ranking of goals focus activities and prevent people from spending time doing inappropriate or unimportant tasks. People who are adequately informed of what is expected of them do not waste time wondering what they are supposed to do. Making time estimates and setting time limits help regulate work flow. Through appropriate planning, problems can be prevented. The decreased amount of time spent in crisis management increases the time available for creative work.

ORGANIZE

The manager structures the agency to accomplish the tasks necessary to meet the agency's goals. Organizational charts help clarify who is responsible to whom and for what. Job descriptions further clarify these matters. Multiple bosses, confusion over who is responsible and who has authority for what, and duplication of tasks can be prevented with planning. Autonomy and independence reduce the amount of time otherwise spent in conflict management. Policies and procedures help clarify expectations.

STAFF

Selection of well-qualified staff is critical for time saving because they require less supervisory time for development and corrective action. Staff development further reduces time lost by better preparing staff to do their jobs. Appropriate use of personnel through assessment of work to be done, careful planning of the number and mix of personnel, and matching staff members' interests and abilities to the job further reduce waste. When nurses' interests are matched to the organizational goals and they feel appreciated, they are likely to have increased job satisfaction. Consequently there is little absenteeism and less turnover. Nurse managers should watch for chronic absenteeism, try to determine the reason, and correct it. They also expect punctuality, because tardiness is a loss of time. If nurse managers find that employees' personal problems are affecting their work, they should refer personnel for appropriate assistance so that they will have more energy to do their jobs.

DIRECT

It is nurse managers' responsibility to delegate what a less qualified, lower-paid person can handle. They identify the task to be delegated, determine the best person to do the job, and communicate the assignment clearly. They allow the staff associate to help determine how the task will be accomplished and keep authority commensurate with responsibility. They set controls, monitor results, and provide support as needed. It is essential that managers teach others how to do the work instead of doing it themselves. They can save considerable time by streamlining communication systems and by not holding any more meetings than necessary. Nurse managers

RESEARCH Perspective 2-3

Data from Stordeur S, D'hoore W, Vandenberghe C: Leadership, organizational stress and emotional exhaustion among hospital nursing staff. *Journal of Advanced Nursing* 35(4):533-542, 2001.

Purpose: The purpose of this study was to examine the effect of work stressors and head nurses' transactional and transformational leadership on the levels of emotional exhaustion experienced among their staff.

Methods: A questionnaire was sent to all nurses of a university hospital. Six hundred twenty-five questionnaires were returned. Correlational analysis and multiple regressions were used to analyze the data.

Results/conclusions: Work stressors explained 22% of the variance in emotional exhaustion, but leadership dimensions explained only 9% of the variance in that outcome measure. Stress emanating from the physical and social environment, role ambiguity, and active management-by-exception were significantly associated with increased levels of emotional exhaustion. Transformational leadership and contingent reward leadership were highly intercorrelated and did not influence emotional exhaustion. Inspirational leadership, individualized consideration, intellectual stimulation, and contingent reward are associated with lower levels of burnout. Assigning tasks, specifying procedures, and clarifying expectations have been shown to result in reduced role ambiguity and increased job satisfaction. Those leaders who are perceived as closely monitoring their nurses in performing their duties to prevent mistakes tend to generate higher levels of emotional exhaustion.

should also facilitate open communications and assertive behavior and handle conflict immediately before it drains time and energy.

CONTROL

Nurse managers set standards, monitor results, and give feedback. They adjust closeness of supervision to the needs of the employee, take disciplinary action as soon as it is justified, and fire personnel who are not meeting minimum standards. Good management conserves time and energy. Lack of it leads to management by crisis.

Chapter Summary

Chapter 2 covered the following:

Stress Management
  Sources of Stress
  Stress Response
  Symptoms of Stress
  Stress Control
    Values clarification
    Goal setting
    Stress avoidance and regulation
    Time blocking
    Time management
    Assertiveness
    Feeling pauses
    Inner shouting
    Anchoring
    Sorting
    Thought stopping
    Compartmentalization
    Environmental changes
    Humor
    Centering
    Nutrition
    Exercise
    Sleep
  Relaxation
    Abdominal breathing
    Massage
    Progressive relaxation
    Biofeedback
    Autogenic training: self-hypnosis
    Meditation
    Visualization and mental imagery
    Poetry
    Music
    Baths
  Enhancing Self-Esteem
  Support Groups
  Protection from Workplace Violence
Time Management
Personal Time Management
Maximize Managerial Time
  Inventory Activities
  Set Goals
  Plan Strategies
  Plan Schedule
  Say No
  Use Transition Times
  Accelerate Learning
  Improve Reading
  Improve Memory
  Critical Thinking
  Streamline Paperwork
  Use Computers for Time Management
  Use Telephone Calls
  Schedule Office Visits
  Control Visit Time
  Use Meetings Effectively
  Delegation
    Reasons for delegating
    The four rights of delegation
    Delegation decision-making process
    Conditions that facilitate delegation
    Responsibility, authority, and accountability
    Cultural considerations for delegation
    Reasons for underdelegating
    Reasons for not accepting delegation
Procrastination
  Reasons for Procrastination
    Emotional reasons
    Nonemotional reasons
  Techniques to Stop Procrastination
Maximize Organization Time
  Plan
  Organize
  Staff
  Direct
  Control

On-line Resources

evolve   Additional critical thinking activities, worksheets, and case studies are available on-line at http://evolve.elsevier.com/Marriner/guide/

References

Allen KR: *Time and information management that really works*, Los Angeles, 1995, Affinity.

Bennis W, Mason RO, Mitroff II: *High-speed management*, San Francisco, 1993, Jossey-Bass.

Covey SR: *First things first*, New York, 1994, Simon & Schuster.

Covey SR: *The 7 habits of highly effective people: Powerful lessons in personal change*, New York, 1989, Simon & Schuster.

Ellis JR, Hartley CL: *Managing and coordinating nursing care*, Philadelphia, 2000, Lippincott.

Grohar-Murray ME, DiCroce HR: *Leadership and management nursing*, ed 3, Upper Saddle River, NJ, 2003, Prentice Hall.

Hansten RI: *Clinical delegation skills: A handbook for professional practice*, ed 2, Gaithersburg, Md, 1998, Aspen.

Lively L: *Managing information overload*, New York, 1996, AMACOM.

Marquis BL, Huston CJ: *Leadership roles and management functions in nursing*, ed 3, Philadelphia, 2000, Lippincott.

Marrelli TM: *The nurse manager's survival guide,* ed 2, St Louis, 1997, Mosby.

Meyer C: *Fast cycle time*, New York, 1993, Free Press.

Sheehan JP: Protect your staff from workplace violence, *Nurs Manage*, pp 24-25, March 2000.

Sullivan EJ, Decker PJ: *Effective leadership and management in nursing*, ed 5, Upper Saddle River, NJ, 2001, Prentice Hall.

Swansburg RC, Swansburg RJ: *Introduction to management and leadership for nurse managers*, ed 3, Boston, 2002, Jones and Bartlett.

Wheatley MJ: *Turning to one another: Simple conversations to restore hope to the future*, San Francisco, 2002, Berrett-Koehler.

Yoder-Wise PS: *Leading and managing in nursing*, ed 2, St Louis, 2003, Mosby.

3

Decision-Making Process and Tools

"Indecision is the graveyard of good intentions."
—Anonymous

Chapter Overview

Chapter 3 outlines the decision-making process, critical thinking, creative
decision making, consultation, ethics, moral reasoning, ethics committees,
decision-making tools, computers, group factors in decision making, and
committee aspects of decision making.

Chapter Objectives

- List the five steps in the decision-making process.
- Describe at least six techniques to increase creativity.
- Compare and contrast at least two ethical positions that can be used to consider
  moral dilemmas.
- Identify at least five decision-making tools.
- Delineate at least three models that can be used to describe phenomena.
- Describe how to use a Gantt chart.
- Discuss how computers can be applied in nursing.
- Compare advantages and disadvantages of group participation in decision making.

Major Concepts and Definitions

Decision-making process the process of selecting one course of action from alternatives
Critical thinking the ability to question philosophically and exercise careful judgment when evaluating a situation
Creativity intellectual inventiveness
Consultation an interactive, helping relationship between two parties
Ethics a moral philosophy that examines how means are related to ends and how to control means to serve human ends
Tool an instrument used to accomplish an end
Model an abstraction or representation of something more complex
Probability the likelihood of an event's occurrence
Simulation an imitation of an event or process
Game theory a simulation of system operations
Gantt chart a tool used to visualize multiple tasks that need to be done
Decision tree graphic tool to visualize alternatives available, chance events, and probable consequences
PERT program evaluation and review technique
CPM critical path method to calculate time estimate for activities
Queuing theory a mathematical technique used to determine efficiency of intermittent services
Linear programming matrix algebra or linear mathematical equations used to determine the best way to use limited resources for maximal results
Computer an electronic machine that performs rapid calculations or compiles, correlates, and selects data by means of stored instructions and information
Vroom and Yetton model a tool used to identify autocratic, consultative, and group decision processes

DECISION-MAKING PROCESS

Decision making, the process of selecting one course of action from alternatives, is a continuing responsibility of nurse managers. They are confronted by a variety of situations. Hospital or agency policies provide guidelines for dealing with routine situations. Exceptional instances, however, can make decisions more difficult and may require a mature sense of judgment. Problem solving is a skill that can be learned, and because staff nurses can learn by observing their leaders, good decision making by the leader may do more than solve immediate problems; more important for the long term, it can foster good decision making by staff nurses.

Decision making relies on the scientific problem-solving process: identifying the problem,

analyzing the situation, exploring alternatives and considering their consequences, choosing the most desirable alternative, implementing the decision, and evaluating the results (Box 3-1).

IDENTIFY THE PROBLEM AND ANALYZE THE SITUATION

The first step in the decision-making process is defining the problem. What is wrong? Where is

---

BOX 3-1 Decision-Making Process

Identify the problem, and analyze the situation.
Explore the alternatives.
Choose the most desirable alternative.
Implement the decision.
Evaluate the results.

improvement needed? Sometimes the problem seems obvious and can be dealt with routinely. If the employee repeatedly reports late to work or abuses the privilege of sick leave, the manager can respond in accordance with agency policies. However, managers who are concerned only with the infraction may be dealing with the effect rather than the cause of the problem. Consequently, similar situations may continue. It is important to define the factors that are causing the problem. For instance, two staff nurses may each complain about the intrusion of the other into her work. Initially the problem may appear to be a personality clash or a political power struggle. However, the cause may be the manager's failure to define the job responsibilities of each nurse. As long as the manager concentrates on the symptom instead of the problem, the difficulties will arise. It is only when the real problem has been identified that effective decision making can be initiated.

Nurse managers can identify the problem by analyzing the situation. All too frequently decisions are made and implemented before all the facts have been gathered. To prevent this the manager should have a questioning attitude. What is the desirable situation? What are the presenting symptoms? What are the discrepancies? Who is involved? When? Where? How? With answers to these questions managers can develop tentative hypotheses and test them against what they know. Progressive elimination of hypotheses that fail to conform to the facts reduces the number of causes to be considered. Feasible hypotheses should be further tested for causal validity. When managers believe they have identified the cause or causes of the problem by analyzing available information, they should begin exploring possible solutions.

EXPLORE THE ALTERNATIVES

There are usually a number of ways to solve a problem. Some may be quick and economical but less effective than their alternatives. Others may be more effective but less economical. If various alternatives are not explored, the course of action is limited.

When solving a problem, managers should determine first whether the situation is covered by policy. If it is not, they must draw on their education and experience for facts and concepts that will help them determine alternatives. Using one's experience is probably the most common approach to solving problems, but it may be inadequate. The more experience the manager has had, the more alternatives may be suggested to solve a variety of problems. However, health care changes rapidly, and solutions to yesterday's problems may not work today. Consequently, managers should look beyond their own experiences and learn how others are solving similar problems. This can be done through continuing education, professional meetings, review of the literature, correspondence, and brainstorming with staff. Inductive reasoning and deductive reasoning are both appropriate.

CHOOSE THE MOST DESIRABLE ALTERNATIVE

The number and quality of alternatives depend largely on the creativity and productivity of managers and their staff. Leadership that prevents immediate acceptance of an apparently obvious solution and facilitates group exploration of decision-making opportunities (such as problems to solve) usually increases the number of alternatives and the quality of problem solving.

Eagerness to reach a decision may lead to premature solutions; on the other hand, considering only a few alternatives in haste blocks good decisions. Avoidance of the real problem, lack of clear problem definition, insufficient data, early statement of attitude by a status figure, mixing of idea generation and idea evaluation, lack of staff commitment because the superior who makes the decision does not implement it, and decisions made by large groups also interfere with reaching effective solutions.

One alternative is not always clearly superior to all others. The manager must try to balance factors such as patient safety, staff acceptance, morale, public acceptance, cost, and risk of failure.

Criteria for calculating the value of decisions are useful. The following questions may be asked: Will this decision accomplish the stated objectives? If it does not, it should not be enforced and another option should be used. Does it maximize effectiveness and efficiency? One should use available resources before seeking outside assistance. Finally, can the decision be implemented? If not, it obviously will not solve the problem.

IMPLEMENT THE DECISION

After a decision has been made, it must be implemented. A decision that is not put into action is useless. The manager will need to communicate the decision to appropriate staff associates in a manner that does not arouse antagonism. The decision and procedures for its implementation can be explained in an effort to win the cooperation of those responsible for its implementation. The manager will need to select the staff associate to implement the decision and provide the direction to initiate action. Managers may need to control the environment so staff associates can function as planned. Once the decision has been implemented, it should be evaluated.

EVALUATE THE RESULTS

The final step of decision making is evaluation of the results of the implementation of the chosen alternative. Evaluative criteria may have to be developed. Audits, checklists, ratings, and rankings can be used to review and analyze the results. Because solutions to old problems sometimes create new problems, making and evaluating additional decisions may be required.

The decision-making and problem-solving models and the nursing process are very similar (Table 3-1). They are all scientific problem solving.

ORGANIZATIONAL MODELS FOR DECISION MAKING

RATIONAL MODEL

The rational model is based on the premises of common goals, technical competence, and sequential process to achieve goals when individual values are consistent with organizational values. It is a deliberate action to select the best solution to achieve the desired outcome. Feedback increases the understanding of causal relations, which can then be used in future decision making. The advantage is that it helps unify associates with the goals of the agency. Disadvantages include unrealistic expectations of how people function, a large amount of time for processing, and narrow thought processes that can become counterproductive.

POLITICAL MODEL

The political model is built on the premises of a win-win situation, diversity of interests, even dispersion of power, and available forums for people with multiple, conflicting values that are protecting their own self-interests. A lobby

TABLE **3-1** Decision-Making and Problem-Solving Models and Nursing Process

DECISION MAKING	PROBLEM SOLVING	NURSING PROCESS
1. Identify the problems, and analyze the situation.	1. Assess—define the problem.	1. Assess.
2. Explore the alternatives.	2. Plan—generate a list of alternatives and evaluate for cost, feasibility, and risk.	2. Select nursing diagnosis.
3. Choose the most desirable alternative.	3. Choose the best solution.	3. Plan care.
4. Implement the decision.	4. Implement the apparent best solution.	4. Implement the care plan.
5. Evaluate the results.	5. Evaluate the effectiveness.	5. Evaluate the outcomes.

majority makes the decisions. Changes are based on negotiations rather than causal links and are unpredictable. Statesmen with political skills provide information to associates who may not share the organizational values. Decisions may be limited to the statesmen's narrow views. This takes less time than consensus models. This model can promote creative solutions with majority support that can be implemented even if there are differences in viewpoints.

COLLEGIAL MODEL

The collegial model involves full participation of a community of peers for decision making. It is based on the premises of group consensus, mutual respect, and adequate time. It is common in an academic community. There are shared responsibilities for organizational goals based on the professional background and interests of the participants. Decisions tend to support general welfare. Feedback is usually informal and dependent on participants' observations and priorities. This shared governance approach with professionals that have diverse and specialized information takes considerable time because of numerous group meetings. When there is consensus, implementation tends to go smoother than when there is no consensus.

BUREAUCRATIC MODEL

The bureaucratic model is common in health care. It is based on the premises of historical norms and operating routines. The value is for operational efficiency based on history and tradition. Implementation of change is through use of routines as determined by policies and procedures that lead to predictable outcomes and only slight adaptations to operations. The hierarchical bureaucracy dictates the key players. Information is from history, tradition, and norms. Time for implementation depends on the efficiency of the operations. This model does not recognize informal channels of communication and ignores political struggles for power. Alternative solutions generated may be limited and depend on the historical success of the agency

and the corporate memory. A past inefficient operation may be perpetuated. If there is a history of efficiency, changes consistent with history and norms may be made with little resistance.

GARBAGE CAN MODEL

The garbage can model is based on the premise of pure accident. Decisions are unplanned and coincidental based on multiple diffuse values. Implementation is incidental with no planning. The outcomes occur by chance and may repeat errors. Key players may be associates that perceive an opportunity and contribute to organization anarchy and adhocracy. Outcomes depend on key player creativity. Because there are no goals or criteria for evaluating outcomes, errors may be repeated. It is also possible to consider creative solutions to problems.

CYBERNETIC MODEL

The cybernetic model has three phases: (1) needs assessment, (2) program implementation, and (3) results assessment. The needs assessment includes determining the desired outputs for the program, nature of the problem, level of goal accomplishment expected, program strategies, goal accomplishment criteria, and construction of a causal chain for program processes and outcomes. Program implementation involves determining that the program is in place and progressing according to the time plan. The results assessment includes determination that the program outcomes were met and that the program outputs justified the costs. The long-term impact on quality of life needs to be determined (Jones, 1996).

CRITICAL THINKING

Elements of reasoning are essential dimensions that provide general logic to reason. They include purpose or goal; central problem or question at issue; point of view or frame of reference; empirical dimension; conceptual dimension; assumptions, implications, and consequences; and inferences and conclusions (Box 3-2).

RESEARCH Perspective 3-1

Data from Daly G: Ethics and economics. *Nursing Economic$* 18(4):194-201, 2000.

Purpose: The purpose of this research was to study the effects of ethics case consultation on use of health care resources.

Methods: This research studied six cases regarding the effects of the use of ethics case consultations and end-of-life support from ethics teams.

Results/conclusions: The decrease in the use of medical interventions and therapies after ethics consultations was consistent in all cases presented, which greatly reduced the cost of health care.

PURPOSE OR GOAL

All reasoning has purpose and requires clarity, significance, achievability, and consistency of purpose.

CENTRAL PROBLEM OR QUESTION AT ISSUE

All reasoning is an attempt to solve a problem, figure something out, or answer a question. To answer a question or solve a problem one must understand what it requires. Clarity, significance, relevance, and answerability of the question are needed.

POINT OF VIEW OR FRAME OF REFERENCE

All reasoning is done from a point of view. Reasoning is improved when multiple relevant points of view are sought and when those points of view are articulated clearly, emphasized logically and fairly, and applied consistently and dispassionately.

EMPIRICAL DIMENSION

Reasoning is only as sound as the evidence on which it is based. The evidence should be clear, relevant, accurate, adequate, fairly gathered and reported, and consistently applied.

CONCEPTUAL DIMENSION

Reasoning is only as relevant, clear, and deep as the concepts that form it. Concepts should be clear, deep, neutral, and relevant.

ASSUMPTIONS

All reasoning is based on assumptions. Reasoning can only be as sound as the assumptions on which it is based. Assumptions should be clear, consistent, and justifiable.

IMPLICATIONS AND CONSEQUENCES

All reasoning has implications, consequences, and direction. Understanding the implications and consequences is important to reason through a decision or issue. One must consider the clarity, completeness, precision, reality, and significance of articulated implications.

INFERENCES AND CONCLUSIONS

All reasoning has inferences by which one draws conclusions and gives meaning to the data.

BOX **3-2** Elements of Critical Thinking and Reasoning

Purpose or goal
Central problem or question at issue
Point of view or frame of reference
Empirical dimension
Conceptual dimension
Assumptions
Implications and consequences
Inferences and conclusions

Data from Paul R: *Critical thinking*, Santa Rosa, Calif, 1993, Foundation of Critical Thinking.

Reasoning is only as sound as the inferences it makes and the conclusions to which it comes. Inferences should be clear and justifiable. Conclusions should be consistent, profound, and reasonable.

CRITICAL THINKING FOR THE NURSING PROCESS

Critical thinking skills used in the assessment phase of the nursing process include observing; distinguishing pertinent and important data from other data; and validating, organizing, and categorizing data. To make the diagnosis, one must find patterns and relationships, make inferences, and state the problem while suspending judgment. To plan the care, one generalizes by transferring knowledge from one situation to another, develops evaluative criteria, and hypothesizes. During implementation of the plan of care, one applies knowledge and tests the hypotheses. To evaluate outcomes, one makes criterion-based evaluations to decide if hypotheses were correct (Sullivan and Decker, 2001).

GROUP DECISION MAKING

GROUP FACTORS

Within an organization, it is unusual for an individual to complete the decision-making process alone. Even if one makes the decision, others will probably be involved in the implementation. Commitment to the decision is important to its implementation and may be increased by participation in the decision-making process. One should be aware that there are always disadvantages as well as advantages to group participation in the decision making.

Advantages

Because of their broader experience, groups have a wider range of knowledge to draw on than does the individual. Participation allows the nurse to express her views and attempt to persuade others, thereby increasing self-expression, innovation, and development. People are more apt to be committed to implementation if they have had the opportunity to share in the decision-making process. Group decisions are time

consuming and expensive. However, if group members have diverse backgrounds, it may be less time consuming for a group to make a decision than for an individual to gather information and analyze it. In the long run, it may be no more expensive than having a higher paid manager make the decision or having to deal with resistance to change because of lack of input.

Disadvantages

Group decisions may result from social pressures. The subordinates may be influenced by a desire for group acceptance or by an attempt to appease their superior. Hierarchical pressures can reduce the subordinate's participation to acquiescence to the manager's desires. Formal status is likely to inhibit interaction even when the supervisor has less expertise than the staff. A competent superior is more likely to possess self-confidence and allow interaction. It is not always easy to determine another's competence, nor can one always expect the level of expertise to match the degree of participation.

Group participants change and so do the problems. A minority may rule if an individual or a few people dominate the group. Members may become more interested in winning an argument than in determining the best alternative. Choosing the most acceptable solution may produce consensus, which is not necessarily the optimal alternative, and may simply serve to foster the status quo.

COMMITTEE/TASK FORCE ASPECTS

A committee is a group of people chosen to deal with a particular topic or problem over time. A task force has a time-limited assignment. The authority delegated to committees and task forces varies widely. A committee may have advisory, informational, coordinating, or decision-making responsibility. A staff committee serves merely in an advisory capacity. A line committee is an executive group responsible for making decisions affecting subordinates. Formal committees are part of the organizational structure and have specific duties and authority. Informal committees have not been delegated authority and are often primarily for discussion. Formal committees tend to be permanent; informal committees are more likely to be temporary. Committees are usually most useful when appointed for a specific purpose. A committee appointed to collect data, analyze it, and make recommendations is an ad hoc committee. There are advantages and disadvantages to decision making by committees.

Advantages

Although the ultimate responsibility for a decision is the top administrator's, that burden can be shared through the use of committees. Group deliberation and judgment can be advantageous for decision making. Complex problems may be more manageable when department heads and specialists participate. Sharing in the decision-making process increases the department head's understanding of the situation and commitment to the decision. Most decisions based on consensus after deliberations are widely satisfactory. The unanimity of committee decisions helps increase the support and confidence of subordinates.

Disadvantages

Although committees can share the top administrator's burden for decision making, more leadership ability is required to conduct business in that manner. Committee decisions may make the manager appear to be a figurehead and decrease the person's prestige in the community. They may in fact control a weak administrator. The manager may use committees to avoid responsibilities or to delay decisions. A committee may have a fixed responsibility, but it is the group rather than the individual that is held accountable, because it is difficult to identify who is responsible for a poor committee decision. A committee decision is a slow, ponderous process that is consequently expensive. Pressure for unanimity may discourage input from more aggressive and creative members. Consensus through compromise may decrease the quality of the decision. Indecisiveness can result in an adjournment without action taken and can contribute to a minority tyranny of the strongest members.

COMMITTEE FUNCTIONING

Despite the obvious disadvantages and misuses of committees, there is an increasing emphasis on group participation. Committee decisions are particularly useful for policy formulation and planning. Consequently, the supervisor should consider how to maximize the use of committees. To build consensus, the chair listens to all committee members, uses the ideas, and gets people onto the team by involving them in critical thinking and realistic critiquing of ideas.

Defining the scope and authority of the committee helps members know what their responsibilities are. Members should know if they are to simply discuss an issue, provide the supervisor with ideas, make recommendations, or be responsible for the decision. Given the above, there is less chance that committee members will waste their time dealing with issues beyond the scope of their responsibility. Moreover, an awareness of the limits placed on them allows committee members to evaluate their work. It may be advisable to review committees periodically, dissolve those no longer needed, consolidate those duplicating responsibilities, and create new ones that are needed.

The size of the committee is important. It should be large enough to facilitate deliberation and have a membership with a breadth of knowledge and expertise. If it is too large, however, that encourages indecision and inefficiency. Effective committee size may range from five to fifteen. Five is considered an ideal size if the five members have adequate knowledge and skill. The larger the group, the more time it takes to allow each member to participate and for the group to reach consensus. Appropriate membership is critical for effective committee functioning. Members need the necessary knowledge and skills, should possess authority, must be suitably representative, and should be able to work well within a group.

Good chairpersonship can increase the effectiveness of a committee. The chairperson can facilitate committee work by preparing agendas, circulating reports before the meeting, making research results available to members, collecting necessary facts before the meeting, defining the proposal for action, and conducting the meeting efficiently. Agendas circulated to members well in advance of meetings allow committee members to know what to expect and to come to the meeting prepared to deal with the subject. There should be an opportunity for members to add to the agenda items at the beginning of a committee meeting. The circulation of reports and other information before the meeting helps prevent the waste of meeting time while members review studies or think aloud. It reduces the chances of a decision being railroaded, a report being meekly accepted, or a decision being postponed until after members have more opportunity to study the proposal.

The chairperson should keep the discussion on the subject and help integrate committee deliberation. Thus, rather than resorting to compromise, members may develop a point of view that differs from the preconceived notions they brought to the meeting. The chairperson should not force members to take a position until after the subject has been fully considered. Members who take a premature stand may feel the need to defend that position for the sake of winning an argument rather than for the quality of the decision. The chairperson can encourage each member to be a critical evaluator and to consider the consequences of the action. Outside experts may be invited in or task forces can be selected to study issues and report back to the committee. It may be useful to have a follow-up meeting after a consensus has been reached to allow for and to deal with any second thoughts.

Committees permit simultaneous participation, and yet people may still leave the meeting with varying interpretations of what happened. Consequently, it is advisable to have a secretary take minutes of the meeting and for the chairperson to circulate the draft for modification before having the minutes approved by the committee. There should be a procedure for keeping a copy of minutes and relevant papers for future reference. The chairperson should also follow up on the decisions made and report her findings to the committee. Was the recommendation implemented? If so, what were the results? If not, why not? (Swansburg and Swansburg, 2002; Young and Cooke, 2002).

CONSENSUS BUILDING VERSUS GROUP THINK

Consensus building is accomplished by bringing people onto the team, listening to their ideas, realistically considering their ideas, using their ideas, and involving them in the critical thinking. It takes time to build consensus. On the other hand, group think seeks fast solutions with little critical thinking or input from group members. People conform rather than challenge ideas, and poor decisions can result (Swansburg and Swansburg, 2002).

CREATIVE DECISION MAKING

THE CREATIVE PROCESS

The creative process has steps similar to those of the problem-solving process, but the emphasis is different (Box 3-3). Decision making stresses choice of a solution, whereas the creative process emphasizes the uniqueness of the solution. Creativity is a latent quality, activated when a person becomes motivated by the need for self-expression or by the stimulation of a problem. Thus the first phase of the creative process is a *felt need*. Similarly, when decision makers are confronted with a problem, they start seeking a solution.

BOX 3-3 Creative Decision-Making Process

Felt need
Preparation
Incubation
Illumination
Verification

The second phase of creative problem solving is a work stage known as *preparation,* from which creative ideas emerge. Innovation partially depends on the number of options considered. By exploring relationships among potential solutions, one may identify additional solutions. Many decisions are made after slight preparation and therefore result in commonplace solutions. Superficial analysis of obvious information does not facilitate creative answers. Extensive use of libraries for data collection is useful; the creative person may take notes on readings, develop them into files with other clippings and ideas, review these materials, and combine the most appropriate aspects of old solutions into new answers.

Incubation, the third phase, is a period for pondering the situation. Repetition of the same thoughts with no new ideas or interpretations is a sign of fatigue and indicates that it is a good time to start the incubation period. Switching one's attention provides a necessary respite, and yet the unconscious mind continues to deal with the problem. A time should be set to reexamine the situation and review the data collected during the preparation phase.

Illumination is the discovery of a solution. It may come to mind in the middle of the night or during the performance of another task. It is recommended that the idea be written down so the details can be preserved. Having paper and pencil readily available at all times (including in the bedside stand) is helpful.

It is rare for an illumination to be ready for adoption. *Verification,* the fifth and final phase of creative decision making, is the period of experimentation when the idea is improved through modification and refinement. The advantages and disadvantages of each alternative must be weighed; resources and constraints such as personnel, finances, facilities, and equipment have to be evaluated, and potential technical and human problems should be considered. Some decisions have failed at implementation because potential problems were not anticipated and dealt with. It would be unfortunate for an otherwise useful alternative to be rejected for a disadvantage that could be easily overcome. By comparing the advantages and disadvantages of the options, the manager can choose the most desirable alternative.

ENCOURAGING CREATIVITY

The thinking mechanism of the human brain has been conceptualized as having two sides. The right side is intuitive and conceptual and is used for uninhibited creative thinking. The left side is analytical and sequential. If we use the analogy of driving a car, the right side of the brain is a green light that keeps us going until we have generated a multiplicity of ideas. The left side is a red light that says stop and questions whether this is worthwhile. The judicial left side of the brain analyzes and evaluates the creative ideas generated by the right side of the brain. We need to use both sides. We are usually socialized to use the left side more than the right side, but the right side can be stimulated. To encourage creativity we can consider how to adapt, combine, eliminate, rearrange, reverse, or substitute ideas or put something to other uses (Grohar-Murray and DiCroce, 2003; Treffinger, Isaksen, and Dorval, 1999). Box 3-4 lists some creative thinking techniques.

Convergent Thinking

The problem is divided into smaller and smaller pieces to find a more manageable perspective (Treffinger, Isaksen, and Dorval, 1999).

Divergent Thinking

One's view of the problem is expanded. The problem is considered in different ways (Treffinger, Isaksen, and Dorval, 1999).

Ladder of Abstraction

A ladder of abstraction helps participants explore the task in broader or narrower ways or at varying levels of abstraction. It encourages making abstract options more concrete, focused, and specific and making specific narrow options broader and more abstract. Then the appropriate level of abstraction can be considered. "Why" questions help broaden an idea, whereas "how"

BOX **3-4** Creative Thinking Techniques

Advantages, limitations, unique qualities, overcome
  limitations (ALUo)
Brainstorming
Brain writing
Collective notebook technique
Convergent thinking
Delphi technique
Divergent thinking
Drawing
Evaluation matrix
Forecasting alternative future scenarios
Highlighting
Ladder of abstraction
Lists
Meditation
Modeling
Morphological matrix
Musts/wants
Paired comparison analysis
Reverse brainstorming
SML
Stepladder technique
Synetics
Visualization
Visually identifying relationships
Visual trek/visual confirmation

questions help to become more specific. Post-its can be used to speed the generation of ideas. If not many ideas are generated, the facilitator may ask, "What is preventing you from accomplishing this task?" (Treffinger, Isaksen, and Dorval, 1999).

Forced Association

The situation requiring improvement is identified. Participants use free association to generate a list of words associated with the situation. Then a list of associated words is generated. The participants look for relationships between the original list and the associated list. The lists are critically analyzed to choose words useful for addressing the situation requiring improvement.

Visual Trek/Visual Confrontation

Visual trekking is good for stretching to generate original and unusual options. The participants make new connections by making a mental journey away from a task and then connecting back to the original task. A word is chosen to create an image and then to stimulate fuzzy connections back to the task, or participants may do a physical journey to find something tangible to stimulate images. Participants may draw pictures rather than use written words. For example, the beach may stimulate people to think about the sun, blue sky, warmth, and good feelings. Fuzzy connections, such as thinking about a sunny, warm work environment with good feelings, could be made. Then more concrete connections are made to find novel options (Treffinger, Isaksen, and Dorval, 1999).

Think Tanks

Five to eight people are gathered together in an exotic or different place to stimulate innovation. A relaxed atmosphere is encouraged to stimulate divergent and unusual ideas. The problem or goal is clearly stated. This is particularly useful for future projections.

Brainstorming

A description of the task may be sent to participants before the brainstorming session so that participants could be brainstorming ideas. It is appropriate to start the brainstorming session by clarifying the task verbally and by writing it so the participants can easily view it. Guidelines for generating options should be clarified. Participants should defer judgment; generate as many ideas as possible and then try to identify a few more ideas; look at how to combine, separate, rearrange, and so on; and focus on quality of decisions. Ideas could be recorded on a chalkboard, flip chart, or Post-its. Using Post-its can speed up the process by having participants write their own ideas on Post-its and having someone collect them and post them rather than having one person record all the ideas. The ideas are easier to move around and to converge, diverge, and rearrange.

Under favorable circumstances a group working together can identify more ideas than an individual or that group of individuals working separately. Brainstorming is a technique leaders can use to create a free flow of ideas. They should encourage the members to contribute a large number of freewheeling ideas without fear of criticism or ridicule. This can improve the quality of ideas offered and result in new combinations through rearrangement, reversal, substitution, and other modifications.

Brainstorming seems to work best for simple and specific problems. Complex problems can be divided into parts that are handled separately. If the problem is too complex, the discussion may lack focus and be very time consuming. Brainstorming may be most useful when group members understand at least part of the problem. Although the session may not produce a viable solution, its stimulation may continue beyond the meeting and cause employees to take another look at their routine activities.

Creativity is probably fostered best in a permissive atmosphere in which mutual respect prevails and people are encouraged to express their views and ideas even if they are at variance with current policies and practices. A free interchange of ideas with considerable borrowing and adaptation fosters the production of creative ideas. This is a divergent way of thinking that apparently generates the largest number of creative ideas when people look for what can be used from "wild" ideas rather than criticizing them because they will not work (Treffinger, Isaksen, and Dorval, 1999).

Reverse Brainstorming

Reverse brainstorming encourages convergent thinking to break down ideas into smaller parts and analyze and focus on a particular problem or part of a problem. It is done verbally and works best for auditory or verbally oriented people.

Brain Writing

Brain writing encourages free association and recording of ideas without verbal interaction. A problem is identified. Participants are given a blank piece of paper and told to write at least four ideas, suggestions, solutions, and so forth. The paper is then passed to someone else. The paper can be systematically passed to the right or left or can be put in the center of the table for selection. Reading others' ideas is intended to stimulate more ideas, which are then written on the page. The process continues until the pages are full, the time period has elapsed, or no one can think of anything else to write (Treffinger, Isaksen, and Dorval, 1999).

Collective Notebook Technique

A problem is identified, and participants are instructed to record thoughts and ideas about the problem for a specified period. Each participant gives her notebook to another person, who reads it, looks for patterns, and synthesizes the content. The participants then meet, analyze the results, and make recommendations to solve the problem.

Stepladder Technique

The stepladder technique structures the entry of group members into the group to ensure that each member contributes to the decision-making process. Initially two group members try to solve a problem. Then a third member joins the core group and presents a preliminary solution to the problem. The entering person's presentation is discussed by all three persons. The process is repeated as group members are added.

Each member is given the group's task and time to think about it before presenting to the group. The entering person presents preliminary solutions before the group comes to a final decision. There is a discussion after each entering person presents. The final decision is delayed until all members of the group have presented and are available to participate in the final decision (Treffinger, Isaksen, and Dorval, 1999).

Morphological Matrix

The morphological matrix helps combine elements from various attributes by creating a framework for new options. Each parameter is listed as a column heading in the matrix. For a patient's diet, appetizer, salad, soup, entrée, vegetable, fruit, dessert, drink, and bread could be listed as parameters. Then specific examples are listed below each parameter. Patients' meals are then individualized. There are numerous different combinations (Treffinger, Isaksen, and Dorval, 1999).

The Delphi Technique

The Delphi technique allows members who are dispersed over a geographical area to participate in decision making without meeting face to face. A problem is identified, and members are asked to suggest potential solutions through the use of a questionnaire. Members anonymously return the first questionnaire, and the results are centrally compiled. Each member is sent a copy of the results; after viewing them, members are asked for their suggestions again. Review of the results of the first questionnaire typically triggers new solutions or stimulates changes in original positions. This process continues until consensus is reached. Little change usually occurs after the second round.

The Delphi technique insulates group members from one another's influence and does not require physical presence, so it is particularly appropriate for scattered groups. Unfortunately, it is time consuming and may not develop as many alternatives as the other techniques.

Lists

The checklist method is used to assemble criteria on a checklist, sort it, prioritize it, eliminate items, and add others. An attribute list records characteristics. They are then rearranged in possible combinations of ideas. The SCAMPER technique lists verbs that are idea generating. SCAMPER is an acronym for substitute, combine, adapt, modify, put to other uses, eliminate, and reverse.

Drawing

Drawings can be used to evoke and record creative insight because intuitive consciousness communicates more readily in symbols and impressions than in words.

Synetics

Synetics is the joining together of apparently irrelevant elements. A problem is identified, and a brief analysis is given. The problem is then simplified to clarify it and reinterpreted in analogy or metaphor. The group then plays with the analogy. The analogy or metaphor chosen to represent the problem is considered in depth. The problem is thus redefined in a new light.

Visualization

Free association can be used to create a big dream approach. First, desired outcomes are visualized and then visually run backward to identify a new approach. Imagine what you would like: a phone that tells you who is calling before you answer it, that shows who is talking to you, that you do not have to touch to answer, that rings wherever you are (office, home, car, beach). Once you have imagined what you want, you can begin dreaming about how to make your dream a reality. This technique allows you to pretend that you already have what you want and facilitates concentration on the outcomes.

Visualization helps one think in pictures, develop imagination, and dream. Meditation allows one to listen to the heart and the creative self. Focus helps one get clear about intention. Visual research by browsing through magazines and pictures stimulates thinking visually. Collage making puts a dream into a tangible form. Poetic wordplay stimulates the right brain, intuitive powers, and creative thinking. Creative journaling can include drawing as well as writing and gives voice to vision.

Capacchione (2000, pp. 33-38) identifies the steps of visioning as follows:

1. Make a wish.

2. Search for images and words.

3. Focus on the vision.

4. Compose the design.

5. Explore and find order in creative chaos.

6. Create the collage.

7. Articulate the vision.

8. Reinforce the dream.

9. Embrace the reality.

10. Celebrate the dream come true.

Visually Identifying Relationships

Visually identifying relationships provides quiet reflective time to generate options. It is particularly good for visual learners. It helps to start with a relaxation exercise and to then show participants a few pictures sequentially. The participants are to record their observations and reactions to each picture on a worksheet. The group then connects their observations back to the task in an effort to generate original ideas. Stepping away helps participants find a new perspective for the task (Treffinger, Isaksen, and Dorval, 1999).

Forecasting Alternative Future Scenarios

The future is often more a matter of choice than of chance. The choice is enhanced by forecasting potential scenarios—status quo, least preferred, most preferred, and not likely—and selecting the most desired. The process includes assessing the present situation, identifying its strengths and weaknesses, recognizing the driving forces in the environment, constructing possible alternative future scenarios, identifying the preferred future, developing a plan of action, implementing the plan, and evaluating the implementation.

Self-Interrogation Checklist

Questions are used to stimulate new perspectives about a situation. Questions help define and refine situations. They help obtain information, assess options, generate new ideas, and make decisions. Questions could include the following: Is it practical? Is it cost effective? Is it efficient? Is it effective? Can we do more? Can we streamline? Can we improve the situation?

Modeling

Look at how others are doing what you wish to do. However, be cautious: what works for someone else, somewhere else, may not work for you here and now. Similarly, what worked for you somewhere else or at some other time may not work now. Seek out what can be used or adapted, given the current situation and the preferred future.

Meditation

The optimal state for peak performance of athletes is relaxed concentration, or "playing loose." Meditation can generate a more focused state of relaxed attention.

Evaluation Matrix

The evaluation matrix structures a way to evaluate several options against specific criteria. The criteria (such as cost, time, legality, ethics, feasibility, risk) label columns across the top of the matrix. Alternatives label rows down the left side of the matrix. A rating scale such as 0 for low and 5 for high is used to specify how well each alternative meets the criteria. Happy or sad faces, colors, or shapes could also be used for evaluating each alternative against the criteria. It is preferable to go down each column rather than across each row for better comparisons when scoring the options. Each group member can complete a matrix. Scores can be averaged or consensus determined before the alternative is evaluated and scored on the primary grid. Then ideas can be generated for ways to strengthen options so that the best option or options can be selected, implemented, and evaluated again (Treffinger, Isaksen, and Dorval, 1999; Yoder-Wise, 2003).

Advantages, Limitations, Unique Qualities, Overcome Limitations (ALUo)

This focusing tool helps evaluate options by identifying the strengths, weaknesses, and unusual qualities. It is particularly useful when choices have been narrowed down to two or three that need further development. Instead of just listing strengths and weaknesses, ask questions such as "How can we overcome the weakness?" By identifying and planning how to overcome weaknesses, novel solutions are generated and supported instead of discounted. The unique qualities are to be preserved (Treffinger, Isaksen, and Dorval, 1999).

Paired Comparison Analysis

The paired comparison analysis is a focusing tool that systematically compares or ranks several options against each other a pair at a time to prioritize them. This helps assess the importance of options. Columns are labeled with options across the top of the matrix. Rows are labeled with the same options down the left side of the matrix. Two decisions are made for each comparison. First, which one is more important? Then, how much more important is one option over the other when total scores are calculated? Total scores help understand the priorities. Let's say a is compared with b and c and outranks both b and c. The letter a is written in the box where a, b, and c converge. We sum the number of a's in the row and get 2. Then we compare b with c. Let's say b outranks c. We have one b in that row. If we now rank a, b, and c, a is first with a score of 2, b is second with a score of 1, and c is third with a score of zero. Each group member can do his or her own paired analysis. Then options can label columns across the top of a grid, and group member names can label rows down the left side of the grid. Their score for each option can be put in the box where the option and their name converge. Total the scores for each option at the bottom of each column to determine the group consensus. Circle or highlight the highest and lowest scores for each option. Have the people giving the highest and lowest scores for each option discuss their reasons for their ranking and how they respond to the other person's rationale. Summarize the outcomes of the conversation, and confirm the group's understanding of the priorities. High scores usually have a higher priority (Treffinger, Isaksen, and Dorval, 1999).

Musts/Wants

Musts and wants is a way to narrow down a large number of alternatives quickly. Make two columns, and label one "musts" and the other "wants." Items that are essential, indispensable, and vital are listed under musts. Desirable and preferable items are listed under wants. Musts are what have to be considered. Failing to consider a must jeopardizes the desired outcome. Wants are nice to consider for polishing or strengthening actions that are not critical to the outcomes. Post-its are a useful tool for categorizing options (Treffinger, Isaksen, and Dorval, 1999).

Highlighting

Highlighting is a focusing tool that condenses a variety of options into themes, consequently compressing a large number of options into a more manageable number of categories. First the best options are identified and called "hits." Screening options from a long list or selecting options for further consideration can do this. Participants can be given bright-colored sticker dots with different colors representing different priorities, colored markers, or gold stars for frequency of selection, or they can draw symbols by the listed items. When more people are doing the hitting, fewer hits per person are recommended. When there are a larger number of options under consideration or more themes, more hits per person are recommended. Then those that are related to each other are clustered into themes called "hot spots." Numbers can be used to cluster options related to each other into hot spots initially. The theme is used to name the category. Each hot spot should have only one theme. Not all hits need to be placed in hot spots. Post-its are an efficient way to put hits into hot spots (Treffinger, Isaksen, and Dorval, 1999).

SML

SML (short, medium, long) is a focusing tool used to determine the order in which options should be deliberated, to compare alternatives in relationship to timing, and to sequence alternatives within time frames. Options could be sequenced

RESEARCH Perspective 3-2

Data from Genrich SJ, Banks JC, Bufton K, Savage ME, Owens MU: Group involvement in decision-making: A pilot study. *The Journal of Continuing Education in Nursing* 32(1):20-26, 2001.

Purpose: The purpose of this study was to determine if leadership could be taught regarding using the appropriate level of group involvement in decision making using the Vroom-Yetton-Jago Leadership Model.

Methods: A convenience sample of 27 health care leaders who attended a 90-minute class offered in one agency were eligible for inclusion in the pretest and posttest on similar case studies for this quasiexperimental study. A paired *t*-test resulted in statistically significant findings.

Results/conclusions: The results indicate that participating in a class on the use of the Vroom-Yetton-Jago Leadership Model may help leaders gain the skill needed to appropriately delegate decision making to groups.

into first, second, and third order for consideration; morning, noon, and nighttime sequencing; short-, medium-, and long-term time frames, and so on. Alternatives can also be sequenced in each time frame. Post-its can facilitate the sequencing process. Some options may span time frames (Treffinger, Isaksen, and Dorval, 1999).

DEVELOPING CREATIVE THINKING ATTITUDES

People need to be open minded about new ideas and the ideas of others. Inquiring minds are never satisfied. Creative people are not unduly concerned about the opinions of others, because many great ideas are first ridiculed and later accepted. People need to put aside critical, analytical, and judicial thinking while working creatively and move beyond their personal habits and attitudes. After numerous ideas have been generated, they can be judged and the best selected. Trust, acceptance, and good humor help create an environment conducive to creative problem solving. Creative people have an inner motivation, mental ability, objectivity, tolerance for complexity, enjoyment of risk taking, and ability to find problems.

BLOCKS TO CREATIVITY

Negative attitudes, self-censorship, inflexibility, lack of confidence, misconceptions, lack of effort, habits, conformity, and reliance on authority all block creativity (Harris, 2002).

CONSULTATION

"Information is not, of course, an end in itself, it is the basic input to decision-making."
—Henry Mintzberg

Consultation is a helping relationship. It is a process of interaction between the consultant, who has the specialized knowledge and skills, and the consultee, who asks for assistance with problem solving. It has a beginning and an end and is a temporary, voluntary, educational relationship. The consultee identifies a problem and seeks help from an expert. Because the consultant is usually not a part of the hierarchical structure of the organization, the consultant is an outsider who advises. Implementation of the recommendations depends on the consultee, thus giving the process a take-it-or-leave-it quality. The consultative process usually involves problem solving, but the consultant may play several roles: helping identify problems, educating staff about related issues, identifying obstacles to problem solving, offering advice about how to solve problems, acting as a change agent, developing interpersonal relationships, mediating conflicts, or performing tasks that organizational members do not have the skill to perform. The consultant typically collects and analyzes data, recommends or intervenes, and then terminates the relationship.

Consultants become known by doing something and telling others about it, volunteering to present workshops and speeches, publishing books and articles, being active in professional organizations, circulating flyers and announcements, and being included in lists of consultants.

An internal consultant knows the system, history, political realities, norms, and language better than an outside consultant and will probably devote more time to the problem. Internal consultants are viewed as less costly because they are usually not compensated extra for consultative services. Unfortunately, there are disadvantages to hiring internal consultants. They may be part of the problem; lack perspective to see the whole; have no independence of movement; have no adequate power base; encounter resistance because of their relationship with the hierarchy, vested interest, or organizational politics; or have a limited background.

An external consultant has a more diverse background, brings new ideas and a different perspective to the situation, is independent of the power structure, and is consequently high powered. Unfortunately, the external consultant does not know the history and politics of the institution and may not care about them.

Once it has been determined that there is a need for consultation, what the purpose is, and who the consultant should be, a contractual agreement is necessary. The agreement may be verbal or written, but it should determine the fee, hours of the consultant's time, expected outcome, and criteria for termination. The fee may be negotiated as a flat fee, a fee based on hours spent at the agency that includes travel and preparation time, or an hourly rate for all the time the consultant spends on the project, including research and report writing. The hours are largely controlled by the compensation structure. The consultant may have a regular schedule or be "on call." In most cases the outcome is accepted whether it is judged acceptable or not. A common outcome is a written analysis with recommendations, decisions reached, systems devised or revised, and projects completed. Usually the termination occurs at a natural closure point, such as the resolution of the problem or completion of the project. However, contingency plans should be made in case there are personality conflicts or the project takes too long and exceeds the budget.

ETHICAL ASPECTS OF DECISION MAKING

"Justice is always violent to the party offending, for every man is innocent in his own eyes."
—*Daniel Defoe*

Ethics is a moral philosophy, a science of judging the relationship of means to ends, and the art of controlling means so they will serve human ends. It involves conflict, choice, and conscience. When there is a conflict, there is a choice between conflicting alternatives. The choice is influenced by values. Values are learned first from important adults and are modified by association with people of different values. Value modification and reinforcement are lifelong processes. A value is consciously prized and cherished, freely chosen from alternatives, and acted on in a variety of ways. Ethical choices must also consider wants, needs, and rights: people may want what they do not need. Someone may want a dessert but not need it; in fact, it may be harmful. People often need what others also need. One who needs food to prevent starvation may have a right to receive food from people who have plenty but not from someone who would starve without it. That would infringe on the other person's rights, and duty and rights are correlated: it is one's duty to protect rights. A legal obligation is legislated, but it may not be ethical. A moral dilemma occurs when a decision has equally unsatisfactory alternatives.

ETHICAL THEORIES

Deontological (from the Greek "deon" or duty) theories focus on the intent of the action and are duty and rights based. Emphasis is on the dignity of human beings. The intention of the action rather than the end of the action is considered.

Teleological (from the Greek "telos" or end) theories derive the rules and norms for conduct from utilitarian consequences of actions. They favor the common good. Right has good consequences, and wrong has bad consequences. The greatest amount of good and the largest amount of happiness are good.

Principlism is an emerging theory that includes ethical principles. The ethical principles control ethical decision making more than the ethical theories. The principles are moral norms, including autonomy, beneficence, fidelity, justice, nonmaleficence, paternalism, respect for others, utility, and veracity. Each principle can be used individually, but they are often used in concert.

Egoism is based on self-interest and self-centeredness. Decisions are made for personal comfort. It is based on the principle that the right decision is the one that brings pleasure to the decision maker.

Obligationism is a theory that tries to balance distributive justice (dividing equally among all citizens regardless of age, gender, race, religion, or socioeconomic status) and beneficence (doing good and not harm). One should do what is good and prevent harm and evil. It is useful for determining public policy.

Social contract theory is based on a concept of original position and considers the least advantaged persons in society as the norm. The determination of what is right or wrong is from the perspective of the least advantaged people, such as children or handicapped people. It is based on distributive justice and supports giving the most to the least advantaged.

Natural law is called the virtue of ethics. Actions are considered right when in accord with human nature. People should do good, avoid evil, and have opportunities to reach their potential. Happiness occurs when people think

rationally and make conscious choices rather than responding to instincts (Catalano, 1995; Simms, Price, and Ervin, 2000; Sullivan and Decker, 2001).

ETHICAL PRINCIPLES

Autonomy involves personal freedom, freedom of choice, and responsibility for one's choices. Informed consent and progressive discipline recognize autonomy.

Beneficence indicates that the actions one takes should be in an effort to promote good. This principle can support providing extensive, painful treatments to increase quantity and quality of life or allowing a person to die without life support. It can be used to promote employees' positive attributes instead of their shortcomings.

Fidelity is keeping one's commitments and promises. One should not make a promise to a patient or worker that cannot be kept.

Justice means treating people equally and fairly. Equals should be treated equally, and unequals should be treated according to their differences. It is useful to apply when making decisions about competition for scarce resources or benefits. Pay raises should reflect performance as well as time of service. Holidays, vacation time, and attendance at conferences should reflect performance as well as who is next on the list.

Distributive justice implies that benefits and burdens should be distributed equally regardless of gender, race, religion, or socioeconomic status. This raises the issue of conflict between cost containment and equal distribution of scarce resources regardless of ability to pay.

Nonmaleficence means if you cannot do good at least do no harm. Nurses may need to remember that even pain and suffering can bring about good for the patient when they are performing painful procedures for the patient's benefit. Performance appraisals should emphasize the employee's good qualities and give positive direction for improved performance instead of destroying self-esteem.

Paternalism allows one to make decisions for another, limits freedom of choice, and is seen as an undesirable principle. Most see it as justified only to keep another person from harm. It is not appropriate for a paternalistic manager to set the personal goals for employees.

Respect for others is considered the highest principle that incorporates all the other principles. Respect for others acknowledges the rights of people to make their own decisions and to live by their decisions. It transcends cultural, gender, and racial issues.

Utility indicates that what is best for the common good outweighs what is best for the individual. It could justify paternalism. One using utility needs to be careful not to become less humanistic.

Veracity indicates that people should tell the truth. It applies to telling patients and staff the truth so they can make well-informed decisions (Grohar-Murray and DiCroce, 2003; Marquis and Huston, 2000; Sullivan and Decker, 2001; Swansburg and Swansburg, 1999; Yoder-Wise, 2003).

ETHICAL POSITIONS

There are several ethical positions that do not solve dilemmas. However, they do provide ways to structure and clarify them.

Utilitarianism is a community-oriented position that focuses on the consequences and prefers the greatest amount of good and happiness for the most people, or the least amount of harm.

In contrast, *egoism* seeks solutions that are best for oneself without regard for others. One's own pleasure is the concern.

Formalism considers the nature of the act and the related principles without thought to personal position or consequences of the actions: be honest; remember the golden rule.

Rule ethics expects obedience to laws, rules, professional codes, and authority.

Fairness considers distribution of benefits and liabilities from the viewpoint of the least advantaged population. Benefit to the least advantaged group is the norm in this type of decision making.

ETHICAL RELATIONSHIPS

There are also models for ethical relationships. In the *priestly model* the manager is paternalistic and makes decisions without considering others' values or seeking others' input. Although nurses may have expertise that qualifies them to make some decisions, they have no right to make moral decisions affecting other people. Autocratic leadership may use the priestly model. The *engineering model* suggests that one person presents facts to another and sets aside her own code of ethics to do what the other wants; staff working for line authority may provide an example of this model. The *contractual model* provides a contract that identifies general obligations and benefits for two or more people. It deals with the morals of both parties and is appropriate for superior-subordinate relationships. In the *collegial model* individuals share mutual goals and reach decisions through discussion and consensus. When there are shared values, this model helps build teams and minimize conflict (Veatch, 1980).*

To make an ethical decision, one must first consider what is intended to be a means and an end and then determine what good or evil is found in the means and the end. If a major evil is intended either as a means or an end, it is an unethical decision.

If the ramifications of the decision are probable but not willed as a means or an end, there are several factors to consider. The good or evil of each alternative should be evaluated: a necessary good outweighs a useful good; paying workers' wages outweighs paying for profit sharing. Urgency increases the necessity; therefore physical needs must be met before self-actualizing needs. An agency should provide adequate wages for food and shelter before providing continuing education. The probability of an outcome should be considered: a possible negative outcome is outweighed by a probable

---

*Robert Veatch's models for ethical medicine are discussed in Aroskar MA: Ethics of nurse-patient relationships, *Nurse Educ* 5:18, 1980.

good; one will work to earn a living even though there is a slight risk of back strain. The intensity of one's influence is considered because one's impact on someone else may have undesirable consequences; for instance, if an employee is fired for incompetence, it may cause a hardship for the employee's family. If the manager did not tell the employee what was expected or how to do the job, the manager would have been a considerable factor in that employee's poor job performance. Firing the employee would seem evil. If, however, the staff associate is frequently tardy or absent through no fault of the manager, the consequences of firing the worker seem justified. If there is no proportionate reason for permitting an evil, the act is unethical. If there is an alternative that provides more good and less risk of evil, it should be chosen; if there is not, there is proportionate reason for risking an evil (Aroskar, 1980).

MORAL REASONING

Levels of moral development have been identified as (1) premoral or preconventional when behavior is motivated by social or biological impulses with no sense of obligation to rules; (2) conventional when the person accepts standards of the group with little critical reflection, uses literal obedience to the rules, and feels obligation; and (3) autonomous when the person thinks and judges for herself, considers the purpose and consequences of the rules, and does not accept the group standards without reflection.

Moral choice involves selecting one of two or more values that conflict. Ten universal moral values are distributive justice, law, liberty, life, property, punishment, roles and concerns of affection, roles and concerns of authority, gender, and truth.

The level of moral development determines what a person finds valuable, how she defines the value, and why she finds it valuable. First, a person considers the power of the person involved. Second, she looks at satisfying her own needs. Third, the individual considers relationships

with others and then sees life as inherently worthwhile aside from other considerations. Moral judgment is necessary but not sufficient for mature moral action. People may do wrong even when they know better.

UNIVERSAL PRINCIPLES OF ETHICS IN A MULTICULTURAL WORLD

Laws tell us what to do, and ethics tell us why. Ethical principles involve both human rights and responsibilities (http://www.unesco.org/opi2/philosophyandethics/intro.htm [accessed 10/27/02]). Personal ethics or morality reflects the general expectations of a person in society. These are instilled in children and are expected of one another. They include concern for the well-being of others, respect for others' autonomy, trustworthiness, honesty, compliance with the law, justice, fairness, benevolence, and preventing harm. Professional ethics have additional responsibilities such as impartiality, objectivity, openness, confidentiality, diligence, fidelity, and avoiding conflict of interest. The principles of global ethics are controversial but may include global justice through international laws, social responsibility, environmental stewardship, interdependence, responsibility for the whole, and reverence for place. The principles only provide guidance and should be considered in the context of universality. There are selective violations of the principles that may be considered acceptable by society. Murder is illegal but may be considered acceptable in war. Lying is wrong but may be considered acceptable to save someone from harm. Most cultures seem to value trustworthiness but have different beliefs about truth telling. Eastern cultures value harmony whereas Western cultures prefer forthrightness. Consequently, misunderstandings can occur because underlying principles are embodied in diverse ways that reflect differences in cultural values. Morality is a matter of opinion, and opinions do vary from culture to culture. However, these principles of ethics, which are recurring patterns of ethically responsible behavior, can serve as landmarks for our consciences (http://www.ethics.ubc.ca/papers/invited/colero.htm [accessed 10/27/02], http://www.studentbmj.com/back_issues/1200/editorials/438.html [accessed 10/27/02]).

ETHICS COMMITTEES

Complex ethical issues regarding patient care and policy making must be addressed. Institutional ethics committees deal with ethical questions that often require painful choices for patients, particularly for infants and those older adults who are unable to make their own decisions.

The following issues must be addressed within the institution's philosophy, both when forming an institutional ethics committee and through ongoing study and evaluation of the existing committee: responsibility; accountability; economic costs; efficacy; role of the committee in patient care decisions; privacy for the patients and families; and committee composition, structure, meetings, and access. Nursing should be represented on the committee. Ethics committees are likely to deal with ethical issues in nursing practice such as do-not-resuscitate orders, patients' rights, professional practice issues, death and dying, and allocation of resources.

AMERICAN NURSES ASSOCIATION'S CODE OF ETHICS FOR NURSES

The American Nurses Association (ANA) House of Delegates approved the new *Code of Ethics for Nurses* at its June 30, 2001 meeting in Washington, DC. In July 2001, the Congress of Nursing Practice and Economics voted to accept the new language of the interpretive statements. The revised *Code of Ethics for Nurses with Interpretive Statements* has the following nine provisions*:

1. The nurse, in all professional relationships, practices with compassion and respect for the inherent dignity, worth and uniqueness of every individual, unrestricted by considerations of social or economic status, personal attributes, or the nature of health problems.

2. The nurse's primary commitment is to the patient, whether an individual, family, group, or community.

3. The nurse promotes, advocates for, and strives to protect the health, safety, and rights of the patient.

4. The nurse is responsible and accountable for individual nursing practice and determines the appropriate delegation of tasks consistent with the nurse's obligation to provide optimum patient care.

5. The nurse owes the same duties to self as to others, including the responsibility to preserve integrity and safety, to maintain competence, and to continue personal and professional growth.

6. The nurse participates in establishing, maintaining, and improving healthcare environments and conditions of employment conducive to the provision of quality health care and consistent with the values of the profession through individual and collective action.

7. The nurse participates in the advancement of the profession through contributions to practice, education, administration, and knowledge development.

8. The nurse collaborates with other health professionals and the public in promoting community, national, and international efforts to meet health needs.

9. The profession of nursing, as represented by associations and their members, is responsible for articulating nursing values, for maintaining the integrity of the profession and its practice, and for shaping social policy.

CANADIAN NURSES ASSOCIATION'S CODE OF ETHICS FOR REGISTERED NURSES

The Canadian Nurses Association's (CNA's) *Code of Ethics for Registered Nurses* provides nurses with direction for ethical decision making and practice in everyday situations as they are influenced by current trends and conditions. This code is organized around eight primary values that are central to ethical nursing practice*:

---

*From http://www.nursingworld.org/ethics/chcode.htm (accessed 10/27/02); American Nurses Association: *Code of ethics for nurses with interpretive statements*, Washington, DC, 2001, American Nurses Publishing.

*From http://www.cna-nurses.ca/pages/ethics.htm (accessed 11/1/02); Reprinted with permission from the Canadian Nurses Association.

1. **Safe, competent and ethical care:** Nurses value the ability to provide safe, competent and ethical care that allows them to fulfill their ethical and professional obligations to the people they serve.

2. **Health and well-being:** Nurses value health promotion and well-being and assisting persons to achieve their optimum level of health in situations of normal health, illness, injury, disability or at the end of life.

3. **Choice:** Nurses respect and promote the autonomy of persons and help them to express their health needs and values, and also to obtain desired information and services so they can make informed decisions.

4. **Dignity:** Nurses recognize and respect the inherent worth of each person and advocate for respectful treatment of all persons.

5. **Confidentiality:** Nurses safeguard information learned in the context of a professional relationship, and ensure it is shared outside the health care team only with the person's informed consent, or as may be legally required, or where the failure to disclose would cause significant harm.

6. **Justice:** Nurses uphold principles of equity and fairness to assist persons in receiving a share of health services and resources proportionate to their needs and in promoting social justice.

7. **Accountability:** Nurses are answerable for their practice, and they act in a manner consistent with their professional responsibilities and standards of practice.

8. **Quality practice environments:** Nurses value and advocate for practice environments that have the organizational structures and resources necessary to ensure safety, support and respect for all persons in the work setting.

INTERNATIONAL COUNCIL OF NURSES' INTERNATIONAL CODE OF ETHICS FOR NURSES

The International Council of Nurses (ICN) first adopted an international code of ethics for nurses in 1953. It has been revised and reaffirmed several times since then. It identifies that the need for nursing is universal and that nurses have four fundamental responsibilities: to promote health, prevent illness, restore health, and alleviate suffering. It reaffirms that nurses give services to the individual, family, and community and coordinate services with related groups unrestricted by age, color, creed, culture, disability or illness, gender, nationality, politics, race, or social status. The 2000 *ICN Code of Ethics for Nurses* has four principal elements that outline the standards of ethical conduct: nurses and people, nurses and practice, nurses and the profession, and nurses and coworkers. They are as follows*:

1. Nurses and people

The nurse's primary professional responsibility is to people requiring nursing care.

In providing care, the nurse promotes an environment in which the human rights, values, customs and spiritual beliefs of the individual, family and community are respected.

The nurse ensures that the individual receives sufficient information on which to base consent for care and related treatment.

The nurse holds in confidence personal information and uses judgment in sharing this information.

The nurse shares with society the responsibility for initiating and supporting action to meet the health and social needs of the public, in particular those of vulnerable populations.

The nurse also shares responsibility to sustain and protect the natural environment from depletion, pollution, degradation and destruction.

2. Nurses and practice

The nurse carries personal responsibility and accountability for nursing practice, and for maintaining competence by continual learning.

The nurse maintains a standard of personal health such that the ability to provide care is not compromised.

The nurse uses judgment regarding individual competence when accepting and delegating responsibility.

The nurse at all times maintains standards of personal conduct which reflect well on the profession and enhance public confidence.

*From http://www.icn.ch/ethics.htm (accessed 11/1/02).

The nurse, in providing care, ensures that uses of technology and scientific advances are compatible with the safety, dignity and rights of people.

3. Nurses and the profession

The nurse assumes the major role in determining and implementing acceptable standards of clinical nursing practice, management, research and education.

The nurse is active in developing a core of research-based professional knowledge.

The nurse, acting through the professional organization, participates in creating and maintaining equitable social and economic working conditions in nursing.

4. Nurses and coworkers

The nurse sustains a cooperative relationship with coworkers in nursing and other fields.

The nurse takes appropriate action to safeguard individuals when their care is endangered by a coworker or any other person.

Copyright © 2000 by ICN—International Council of Nurses, 3, place Jean-Marteau, 1201 Geneva (Switzerland) http://www.icn.ch/

DECISION-MAKING TOOLS

"Choices are the spice of life." —Anonymous

Most decisions involve varying degrees of uncertainty. Leaders and managers use research of various kinds to minimize the uncertainty of their decisions.

PROBABILITY THEORY

Probability theory can be applied when risk or uncertainty is present in a decision. It operates on the assumption that factors occur in accordance with a predictable pattern. For example, if a person tosses a coin 200 times, we can predict that it will show heads 100 times and tails 100 times. Deviations can be set within a predictable margin. Inferences based on statistical analysis of existing data can be used to predict results.

Sometimes a sample of the population may be analyzed. Measures of probable error become increasingly important when one is dealing with a sample because the smaller the probable error, the greater the amount of confidence that can be put in the findings. One must consider the reliability of sampling and the additional time and expense involved in collecting more information. Probability can become a substitute for otherwise unknown information: when probabilities can be substituted for unknowns, the margin of error for the solution may be limited but not completely removed.

There are three criteria that assume that previous experience is necessary to work with probability. In the "maximax" criterion managers maximize the maximum possible gain. Managers are optimistic about the factors influencing their decisions and select the option from which they can achieve the best results. This is a dangerous criterion in that it does not consider possible complications. When applying the "maximin" criterion, managers are pessimistic and expect the worst possible results. They select the option that allows them to maximize the least favorable results. They consider what complications can occur for each option, assume that everything that can go wrong will go wrong, and select the alternative that offers the best results when everything possible goes wrong. The "minimax" criterion can be applied when managers have made a decision they regret. Something unexpected prevented them from achieving the most favorable results; managers then subtract the complication from the most favorable results and try to minimize their regrets.

Uncertainty arises when the manager has to make a decision for which there are no historical data on which to calculate probabilities. Under uncertain conditions there is no best criterion to apply. The manager considers objective and subjective options according to her own optimistic or pessimistic philosophy and guesses which alternative will render the most desirable results.

SIMULATION, MODELS, AND GAMES

Simulation is a way of using models and games to simplify problems by identifying the basic components and using trial and error to determine a solution. Through simulation the manager may compare alternatives and their consequences. The computer may be used to help solve simulations. These methods may be used to study organizational changes, scheduling, assembly line management, and time sequences.

A model represents something else, most commonly objects, events, processes, or systems. It is a technique of abstraction and simplification for studying something under varying conditions. Manipulation is used to test the impact of proposed changes on the system without disturbing the subject of the model. Almost all quantitative methods used to guide decision making are models. They are particularly useful because of their convenience and low cost compared with manipulating real occurrences. Although models vary considerably in the accuracy with which they represent real situations, they increase predictive capabilities over such methods as guesswork and intuition.

Models are developed to describe, explain, and predict phenomena. The critical element of model building is conceptualization. Consequently, models can provide abstractions that facilitate communication. Models vary in the degree of abstraction used: a life-size mannequin is a realistic model that nursing students use to learn to make occupied beds; a model of a building or a piece of equipment built to scale is quite concrete, whereas blueprints or photographs, organizational charts, and mathematical models are abstract.

The more variables added to the model, the more realistic but cumbersome it becomes. The objective of modeling is to provide a simplified, abstract version of reality. Managers must strive for the appropriate level of abstractness. They may base their decision on an oversimplified model if they do not attempt to expand their knowledge of the situation. Simplified models may be useful for quantitative analysis and prediction, but one must be cautious, because a person with the least knowledge of a situation may be the most certain about how to solve the problem. If description and understanding are important, more comprehensive models should be developed. Continuing to research a problem may contribute to a more realistic model, but it may also delay the decision too long. The cost of gathering additional information may be prohibitive; therefore balancing the cost of model refinement against the benefits obtained is required.

Game theory is a simulation of system operations. The player tries to develop a strategy that will maximize gains and minimize losses, regardless of what the competitor does. War games are commonly used to train personnel and to test plans and equipment under field conditions. Management games are used primarily to train personnel rather than to solve competitive problems. They are particularly useful for training in decision making by simulating real-life operations in a laboratory setting.

GANTT CHART

Gantt charts, named for their developer, Henry Gantt, are highly developed schedules that allow one to visualize multiple tasks that have to be done. A Gantt chart (Figure 3-1) is a grid with columns for tasks, assigned responsibility, and time frame, which may be minutes, hours, days, weeks, months, years, or decades, depending on the longevity of the project. A line is drawn through the time frame while a task is in process. An X is put at the point where that task is completed. One typically works backward from due dates.

A person is told on Monday that a report is due Friday at 4 PM. The person needs to collect information, type the report on the computer, revise the report, and submit it. The person will use 3 days to collect the information and 1 day to type or word process it, incubate the ideas overnight, do any revision needed Friday morning, and submit the report Friday afternoon.

DECISION TREES

A decision tree (Figure 3-2) is a graphic method that can help managers visualize the alternatives

Task	Responsible	Mon	Tue	Wed	Th	Fr
Collect information	ME	– – – – – – – – – ·				
Type report	ME				X	
Revise report	ME					X
Submit report	ME					X

Figure 3-1   Gantt chart.

available, outcomes, risks, and information needs for a specific problem over a period of time. It helps them to see the possible directions that actions may take from each decision point and to evaluate the consequences of a series of decisions. The process begins with a primary decision having at least two alternatives. Then the predicted outcome for each decision is considered, and the need for further decisions is contemplated. The matrix resembles a tree as the decision points are diagrammed.

The results diagrammed on the tree are founded on the manager's experience and judgment but may be supported by computational data. For complex problems probability statistics may be used to explore further factors that favor or oppose expected events. Although the decision tree does not depict an obviously correct decision, it allows managers to base their decision on a consideration of various alternatives and probable consequences. It helps them realize that subsequent decisions may depend on future events. Decision trees are useful for short- and medium-range planning, as well as for decision making. Unfortunately, decision trees for longer than 2 or 3 years become cumbersome and speculative.

In Figure 3-3 the nursing staff decides to have a ward picnic for the psychiatric patients. The alternatives are to hold the picnic indoors or outdoors, and the chance events are rain or no rain. If the picnic is scheduled indoors and it rains, the patients may be crowded but dry; there

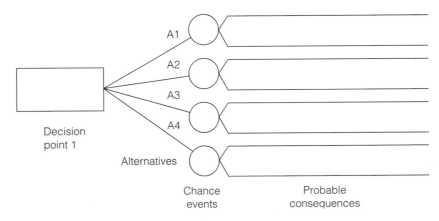

Figure 3-2   Decision tree.

will be no bugs; and the staff will be proud of their decision. If the picnic is scheduled indoors and it does not rain, the patients may feel crowded; the room may seem stuffy; the party will lack a picnic atmosphere; and the staff may regret not scheduling it outside. On the other hand, if the picnic is scheduled outdoors and it rains, the participants will get wet; the food will be ruined; and spirits will be dampened. If the picnic is scheduled outdoors and it does not rain, it will be a pleasant experience (Marquis and Huston, 2000; Umiker, 1998).

PROGRAM EVALUATION AND REVIEW TECHNIQUE

Program evaluation and review technique (PERT) is a network system model for planning and control under uncertain conditions. It involves identifying the key activities in a project, sequencing the activities in a flow diagram, and assigning the duration of each phase of the work. It is particularly appropriate for one-of-a-kind projects that involve extensive research and development.

PERT recognizes that certain tasks must be completed before the total project can be completed and, further, that subtasks must be completed before others can be started. The key events are identified, numbered, labeled, or numbered and labeled on the flow chart. The activities that cause the progress from one event to another are indicated by arrows, with the direction of the arrow showing the direction of the work flow.

PERT also deals with the problem of uncertainty with respect to time by estimating the time variances associated with the expected time of completion of the subtasks. Three projected times are determined: (1) the optimistic time (t_o), which estimates the completion time without complications; (2) the most likely time (t_m), which estimates the completion time with normal problems; and (3) the pessimistic time (t_p), which estimates the completion time given numerous problems. Thus the shortest, average, and longest times needed to complete an activity are calculated. The expected time (t_e) is calculated from these figures by the following formula:

$$t_e = \frac{t_o + 4(t_m) + t_p}{6}$$

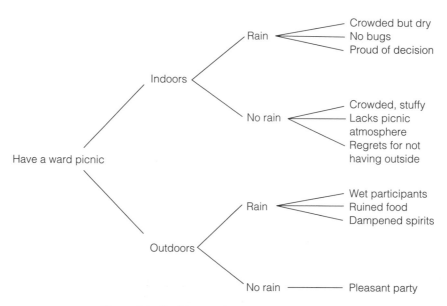

Figure 3-3 Decision tree for psychiatric ward picnic.

If the optimistic time is 2 weeks, the most likely time 4 weeks, and the pessimistic time 6 weeks, the expected time is as follows:

$$t_e = \frac{2 \text{ weeks} + 4(4 \text{ weeks}) + 6 \text{ weeks}}{6} =$$

$$\frac{24 \text{ weeks}}{6} = 4 \text{ weeks}$$

The PERT model helps the manager determine priorities (Figure 3-4). Use of resources can be considered when setting priorities. Assignments may be changed temporarily, overtime may be allowed, or temporary help may be hired to facilitate the activity flow and to manipulate the time required to move from one event to another (Marquis and Huston, 2000).

CRITICAL PATH METHOD

Critical path method (CPM), closely related to PERT, calculates a single time estimate for each activity, the longest possible time. A cost estimate is figured for both normal and crash operating conditions. Normal means the least-cost method, and crash refers to conditions in less-than-normal time. Simple sequences can be worked out manually and more complex ones by computer. CPM is particularly useful where cost is a significant factor and experience provides a basis for estimating time and cost. Managers can observe the critical path and compare the progress with the projected dates.

Network analysis techniques facilitate planning and result in objective plans by making it possible to identify the critical path and show interrelationships among parts, thus facilitating improvements in structure and communications. They are particularly useful for task force or project forms of organization and for projects.

QUEUING THEORY

Queuing theory deals with waiting lines or intermittent servicing problems. It is a mathematical technique for determining the most efficient balance of factors related to intermittent service. It is particularly applicable when units to receive service arrive in a random fashion but the time required for service is predictable. It balances the cost of waiting versus the prevention of waiting by increasing service; it acknowledges that although delays are costly, eliminating them may be even more costly. Decreasing or eliminating the waiting line to reduce waiting line costs causes an increase in cost of labor and physical facilities. The time of arrival is an important factor in determining the optimal size of facilities and staffing. Sometimes actual observations may be made, and tallies kept, of how many units or patients require service each hour of the workday or during certain seasons. For example, through observation one may determine that many junior and senior high school students attend sexually transmitted disease

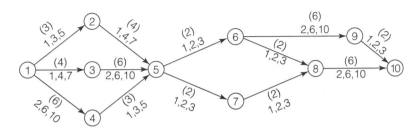

Figure 3-4 Program evaluation and review technique (PERT) model. This PERT model indicates that subtask 1 must be completed before 2, 3, and 4 can be done; 2, 3, and 4 before 5; 5 before 6 and 7; 6 before 9; 6 and 7 before 8; and 8 and 9 before 10. A coding system can be used to determine what the numbers mean. For example, 1 = program planned, 2 = staff informed. Arrows show direction of work flow. Optimistic, most likely, pessimistic, and expected times are recorded for each activity. The expected time is in parentheses.

(STD) or family planning clinics during after-school hours. The STD or family planning clinics in a small college community may have fewer demands for service during holiday seasons and summer vacation because many students have returned to their hometowns. The manager may adjust staffing accordingly. In the hospital setting the manager may choose to use part-time people or split shifts to help compensate for an increased workload during the morning, when most patients are bathed and once-a-day treatments are given, and again during late afternoon or early evening, when most patients are admitted.

When observations cannot be made for an extended period to determine a stable pattern of workload, the Monte Carlo technique may be applied. It provides a large sample of random numbers that may be generated by a computer to determine rather precise predictions of servicing load per hour.

LINEAR PROGRAMMING

Linear programming uses matrix algebra or linear mathematical equations to determine the best way to use limited resources to achieve maximal results. The technique is based on the assumption that a linear relationship exists among the variables and that the limits of the variations can be calculated. Three conditions are necessary for linear programming. First, either a maximal or minimal value is sought to optimize the objective. The value may be expressed as cost, time, or quantity. The manager may wish to minimize time and expense while maximizing quantity and quality of production. She may wish to reduce the time lost through inefficient allocation of resources or minimize the number of people required to do a job. Second, the variables affecting the goal must have a linear relationship; the ratio of change in one variable to the change in another variable must be constant. If it takes 3 minutes to do a task, it should take 15 minutes to do the task five times. Third, constraints or obstacles to the relationships of the variables exist. Linear programming would not be needed if there were no restrictions.

Simple allocations can often be made by observation and experience, but in large operations the problems may be complex and involve thousands of possible choices. Linear programming is a sophisticated shortcut technique in which a computer can be used to determine solutions. It may be used to determine a minimal-cost diet for meeting certain nutritional standards or for assigning community health nurses to territories. A school of nursing might use this technique to determine class sizes, class hours, and instructors by feeding information into a computer equation containing such variables as a student's desire or requirement to enroll in particular classes, number of students, number of professors qualified to teach the course, and the hours available to conduct the course. Because linear programming depends on linear relationships and many decisions do not involve them, the manager may need to apply nonlinear programming.

ADVANTAGES AND LIMITATIONS OF QUANTITATIVE TOOLS FOR DECISION MAKING

Quantitative tools lend themselves to a rational, systematic approach to problem solving for decisions that can be expressed mathematically. They encourage disciplined thinking. They are not limited to the six or seven variables the human mind can consider at one time, and they may evaluate thousands of interrelationships simultaneously. Decisions made with the use of quantitative tools are likely to be superior to those that rely heavily on judgment. Unfortunately, many managerial problems involve intangible, nonmeasurable factors that reduce the effectiveness of the tools. The mathematical expressions are based on assumptions; if those assumptions are not true for a given situation, the tool becomes useless.

COMPUTERS

Computers provide several advantages over paper-based record systems. Information can be stored in smaller areas, search and analytical

RESEARCH Perspective 3-3

Data from Issel LM, Anderson RA: Intensity of case managers' participation in organizational decision making. *Research in Nursing and Health* 24:361-372, 2001.

Purpose: The purpose of this research was to study if registered nurse participation in decision making is related to better outcomes in nursing homes and hospitals.

Methods: A purposive sample of case managers, case manager aides, and program supervisors in one Midwestern state was invited to participate. The sample was drawn from all 120 Medicaid-approved prenatal-care case management programs in that state. Sixty-eight usable surveys were returned. The measure of intensity used the intensity subscale of the Nursing Participation in Decision Making Instrument (NPDMI). Repeated-measures multivariate analysis of variance was used to analyze data. Pairwise comparisons, performed post hoc using paired-sample *t*-tests were adjusted using Bonferroni's adjustment to alpha for a potential increased rate of Type I errors. Stepwise multiple regressions were used to identify which activities and mechanisms predict case managers' influence on final choices.

Results/conclusions: Case managers were most involved in the activity of "raising the issue" and least involved in "choosing the alternative." "Choosing the alternative" was the strongest predictor of perceived influence over the final choice.

tasks can be performed, and information can be obtained quickly and efficiently. Unfortunately, if used improperly, computers can magnify weaknesses in an organization.

Computers can be applied in nursing in three major categories: (1) clinical systems, (2) management information systems, and (3) educational systems. In clinical systems, computers help with patient histories, medical records, and patient monitoring. Computerized record systems can improve the usability of patient information because data from the chart can be rearranged to be useful to various health care professionals. Physicians can enter their diagnoses, protocols, and notes directly into the computer, saving nurses transcribing time. The instructions can be printed out at the appropriate auxiliary department. Nurses can also record their notes directly into the computer and spend less time and energy accumulating and summarizing data to develop care plans. Standard screens with standard choices increase efficiency for recording observations and doing care plans. Nurses are made aware of changes that require their

intervention quickly because information from ancillary departments can be sent automatically to the nursing station terminal. The computer can sort and analyze data and facilitate communication about the patients among health care providers.

An integrated clinical system allows patient data to be quickly available to health care providers. The system should be easy to use, have standardized data elements, have data repositories and archival systems for information that should be retained long term, and have stand-alone or departmental system accessibility to patient information.

Emergency department systems can triage patients based on assessment criteria. The system can calculate the level of severity based on the assessment and historical data entered by the triage person. The data can be readily available to all clinical personnel, such as those in the laboratory, pharmacy, and radiology departments. The marketing and planning departments can use the statistics to evaluate the market share information. The *laboratory system* allows ordering, collecting, analyzing, and storing of laboratory information, as well as reporting of results. *Pharmacy systems* can be used to order, check allergies, check dosage based on the patient's height and weight, check drug-to-drug interactions, check drug-to-food interactions, label medications, do inventory control, do drug utilization monitoring, and dispense medications. It allows medication cart fill, update, and check functions; printing of written orders; electronic recording of administration of medications; and an alert system for when medications are overdue. *Radiology systems* allow for ordering, scheduling, recording results, and tracking radiology exams. They can generate notices to send to patients and schedule repeat exams. Transcription can be done electronically with an electronically attached signature. Some transcription systems allow for filling in the blanks to eliminate excessive typing. The systems can also track the location of various exam results and has the capability to store images directly on the radiology system, making digitized images readily available. *Cardiology systems* are similar to radiology systems and can be used for the collection, analysis, and reporting of cardiology exams. Transcription capabilities, ability to display and store digitized images, and telemedicine to transmit the report to physicians are desirable.

Dietary systems can assess nutritional status and facilitate ordering and preparing diets. They can create, maintain, and print menus; enter modifiers about restrictions or limitations to basic diets; place a diet on hold for a period of time; print a worksheet for the tray preparation area; and print out diet information for patient and family education.

Respiratory therapy systems can be used to order equipment and treatments, schedule procedures, document responses to treatments, and record interventions. The system can track routine cleaning and maintenance of equipment and disposable and reusable equipment and supplies.

Computer systems can also be used in *operating rooms, ambulatory clinics, physician offices,* and *case management systems.* They are good for scheduling and materials management. Transcription and patient billing are useful functions. Systems can handle scheduling of appointments with several different services with one phone call, which can also obtain basic data, such as insurance information, which can be verified later. They can track missed appointments.

Patient care documentation systems are the largest application of computer systems in health care. Point of care or bedside systems document patient assessments, treatments, medication administration, response to treatments and medications, and other progress notes. They can be used in home care as well as critical care. They allow for integration of care by several care providers.

Patient monitoring systems record patient responses and can alert nurses to changes. Computers can record the patient's progress on paper or on the monitor, sound an alarm, and often transmit information from the patient's bedside to monitors at the nursing station. In addition to monitoring patients continuously and detecting changes, computers can analyze and interpret the data. Through computer monitoring, nurses can respond quickly to changes in patients' conditions.

Computers have many applications in management information systems. They can be used for tracking patient acuity and calculating patient care requirements and for patient classification systems, inventory control, supplies and material management, staff scheduling, policy and procedure changes and announcements, patient charges, budget information and management, personnel records, statistical reports, administrative reports, memos, and record location and tracking.

In educational systems computer-assisted instruction allows students to proceed at their own speed, provides immediate feedback, and allows dissemination of information to remote areas.

When using computers as decision-making tools, nurses should take advantage of good commercial software that is available and should investigate the possibility of using existing systems. Securing the confidentiality of patient and personnel records by carefully locking up diskettes or by constructing a password system is very important (Kreider and Hasselton, 1997).

The Vroom and Jago model (1988) is a computer-friendly revision of the Vroom and Yetton model (1973) (Box 3-5). It provides an additional number of problem attributes, deletes the decision rules, changes dichotomous variables to continuous variables, and provides mathematical formulas to determine decisions.

"The only exercise some minds get is jumping to conclusions!" —Pansy Torrance

---

BOX **3-5** Vroom and Yetton Normative Model

Vroom and Yetton address decision making as a social process and emphasize how managers do rather than should behave in their normative model. They identify the following alternative decision processes: A = autocratic, C = consultative, G = group, I = first variant, and II = second variant.

TYPES OF MANAGEMENT DECISION STYLES*

AI You solve the problem or make the decision yourself, using information available to you at that time.

AII You obtain the necessary information from your subordinate(s), then decide on the solution to the problem yourself. You may or may not tell your subordinates what the problem is in getting the information from them. The role played by your subordinates in making the decision is clearly one of providing the necessary information to you, rather than generating or evaluating alternative solutions.

CI You share the problem with relevant subordinates individually, getting their ideas and suggestions without bringing them together as a group. Then you make the decision that may or may not reflect your subordinates' influence.

CII You share the problem with your subordinates as a group, collectively obtaining their ideas and suggestions. Then you make the decision that may or may not reflect your subordinates' influence.

GII You share a problem with your subordinates as a group. Together you generate and evaluate alternatives and attempt to reach agreement (consensus) on a solution. Your role is much like that of chairperson. You do not try to influence the group to adopt "your" solution, and you are willing to accept and implement any solution that has the support of the entire group.

(GI is omitted because it applies only to more comprehensive models outside the scope of the article.)

DECISION RULES

Vroom identifies seven rules that do most of the work of the model. Three rules protect decision quality, and four protect acceptance.*

1. The information rule

If the quality of the decision is important and if the leader does not possess enough information or expertise to solve the problem by herself, AI is eliminated from the feasible set. (Its use risks a low-quality decision.)

2. The goal congruence rule

If the quality of the decision is important and if the subordinates do not share the organizational goals to be obtained in solving the problem, GII is eliminated from the feasible set. (Alternatives that eliminate the leader's final control over the decision reached may jeopardize the quality of the decision.)

3. The unstructured problem rule

In decisions in which the quality of the decision is important, if the leader lacks the necessary information or expertise to solve the problem by herself, and if the problem is unstructured (that is, she does not know exactly what information is needed and where it is located), the method used must provide for her not only to collect the information but also to do so in an efficient and effective manner. Methods that involve interaction

Continued

BOX **3-5** Vroom and Yetton Normative Model (Cont'd)

among all subordinates with full knowledge of the problem are likely to be both more efficient and more likely to generate a high-quality solution to the problem. Under these conditions AI, AII, and CI are eliminated from the feasible set. (AI does not provide for her to collect the necessary information, and AII and CI represent more cumbersome, less effective, and less efficient means of bringing the necessary information to bear on the solution of the problem than methods that do permit those with the necessary information to interact.)

4. The acceptance rule

If the acceptance of the decision by subordinates is critical to effective implementation, and if it is not certain that an autocratic decision made by the leader would receive that acceptance, AI and AII are eliminated from the feasible set. (Neither provides an opportunity for subordinates to participate in the decision, and both risk the necessary acceptance.)

5. The conflict rule

If the acceptance of the decision is critical, and an autocratic decision is not certain to be accepted, and subordinates are likely to be in conflict or disagreement over the appropriate solution, AI, AII, and CI are eliminated from the feasible set. (The method used in solving the problem should enable those in disagreement to resolve their differences with full knowledge of the problem. Accordingly, under these conditions, AI, AII, and CI, which involve no interaction or only one-on-one relationships and therefore provide no opportunity for those in control to resolve their differences, are eliminated from the feasible set. Their use runs the risk of leaving some of the subordinates with less than the necessary commitment to the final decision.)

6. The fairness rule

If the quality of the decision is unimportant and if acceptance is critical and not certain to result from an autocratic decision, AI, AII, CI, and CII are eliminated from the feasible set. (The method used should maximize the probability of acceptance because this is the only relevant consideration in determining the effectiveness of the decision. Under these circumstances, AI, AII, CI, and CII, which create less acceptance or commitment than GII, are eliminated from the feasible set. To use them is to run the risk of getting less than the needed acceptance of the decision.

7. The acceptance priority rule

If acceptance is critical and not ensured by an autocratic decision, and if subordinates can be trusted, AI, AII, CI, and CII are eliminated from the feasible set. (Methods that provide equal partnership in the decision-making process can provide greater acceptance without risking decision quality. Use of any method other than GII results in an unnecessary risk that the decision will not be fully accepted or receive the necessary commitment on the part of subordinates.)

As one asks the diagnostic questions and applies the rules to specific situations, one may eliminate all but one decision style from the feasibility set. However, it is more likely that several decision styles could be used and still protect both the decision quality and acceptance requirements. Then the time factor is used to determine which of the feasible options will require the least time.

Vroom and Yetton focus on three classes of outcomes that influence the ultimate effectiveness of decisions: (1) the quality of the decision, (2) acceptance of the decision by the subordinates, and (3) available time needed to make the decision. The authors found that managers can diagnose a situation quickly and accurately by answering the following seven questions*:

PROBLEM ATTRIBUTES	DIAGNOSTIC QUESTIONS
A. The importance of the quality of the decision	Is there a quality requirement such that one solution is likely to be more rational than another?
B. The extent to which the leader possesses sufficient information/expertise to make a high-quality decision by herself	Do you have sufficient information to make a high-quality decision?
C. The extent to which the problem is structured	Is the problem structured?

BOX **3-5** Vroom and Yetton Normative Model (Cont'd)

D. The extent to which acceptance or commitment on the part of subordinates is critical to the effective implementation of the decision

Do you need the acceptance and commitment of others to implement the decision?

E. The prior probability that the leader's autocratic decision will receive acceptance by subordinates

If you were to make the decision by yourself, is it reasonably certain that it would be accepted by your subordinates?

F. The extent to which subordinates are motivated to attain the organizational goals as represented in the objectives explicit in the statement of the problem

Do subordinates share the organizational goals to be obtained in solving this problem?

G. The extent to which subordinates are likely to be in conflict over preferred solutions

Is conflict among subordinates likely in preferred solutions?

*Reprinted from *Organizational Dynamics,* Spring 1973. Copyright © 1973 American Management Association International. Reprinted by permission of American Management Association International, New York. All rights reserved. http://www.amanet.org.

Chapter Summary

Chapter 3 covered the following:
Decision-Making Process
    Identify the Problem and Analyze the Situation
    Explore the Alternatives
    Choose the Most Desirable Alternative
    Implement the Decision
    Evaluate the Results
Organizational Models for Decision Making
    Rational Model
    Political Model
    Collegial Model
    Bureaucratic Model
    Garbage Can Model
    Cybernetic Model
Critical Thinking
    Purpose or Goal
    Central Problem or Question at Issue
    Point of View or Frame of Reference
    Empirical Dimension
    Conceptual Dimension
    Assumptions
    Implications and Consequences
    Inferences and Conclusions
    Critical Thinking for the Nursing Process
Group Decision Making
    Group Factors
        Advantages
        Disadvantages

Committee/Task Force Aspects
    Advantages
    Disadvantages
    Committee Functioning
    Consensus Building Versus Group Think
Creative Decision Making
    The Creative Process
    Encouraging Creativity
        Convergent thinking
        Divergent thinking
        Ladder of abstraction
        Forced association
        Visual trek/visual confrontation
        Think tanks
        Brainstorming
        Reverse brainstorming
        Brain writing
        Collective notebook technique
        Stepladder technique
        Morphological matrix
        The Delphi technique
        Lists
        Drawing
        Synetics
        Visualization
        Visually identifying relationships
        Forecasting alternative future scenarios
        Self-interrogation checklist
        Modeling

Meditation
Evaluation matrix
Advantages, limitations, unique qualities, overcome limitations (ALUo)
Paired comparison analysis
Musts/wants
Highlighting
SML
Developing Creative Thinking Attitudes
Blocks to Creativity
Consultation
Ethical Aspects of Decision Making
Ethical Theories
Ethical Principles
Ethical Positions
Ethical Relationships
Moral Reasoning
Universal Principles of Ethics in a Multicultural World
Ethics Committees
American Nurses Association's Code of Ethics for Nurses
Canadian Nurses Association's Code of Ethics for Registered Nurses
International Council of Nurses' International Code of Ethics for Nurses
Decision-Making Tools
Probability Theory
Simulation, Models, and Games
Gantt Chart
Decision Trees
Program Evaluation and Review Technique
Critical Path Method
Queuing Theory
Linear Programming
Advantages and Limitations of Quantitative Tools for Decision Making
Computers

On-line Resources

evolve Additional critical thinking activities, worksheets, and case studies are available on-line at http://evolve.elsevier.com/Marriner/guide/

References

Aroskar MA: Ethics of nurse-patient relationships, *Nurse Educ* 5:18, 1980.

Capacchione L: *Visioning*, New York, 2000, Tarcher/Putnam.

Catalano JT: *Ethical and legal aspects of nursing*, Springhouse, Pa, 1995, Springhouse.

Grohar-Murray ME, DiCroce HR: *Leadership and management in nursing,* ed 3, Stamford, Conn, 2003, Appleton & Lange.

Harris RA: *Creative problem solving: A step-by-step approach,* Los Angeles, 2002, Pyrczak.

Jones RAP: *Decision making in nursing*, Albany, NY, 1996, Delmar.

Kreider NA, Hasselton BJ: *The systems challenge*, Chicago, 1997, American Hospital Association.

Marquis BL, Huston CJ: *Leadership roles and management functions in nursing: Theory and application*, Philadelphia, 2000, Lippincott.

Paul R: *Critical thinking*, Santa Rosa, Calif, 1993, Foundation of Critical Thinking.

Simms LM, Price SA, Ervin NE: *Professional practice of nursing administration,* ed 3, Albany, NY, 2000, Delmar.

Sullivan EJ, Decker PJ: *Effective leadership and management in nursing,* ed 5, Upper Saddle River, NJ, 2001, Prentice Hall.

Swansburg RC, Swansburg RJ: *Introduction to management and leadership for nurse managers,* ed 3, Boston, 2002, Jones & Bartlett.

Swansburg RC, Swansburg RJ: *Introductory management and leadership for nurses,* Boston, 1999, Jones & Bartlett.

Treffinger DJ, Isaksen SG, Dorval KB: *Creative problem solving: An introduction*, 1999.

Umiker W: *Management skills for the new health care supervisor,* ed 3, Gaithersburg, Md, 1998, Aspen.

Vroom VH, Jago AG: *The new leadership: Managing participation in organizations*, Englewood Cliffs, NJ, 1988, Prentice Hall.

Vroom VH, Yetton PW: *Leadership and decision-making*, Pittsburgh, 1973, University of Pittsburgh.

Yoder-Wise PS: *Leading and managing in nursing*, St Louis, 2003, Mosby.

Young AP, Cooke M: *Managing and implementing decisions in health care*, Edinburgh, 2002, Baillière Tindall & Royal College of Nursing.

4

Motivation and Morale

*"Whether you think that you can, or that you can't,
you are usually right."* —Henry Ford

Chapter Overview

Chapter 4 explains theories of motivation, including Taylor's monistic
theory, Maslow's hierarchy of needs theory, Alderfer's modified need
hierarchy, McClelland's basic needs theory, Herzberg's motivation hygiene
(two-factor) theory, Argyris's psychological energy theory, Vroom's
expectancy theory, Skinner's positive reinforcement theory, equity theory,
intrinsic motivation, McGregor's Theory X and Theory Y, Likert's
participative management theory, and Theory Z. Historical development of
motivation theory, morale, burnout, and job satisfaction are discussed.

Chapter Objectives

- Put Maslow's five needs into Alderfer's three categories of existence, relatedness,
  and growth needs.
- Identify at least five hygiene and five motivation factors in Herzberg's theory.
- Describe Vroom's expectancy theory.
- Explain how Skinner's positive reinforcement theory works.
- Describe ways people deal with perceived inequities.
- List at least three beliefs each for McGregor's Theory X and Theory Y.

MOTIVATION

Why do people work? Why do some employees achieve high productivity whereas others are content with mediocrity or less? What can a manager do to stimulate intrinsic and extrinsic motivation? These questions are important to the manager. They elicit complex and uncertain answers. Unfortunately, there are no simple rules that a manager can follow to stimulate the staff.

TAYLOR'S MONISTIC THEORY

Monistic theory is derived from the principles of scientific management. Frederick Taylor, a pioneer in this field, believed that if energetic people with high productivity learn that they earn no more than a lazy worker who does as little as possible, they will lose interest in giving optimal performance. Taylor argued that an incentive is needed to prevent this loss. It should be possible to earn more by producing more, so that pay would depend on productivity. Incentives such as merit increases, bonus systems, profit sharing, savings sharing, and piece rates are examples of monistic methods. With implementation of payment by piece rate, the employer must be certain that wage costs do not increase more rapidly than production. This system can place considerable pressure on the worker and create tensions that lead to undesirable behavior. Payment by piece rate almost certainly guarantees that some workers will be paid more than others. A larger paycheck may increase one's self-esteem and even serve as a status symbol, but the amount of motivation provided by money is questionable.

MASLOW'S HIERARCHY OF NEEDS

In contrast to Taylor's belief that money is a primary motivator, Abraham Maslow maintained that people are motivated by a desire to satisfy a hierarchy of needs. Maslow hypothesized that satisfaction of the basic physiological needs triggers the emergence of more abstract needs and that a satisfied need is no longer a motivator. The five basic needs he identified are physiological, safety/security, social/belonging, esteem, and self-actualization (Figure 4-1).

Physiological Needs

The body needs water, food, oxygen, elimination, rest, exercise, sex, shelter, and protection from the elements. People have a strong drive for self-preservation, and whenever their basic physiological needs are threatened, the needs become prepotent. These needs are relatively independent and must be met repeatedly to remain fulfilled. In an affluent society physiological needs are probably not the most common motivators. The nurse manager should determine whether physiological needs are being met. Personnel should not be overworked. Meal breaks and rest breaks should be provided. Pay should be adequate for food, shelter, health care, and recreation.

Safety/Security Needs

People need physical, emotional, and financial safety. They need a stable environment in which

R:SEARCH Perspective 4-1

Data from Ingersoll GL, Olsan T, Drew-Cates J, DeVinney BC, Davies J: Nurses' job satisfaction, organizational commitment, and career intent. *JONA* 32(5):250-263, 2002.

Purpose: The purpose of this survey was to define the characteristics of the nursing work force of a mixed urban/rural region of New York State and to determine the nurses' level of job satisfaction and commitment to the work setting.

Methods: A random sample survey was mailed to 4000 registered nurses in the Finger Lakes region of New York State in June 2000. Forty-six percent of the sample returned completed questionnaires. Organizational Commitment Questionnaire and Index to Work Satisfaction were used. Items in the questionnaire addressed nurse characteristics, reasons for leaving or staying with an employing agency, 1- and 5-year career intent, and level of job satisfaction and organizational commitment. Descriptive statistics, analysis of variance, chi-square, and multiple regression techniques were used to analyze the data to detect differences in perceptions and career intent according to respondent characteristics.

Results/conclusions: Findings indicated that the organizational and personal characteristics of currently employed registered nurses affect their current job satisfaction, organizational commitment, and plans for continuing as a nurse. Characteristics of satisfied nurses were older than 50 years of age; master's prepared; employed by school of nursing or by home care agencies; appointed as administrators, educators, or advanced practice nurses; and specialized in pediatrics, community health, family health, occupational health, or education. Characteristics of nurses committed to their organization were older than 50 years of age; worked in primarily rural areas; employed by schools of nursing, home care agencies, or non–health-related facilities; appointed as administrators or as educators; specialized in community health, family health, occupational health, education, or non–health-related fields. Many of the most satisfied and committed nurses reported their intent to leave nursing within the next 5 years.

they are protected against the threats of danger and deprivation. People do not want to worry about inadequate income because of loss of job, accident, or old age. Arbitrary management actions, favoritism toward or discrimination against employees, and unpredictable administration of policies are dangerous to safety needs and should be avoided.

Social/Belonging Needs

Social needs include a feeling of belonging, acceptance by one's peers, recognition as an accepted member of a group, being an integral part of the operation, giving and receiving friendship, and affectionate relations with others. A cohesive work group is likely to be more effective than an equal number of people working separately. Yet management, fearing hostility toward its objectives, may control situations to prevent *esprit de corps*. Thwarting of the social needs, however, may stimulate resistance and antagonism that further defeat management's objectives.

Esteem Needs

Achievement, competence, knowledge, independence, status, recognition, prestige, appreciation, reputation, and respect contribute to one's self-confidence and self-esteem. Management can help meet these needs by giving praise when it is deserved and through the use of constructive evaluations, pay raises, and titles. Unlike the

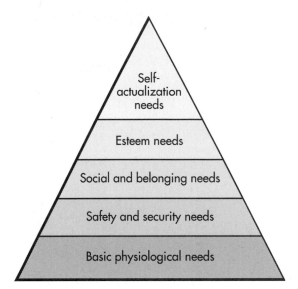

Figure 4-1 Maslow's hierarchy of needs. (Modified from Maslow AH: *Motivation and personality.* © 1954, 1987, 1970 by Abraham H. Maslow. Modified by permission of Prentice-Hall, Upper Saddle River, NJ.)

lower physiological and safety needs, the esteem needs are not so easily satisfied.

Self-Actualization Needs

It is doubtful that one ever achieves all that of which one is capable. Feelings of accomplishment, responsibility, importance, challenge, advancement, and new experiences and opportunities for growth contribute to self-fulfillment.

ALDERFER'S MODIFIED NEED HIERARCHY

Clayton Alderfer proposes a modified need hierarchy theory that collapses Maslow's five hierarchical levels into three (Box 4-1). His existence-relatedness-growth (ERG) theory suggests that in addition to a satisfaction-progression process,

BOX **4-1** Alderfer's Modified Need Hierarchy

Existence needs
Relatedness needs
Growth needs.

in which people are constantly frustrated in their attempts to satisfy one level of needs, they can redirect their energy toward a lower-level need. Alderfer's model is less rigid than Maslow's and suggests that more than one need may be operative (Table 4-1).

McCLELLAND'S BASIC NEEDS THEORY

David McClelland has identified three basic needs that all people have in varying degrees: the need for achievement, power, and affiliation (Box 4-2). The need for achievement involves a desire to make a contribution, to excel, and to succeed. People with high achievement needs are eager for responsibility, take calculated risks, and desire feedback about their performance. People who have a high need for power want to be in control and desire influence over others. They are more interested in personal prestige and power than effective performance. For contrast, people with high affiliation needs desire working in human environments and seek out meaningful friendships. They want to be respected and avoid decisions or actions that oppose group norms. They are more interested in high morale than productivity. Managers should match personnel needs with assignments. If a project has well-defined objectives and specific tasks, a person with a high achievement need may be appropriate. If a project involves unpleasant tasks with personnel (such as retrenchment), a person with high power needs may do the job best. A person with high affiliation needs would not want to make decisions that would alienate peers but would be good for fostering morale.

TABLE 4-1 Comparison of Maslow's Hierarchy of Needs and Alderfer's Existence, Relatedness, and Growth

MASLOW	ALDERFER
Self-actualization needs Esteem needs	Growth needs
Social/belonging needs	Relatedness needs
Safety/security needs Physiological needs	Existence needs

HERZBERG'S MOTIVATION HYGIENE (TWO-FACTOR) THEORY

"Obstacles are those frightful things you see when you take your eyes off your goal." —Henry Ford

Frederick Herzberg found that work motivators include achievement, growth, responsibility, advancement, recognition, and the job itself. According to Herzberg, if people are satisfied with their job, they are receiving positive feedback, developing skills, and improving their performance. Herzberg maintains that employees can be motivated by giving them challenging work in which they can assume responsibility (Figure 4-2 and Box 4-3).

Dissatisfaction results when people perceive that they are being treated unfairly in pay, benefits, status, job security, supervision, and interpersonal relationships. Herzberg classifies all of the above as hygiene factors and argues that they are not motivators because they do not cause any improvement in attitudes or performance. They can only prevent dissatisfaction and poor morale. Hygiene factors do not make a job more interesting. If people are highly motivated and find their job interesting and challenging, they can tolerate dissatisfaction with hygiene factors (Figures 4-3 and 4-4).

ARGYRIS'S PSYCHOLOGICAL ENERGY THEORY

Chris Argyris believes that people will exert more energy to meet their own needs than those of the organization. The greater the disparity

Figure 4-2 Herzberg's two-factor motivation hygiene theory of needs motivation. (From Claus KE, Bailey JT: *Power and influence in health care*, St Louis, 1977, Mosby.)

BOX **4-3** Herzberg's Motivation Hygiene Theory

MAINTENANCE FACTORS	MOTIVATIONAL FACTORS
Dissatisfiers	Satisfiers
Hygiene factors	Motivators
Job contest	Job content
Extrinsic factors	Intrinsic factors

between the individual's and the organization's goals, the more likely it is that the employee will feel dissatisfaction, tension, conflict, apathy, or subversion. Argyris suggests that management match personnel and jobs by taking advantage of people's talents and interests, make jobs interesting and challenging, help personnel satisfy their needs for self-actualization, improve interpersonal relationships, and use a management style consistent with Theory Y (which will be discussed later).

VROOM'S EXPECTANCY THEORY

"There's nothing either good or bad, but thinking makes it so." —William Shakespeare

Victor Vroom popularized the expectancy theory during the 1960s. It is based on Kurt Lewin's field theory and has been expanded by Lyman Porter and others. Expectancy theory states that motivation depends on how much people want something and their estimate of the probability of getting it (Figure 4-5).

Valence is the strength of a person's preference for something. It may be negative or positive from −1 to +1. If the person does not want something, there is a negative valence. If the person is indifferent, the valence is zero. A positive valence indicates a desire for something (Figure 4-6, *A*).

Expectancy is the probability of getting something through specific actions. If a person believes that an action will result in an outcome, expectancy has a value of 1. If no probability is perceived, the expectancy is zero. Expectancy varies from one situation to another (Figure 4-6, *B*).

If someone has a high valence and a high expectancy, the motivation will be high. If there is a low valence and a low expectancy, the motivation will be low. If one is high and the other low, moderate motivation will result.

The expectancy theory has been further developed to include the value of the outcome factor. To be highly motivated, a person needs to find an outcome attractive, believe that certain actions will lead to the desired outcome, and assess that the result is worth the effort.

Figure 4-3 Comparison of the Maslow and Herzberg models. (From Donnelly JH Jr, Gibson JL, Ivancevich JM: *Fundamentals of management: Functions, behavior, models,* ed 4, Dallas, 1990, Business Publications. © by Business Publications.)

Figure 4-4 Maintenance and motivational factors.

Consequently, to motivate personnel, managers should clarify connections between work and outcome and should reward desirable behavior.

SKINNER'S POSITIVE REINFORCEMENT THEORY

Operant conditioning and behavior modification are other names for B.F. Skinner's positive reinforcement theory. Behavior may be strengthened or weakened depending on what follows it. Positive reinforcement strengthens behavior. Withholding positive reinforcers weakens behavior, whereas intermittent reinforcement increases resistance to extinction. Punishment will help reduce behavior, but it cannot teach new behaviors, and it may condition avoidance.

Accentuating the positive with plenty of praise and positive feedback may increase the frequency of desired behavior. If, however, a subordinate admits to less than desirable behavior, the manager may respond, "I appreciate your honesty," while reminding the worker of the goal.

When desired results are not obtained, managers should analyze the situation. First, they should assess the working environment for interference. Do the employees have adequate time to complete the task? Does the system allow nurses to maximize their efficiency, or must they spend most of their time running to central supply to gather materials that should have been readily available? If managers do not locate the cause of the problem in the environment, they must ask themselves if the employees have been properly utilized. Do they have the knowledge and skills necessary to do the job? If not, can they be taught? If they cannot be taught, can they be replaced and assigned other duties?

EQUITY THEORY

"Argue for your limitations, and sure enough they're yours." —Richard Bach

During the 1960s Jo Stacy Adams and others studied perceptions of equity and inequity. They found that employees assess fairness by considering their input and the psychological, social, and financial rewards in comparison with those of others. Perceived inequity causes tension. The amount of the tension was found to be proportional to the magnitude of the perceived inequity. Tension motivates people to reduce its cause. Consequently, the strength of the motivation to reduce the perceived inequity is proportional to the cognitive dissonance. To reduce the inequity, people may alter input or output, cognitively distort input or output, change the basis for comparison, or leave. If people feel overworked and underpaid, they are likely to decrease their productivity. Less often, employees feel overrewarded and strive to improve their performance. People resist changing their bases of comparison or distorting their perceptions. People do not usually leave an organization unless there is extreme inequity. If the comparison is equal, people feel that they are treated fairly. If not, they are motivated to take corrective action. Managers should be attentive to the perceived equity of the reward system (Box 4-4).

INTRINSIC MOTIVATION

Edward Deci has studied intrinsic motivation. He found that some activities are ends in themselves, not just means to ends. There is no apparent

Figure 4-5 Expectancy theory.

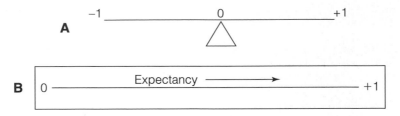

Figure 4-6 Ranges of valence and expectancy. **A**, Valence. **B**, Expectancy.

reward except the activity itself. Intrinsically motivated behavior seems to be stimulated by people's needs for feeling competent and self-determining. When there is no stimulation, people will seek it. When they are overstimulated, they back away, regroup, and reaffirm competence. People engage in a process of seeking and conquering to feel competent and self-determined. When people's feelings of competence and self-determination are enhanced, their intrinsic motivation will increase. If their perceptions of competence and self-determination are diminished, their intrinsic motivation will decrease. Extrinsic rewards have a controlling aspect that may decrease intrinsic rewards. Insufficient extrinsic rewards tend to increase intrinsic motivation because people try to reduce cognitive dissonance. Consequently, managers should foster

stimulation through means such as continuing education and special projects.

McGREGOR'S THEORY X AND THEORY Y

Douglas McGregor has classified traditional management theories as Theory X. They are based on the assumption that people will avoid work if possible because they dislike it; consequently, most people must be directed, controlled, coerced, and threatened. Theory X assumes that people want direction, have little ambition, avoid responsibility, but want security. A manager with a Theory X philosophy would probably use fear and threats to motivate personnel, supervise closely, delegate little responsibility, and not consider personnel participation in planning.

McGregor maintains that if people behave as described in Theory X it is because of what the system has done to them—not because of their inherent nature. He believes that as long as managerial strategies are based on Theory X, managers will fail to discover, let alone use, the potentials of their personnel.

McGregor classifies the newer developments in management as Theory Y. In this theory McGregor makes the assumption that people like and enjoy work, are self-directed, and seek responsibility. It maintains that most people have imagination, ingenuity, creativity, and other intellectual capacities that are only partially utilized. A manager with a Theory Y philosophy will use positive incentives such as praise and recognition, give general supervision, provide opportunities for individual growth, delegate responsibilities, and encourage participation in problem solving. Job enlargement and decentralization are additional

---

BOX 4-4 Equity Theory

A person compares her input/output with and perceives relation to a reference person.

IP = IRP
OP = ORP $\Big\}$ Equity

IP < IRP
OP < ORP $\Big\}$ Inequity

IP > IRP
OP > ORP $\Big\}$ Inequity

IP = Inputs of the person
OP = Outputs of the person
IRP = Inputs of reference person
ORP = Outputs of reference person

motivational techniques that may stimulate personnel's performance to the extent that it exceeds the requirements stated in the job description (Table 4-2).

LIKERT'S PARTICIPATIVE MANAGEMENT THEORY

Rensis Likert believes that effective managers are highly sensitive to their staff associates, use communication to keep the group working as a unit, and foster supportive relationships among all group members. Participative management is a human relations theory that may use management by objectives and job-enrichment approaches.

THEORY Z

The Japanese form of participative management is known as Theory Z. The major firms of Japan are organized into *zaibatsu,* small groups of 20 to 30 firms representing each important industrial sector. Each firm hosts satellite companies that provide a service or manufacture a subassembly for the host firm. Employees are hired to work for the host firm until retirement. After slow evaluation and promotion in nonspecialized careers, employees retire at age 55 years. They then work on a part-time basis for a satellite company. Women work temporarily and serve as a buffer to the job security of the male work force. Their schedules are flexible so they can care for their families, and they are laid off in slack periods.

Concern for the worker is apparent. Japanese companies form inclusive personal and professional relationships and provide social support. Because personnel anticipate lifetime relationships, they are cautious about interpersonal conflicts. Cooperation is stressed. Collective decision making is practiced. Through the ritual *ofringi,* ideas pass from manager to manager for approval. This helps establish trust and cooperation. Objectives and the procedures to achieve them are implicitly described. Quality circles are formed when two to ten employees meet to identify problems, explore options, and make decisions. Quality circles have increased worker productivity, enhanced job satisfaction, and reduced turnover in addition to solving identified problems. Decisions are made by consensus. Because it takes so much time to reach a consensus, only policy and behavior changes are dealt with. Responsibility is also collective. An emphasis is placed on developing all aspects of the employees, and they are rewarded with regular pay bonuses based on the company's performance.

The Japanese Theory Z managers focus on the four soft *S*'s of management: staff, skills, style, and superordinate goals. Staff is the workers. Skills are the capabilities of the organization or key personnel. Style refers to the cultural style of the organization or how managers achieve goals. The superordinate goals are the guideposts as determined by the personnel.

Less attention is given to the hard *S*'s: system, structure, and strategy. The system is the mechanism whereby information circulates through the organization. Structure is the organization, and strategy is the plan of action.

HISTORICAL DEVELOPMENT OF MOTIVATION THEORY

Traditional management theory is based on McGregor's Theory X. Traditional theory

TABLE **4-2** McGregor's Theory X and Theory Y

X	Y
People dislike work.	Work is natural.
People must be directed to do work.	People will exercise self-control.
People want to avoid responsibility.	People enjoy responsibility.
People believe that achievement is irrelevant.	People value achievement.
People are dull and uncreative.	People have potential, imagination, and creativity.
Money is the reason for working.	Money is only one reason for working.
People lack desire to improve quality.	People want to improve quality.

addresses itself to Maslow's primary physiological and safety needs and employs the monistic theory for reinforcement. The latter, according to Herzberg, helps meet some of the hygiene needs but does not provide motivation.

Newer developments in management are based on McGregor's Theory Y. Maslow's secondary needs of belonging, esteem, and self-actualization are more prepotent than the primary needs for most personnel. Because a satisfied need is no longer a motivator, hygiene factors such as money and working conditions do not serve as motivators. People are more interested in autonomy, responsibility, achievement, recognition, variety in work, and efforts for self-actualization. Argyris has suggested that personnel may become more self-actualized if their personal goals are consistent with the goals of the organization. Talents and interests should be considered when assigning jobs. And then, according to Skinner, positive reinforcement will further increase desired behaviors.

Participation is a major factor in newer management techniques. Personnel are encouraged to contribute to decisions, goals, and plans. Decentralization is supported to the point of management by objectives, allowing personnel to define their own objectives and to determine how they plan to achieve them. The supervisor approves the goals, makes sure they are consistent with the organization's goals, and evaluates personnel using their own objectives as the standard. Modern managers delegate duties and assist others to work more effectively. They help each person develop her own talents and try to maintain a close relationship between the interests and skills of the individual and the requirements of the job. Job enrichment and job rotation may be used to help develop personnel fully. When personnel are actively striving toward esteem and self-actualization and when their goals are consistent with those of the organization, there is likely to be a noticeable effect on the accomplishment of the organization's goals and productivity.

EMOTIONAL INTELLIGENCE

HISTORY OF EMOTIONAL INTELLIGENCE

From 1900 to 1969, intelligence and emotions were viewed as separate narrow fields. However, the renowned psychologist E.L. Thorndike (1935) did write about social intelligence. David Wechsler (1952) continued to develop his intelligence quotient (IQ) test but did consider affective capacities as part of the human repertoire of capabilities. The decades from 1970 to 1989 contained precursors to emotional intelligence as the field of cognition and affect emerged to examine how emotions interacted with thoughts. The field of nonverbal communications developed. Gardner (1983) proposed a new theory of multiple intelligences including an intrapersonal and interpersonal intelligence that included the capacity to perceive and symbolize emotions. Social skills and empathy were studied as social intelligence. Brain research started separating out connections between emotion and cognition. Reuven Bar-On (1988) developed attempts to assess emotional intelligence in terms of a measure of well-being. Emotional intelligence emerged during 1990 to 1993, particularly in the brain sciences. Salovey and Mayer published the seminal article "Emotional Intelligence" in 1990. The popularization and broadening occurred from 1994 to 1997, especially with the publication of Daniel Goleman's worldwide bestselling book, *Emotional Intelligence*, in 1995. Bar-On (1997) identified the five main domains in his model as intrapersonal skills, interpersonal skills, adaptability, stress management, and general mood. A number of personality scales were developed and published under the name of emotional intelligence. Research on and institutionalization of emotional intelligence have occurred since 1998 (Bar-On and Parker, 2000; Cherniss and Adler, 2000; Cherniss and Goleman, 2001).

COMPETENCIES OF EMOTIONAL INTELLIGENCE

Goleman (1995) indicates that how well we handle each other and ourselves is even more important than IQ or advanced degrees for success in organizations. He says star performers

RESEARCH Perspective 4-2

Data from Laschinger HKS, Shamian J, Thomson D: Impact of magnet hospital in characteristics on nurses' perceptions of trust, burnout, quality of care and work satisfaction. *Nursing Economics* 19(5):209-219, 2001.

Purpose: The purpose of this survey was to explore what influences nurses' perceptions of trust, burnout, quality of care, and work satisfaction.

Methods: A subset from a larger study designed to explore relationships among hospital work environment characteristics, nurse staffing, and nurse and patient outcomes was used to assess nurses' perceptions of autonomy, control, physician relationships, faith and confidence in peers and managers, emotional exhaustion, job satisfaction, and the quality of patient care. A stratified random sample of nurses who worked in the medical-surgical setting was drawn from the registry list of College of Nurses of Ontario. Three thousand sixteen staff nurses from 135 hospitals from the larger study completed additional items related to organizational trust. Nursing Work

Index was used to study organizational attributes of the work setting. The Interpersonal Trust at Work Scale measured trust and confidence in management of peers. The Human Services Survey measured burnout. A one-item scale asking respondents to rate their satisfaction with their present job on a four-point Likert scale measured job satisfaction. Descriptive statistics and internal consistency reliability analyses were conducted on the aggregated data. Path analyses and structural equation modeling were used. Chi square was used to evaluate the relative differences in fit among competing models.

Results/conclusions: The findings suggest that perceived autonomy, control, and physician relationships influence the trust, job satisfaction, and perceived quality of patient care.

---

have a capacity to work well with individuals and teams as well as have personal achievement whereas people who are isolated or explosive can be toxic to the whole organization. He labels that ability to work with individuals and groups as emotional intelligence and identifies the five components of emotional intelligence as self-awareness, self-regulation, motivation, empathy, and social skills. These are divided into personal competence and social competence (Goleman, 1998) (Box 4-5).

Personal competence influences how we manage ourselves. Self-awareness involves doing an accurate self-assessment to know our strengths and weaknesses and an emotional awareness of our emotions and their effects. That helps ensure self-confidence about our self-worth and capabilities.

Self-regulation involves keeping our disruptive emotions and impulses under control, maintaining honesty and integrity, taking responsibility for our own performance, being flexible for handling change, and becoming comfortable with new information and approaches.

Motivation can help us reach goals by striving to meet a standard of excellence, aligning our personal goals with the group and organizational goals, taking advantage of opportunities, and keeping a positive attitude about pursuing goals despite obstacles and setbacks.

Social competence determines how we handle relationships. Empathy involves taking an interest in others' concerns and understanding them, developing others' abilities, anticipating and meeting customers' needs, leveraging diversity to cultivate opportunities, and political awareness.

BOX **4-5** Emotional Intelligence

Personal competence
  Self-awareness
    Emotional awareness
    Accurate self-assessment
    Self-confidence
  Self-regulation
    Self-control
    Trustworthiness
    Conscientiousness
    Adaptability
    Innovation
  Motivation
    Achievement drive
    Commitment
    Initiative
    Optimism
Self-competence
  Empathy
    Understanding others
    Developing others
    Service orientation
    Leveraging diversity
    Political awareness
  Social skills
    Influence
    Communications
    Conflict management
    Leadership
    Change catalyst
    Building bonds
    Collaboration and cooperation
    Team capabilities

From Goleman D: *Working with emotional intelligence*, New York, 1998, Bantam Books.

Social skills are an adeptness at inducing desirable responses in people through influence, listening and sending convincing messages, resolving disagreements, inspiring others, managing change, nurturing relationships, collaborating and cooperating toward shared goals, and creating group synergy through team development (Goleman, 1998).

Goleman (1998) reports that there are more similarities between groups of men and women than differences. Although on the average women may be better than men at some emotional skills, some men are better than most women.

Women may be able to detect fleeting feelings in others better than men, but the gender gap in reading emotions closes when emotional cues are less easy to control than facial expression, such as tone of voice or body language. There appears to be no gender difference in being able to sense someone's specific thoughts. That empathic accuracy integrates both cognitive and affective skills (Goleman, 1998).

PROMOTING EMOTIONAL INTELLIGENCE

In *Promoting Emotional Intelligence in Organizations: Make Training in Emotional Intelligence Effective*, Cherniss and Adler (2000) describe several model programs such as conflict management training, self-management training, stress management training, emotional competence training, empathy training, human relations training, caregiver support program, achievement motivation training, supervisory training, executive coaching, and leadership lab. Key competencies to be taught as identified in *The Handbook of Emotional Intelligence* by Bar-On and Parker (2000, p. 400) are:

1. awareness of self and others,

2. positive attitudes and values

3. responsible decision making

4. communication skills

5. social skills

Segal (1997, pp. 215-216) outlines a 10-step curriculum for emotional wisdom:

1. Make care of your body a priority.

2. Search for feeling in your body, not your head.

3. Build emotional muscle every day by taking time to focus on emotional experience.

4. Be accepting of all that you feel.

5. Open your heart to others.

6. Take action—do things that make you feel useful and relevant.

7. Listen with your empathy.

8. Tell them how you feel.

9. Use change as an opportunity to grow.

10. Take a dose of humor with you wherever you go.

Saarni (1997, pp. 47-58) identified the following relevant skills and capabilities of emotional competence from a review of research studies and published them in *Emotional Development and Emotional Intelligence* edited by Salovey and Sluyter:

1. Awareness of one's emotional state, including the possibility that one is experiencing multiple emotions, and at even more mature levels, awareness that one might also not be consciously aware of one's feelings because of unconscious dynamics or selective inattention

2. Ability to discern others' emotions, based on situational and expressive cues that have some degree of cultural consensus as to their emotional meaning

3. Ability to use the vocabulary of emotion and expression terms commonly available in one's (sub)culture and at more mature levels to acquire cultural scripts that link emotion with social roles

4. Capacity for empathic and sympathetic involvement in others' emotional experiences

5. Ability to realize that an inner emotional state need not correspond to outer expression, both in oneself and in others, and at more mature levels the ability to understand that one's emotional-expressive behavior may impact on another and to take this into account in one's self-presentation strategies

6. Capacity for adaptive coping with aversive or distressing emotions by using self-regulatory strategies that ameliorate the intensity or temporal duration of such emotional states (e.g., "stress hardiness")

7. Awareness that the structure or nature of relationships is in part defined by the quality of emotional communication within the relationship

8. Capacity for emotional self-efficacy: The individual views herself as feeling, overall, the way she wants to feel.

Cherniss and Adler (2000) identified a four-phase model for promoting emotional intelligence–based learning in work organizations as follows:

1. Phase 1
   a. Securing organizational support by moving when the timing is right
   b. Finding a powerful sponsor
   c. Linking emotional intelligence to business needs
   d. Recruiting emotionally intelligent leadership
   e. Giving the initiative plenty of autonomy
   f. Using research
   g. Maintaining high quality
   h. Infusing emotional intelligence training throughout the organization

2. Phase 2
   a. Preparing for change by assessing organizational needs
   b. Assessing individuals and delivering results with care
   c. Gauging readiness of learners
   d. Setting clear, meaningful, manageable goals
   e. Making learning self-directed
   f. Building positive expectations

3. Phase 3
   a. Training and development by fostering a positive relationship between trainer and learner
   b. Using live models
   c. Relying on experiential methods
   d. Providing practice and feedback
   e. Inoculating against setbacks

4. Phase 4
   a. Encouraging, maintaining, and evaluating change by building in support
   b. Creating an encouraging environment
   c. Conducting ongoing evaluation and research

Ryback (1998, p. 64) outlined five dynamic interactive principles of the new team ethic that he developed inductively from years of consulting as follows:

1. Building trusting relationships and effective communication through risk taking, openness, effective listening skills, and learning to respect differences of opinion while building on a consensus that proves worthwhile

2. Creative innovation through group discussions that foster openness and playful opposition

3. Fostering a sense of self-appreciation and team pride through group discussion focused on patterns of successful decision making and appropriate actions based on emotional insights

4. Learning to distinguish between decisions based on fact and those based on emotion, as well as the most effective balance between the two for each particular individual

5. Reducing stress through the encouragement of healthy fitness habits and relaxation techniques

These principles should help develop emotional intelligence in the team members.

Ciarrochi, Forgas, and Mayer (2001) outline the history of the emergence of the emotional intelligence concept and discuss the applications of emotional intelligence research to everyday life while Feldman (1999) provides a hands-on guide to understanding and applying the 10 skills of emotionally intelligent leadership and a 50-question self-assessment.

MORALE

Morale is a state of mind related to cheerfulness, confidence, and discipline. A person who works confidently, courageously, and with discipline demonstrates high morale. A person who is cowardly, disorderly, devious, fearful, and rebellious demonstrates low morale. Morale is related to productivity, quality, job satisfaction, and motivation. Morale is related to leadership style and the interpersonal and communication skills of the leader. Recognition and praise contribute to high morale.

Replacing competition with an effort to outdo one's own previous accomplishments is helpful. That leads to continuous improvement. One sees others as benchmarks while trying to improve one's own performance and appreciates one's own importance. This replaces the old competitive paradigm of the game where the goal is winning; the others are enemies; and I am separate and

better than they. The transformational leader helps others gain enthusiasm from shared accomplishments and permission to take risks. This encourages initiating, asserting, engaging, collaborating, appreciating, and supporting toward a high-focused energy.

Organizational morale is the attitudes of the workers toward the quality of their work lives. Each work environment is unique, and each worker's view of the quality of life is uniquely related to how it satisfies one's needs. Managers should survey workers' perceptions of the importance of job factors and their satisfaction with those factors. Common factors affecting morale, in alphabetical order, are as follows (Morrison, 1993, p. 301):

Absence of apathy
Absence of undue stress associated with the job
Advancement based on merit
Career goal progress
Confidence in the management
Development and utilization of skills, talents, and abilities
Economic well-being (salary, benefits)
Employee commitment, involvement, and influence
Employee state of mind
Impact of job on personal life
Physical working environment
Relations with supervisor and work group
Respect for the individual
Union-management relations

Because both the individual worker and the work environment are changing, managers need to constantly monitor the work environment regarding morale and job satisfaction. Increased interpersonal conflict; criticism of policies, procedures, and rules and disregard of rules; decreased productivity; decreased quality of work; and increased lateness, absenteeism, and job turnover are signs of low morale. Managers can observe, listen, and ask related questions to assess morale.

There are age-related differences related to morale. Younger people make commitments to the job more slowly than older adults do. They are concerned about career decisions rather than just working. Because they often have been raised under more permissive conditions than older people have, they respond well to participative leadership styles rather than an autocratic environment. Challenge, opportunity to learn, and involvement are more important to the younger worker, whereas security becomes increasingly important as the worker grows older. Money is important but is not always the most important factor. Automation has eliminated most of the needs for physical labor and endurance that were important in the past. Young people tend to be loyal to their profession but not necessarily to the job or boss. They tend to want to prove themselves, push for opportunities, and be recognized.

It is natural for older workers to refer to how it was done in the past. They need consistent and frequent feedback to help them through change. They have been through a variety of leadership styles, may be suspicious of new leadership, and need open and direct communication. It is preferable to ask them for what the manager wants and needs specifically. They seem to respect high standards. They respond favorably to having their knowledge and experience used. They like to know that seniority counts. Habits, routines, and work schedules may be ingrained and difficult to change.

Manager morale is important too. The first 3 months on a new job are very important for setting an impression. Projecting confidence and enthusiasm and building relationships are important. Each worker should be respected and treated fairly and equally to develop credibility. Managers should act as a buffer for outside stressors, should save time for planning, and should not make changes too quickly. Managers should involve people in decisions and slowly introduce innovations to help maintain good morale. They should get to know the business and the people; communicate the goals and expectations clearly; clarify values and priorities; and motivate, delegate to, and reward people. It is very important for managers to replenish their energy by eating a balanced diet, exercising, resting, and relaxing to help maintain their morale.

RESEARCH Perspective 4-3

Data from MacPhee M, Scott J: The role of social support networks for rural hospital nurses: Supporting and sustaining the rural nursing work force. *JONA* 32(5):264-272, 2002.

Purpose: The purpose of this survey was to describe the workplace social support networks of rural hospital nurses in one geographic region in Colorado.

Methods: The Social Network Questionnaire was mailed to all nurses within one rural region of Colorado. Descriptive, correlational, and comparative statistics were used to evaluate the structure and function of these nurses' networks.

Results/conclusions: The nurses' networks were predominantly peer based, but managers provided significant functional support. The type of support provided by managers depended on the mangers' placement in the nurses' networks. First-line managers offered physical assistance and emotional support. Upper management provided only performance feedback. Communication of roles and expectations between staff and management can enhance nursing satisfaction in the workplace setting.

BURNOUT

Burnout is a syndrome of physical and emotional exhaustion that leads to negative attitudes and behaviors. The major cause is stress. It leads to the signs of low morale and job dissatisfaction. Prevention is the best strategy. Managers should try to prevent overwhelming situations. One should appraise the situation, set priorities, and focus on what work needs to be done. Meeting goals can reduce stress. When one is busy doing what one can, achieving goals, feeling comfortable with what one is doing, and getting recognition for work well done, one will probably use less energy for being stressed. Open communications, identifying negative feelings and talking them through, good nutrition, physical exercise, rest and relaxation, and stress management should help prevent burnout. The manager can help create a pleasant work environment; set realistic goals; make realistic demands on self and others; acknowledge people's good work; prioritize; identify and talk about negative feelings; rotate undesirable, popular, and unpopular tasks; and facilitate good nutrition, exercise, rest and recreation, and various relaxation and stress management techniques (Morrison, 1993).

Personal hardiness through commitment, control, and challenge helps prevent burnout. Commitment is a tendency to involve oneself in whatever one does to find purpose and meaning in events, things, and people. Control is influence over the surroundings, events, and people. One believes one can influence life events rather than feel helpless. Challenge is anticipation of change as an opportunity instead of a threat. Stress management techniques help prevent burnout. Exercise, good nutrition, rest, and relaxation are helpful. Setting limits on commitment to work and giving attention to meaningful relationships and satisfying activities are important.

Burnout is a state of emotional exhaustion. It is characterized by depletion of energies, disillusionment, doubts, depersonalization, and frustration, leading to loss of purpose, ideas, and energy. A person with burnout may feel alienated, apathetic, and exhausted. The person is at high risk of developing symptoms of stress, including backaches, headaches, indigestion, and lowered resistance. Family difficulties and social problems may develop. Burnout leads to excessive absenteeism and turnover.

Factors contributing to burnout include but are not limited to long hours, dissatisfaction with quality of work, lots of paperwork, lack of appreciation, lack of support, low pay, sense of powerlessness, and few advancement opportunities.

Improving job design, personnel policies, and staff relationships is appropriate. A stress management workshop including delegation, time management, meditation, relaxation techniques, and yoga could help. A multifaceted worker-support program including exercise programs; nutrition instruction; stress management; health promotion education such as hypertension screening, stop-smoking activities, and weight loss plans; and individual counseling helps.

JOB SATISFACTION

"He who seeks only for applause from without has all his happiness in another's keeping."
—Oliver Goldsmith

Job dissatisfaction contributes to higher turnover rates and decreased productivity. Considerable time and money are required to recruit and select a replacement for someone who leaves a position. It takes time to socialize the new employee to the organization's norms. This orientation period is expensive because of educational expenses and decreased productivity. Other employees must carry more than their share of the load until the new individual can work to capacity, and group redevelopment is necessary after each change in membership. For all these reasons job satisfaction is a concern for nursing administrators.

Job dissatisfaction has been shown to be correlated with absenteeism and turnover.

Herzberg maintains that satisfiers and dissatisfiers are mutually exclusive; he classifies the sense of achievement, recognition for achievement, the work itself, responsibility, advancement potential, and possibility of growth as motivators or satisfiers; matters such as working conditions, policies, supervision, interpersonal relations, salary, status, and job security are classified as hygiene factors or dissatisfiers. He concludes that hygiene factors cannot motivate employees but can only prevent dissatisfaction. Herzberg's work remains controversial.

Maslow's theory shows insight into Herzberg's findings. It suggests that hygiene factors can be motivators and that only when hygiene factors are satisfied do satisfiers such as responsibility become motivators. Several research studies have indicated that people at lower educational, socioeconomic, and occupational levels and minority members tend to place more emphasis on hygiene or extrinsic job factors, whereas people at higher educational, socioeconomic, and occupational levels and Caucasian Americans are more concerned with motivators or intrinsic factors. In accordance with Maslow's theory, physiological and safety needs are apparently prepotent for lower socioeconomic groups, whereas these needs have probably been satisfied for people at higher educational and occupational levels, such as nurses, for whom esteem and self-actualization needs have become prepotent.

Researchers disagree about the effects of supervision on job satisfaction. Employees' attitudes toward supervision are influenced by their perception of the supervisor's role, their self-perception, and their level of development. These individual differences necessitate that supervision be an adaptive leadership process.

The desire for influence in decision making is also affected by individual differences. Even though people presumably desire some control over their environment, this desire is not equally strong for all people. Vroom (1960) found that authoritarians are relatively unaffected by participating in decision making but that participation in decision making generally has a favorable effect on job satisfaction. Role ambiguity, the result of a failure to inform an individual of what is needed to do the job, is relatively common. Even if the role is clear, an employee in that role may resign if role conflict is present and persists. Role conflicts may result from a number of factors and are affected by individual differences. Likewise, job satisfaction is multidimensional and subject to individual differences.

Women seem to show more variation than men in their job attitudes. Women emphasize working conditions, hours and ease of work, supervision, and social aspects of the job, whereas men emphasize wages, opportunity for advancement, company management and policies, and task interest. College-educated women rank the importance of motivators such as achievement, recognition, and responsibility significantly higher than female clerical workers without college degrees. People tend to have more job satisfaction before the age of 20 years and after the age of 35 years than during the period between. Younger people tend to be more interested in income, whereas older people are more interested in security.

Nurses surveyed about their sources of satisfaction identify a sense of achievement, recognition, challenging work, responsibility, advancement potential, autonomy, authority, pleasant work environment, agreeable working hours, and adequate staffing all as satisfiers. Nurses stress the importance of respected hospital administrators, supportive nursing administrators, trustful managers, fair evaluations, and adequate feedback. Poor planning, poor communication, inadequate explanations of decisions affecting jobs, unclear rules and regulations, unreasonable pressure, excessive work, workload negatively affecting work quality, understaffing, uncooperative physicians, nonnursing duties, and unqualified managers are all sources of dissatisfaction. Reduced productivity, increased absenteeism, and rapid turnover are expensive consequences of job dissatisfaction but can be reduced if the nursing administrator fosters job satisfaction through organization and management (Marriner, 1982).

RESEARCH Perspective 4-4

Data from Shader K, Broome ME, Broome CD, West ME, Nash M: Factors influencing satisfaction and anticipated turnover for nurses in an academic medical center. *JONA* 31(4):210-216, 2001.

Purpose: The purpose of this survey was to examine the relationships among work satisfaction, stress, age, cohesion, work schedule, and anticipated turnover in an academic medical center.

Methods: This study used a cross-sectional survey design in which nurses from 12 units in a 908-bed university hospital in the southeastern United States completed questionnaires on one occasion. The sample was composed of five nurse managers and 241 staff nurses. The Index of Work Satisfaction was used to measure nurses' satisfaction with their job. Group cohesion was measured with a six-item Bryne Group Cohesion Scale. Anticipated Turnover Scale measured nurses' intention to leave their current job.

A retrospective turnover rate was calculated. Demographic information was collected. Pearson's correlation analysis was performed on all major study variables.

Results/conclusions: The more stable the schedule the less work-related stress, the lower the anticipated turnover, the higher group cohesion, and the higher work satisfaction. Work satisfaction, weekend overtime, job stress, and group cohesion were all predictors of the anticipated turnover. For the nurse who was 51 years or older, there were no significant predictors of turnover. Scores on the Anticipated Turnover Scale were positively correlated with the past unit turnover rate. Job stress and anticipated turnover decrease as levels of job satisfaction and group cohesion increase.

Chapter Summary

Chapter 4 covered the following:
Motivation
  Taylor's Monistic Theory
  Maslow's Hierarchy of Needs
    Physiological needs
    Safety/security needs
    Social/belonging needs
    Esteem needs
    Self-actualization needs
  Alderfer's Modified Need Hierarchy
  McClelland's Basic Needs Theory
  Herzberg's Motivation Hygiene (Two-Factor)
    Theory
  Argyris's Psychological Energy Theory
  Vroom's Expectancy Theory
  Skinner's Positive Reinforcement Theory
  Equity Theory
  Intrinsic Motivation
  McGregor's Theory X and Theory Y

  Likert's Participative Management Theory
    Theory Z
  Historical Development of Motivation Theory
Emotional Intelligence
  History of Emotional Intelligence
  Competencies of Emotional Intelligence
  Promoting Emotional Intelligence
Morale
Burnout
Job Satisfaction

On-line Resources

evolve   Additional critical thinking activities, worksheets, and case studies are available on-line at http://evolve.elsevier.com/Marriner/guide/

References

Bar-On R: *Development of a concept of psychological well-being* Unpublished doctoral dissertation, 1988. Rhodes University, South Africa.

Bar-On R: *The emotional quotient inventory (RQ-I): Technical manual,* Toronto, 1997, Multi-Health Systems.

Bar-On R, Parker JDA, editors: *The handbook of emotional intelligence: Theory, development, assessment and application at home, school and in the workplace,* San Francisco, 2000, Jossey-Bass.

Cherniss C, Adler M: *Promoting emotional intelligence in organizations: Make training in emotional intelligence effective,* Alexandria, Va, 2000, American Society for Training & Development.

Cherniss C, Goleman D: *The emotionally intelligent workplace: How to select for, measure, and improve emotional intelligence in individuals, groups, and organizations,* San Francisco, 2001, Jossey-Bass.

Ciarrochi J, Forgas JP, Mayer JD, editors: *Emotional intelligence in everyday life: A scientific inquiry,* Philadelphia, 2001, Psychology Press.

Feldman DA: *The handbook of emotionally intelligent leadership: Inspiring others to achieve results,* 1999, Falls Church, Virginia: Leadership Performance Solutions Press.

Gardner H: *Frames of mind: The theory of multiple intelligences,* New York, 1983, Basic Books.

Goleman D: *Emotional intelligence: Why it can matter more than IQ,* New York, 1995, Bantam Books.

Goleman D: *Working with emotional intelligence,* New York, 1998, Bantam Books.

Marriner A: *Contemporary nursing management,* St Louis, 1982, Mosby.

Maslow AH II: *Motivation and personality,* ed 3, Upper Saddle River, NJ, 1987, Prentice Hall.

Morrison M: *Professional skills for leadership: Foundation of a successful career,* St Louis, 1993, Mosby.

Ryback D: *Putting emotional intelligence to work: Successful leadership is more than IQ,* Boston, 1998, Butterworth-Heinemann.

Saarni C: Emotional competence and self-regulation in childhood. In Salovey P, Sluyter DJ, editors: *Emotional development and emotional intelligence: Implications for educators,* New York, 1997, Basic Books.

Salovey, P., Mayer, J.D. (1989-1990). Emotional intelligence. *Imagination, cognition, and personality,* 9, 185-211.

Salovey P, Sluyter DJ, editors: *Emotional development and emotional intelligence: Educational implications,* New York, 1997, Basic Books.

Segal J: *Raising your emotional intelligence: A practical guide,* New York, 1997, Henry Holt.

Thorndike EL: *The psychology of wants, interests, and attitudes,* New York, 1935, Appleton-Century-Crofts.

Vroom, VH: *Some personality determinants of the effects of participation.* Englewood Cliffs, NJ, 1960, Prentice-Hall, Inc.

Power, Politics, Negotiations, and Labor Relations

> *"Diplomacy is the art of letting someone else have your way."* —Daniele Vare

Chapter Overview

Chapter 5 describes power, authority, politics, sources of power, power relations, kinds of power, negotiations, labor relations, labor laws, unionization, nurse managers' role in collective bargaining, and advantages and disadvantages of collective bargaining.

Chapter Objectives

- Identify at least five sources of power.
- Discuss ways to communicate with legislators.
- Outline the process by which a bill becomes a law.
- Describe principled negotiations.
- Compare hard and soft negotiation tactics.
- Discuss the four phases of unionization.
- Explain the decertification process.
- Identify advantages and disadvantages of collective bargaining.

Major Concepts and Definitions

Power one's capacity to influence others
Formal power power related to position
Informal power power related to personal power
Reward something given in recompense for a good deed
Coercive restraining, constraining, or curbing in nature
Legitimate logically correct
Referent a type of power based on identification with a leader and what that leader symbolizes
Expert skillful, having knowledge and training
Information knowledge, access to information
Connection coalition
Authority legitimate power determined by structure
Politics authoritative allocation of scarce resources
Negotiation bargaining process
Labor relations relations between the workers and management
Unionization organization of workers
Collective bargaining organization of workers to bargain for working conditions
Synergy the sum is greater than the individual parts

POWER, AUTHORITY, AND POLITICS

Power and authority are closely related and often confused. Power is one's capacity to influence others, whereas authority is the right to direct others. One's power may be greater or less than the authority of the position. Authority is obtained through position power, but several other sources of power exist (Box 5-1). Politics uses legitimate power.

SOURCES OF POWER
Reward

Much of a manager's power comes from the ability to reward others for complying. When a

BOX **5-1** Sources of Power

Reward
Coercive
Legitimate
Referent
Expert
Information and connection

staff associate perceives that managers have the ability to provide something valued, the manager has reward power. Sources of reward power include money, desired assignments, provision of personal space, or the acknowledgment of accomplishments. Rewards contribute to an independent system.

Coercive Power

Coercive power is the opposite of reward power and is based on fear of punishment if one fails to conform. Undesired assignments, embarrassment in front of others, withheld pay increases, and termination are sources of coercive power that contribute to a dependent system.

Legitimate Power

Their official positions in the organizational hierarchy give managers legitimate power. Legitimate power gives the manager the right to influence and the staff associate an obligation to accept that influence. The director of nursing has more legitimate power than the manager, who in turn has more legitimate power than the head nurse. Cultural values that give a person the right to prescribe appropriate behavior for another (such as parents for children), social structures involving a hierarchy of authority, and election processes to legitimize a person's right to an office are bases for legitimate power.

Referent Power

Referent power is based on identification with a leader and what that leader symbolizes. The leader is admired and exerts influence because the followers desire to be like the leader.

Expert Power

People gain expert power through knowledge, skills, and information. Their expertise gains them respect and compliance. Knowledge of the organization and its rules, regulations, and work flow helps one to acquire power over others who need the knowledge to meet their responsibilities (Loveridge and Cummings, 1996).

Information

Information power comes from knowledge and access to information.

Connection

Connection power comes from coalitions and interpersonal relations.

SOURCES OF PERSONAL POWER

Expand your personal resources. Start by taking good care of yourself. Eat a well-balanced diet. Rest. Relax. Exercise. Develop relationships. Develop hobbies and interests. Have fun. Develop and focus on your goals. Recognize opportunities. Be assertive. Learn how to collect and review accurate information. Be a proactive decision maker. Expand your personal resources by broadening your skill base and continuing your education. Show up to do networking and develop political alliances and coalitions. Ninety percent of success may be showing up and volunteering.

SOURCES OF INTERPERSONAL POWER
Connection Power

This is a power based on connections with a powerful person or others as a way to get

accurate and reliable information. One can expand the network of communication contacts to increase connection power by joining listservs and professional organizations and volunteering for committee work.

Information Power

Information is power if used strategically. Increase information power through connections, and try to get on routing lists.

Group Decision-Making Power

Synergy can be created when people come together to make decisions and go forth as a united front. Increase decision-making power by volunteering for problem-solving task forces.

SOURCES OF POSITION POWER
Centrality

Access to information in a communication network increases position power. Increase centrality power by getting centrally located and by having information routed through you.

Criticality

Criticality increases position power. It is determined by (1) how dependent others are on the work performed by the position, (2) the number of others performing the same tasks, and (3) the level of knowledge and skills required by the position. General-purpose positions have less power than highly technical and specialized positions, which fewer people can do. One can increase criticality by increasing technical sophistication of one's job, by making part of one's job responsibilities unique, and by taking on tasks that are critical to the work processing.

Flexibility

Flexibility or discretion allows one to exercise judgment. It is associated with the life cycle of a position. It is more difficult to make new tasks routine than it is to make old tasks routine. The number of rules governing a position increases with the number of people occupying the position over time. Flexibility is associated with novelty and variety. The more routine the work and the fewer tasks assigned to a person the easier it is to establish routines, and the less powerful the position is. One can increase flexibility power by getting involved in new projects, participating in decision-making processes, initiating new ideas, reducing the percentage of routine activities in one's job, expanding task novelty and variety, and seeking unusual jobs rather than maintenance-oriented, repetitive jobs.

Relevance

Positions related to central objectives and issues of the organization have more position power. The trainer or mentor, evaluator, and advocate or representative are relevantly powerful positions. Trainers reduce uncertainty for new employees and tend to be appreciated by those who have benefited from the training. Evaluators are powerful by virtue of the dependence on good evaluations for organizational rewards. Advocacy identifies a person with important causes. One can increase relevance power by becoming involved in activities central to the priorities of the organization and by expanding one's work domain.

Visibility

A key to success is excellent performance multiplied by visibility. Direct contact with face-to-face communication is a way to have visibility. A good presentation of a report will get more visibility than writing the report. Participating in problem-solving task forces gives one visibility. Name recognition gives visibility and can be addressed by introducing oneself to others, using business cards, sending out information with a signed cover note, sending a note of congratulations or appreciation to colleagues as appropriate, and sharing good ideas with appropriate parties in person with a follow-up memo.

INFORMAL SOURCES OF POWER

Informal sources of power are related to one's personal power rather than position power. Some people have situational power because

they happen to be in the right place at the right time. Others have personal power because of their unique characteristics.

Education, experience, drive, and decisiveness are viewed positively and help establish credibility. The person with these qualities may be viewed as reliable, and therefore others are willing to cooperate. Attractiveness gains an individual access to people who will help promote the cause, because people enjoy being around others who have a happy temperament, generate a sense of well-being, and foster goodwill in others. Personal appearance, good manners, body language, posture, gestures, eye contact, and speech with a firm, confident voice contribute to personal power. Location also influences others, because individuals communicate more with people who are located near them in the organization, and communication increases their opportunities to influence. For instance, full voting membership on powerful committees places one in close proximity for persuading other members and provides the opportunity to confront, negotiate, and solve problems. In general, people are most comfortable with others who have similar values, beliefs, and customs. Social pressure from people who share social norms encourages others to conform to those norms. Coalitions strengthen one's power base. Consequently, friendships and associations with people can be a source of power.

Interpersonal relationships also provide access to the informal communication network. Doing favors for others so that they owe you favors creates an obligation-based power. One may gain power by default when there is no one else available or by autonomy when the decision is one's own to make. Control of resources, such as information, procedures, equipment, and personnel, also strengthens one's power base. Religion, politics, race, and national origin are bases for establishing power in some situations but interfere with power bases in others. For example, a nurse of a certain faith may be given priority for a job on the staff of an institute run by that faith, but religion may be held against the person seeking a position at a hospital affiliated with another religion or denomination.

Organizational informal power is enhanced by expertise, career goal setting, and communication skills plus understanding the organization, a sense of unity with the organizational goals, mentoring, networking, coalition building, negotiating, collaborating, fostering collegiality, and using an empowering attitude.

POWER RELATIONS

"It is certainly more agreeable to have power to give than to receive." —*Winston Churchill*

Power is interpersonal. It is a dependence relationship. Person x has power over person y to the extent that y depends on x for goal attainment. The power varies inversely to the availability of goals outside the particular interpersonal relationship. If nurses want to work for a hospital but do not care whether they work for one manager or another, they reduce the manager's power. Motivational investment in the goals being mediated is a variable. The nurse who wants to work in intensive coronary care depends far more on one manager than the nurse who is willing to work on several units. Cost of goal achievement is also a factor. Nurses may not be willing to work straight nights to work on the unit of their choice. A staff nurse may not be willing to hassle with a grievance procedure to get what is deserved. Sources of dependence are numerous: knowledge, skills, interpersonal relations, and organizational authority.

Predictable behaviors occur when there is a conflict of interest between people with power. Coalition is a technique to strengthen one's power. It involves uniting to gain a sense of strength. Whether coalition occurs or not, there will probably be bargaining in an attempt to negotiate the conflict. One may leave the situation if bargaining is ineffective or adjust to lessened power if alternative positions are not readily available.

It is useful to assess one's power in a relationship before engaging in conflict. Although there is no magic formula to assess one's power, there are considerations that help identify one's power in relation to that of others. Who is the most powerful? The person who appears the most powerful may not be. Communication patterns help assess who actually has the power. The person who structures the options has more power, whereas the person who does more accommodating probably has less power. The person with the least interest in maintaining the relationship has more power. Those who gain the most from ritualized patterns have the most power, because institutionalized norms reinforce the existing power structure, and people who try to maintain the status quo are probably protecting their own power. People who are aware of their sources of power can use that knowledge, but people are often unaware of their sources of power and consequently are unable to use those sources effectively.

KINDS OF POWER

In *Power and Innocence,* Rollo May (1972) identified five kinds of power. Exploitative power is the most destructive type. It subjects people to whatever use the power holder chooses. Slavery is an example. Manipulative power is influence over another person that may have been invited because of the person's desperation and anxiety. Operant conditioning is an example of manipulative power. Competitive power is energy used against another. One person wins and another loses, although neither the gain nor the loss is necessarily related to merit. An example is the competition of several people for one position. One person wins, and the others lose—even if they were well qualified for the job. Nutrient power, such as parents' caring for their children, teachers' caring for students, and politicians' caring for their constituents, is influence used for others. Integrative power is cooperative power with others. A person can possess the five types of power at different times (Box 5-2).

BOX 5-2 Kinds of Power

Exploitative
Manipulative
Competitive
Nutrient
Integrative

AUTHORITY

Authority is legitimate power. It is determined by structure, which involves rules, roles, and relations. Rules legitimize authority and tend to suspend the subordinate's critical faculties. Subordinates tend to do unquestioningly what the superior with legitimate authority tells them to do. Role is position or office. Authority is inherent in the position, not in the person. Relations are related to credibility, which is obtained through knowledge and expertise.

Authority is traditionally structured as line or staff. Line authority refers to levels of authority and superior-subordinate relationships, and it therefore provides the framework for the organization. Staff authority has no command privileges. It has only the right to advise or assist managers in the performance of their duties. Staff members provide assistance when requested, must sell their ideas to the manager over whom they have no authority, and must sell their ideas up the line to managers who have the line authority to implement the ideas. More recently, functional authority, or authority of the specialist, has emerged. Functional authority is normally limited to the performance of defined duties for a limited period.

It is preferable for a manager's power to be equal to the authority of the position. Knowledge, experience, drive, and decisiveness help achieve power. Being attractive, being visible, and being available are sources of informal power. More formal sources of power available to nurse managers are control of resources, reward and coercive power, association with other powerful people, and legitimate power derived from the managerial position. The nurse manager's

knowledge of sources of power can help her assess and use them.

POWER AND GENDER

Gender differences are noted in relation to power. There has been a tendency to socialize women into family and societal roles to facilitate others' success. Men have generally been socialized to relate to others' rank and status. Power is likely to be perceived within the nursing profession differently from outside the profession. Nurses are commonly stereotyped as "superwomen," "iron maidens," or "mothers." Superwomen often are isolated and overcommitted, demanding perfection and refusing to delegate. Iron maidens tend to be distant, competitive, and controlling. They may critically sabotage collaboration. Mothers tend to be passive, sacrificing peacemakers who foster dependence. These roles may be perceived as dysfunctional in a male-dominated organization (Cummings, 1995).

Gendering of occupations is apparent in health care, with most physicians being men and most nurses being women. Men had limited opportunities in nursing until after World War II. Then nursing education for men was facilitated through financial support from GI bills. Men in nursing have often experienced role strain. Female nurses have often expected male nurses to function like orderlies by assisting with lifting and transferring patients and by doing male procedures. As society begins to challenge gender-specific occupations, we may begin to see more men in nursing (Hein, 1998).

EMPOWERMENT

Empowerment is the process of gaining control. One can use physical, psychological, and material resources to empower oneself. Maintaining one's physical health provides a basis for personal power. A balanced diet, exercise, rest, and relaxation help one maintain good health, making it easier to become more powerful.

Personal psychological resources are also important for gaining control. One should schedule activities to maintain one's mental

RESEARCH Perspective 5-1

Data from Finegan JE, Laschinger HKS: The antecedents and consequences of empowerment, *JONA* 31(10):489-497, 2001.

Purpose: The purpose of this study was to explore the possibility of gender differences in empowerment.

Methods: Kanter's conceptualization of empowerment as three separate sources (formal power, informal power, access to certain organizational structures) was used as the theoretical framework. A nonexperimental predictive survey design was used. A questionnaire was mailed to 300 men and 300 women; 412 were useable: 195 (70.1%) from men and 217 (75.6%) from women. Items were summed and averaged on a five-point Likert scale. Structural equation modeling was used to determine whether the model derived from Kanter's work worked equally for men and women. The AMO statistical package within SPSS-PC was used. Independent *t*-tests were run on all variables used in the mode.

Results/Conclusions: Empowerment influenced affective commitment indirectly through its impact on trust in management. The amount of variance explained in affective commitment was 26%. Men's responses were similar to that based on the women's responses. Empowerment influenced affective commitment both directly and indirectly through trust. Empowerment did not predict continuance commitment strongly for either men or women. This suggests that the impact of work conditions on continuance commitment is mediated by trust in management. Empowerment might be more important to people with a need for achievement. These people might be more likely to desire and achieve formal and informal power. Both trust and empowerment will lead to increased affective commitment.

health and emotional balance. One needs a strong self-concept and a clear understanding of one's strengths and weaknesses. Effective decision making and creative problem solving demonstrate power. One needs to be able to admit mistakes and look for solutions instead of someone to blame. Maintaining a positive outlook is important to one's power.

Material resources may include money, clothing, supplies, or personnel. Much power is derived from control of material resources. An awareness of what material resources are needed and how to get them is important to empowerment.

One can help empower oneself by developing expertise through formal education, continuing education, in-service classes, and reading. Joining a professional organization, attending meetings, and reading professional journals help

develop both information and connection power. One can seek legitimate power by seeking a position or promotion to a position with greater authority and to where one can use reward or perhaps coercive power.

Empowerment means providing freedom that allows people to successfully do what they want to do rather than getting them to do what the managers want them to do. Removing controls and constraints empowers people. Managers design work situations to energize and stimulate intrinsic encouragement. People then perform because of intrinsic motivation instead of external rewards. Empowered employees tend to be more satisfied, productive, and innovative. They are likely to produce higher quality products and services than nonempowered employees. Nurse managers can empower employees by letting those closest to the situation do the decision making, encouraging personal growth and achievement of organizational goals, recognizing excellence and expertise, and emphasizing the importance of contributions of individuals. This may help develop self-confidence and higher self-esteem. Patients can be given cognitive and decisional control too. Clients can be informed of what is happening and what is expected in the future. They can be allowed to make decisions based on information and their goals.

Managers and nurses may have difficulty empowering others because of negative attitudes about others, personal insecurities, or a desire for power. Some managers may think that subordinates avoid work, are not competent, are not interested, and will not accept responsibility. The manager may fear subordinates' making mistakes, getting the recognition, or even doing better than the manager could do. Some people have a high need to control and direct and may fear confusion if they do not closely "snoopervise." And then empowerment is not completely controlled by the manager; some people refuse to feel empowered no matter how much a manager does to empower others.

David Whetten and Kim Cameron (1998) have identified five dimensions of empowerment based on research by Gretchen Spreitzer (1992) and Aneil Mishra (1992): a sense of (1) self-efficacy, (2) self-determination, (3) personal consequences, (4) meaning, and (5) trust. When people have self-efficacy, they feel competent and confident. People need to believe that they have the ability and the necessary effort and support to do the task. Having a choice is necessary for self-determination. A sense of self-control is a desired personal consequence. People need to make a sense of meaning out of a task to get committed to it. Then people get a sense of trust and feel they will be treated fairly.

Whetten and Cameron (1998, p. 387) have identified nine prescriptions for fostering empowerment as follows: (1) articulating a clear vision and goals, (2) fostering personal mastery experiences, (3) modeling, (4) providing support, (5) creating emotional arousal, (6) providing necessary information, (7) providing necessary resources, (8) connecting to outcomes, and (9) creating confidence. The best ways to articulate a vision are through metaphors, real-life examples, stories, and word pictures. SMART goals are specific, measurable, aligned, reachable, and time bound. Vision and goals should be associated with personal values. Success breeds success. Managers need to help employees develop an awareness and belief that they can succeed. Finding opportunities for small successes or a small-wins strategy can help build self-confidence and lead to bigger successes. Managers can divide large problems into smaller ones and assign simpler tasks before more complex ones. Managers can role model by demonstrating correct and desirable behavior and can give recognition to others' successes. Feedback about good performance, praise, thank-you notes, and recognition ceremonies provide support. It is also important to provide social and emotional support. Counseling and training can help empower people through changes. They can also help replace negative emotions such as anxiety, fear, and complaints with positive emotions such as anticipation, excitement, and passion. Information is a power tool that helps empower people with self-determination, personal control, and trust to work more productively in harmony with the manager's goals. If people are given relevant information instead of too much information, overload is less likely to occur. People need task-related information and the resources necessary to do their jobs. Connecting an individual's work with organizational outcomes helps develop a sense of self-efficacy and personal consequence. According to Whetten and Cameron (1998, p. 394), (1) reliability, (2) fairness, (3) caring, (4) openness, and (5) competence contribute to a sense of confidence and trustworthiness. Authentic, honorable, and trustworthy behavior contributes to confidence in employees and managers.

EMPOWERED DELEGATION

Research results show a positive correlation between participation and acceptance of change, commitment, desire for more work, productivity, and satisfaction. Quality of decisions can be improved through empowered delegation by using more information closer to the problem than the manager alone has. Whetten and Cameron (1998, p. 397) have identified "five dimensions of empowerment: a sense of competence, choice, impact, value, and security." Unfortunately, when poorly done, delegation can have negative consequences that inhibit empowerment, subvert the ability to get the tasks accomplished, take more time, increase frustration and stress, and create chaos. Managers need to consider when to delegate to whom and how.

Based on work by Victor Vroom and Philip Yetton (1973) and Vroom and Arthur Jago (1974), Whetten and Cameron (1998, p. 398) identified five questions managers should ask when making delegation decisions:

1. Do subordinates have the necessary (or superior) information or expertise?

2. Is the commitment of subordinates critical to successful implementation?

3. Will subordinates' capabilities be expanded by the assignment?

4. Do subordinates share with management and each other common values and perspectives?

5. Is there sufficient time to do an effective job of delegating?

Also ask, who can ensure the necessary quality?

A manager may make an autocratic decision (tell and sell) when she knows the relevant information, especially if others do not; when the workers do not share the same values and goals and their commitment is not necessary; when time is limited; and when the manager can address the necessary quality. Managers may consult with others but make the decision with or without incorporating ideas expressed (tell and listen) when interaction helps clarify the situation; the interaction will increase commitment; dysfunctional conflicts are unlikely; and time is not critical. The manager may participate in group decisions when the manager has important information to share; no one else could provide the necessary leadership; the manager's presence does not interfere with the expression of ideas; and the time is well spent developing others. The manager may delegate when the group collectively has the necessary information; its commitment is important; it has the same goals as management; it can ensure the necessary quality; and time is not critical.

Whetten and Cameron (1998, pp. 400-403) also have identified the following 10 principles regarding how to delegate:

1. "Begin with the end in mind." It is important for the manager to specify the results desired from the delegation. It is motivating to specify the importance of the task.

2. "Delegate completely." The manager should be clear about to whom accountability is being assigned; for what task; when the work is to be completed; and how and to whom the results are to be reported. The level of initiative should be clarified when the assignment is made. Does the worker need to wait to be told what to do? This is not very empowering. Can the worker formulate ideas and ask permission to implement the ideas? Empowerment is constrained. Can the worker collect information, determine courses of action, and present options to the manager to decide or make recommendations for approval? This is progressively more empowering. Can workers act and then report what was done? Can mature workers initiate action and then report routinely? This is the most empowering and most likely to produce high motivation and satisfaction with quality results if the workers are mature problem solvers.

3. "Allow participation in the delegation of assignments." When workers understand the assignment and its importance to the organizational goals; have the knowledge and skills necessary to do the job; find the assignment consistent with their values and interests; and have input into what is delegated to them

when, they are more likely to willingly accept delegated tasks.

4. "Establish parity between authority and responsibility." Balance responsibility with authority to do the job.

5. "Work within the organizational structure." Delegate down through the hierarchy. Do not skip people with line authority to get to the people closest to the situation.

6. "Provide adequate support for delegated tasks." Give people what they need to do the job or explain why desired resources are not available.

7. "Focus accountability on results." Close monitoring of the process "destroys the five dimensions of empowerment: self-efficacy, self-determination, personal control, meaningfulness, and trust."

8. "Delegate consistently." Use delegation to empower and develop others, not to get rid of unpleasant tasks.

9. "Avoid upward delegation." Ask workers to make recommendations rather than to ask for advice or assistance. If asked for advice, respond with questions such as "What do you think we should do?"

10. "Clarify consequences." Identify the impact the task has had on the organization and consumers. Give rewards for success even if they are as simple as a thank you for a job well done.

Not all employees want to be empowered. Some resist delegation. One might ask oneself if the request is delegation or dumping. Has the employee been taught how to do what was delegated? Has there been recent practice? Is there a reward for not doing the task? Is there punishment for doing the delegated task? Once those issues have been satisfied and the employee is performing at or above the minimum standard, there is little the manager can do except give attention to other employees. The resistant employee is likely not to receive additional delegations or new assignments, thus forfeiting learning opportunities, and will become self-limited for promotional opportunities (Hein, 1998).

POLITICS

Politics is the authoritative allocation of scarce resources. It requires legitimate power to distribute goods, services, and other resources that are less abundant than desired. A political system is a social system that gets people to do what they would not ordinarily want to do. There are several theories that help explain the dynamics of political systems. According to *game theory*, politics is a fascinating game with rules, referees, and players on opposing sides. *Elite theory* purports that political power is concentrated with people who hold top positions in large, centralized institutions. These people tend to have a unified purpose because of similar social backgrounds and interests and consequently have stable power. *Pluralist theory* explains that political life is based on competition between interest groups. The influence of political groups is determined by their political organization, strategies, and leadership. These competitive relationships are unstable because interest groups and related alliances are short-lived and new coalitions and interest groups develop as old ones decline. The power of interest groups is limited by dependence on other groups and the need for compromises. *Exchange theory* states that political behavior is based on the exchange of resources. People decide what they want, what it will cost, and whether they have the resources to exchange for it.

Stages of Political Development

The following are stages of political development and activism for individual nurses and the profession of nursing (Cohen, Mason, Kovner, et al., 1996; Yoder-Wise, 2003):

- Apathy—The nurse has little to no interest in politics and does not belong to a professional organization.
- Buy-in—The nurse recognizes the importance of activism within professional organizations and may join a professional organization but is not active.
- Self-interest—The nurse uses professional organizations for networking to further her own career and the interests of the profession.

- Political sophistication—The nurse moves beyond self-interest to activism on behalf of the public through holding offices in professional organizations at local and state levels.
- Leading the way—The nurse provides leadership on broad issues, often by serving in elected and appointed positions in professional organizations.

Levels of Political Participation

There are levels of political participation ranging from apathetic inactivists who engage in no political activity to complete activists who engage in numerous activities. As nurses become involved in politics, they can expand their influence beyond a single vote. Spectator political activities include gathering political information, displaying bumper stickers or wearing buttons, initiating political discussions, trying to persuade others, and voting. As one becomes increasingly involved, one can make financial contributions, attend political meetings, and contact political leaders. Activists become active members in political parties, attend caucus meetings, contribute time to political campaigns, solicit funds, and run for offices.

Mason, Leavitt, and Chaffee (2002) identified four spheres of political action in which nurses can effect change as follows: (1) workplace, (2) government, (3) professional organizations, and (4) community. Magnet institutions involve nurses at all levels of the organization and give nurses a voice in policy formation. Policy and procedure manuals are common in health care organizations. Important workplace policy issues include but are not limited to working conditions, mandatory overtime, substitution of unlicensed personnel for registered nurses, clinical ladder, smoking areas, family visiting privileges, and referral process for home health care. The government sphere is extensive and includes such issues as where alcohol and tobacco products can be advertised and used, reproductive rights, distribution of condoms to prevent the spread of sexually transmitted diseases (STDs), clean needles for drug users to prevent the spread of blood-borne pathogens, treatment for violence, pollution, and low-income housing. Professional organizations develop standards of practice, advocate change for health care, and facilitate collective action. The national organization should have a national presence, and the local organization should have visibility in the local community. Organizations should identify issues of health care importance, bring those issues to the attention of the public, and take leadership in the development of related policies. Collective action in a specific direction increases power. The community can be the workplace, government, professional organization, neighborhood, social unit, or international online group where there is a special interest. There are interrelationships among all four spheres. It takes time and effort to develop influence in all of the spheres, and networking and collaborating with others are critically important to that process.

Nurse managers can encourage others to become more politically active by educating them in issues, posting and circulating information, and encouraging staff discussion of political topics. They can educate and encourage others to work with legislators by providing formal classes on the legislative process, a list of key contacts, and information about voting records. The nurse manager can encourage participation in professional organizations, consumer groups, boards, legislative committee meetings and hearings, and political functions. Staff members can be sent to testify at hearings and be assigned to attend political activities. The manager can generally support political activities, exemplify political involvement, encourage others to vote, and grant release time for political participation.

"One enemy can harm you more than a hundred friends can do you good." —German saying

---

Communicating with Legislators

Nurse administrators have found that communicating with legislators, building coalitions, being knowledgeable about current issues, providing testimony, solving problems, educating and involving other nurses, and knowing the legislator before needing help are the most successful political strategies. Less effective political strategies include mass mailings, petitions, demonstrations, and reliance on others to protect nurses' interests. Factors that have contributed to unsuccessful political outcomes include emotionalism, lack of preparation, lack of unity among nurses, failure to build an adequate power base, failure to attend political meetings, failure to contact policy makers until too late, lack of publicity, and lack of feedback from politicians, other nurses, and community members.

Legislators spend so much time in sessions and at committee meetings that it can be difficult to reach them by telephone. A letter is a written record that requires a written reply and is more likely to reach the legislator. Letters should be kept brief, preferably one and not more than two pages. A personal letter is more effective than a form letter or a petition. The title and number of the bill one is addressing and a brief interpretation of it should be included. One's position should be stated succinctly. The name and address of the writer should be legible, and when possible writers should identify themselves as nurses and voters in the legislator's district. One must use discretion in selecting a time to discuss an interest with a legislator. It is preferable not to talk to legislators who are engrossed in activities related to another bill; one should wait until they can give their full attention to one's concerns. Appointments are set up ahead of time. The nurse should prepare a short, well-written statement of what legislative action is preferred and why, specifying the direct impact it will have on the legislator's constituents. The points should be concise and accompanied with news clippings, research reports, and other supportive documentation. It is preferable to deal with one issue at a time.

One should know the party of which the legislator is a member and address him or her as a representative or senator, as appropriate, to show respect. One should be specific and reasonable about what is wanted and should ask legislators to do only what is within their power. A dialogue can be continued by writing to express gratitude for the meeting and by sending new information as it becomes available.

Organizing Political Meetings

Nurse managers can take the initiative to organize political meetings. It is best to start with a small group with political and organizing experience. The group should include all organizations and important people willing to be involved. One should compile lists of members of organizations, agency directories, officers, names from newspaper articles, and so on. Personal time and money will be needed to type, copy, and mail invitations, as well as for refreshments, room rental, supplies such as name tags and agendas, and follow-up correspondence.

The meeting should be held at a neutral meeting site. A map should be included with the invitation. A self-addressed, stamped response postcard and request for correction of address and telephone number should also be enclosed. Brief handouts and name tags should be prepared in advance of the meeting. A minimum of food should be served. The atmosphere of the political meeting should be kept comfortable and professional.*

The Legislative Process

Because the legislative process is complex and technical, nurses need to know the process to determine when to intervene. The state legislative process is similar to the national process that follows. First, legislation is introduced. These legislative proposals originate in a number of ways, but most originate in the executive branch. However, either individuals such as members of Congress or groups such as interest groups may introduce legislation.

---

*From Davis CK, Oakley D, Sochalski JA: Leadership for expanding nursing influence on health policy, *JONA* 12:15-21, Jan 1982.

Next, there is committee referral. A bill is considered read for the first time when it is referred to a committee. Only a member of Congress can introduce legislation in the committee. There is no limit to the number of bills a member may introduce. In the House of Representatives and the Senate, a bill is numbered according to its place in the order of introduction, referred to committee, labeled with the sponsor's name, and printed by the Government Printing Office. Bills are prefixed with HR when introduced in the House of Representatives and S when introduced in the Senate. After referral to a standing committee, most legislation is referred to a subcommittee. Most bills go no further. Each bill introduced must pass the House of Representatives and the Senate in identical form within 2 years to become a law.

After referral to a standing committee and a subcommittee, hearings are held by the subcommittee. Often only a few members of the subcommittee who have a special interest in the subject will participate in the hearings. The chairperson uses the agenda, funds, and staff to expedite, delay, or modify legislation. The subcommittee usually schedules public hearings and invites testimony from private and public witnesses. Interested individuals submit written requests to testify. Once they are informed of when to testify, rescheduling is not allowed. If one cannot be present at the designated time, one may file a written statement for the record of the hearing. Witnesses who share common positions are urged to consolidate testimony and designate a single spokesperson. Groups with similar concerns that are unwilling to have a single spokesperson may form panels. Panelists are allowed a 6-minute presentation of the key points in their written documents and are urged to avoid repeating other presentations. All witnesses are required to file a written statement with the committee at least 1 day before the scheduled appearance or the preceding Friday if the testimony is to be on Monday or Tuesday. The statement should be typed on letter-size paper and include a summary of the principal points. Witnesses should not read their written statements but should summarize the key points in no more than 6 minutes. Once the testimony has been given, each subcommittee member may ask questions.

If, after the hearing, the subcommittee members decide the legislation should go further, they consider the language line by line and section by section to determine the language of the final bill, which is then recommended to the full committee.

When presenting the bill to the floor of the House or Senate, the full committee justifies its actions in a written report that accompanies the bill. Bills that are unanimously voted out of committee have a good chance on the floor. However, dispute is likely to occur on the floor if there has been a divided committee.

After a bill has passed one house, it is sent to the other, where the same process takes place. If the second house approves the bill as it was passed by the first, it is sent to the president for his signature. However, if the bill was revised or amendments added, the bill must be returned to the originating chamber for approval of the changes. If that body refuses to approve the revised bill, both versions are sent to a conference committee. The bill is sent to the president for signature or veto after the differences are reconciled and there is a final vote of acceptance by the conference committee. In the case of a presidential veto, both houses can override the veto to make the bill law.*

NEGOTIATION

Two major ways of negotiating have been identified: hard and soft. The hard negotiator wants to win and believes that the side that takes an extreme position and holds out longer benefits more. Unfortunately, hard negotiators often exhaust themselves and their resources and

---

*The legislative process is discussed in more detail in Kalisch BJ, Kalisch PA: *Politics of nursing*, Philadelphia, 1982, Lippincott.

harm relationships. On the other hand, the soft negotiator prevents conflict and makes concessions quickly to reach an agreement. The soft negotiator ultimately feels exploited and bitter.

Positional bargaining is typical; each side takes a position and argues for it. Negotiations then involve taking and giving up positions successively. The more one defends a position, the more committed one becomes to it and the more difficult it becomes to revise the position. Egos become involved, and "saving face" is an issue. Besides producing unwise agreements, positional bargaining is inefficient. The more extreme the opening position and the smaller the concessions, the longer it takes to reach an agreement. Positional bargaining also damages ongoing relationships.

Principled negotiation is another option for negotiation that is neither hard nor soft. This method decides issues on their merits, looks for mutual gains, and insists on fair standards. It is hard on merits and soft on people. There are four basic points to principled negotiations: (1) separate the people from the problem, (2) focus on interests instead of positions, (3) generate a variety of options before deciding what to do, and (4) insist that the result be based on an objective standard (Box 5-3). Roger Fisher and William Ury (1991) discuss these strategies in detail in *Getting to Yes.*

During the analysis phase one tries to gather and organize data and to diagnose the situation. One notes the people problems, hostile emotions, unclear communications, interests, and options and standards already identified. During the planning phase each of the four principles is again considered and additional options and

criteria are generated. During discussions differences in perceptions, feelings such as frustration and anger, and difficulties in communication can be identified and addressed. There can be mutual exploration of how to meet each party's concerns by using objective standards. Negotiations that focus on interests, mutually satisfying options, and fair standards are likely to reach sound agreements.

When separating the people from the problem, understanding others' thinking is critical because that thinking is the problem. Activities include discussing each other's perceptions, trying to put yourself in others' shoes, avoiding blaming them for your problem, getting them involved and committed through participation, and making your proposal consistent with their values. It is also important to understand both your and their emotions; make the emotions explicit and acknowledge them as legitimate; let them ventilate; do not react to their emotional outbursts; and use symbolic gestures of friendship, such as shaking hands, embracing, eating together, apologizing, and sending a note of congratulations or sympathy.

Communications are critical to negotiations. Listen actively, and acknowledge what is being said. Speak calmly to be understood. Speak about yourself instead of about them. Speak with a purpose. Build working relationships, and face the problem, not the people.

Focus on interests instead of positions, because the conflicts among needs, desires, concerns, and fears are the problem. Look for shared and compatible interests, as well as conflicting ones. Realize that each side has multiple interests and that the most powerful interests are the basic human needs for security, belonging, recognition, and control.

Next, invent options for mutual gain. Separate inventing options from judging them. During brainstorming, generate as many ideas as possible without judging them. After brainstorming, note the most promising ideas and invent improvements on them. Later, evaluate the ideas and the ramifications of implementing

---

BOX 5-3 Principled Negotiations

1. Separate the people from the problem.
2. Focus on interests, not positions.
3. Generate a variety of options before deciding what to do.
4. Insist on objective data.

them. Then decide on the best options. Each side may want different things from the same item, so look for ways to dovetail differing interests. Try to make the desired option so appealing that the decision is easy.

Finally, insist on objective criteria for reaching wise agreements amicably and efficiently. Look for fair standards and fair procedures, such as parliamentary procedure.

Some players will not play fairly. Some assert their position, attack your ideas, and even attack you. First, do not attack the idea; look behind it to see what the person's interest is. Second, do not defend your idea; invite criticism and advice instead. Third, reframe the attack on you as an attack on the problem. When attacked, do not counterattack. Break the vicious cycle by refusing to attack. Avoid pitting your strength against theirs directly. Instead of resisting their force, channel their energy into exploring interests, generating options that are mutually acceptable, and finding independent standards. Some negotiators use dirty tricks such as deliberate deception by misrepresenting the facts, using ambiguous authority, and seeking dubious intentions. They employ psychological warfare by using stressful situations, personal attacks, and threats.

Positional pressure tactics, such as refusal to negotiate, extreme demands, escalating demands, and calculated delay, are also common devices. Other dirty tricks include ridicule to undermine the psychological space of others. To counter ridicule, try to keep a relaxed body posture, pleasant smile, and steady gaze. "Smoke screen" uses ambiguous or inappropriate questioning. Simply state that the question is irrelevant to the issue. "Over the barrel" is when one uses the weaknesses of the other to force concessions. Attempt to hide weak spots and desensitize areas of vulnerability. Seduction implies future promises that something good will happen. Flattery is a form of seduction that causes a loss of power. However, exchanging pleasant opening statements before negotiating is acceptable. Gender can be used as a weapon. Illness

and helplessness bring out an impulse to help. Guilt causes discomfort. A definitive statement such as "I know you are an intelligent person" limits the freedom of another person. Self-definition, such as "I am an abused person," is an excuse for not taking responsibility for one's own behavior. Paternalism is an attempt to convince the other party that the action will be for that person's good. Favors, flattery, and gifts are forms of ingratiation. Aggressive takeover is when someone assumes authority and rapidly makes a decision. Saying "I need time to think about this" helps stop an aggressive takeover. Pacifists win because they refuse to fight (Marquis and Huston, 2000). There are three steps in negotiating the rules when the other side uses dirty tricks (Box 5-4): (1) recognize the tactic, (2) raise the issue explicitly, and (3) question the tactic's legitimacy and desirability by using principled negotiations. Again, separate the people from the problem. Focus on interests instead of positions. Invent options for mutual gain, and insist on objective criteria (Fisher and Ertel, 1995; Fisher and Ury, 1991).

Ury (1991) described a five-step method of breakthrough negotiation in *Getting Past No*. The breakthrough strategy is counterintuitive because it requires one to do the opposite of what one might naturally do in difficult situations. Natural reactions are to strike back, give in, or break off. The five steps to breakthrough negotiations are (1) do not react, (2) disarm them, (3) change the game, (4) build them a golden bridge, and (5) make it hard to say no. The first step is to control one's own behavior. One needs to break through one's own defensiveness, fear, suspicion, and hostility so one can listen to the other party and break the vicious cycle of action and reaction. One needs to identify one's own

---

BOX **5-4** Three Steps in Negotiating

1. Recognize the tactic.
2. Raise the issue explicitly.
3. Question the tactic's legitimacy and desirability.

interests and one's best alternative to a negotiated agreement (BATNA) without the other's agreement. That can be used to evaluate any potential agreements. If one's BATNA is better than anything that can be negotiated, one may decide not to negotiate. Stay focused on the goal, recognize the tactic being used, and name it. Dirty tricks are often obstructive, similar to stone walls that refuse to budge; offensive, such as attackers using pressure tactics to intimidate; and tricks, such as manipulating data, assuming more legitimate power than one has, and adding on a last-minute demand after one thought the agreement had been reached. Know your hot buttons, buy time to think, pause and say nothing, rewind the tape and review the discussion, take time-outs to cool off, do not make important decisions on the spot, and do not get mad or even, get what you want.

Disarm your opponent by listening, paraphrasing, and asking for corrections; acknowledge points made and the opponent's feelings; offer an apology when appropriate; and project confidence. Agree when you can without conceding. Send a subtle message of "I am like you" by imitating your opponent's communicative manner—speed of speech, loudness or softness, and body position. Acknowledge the opponent's authority and competence to build a working relationship. Express your views without provoking by saying "yes and" instead of "but" and using "I" statements instead of "you" statements; and acknowledge the differences with optimism to create a favorable climate for negotiation.

Change the game by reframing instead of rejecting. Ask why, why not, and what if; and ask for the opponent's advice to facilitate problem solving. Ask open-ended questions such as "What makes that fair?" Reframe tactics. You can go around a stone wall by ignoring it (keep talking like you did not hear the comment or change the subject), reinterpreting it (reinterpret an ultimatum as a target), or testing it (ask questions to look for flexibility, or turn it to your advantage: "I'd like to work this out but I can't in that time frame." Deflect attacks by ignoring the attack

(pretend you did not hear the attack and continue discussing the problem); reframe the personal attack as an attack on the problem, such as "How would you deal with the situation?" You can reframe a personal attack in a friendly manner with "Thank you for your concern." It is also possible to reframe past wrongs to future remedies by changing the blame to joint responsibility to deal with the problem: "How can we make sure that never happens again?" "You" and "me" can be reframed to "we."

Reframing tricks is challenging but can be done by asking clarifying questions to clarify the opponent's assertions; for example, "You must have good reasons for concluding that. I'd be interested in knowing why you believe that." When you identify a contradiction you can act confused and say, "I don't understand. Could you explain how that relates to what you said?" Clarify authority early by asking, "Am I correct in assuming that you have the authority to make this decision?" Be sure to get a specific answer, and find out who else must agree and how long it will take to get a decision. When given a last-minute demand after you thought an agreement had been reached, ask, "Are you suggesting that we reopen the negotiation? If not, I think we should just stick to the agreement we reached." Do a reasonable request test by requesting that the opponent live up to his or her pretense of cooperation or drop the sham. You can also turn the trick to your advantage by stipulating consequences. It is appropriate to name the trick and negotiate about negotiations. The turning point of the breakthrough strategy is when players change from positional bargaining to problem-solving negotiation.

Step four is to make it easy to say yes. Some obstacles to agreement are that it is not the opponent's idea, interests are unmet, there is fear of losing face, and the decision seems overwhelming. It is important that both parties develop an agreement together rather than for one to announce the plan. The opponent can be asked for ideas. You can acknowledge and build on those ideas, ask for constructive criticism, and offer a recommendation. Try to identify your opponent's unmet needs without considering the person irrational. Do not assume a zero sum fixed pie (the more one person gets, the less for the other party). Look for low-cost, high-benefit solutions. Ask "if then, what" questions. Help your opponent save face by backing away without backing down. You can indicate how circumstances have changed, ask for a third-party mediator's recommendation, or point to a standard of fairness. Then you can help your opponent write a victory speech. Go slow to go fast. When the situation seems overwhelming, break the agreement into smaller parts and proceed step by step. Do not rush to the finish, and do not ask for a final agreement until the end.

Step five is to make it hard to say no by bringing the opponents to their senses, not their knees. Use your power to educate the opponent about the consequences of decisions. You can help opponents educate themselves by asking reality-testing questions such as "What do you think will happen if we reach agreement?" "What do you think I will do?" "What do you think you will do?" Warn, but do not threaten. The more power you use, the more resistance you are likely to get. Legitimate power depersonalizes the use of power and gets less resistance. Rather than counterattacking the opponent's power, try to neutralize the attack without striking back. Keep sharpening your opponent's choice. Let opponents know they have a way out. Let your opponents choose from options and potential consequences. Craft a lasting agreement, keeping implementation in mind. Design the agreement to minimize risks. Build in a dispute resolution procedure, reaffirm the relationship, and aim for mutual satisfaction not victory (Ury, 1991).

Fisher and Brown (1988) indicate that a balance of reason and emotion, understanding, good communication, reliability, and persuasion rather than coercion helps parties deal with differences. Approval and shared values are not necessary. We need to develop an awareness of others and our emotions. Taking a break and

counting to 10 before we act are wise. It is appropriate to accept responsibility for our emotions and apologize for them rather than to blame others. Assertive communications would say, "I am feeling angry" instead of "You made me mad." We cannot solve differences without understanding them so it is important to explore the opponent's views. What does the adversary want? What is the adversary's perceived choice? Consult to promote two-way communication, to be more reliable, and to establish acceptance instead of coercion before making a decision. Be wholly trustworthy but not wholly trusting.

Peter Block (1987, 1991) describes negotiating with allies and adversaries in *The Empowered Manager*. He presents a grid with agreement increasing up the vertical axis and trust increasing to the right along the horizontal axis (Figure 5-1). Adversaries are represented by low agreement and low trust in the lower left quadrant; opponents are represented by low agreement and high trust in the lower right quadrant. Allies are indicated by high agreement and high trust in the upper right quadrant, and bedfellows are indicated by high agreement and low trust in the upper left quadrant. Fence sitters are represented by low trust and medium agreement between adversaries and bedfellows on the left side of the grid.

Adversaries, with whom we have low agreement and low trust, use much of our time and psychic energy. They become adversaries only after our attempts to negotiate agreement and trust have failed. Steps in dealing with adversaries include the following: (1) state your vision of the project; (2) state in a neutral way your best understanding of the adversary's position; (3) identify your own contribution to the problem, such as having lobbied against them, discounted their position, gone around them, or talked to a higher authority; and (4) end the meeting with your plans and no demand.

Opponents are people whom we trust but who disagree with our goals and purposes. Opponents can bring out the best in us by challenging us and making us clarify our beliefs and strategies.

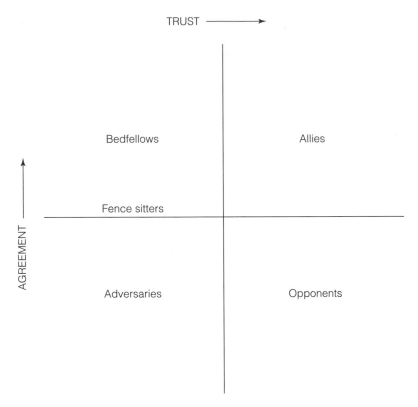

Figure 5-1 Negotiating with allies and adversaries. (Modified from Block P: *The empowered manager*, San Francisco, 1987, 1991, Jossey-Bass.)

The steps for dealing with opponents are as follows: (1) reaffirm the quality of your relationship and mutual trust; (2) state your position; (3) state in a neutral way what you think your opponent's position is; and (4) do problem solving.

One has high agreement and high trust with *allies.* They should be treated as friends; one can discuss doubts and vulnerabilities with them. The basic strategy when dealing with allies is to bring them into the organization and treat them as members. Steps include the following: (1) affirm agreement; (2) reaffirm the quality of the trusting relationship; (3) acknowledge doubts and vulnerabilities related to the project; and (4) ask for advice and support.

One has high agreement and low trust with *bedfellows.* There is a tendency to become manipulative toward people we do not trust. One is careful about how much information to share. The issue is trust, not agreement. To work with bedfellows, (1) reaffirm the agreement; (2) acknowledge caution; (3) be clear about what one wants from the bedfellow, such as keeping one informed; (4) ask what the bedfellow wants and expects; and (5) try to agree about how to work together.

Fence sitters do not take a stand for or against us; they exhibit doubt, risk, and uncertainty. To deal with fence sitters, (1) state your position; (2) ask for the fence sitter's position; (3) apply gentle pressure to get a decision and express frustration with neutrality; and (4) ask what it would take to get the fence sitter's support (Block, 1987, 1991).

Using our power in organizations and politics through principled negotiations with people with whom we have more or less agreement and trust can advance nursing.

"Speak when you are angry and you will make the best speech you will ever regret."
—Ambrose Bierce

NEGOTIATION PROCESS

Negotiations may result around emotional issues such as anxiety, fear of rejection, need for recognition or status, and personal need deprivation. Substantive issues concern policies, rules, and regulations. To do negotiations, parties must recognize that a conflict of interest or incompatibility exists. The relationship should be voluntary, and both parties should desire an agreement that satisfies both parties.

One starts negotiations by creating a dialogue. Exchanging ideas and information helps make the negotiating process a collaborative problem-solving process allowing parties to communicate openly, seek to understand each other, and identify mutually agreeable solutions. Even though it may be impossible to reach total agreement, dialogue increases the chances of producing productive and viable options. To create the dialogue, one needs to probe, offer ideas, build on ideas, and constructively criticize. Probing asks questions to get information from the other party, determine the other party's ideas and needs, ensure understanding, and respond to the concerns. By discovering and understanding the needs of the other party, it becomes possible to work toward mutually acceptable solutions instead of becoming locked into a fixed position. Probing helps avoid miscommunications and is useful when one needs to verify or uncover information or to make a decision based on what was said. A probe is a statement or question used to get more information. Open probes encourage people to speak freely. They are often who, what, when, where, why, how questions or "explain to me" or "tell me" statements. Closed probes elicit a yes or no response and often include words such as *could, would, are, is,* or *will.* Open probes are

better for identifying others' needs and ideas and clarifying when one is not sure what the other person is meaning. Closed probes can be used to ensure understanding by stating your understanding and then using a closed probe to ask for confirmation.

There are two steps to offer ideas so they will more likely be heard. First, indicate your intent, and then present your reasons before your conclusions. Your intent may be that you want to introduce or present an idea or support an idea. Indicating intent gives you time to prepare what you want to say before you say it and prepares the other person to hear what you are about to say. You might say, "I have a question" or "I would like to make a suggestion." However, do not state your intent if you plan to offer a criticism or opposing idea, because that would greatly reduce the chances of the other person listening. Because most people stop listening when they hear the bottom line, you should give your reasons before your conclusions. That way the other person is more likely to hear your rationale for your opinions.

There are two steps to build on another person's idea when you want to increase its usefulness. First, acknowledge the connection, and then add value. You might say, "Your comment made me think about …." Then you can add value by suggesting a modification or a different approach to the other person's idea. You retain a significant part of the content or intent of the other person's idea rather than dismissing it for your own idea.

When you disagree with the other person's idea or opinion, you may want to constructively criticize. First, you state the merits, and then you state your concerns. Then ask for ways to retain the merits and eliminate the concerns. For example, if you were negotiating the redecorating of a wing of a building or a room in your home and you liked the decorator's ideas but thought the cost was too high, you might say, "I love the color scheme and the furnishing. However, the price estimates are about 20% over the budget. Can you think of ways to cut back on the costs?"

It is not uncommon to encounter obstacles, impasses, and even counterproductive tactics. You should break an impasse by stating your desire to continue and by initiating a change of pace; for example, you can say, "Let's take a 5-minute break and then continue trying to resolve this problem," or "Let's meet again after lunch." Maintain a positive and collaborative tone.

Counterproductive tactics should be confronted. Counterproductive tactics or dirty tricks are underhanded and adversarial to negotiation. They are attempts to strengthen one's position while weakening the other person's position. They undermine the relationship between the parties and the agreement. They are numerous and have been previously discussed. When confronting counterproductive tactics, first confirm the behavior, and then express the impact on you or the negotiation. Make sure you are confirming the person's behavior, not your judgment of that behavior. Express how the behavior makes you feel. Speak to how it affects the negotiation process. Express the impact in ways that allow the other person to change without losing face.

To plan your strategy, analyze the situation. Identify the who, what, when, and where. Determine the facts about the issue, and consider the relationship. Next, organize the information by anticipating the needs and identifying the common ground and options. Then synthesize the approach by examining consequences of options and planning the discussion.

When negotiating, state the purpose and review the situation. Then explore the ideas and needs. Examine ideas from both points of view. Combine ideas. Rework solutions. Reverse perspectives. Uncover dissatisfactions. Restate the desire to satisfy needs. Determine the best alternative. Set terms and conditions. Summarize the agreement, and confirm the next steps (*Negotiating Self-Taught*, 1984). Then write a follow-up letter specifying your understanding of the agreement.

ESSENTIAL RULES OF NEGOTIATION

Steinberg and D'Orso (1998, p. 225) identify 12 essential rules of negotiation:

1. Align yourself with people who share your values.
2. Learn all you can about the other party.
3. Convince the other party that you have an option...
4. Set your limits before the negotiation begins.
5. Establish a climate of cooperation, not conflict.
6. In the face of intimidation, show no fear.
7. Learn to listen.
8. Be comfortable.
9. Avoid playing split-the-difference.
10. Emphasize your concessions; minimize the other party's.
11. Never push a losing argument to the end.
12. Develop relationships, not conquests.

Cleary (2001) reminds us that everything is negotiable and negotiations are a process. One needs to be patient and persistent. There is a lot of noise in the process. "No" does not mean "no" and, "final" does not mean "final." We should be aware that our actions speak louder than our words, be aware of what is going on away from the table, and take a long view of the negotiations for a continuing relationship. We should probe our counterpart's priorities, ask "what if's," ask "whose interest is this?" clarify interests, and pick up points by making concessions.

"Know when to hold them, when to fold them, know when to walk away and know when to run."
—Don Schlitz (sung by Kenny Rogers)

LABOR RELATIONS

WHY EMPLOYEES JOIN UNIONS

Employees join a union essentially to increase their power to get certain responses from management. Management's actions or inactions have probably caused the employees to reach their limit of tolerance. Poor working conditions and job inequities in wage increments, promotion, and benefits cause distress. Poor quality of immediate supervision, arbitrary treatment from management, and poor communications between employer and employee are major reasons for unionization. Instead of quitting their jobs and giving up their seniority, security, and friends to move to another job, employees form a union.

LABOR LAW

In 1935 the National Labor Relations Act (NLRA), or the Wagner Act, was passed in an effort to end the depression. It prevented some employers from cutting wages in the hopes that higher worker incomes and increased spending would lessen the severity of the economic depression. Unfortunately, some employers went bankrupt because they could not reduce wages. Employers could not legally fire employees who sought unionization. The NLRA created the National Labor Relations Board (NLRB) to investigate and initiate administrative proceedings against employers who violated a law that listed employer violations only.

In 1887 the Nurses' Associated Alumnae of the United States and Canada was formed, and in 1911 it became the American Nurses Association (ANA). In 1946 the ANA started the Economic Security Program to help state associations bargain collectively. The "no strike" pledge adopted at the start of the program hampered nurses' bargaining position. The "no strike" policy was rescinded in 1968 (Decker and Sullivan, 1992).

Because the NLRA was biased toward unions, it was amended in 1947 by the Taft-Hartley Act, or Labor Management Relations Act. It listed union restrictions to restore equality between employers and employees. Nonprofit health care institutions, however, were exempted from the law. The unions developed public relations

problems when some of them went on strike during the war and when unions were blamed for the postwar inflation (Dienemann, 1990).

In 1959 the laws were further modified by the Landrum-Griffin Act, or Labor-Management Reporting and Disclosure Act, to safeguard against corrupt financial and election procedures used by some unions. The Union Members' Bill of Rights resulted.

The Equal Pay Act of 1963 established that men and women performing equal work should receive equal compensation.

The Civil Rights Act of 1964 prohibits discrimination and promotes employment based on ability and merit. It specifically mentions race, color, religion, gender, and national origin. Equal employment opportunity legislation is to prevent discrimination. Affirmative action plans are to actively seek to correct past injustices.

The Age Discrimination in Employment Act (ADEA) of 1967 promotes employment of older people based on their ability rather than age, and the 1978 amendment increased the protected age to 70 years. Although statistics show a trend toward earlier retirement, Congress voted to remove the age restriction except in certain categories in 1987.

The Rehabilitation Act of 1973 provides affirmative action to recruit, hire, and advance qualified handicapped people. Congress passed the Americans With Disabilities Act (ADA) in 1990 to eliminate discrimination against people with physical or mental impairments, including physical disabilities, cancer, diabetes, and human immunodeficiency virus, and persons recovering from alcoholism and drug use.

The Vietnam Veterans Act of 1973/1974 addressed employment rights and privileges for veterans. It allowed some nurses to get reemployed after serving in the Persian Gulf War even though there was a nursing surplus at the time.

In 1974, Public Law 93-360, the Nonprofit Health Care Amendments to the Taft-Hartley Act, extended federal collective bargaining rights to private sector employees. It created notification procedures that must precede a strike and ensured employees of the right to join, or refrain from joining, a union. The 1974 amendments to the NLRA resulted in the following changes:

- Required unions to give a 10-day prestrike notice
- Did not permit a strike or lockout during the notice period
- Required unions to give advance written notice of contract termination or modification to the employer and to a federal mediator and conciliation service
- Required mediation by a federal mediator and conciliation service
- Allowed a board of inquiry to be established to settle disputes
- Allowed employees to be held exempt from a requirement to join or financially support a union for bona fide religious grounds

This extended the legal protection of nurses for collective bargaining. Because of declining union membership in manufacturing industries, unions welcomed the expanded market (Gillies, 1994; Vestal, 1995).

Taft-Hartley Amendments give the NLRB the responsibility to determine the composition and size of bargaining units. However, all NLRB decisions are subject to review by 12 federal circuit courts of appeal, which did reject separate bargaining units for registered nurses. In 1984 the NLRB made a landmark decision to recognize two broad units of professional and nonprofessional employees (St. Francis Hospital II NLRB 948, 1984), which the federal court of appeals overturned in 1987. In 1987 the NLRB designated eight bargaining units: registered nurses, employed physicians, all other professionals, technical employees, skilled maintenance employees, business office and clerical staff, security guards, and all other nonprofessional employees. Nursing homes, psychiatric hospitals, and rehabilitation facilities were exempt. The NLRB had never used its rulemaking power to establish bargaining units

before. In May 1989 the American Hospital got injunctive relief against the rules, and the Chicago Federal District Court issued a permanent injunction against the rule in July 1989. However, in April 1990 the U.S. Court of Appeals for the Seventh Circuit reversed the lower court's decision. In 1991 the U.S. Supreme Court upheld the NLRB ruling that unions can organize eight separate groups of hospital employees. This opened the market of the minimally unionized health care industry to unions (Grohar-Murray and DiCroce, 1997; Management Science Associates, 1997; Marquis and Huston, 2000; National Labor Relations Act, 1935; Tappen, 1995; Vestal, 1995).

The Family and Medical Leave Act (FMLA) of 1993 was intended to cover pregnancy and maternity leave but became very broad. The act requires employers with 50 or more employees to provide up to 12 weeks per year of unpaid, job-protected leave. Eligible workers must have been employed for at least 12 months and completed 1250 hours of service during the 12 months immediately preceding the leave. A worker is entitled to a leave for the following circumstances: (1) for the birth of the worker's child, (2) for adoption or foster placement of a child with the worker, (3) to provide care for a child, spouse, or parent with a serious health condition, and (4) when the worker is unable to perform functions of the job position because of a serious health condition. The worker then has the right to return to work in the same or an equivalent position with equivalent benefits, compensation, and conditions of employment and to take leave on a reduced time or intermittent basis if medically necessary for a serious health condition of the worker, child, spouse, or parent. The employer can require the worker to use accrued paid vacation and sick leave time in lieu of part of the 12 weeks of unpaid leave. The employer must continue to pay health benefits for the duration of the leave. Records are to be maintained with the medical information and kept confidential and separate from the personnel file (Grohar-Murray and DiCroce, 1997).

In 1994 the U.S. Supreme Court decision in *National Labor Relations Board (NLRB)* v. *Health Care and Retirement Corporation of America* was that licensed practical nurses employed by Heartland Nursing Home in Urbana, Ohio, were considered "supervisors" who acted in the interest of their employer when performing patient care duties and were consequently not eligible for protection under the amended NLRA. In 1996 the NLRB did a reinterpretation of the NLRA and issued a decision containing a detailed analysis of nursing duties defining true supervisory work according to labor law. In the NLRB decision (not the Supreme Court decision), non-supervisory employees continue to have the right to organize for collective bargaining purposes (Grohar-Murray and DiCroce, 1997; Hein, 1998; Marquis and Huston, 1998).

NLRA Section 7 about employee rights states the following:

Employees shall have the right to self-organization, to form, join, or assist labor organizations, to bargain collectively through activities for the purpose of collective bargaining or other mutual aid or protection, and shall also have the right to refrain from any or all such activities except to the extent that such right may be affected by an agreement requiring membership in a labor organization as a condition of employment as authorized in section 8(a)(3).

NLRA Section 2(11) defines supervisor as follows:

The term "Supervisor" means any individual having authority, in the interest of the employer, to hire, transfer, suspend, lay off, recall, promote, discharge, assign, reward or discipline other employees, or responsibility to direct them, or to adjust their grievances, or effectively to recommend such action, if in connection with the foregoing the exercise of such authority is not of a merely routine clerical nature, but requires the use of independent judgment.

This has implications for nursing, particularly since registered nurses are supervising more and more unlicensed personnel. This eliminates many nurses from bargaining units.

Title VII prohibits an employer from engaging in conduct that creates a hostile or offensive working environment on the basis of race, religion, gender, or national origin. To state a claim of harassment or discrimination, a plaintiff must establish that the behavior endured by her at her place of work was severe and pervasive enough to alter the conditions of her employment and to create an abusive working environment. The behavior complained to be harassment or discrimination usually takes the form of an action or inaction by a supervisor. The U.S. Supreme Court placed vicarious liability on employers for the actions or inactions of their supervisors in the context of sexual harassment. If an employee is being harassed by anyone who is a supervisor, the employer is vicariously liable for the harassment. This is true whether the harassment is in the form of sexual favors or jokes or tangible job detriment, such as a cut in pay, termination, or demotion. The only defense the employer will have is claiming an effective antiharassment policy was in place and that the employees failed to use the policy or to avoid harm otherwise. These rulings have not been extended beyond the areas of sexual discrimination as of 1999. Supervisors are not individually liable for Title VII, ADA, or ADEA violations because they are not "employers" as that term is defined in Title VII, ADA, or ADEA (McCrory, 1999).

The 1999 ANA House of Delegates supported affiliation with the American Federation of Labor Congress of Industrial Organizations (AFL-CIO), a federation of trade and professional unions. The AFL-CIO's constitution requires that federation members do not raid other federation unions. That would provide the state nurses associations (SNAs) some protection and allow more time and resources for educating, organizing, and representing registered nurses instead of fending off other unions. The 1999 ANA House of Delegates also recommended establishment and funding of a Task Force on Workplace Advocacy to develop and evaluate models by which the ANA and SNAs could ensure that nurses not represented by a collective bargaining unit will have access to workplace advocacy (ANA House of Delegates conference materials, 1999).

Unfair Labor Practices by Management

The NLRA's section 8(a) prohibitions on management are known as the unfair labor practices. They include interference, 8(a)(1); domination, 8(a)(2); discrimination, 8(a)(3); discrimination, 8(a)(4); and refusal to bargain, 8(a)(5). Restraining, coercing, or otherwise interfering with employees during the exercise of their right to organize is an unfair labor practice. Management may not contribute financial or other support or otherwise dominate or interfere during the development or administration of a labor organization. The employer may not discriminate in hiring or tenure or other terms of employment to encourage or discourage membership in a labor organization. Nor can the employer discriminate against an employee for filing charges or giving testimony. The employer is also forbidden to refuse to bargain with representatives of the employees.

Unfair Labor Practices by Unions

Before 1935 management's power had few limitations. From 1935 to 1947 managers had to contend with unfair labor practice limitations, but no such unfair labor practices were defined for labor organizations. In 1947 the Labor Management Relations Act amended the NLRA and added restrictions for labor organizations. These include interference, 8(b)(1); induced discrimination, 8(b)(2); refusal to bargain, 8(b)(3); strikes and boycotts, 8(b)(4); initiation fee, 8(b)(5); featherbedding, 8(b)(6); and recognition picketing, 8(b)(7). Labor organizations may not restrain or coerce an employer in the selection of a representative for collective bargaining. The union may not cause an employer to discriminate against an employee who is not a member of the union. Nor can a union representative of the employees refuse to bargain with the employer. With adherence to required notification procedures, an employee organization may strike against the employer when negotiations have failed.

A primary boycott is a strike action taken by union members against their employer. The illegal or protected status of strikes or boycotts depends on the union objectives and the tactics used. Labor unions may not force an employer to join any organization or cease using specific products or doing business with someone, thus making "hot cargo" clauses illegal. Hot cargo agreements are stipulations on the employer's use of products that give the union power over other organizations. A secondary boycott that is directed at a customer or supplier of the employer is also illegal. An employee group may not force an employer to bargain with them if the employees are represented by another bargaining agent. Labor organizations may not force "any employer to assign particular work to employees in a particular labor organization ... rather than to employees in another labor organization," and they may not honor strike lines against other employers by refusing to cross the picket lines. Informational picketing is not barred because it does not disrupt the employer's operation. Recognition picketing to get an employer to recognize an employee group is lawful except when the employer has recognized another labor organization, when it is within 12 months preceding a valid election, and when picketing has been conducted without a petition. The union may not charge discriminatory or excessive initiation fees or cause an employer to pay for services not performed, a practice called featherbedding.

UNIONIZATION

ORGANIZING PHASE

To form a union, an organizer must establish internal contacts. In a hospital or other health care agency the organizer needs at least one nurse on each shift to assist with unionization. The organizer should be known by a majority of the nurses, be knowledgeable about related laws, and be able to use free time for organizing. The organizers ascertain the level of interest informally by listening, asking questions, and

RESEARCH Perspective 5-2

Data from Laschinger HKS, Finegan J, Shamian J, Wilk P: Impact of structural and psychological empowerment on job strain in nursing work settings, *JONA* 31(5):260-272, 2001.

Purpose: This study tested a model derived from Kanter's theory linking staff nurse work empowerment to job strain and work satisfaction.

Methods: A predictive nonexperimental design was used to test the model in a random sample of 404 Canadian staff nurses. The Conditions of Work Effectiveness Questionnaire, the Psychological Empowerment Questionnaire, the Job Content Questionnaire, and the Global Satisfaction Scale were used to measure the major study variables.

Results/Conclusions: Staff nurses felt that structural empowerment in their workplace resulted in higher levels of psychological empowerment. These heightened feelings of psychological empowerment in turn strongly influenced job strain and work satisfaction. However, job strain did not have a direct effect on work satisfaction. Although structural empowerment has been empirically associated with job satisfaction in several studies, this study is the first to demonstrate the intervening role of psychological empowerment. Because satisfied employees are more likely to rise to the challenges of organizational restructuring and to be more resistant to job strain and burnout, the results suggest that managerial interventions that increase feelings of empowerment in employees will facilitate employees' effective response to the demands of their work environment.

---

supplying information. After an assessment period, the organizers meet, discuss the prevailing climate, identify the frustration level, enumerate the kinds and extent of employment problems, and assess the nurses' interest in unionization. If interest is minimal, further organizing efforts should be postponed. If nurses show interest in organizing, the campaign is planned.

There must be commitment from the nurses before a formal organization can be established. To achieve this, the organizers hold informational meetings. Coordination of efforts, development of unity, identification of problems and concerns, education about collective bargaining, and active participation of nurses are the tasks to be accomplished in the organizing meetings. The organizers should work in nonwork areas on their own time. The organizers contact the labor organization that they want to represent them for information and authorization cards.

The labor organization can send a letter to the employer informing management that the nurses within that agency are organizing and that the activity is protected by law. Box 5-5 lists questions that the manager can ask to help determine whether staff members are in the organizing phase.

RECOGNITION PHASE

The organizers must get at least 30% of the nurses to be represented to sign individual authorization cards before the labor organization can act on behalf of the group. Handing out authorization cards is solicitation but cannot be prohibited by management anywhere in the agency during nonworking time. Recognition of the labor organization by the employer is necessary before collective bargaining can begin. Some employers will recognize the labor organization on a voluntary basis when given

---

BOX 5-5 Questions to Help Determine Whether Staff Are in the Organizing Phase

A "yes" answer to the following questions may indicate that personnel are in the organizing phase:

- Have you seen union authorization cards anywhere on the agency premises?
- Have you heard of any union-sponsored meetings outside the organization?
- Have you heard of any employee meetings being held at an employee's home?
- Has there been an increase in the number of peer work social activities?
- Have you noticed a repeated presence of strangers or ex-employees mingling with employees outside the agency as employees are coming to and going from work?
- Have employees been forming into groups that include people who do not normally associate with one another?
- Are you finding employees in work areas where they do not/should not visit normally?
- Have you seen employees talking together in small groups and either breaking up their conversation and walking away or becoming silent as you or other members of management approach?
- Have employees who are usually friendly toward supervisors become "cool" toward them?
- Has there been any significant increase in the number of employee complaints about wages or conditions of employment?
- Has there been an increase in employee complaints regarding schedules, staffing levels, content or frequency of in-service education programs, or unclear and overlapping job classifications?
- Has there been an increase in the number of argumentative questions asked during meetings?
- Has there been an increase in graffiti or cartoons that direct humorous hostility toward management?
- Are local or national news items about unions or union settlements put up on bulletin boards?
- Has there been a change in the rate of turnover?
- Are you aware of any other factors that appear to be out of the ordinary and seem to be separating administration from employees?

---

proof of the majority representative status. However, employers often refuse to recognize the labor organization voluntarily on the basis of a good faith doubt of majority representation.

Thus it becomes necessary to obtain certification from the NLRB.

The NLRB does not start an election until requested to do so by an employee organization. A *petition* for an election must be accompanied by designation cards signed by 30% of the employees in the bargaining group to indicate a substantial show of interest. Labor organizations usually obtain signatures from at least 50% of the potential members before they file a petition.

A *preliminary hearing* is held before an election is scheduled. This provides participants an opportunity to express their opinions. The regional director of the NLRB assesses that the employer is under the board's jurisdiction; determines that other criteria are met; determines the bargaining unit and voter eligibility; and sets the date, hours, and place for the *election*. The election usually takes place during working hours on the employer's premises about 1 month after the hearing. All employees in the bargaining unit who were on the employer's payroll during a given payroll period in the recent past are allowed to vote. This rule prevents hiring people to vote in the election.

The number of bargaining units within an agency is held to a minimum. Appropriate bargaining units include the following: (1) technical employees, such as x-ray technicians, surgical technicians, and licensed practical nurses; (2) service and maintenance employees, such as employees doing kitchen work, laundry, and housekeeping; (3) business office clerical employees, such as receptionists, clerks, and switchboard operators; and (4) professional employees, such as nurses.

Spouses and children of the employers, temporary employees, and managerial employees are not eligible to vote. People who have the authority to hire, fire, and direct others are considered managers. This may include nurse managers, head nurses, and charge nurses. As a member of management, the director of nursing is ineligible to vote.

During the preelection period, the employer is required to post NLRB election notices stating the time, date, and place of the election. On election day the field examiner from the regional board sets up the election machinery and does not allow electioneering around the polling place. Eligible employees cast secret ballots. Ballots are counted in the regional office. The tabulation of votes is forwarded to the office of the General Counsel in Washington, D.C., and the General Counsel decides the election. If employees no longer want to be represented by the labor organization, they can initiate a decertification election with a requisite 30% show of interest. If a bargaining unit is denied because of the vote tabulation, the labor organization is not permitted to seek certification among the same people until after a 12-month moratorium, and the management group should rectify the problems identified during the organization. If a union wins the election, both parties prepare to negotiate.

CONTRACT NEGOTIATION PHASE

The piecemeal, total, and combination approaches are used for contract negotiations. The piecemeal is a step-by-step approach that tries to settle the issues one by one. The total approach considers nothing settled until everything is settled. This allows for calculation of the effects of the interdependent variables on each other. The combination method uses both approaches. The step-by-step method is used to progress from the easy to the hard issues. The decisions are not irrevocable, trading takes place, and decisions are reworked until negotiations are acceptable to both parties. The union representatives present the solutions to the members for a ratification vote to accept or reject the offer. If the solutions are accepted, the employee and management representatives sign the agreement, and it becomes binding. If they are rejected, the representatives reassemble to continue negotiating the contract.

During contract negotiations the union is on the offensive and management is on the defensive. The union makes most of the demands, whereas management defends itself against them

and prepares for a strike. The threat of a strike strengthens the union negotiator's position.

Strikes in the health care field require more special and elaborate notification procedures than those in other industries. This allows for the delay of new admissions or referral to other facilities. Alternative health care plans are made for ambulatory patients. Some hospitalized patients may be transferred to other agencies, and supervisory personnel are scheduled to care for the remaining patients.

The NLRB categorizes collective bargaining into three groups: illegal, voluntary, and mandatory. Illegal topics violate the NLRA and other laws. Voluntary subjects need not be negotiated unless both sides consent to do so. Voluntary issues include size of the bargaining team, union dues, management salaries, and patient charges. Mandatory subjects are related to conditions of employment, work hours, and remuneration.

Contracts often start with a preamble that states both parties' objectives and a pledge of cooperation. Near the beginning there is a statement of the employer's recognition of the union as the bargaining representative for specific employees with specification of employees who are excluded.

A union security clause requires new workers to join the union. Union security is protected by establishing a closed shop, union shop, agency shop, or maintenance-of-membership arrangement in the contract. The closed shop requires the employer to hire and retain only union members in good standing. However, this is prohibited by the Labor Management Relations Act of 1947 for employers and employees in industries affecting interstate commerce. A union shop requires all employees to become members of the union within a specific time after hiring (usually 30 to 60 days) and to maintain membership as a condition of employment. An agency shop requires all employees in the negotiating unit who do not join the union to pay a fixed amount equivalent to organization dues on a regular basis as a condition of employment. The money may go to the organization's welfare fund or to a charity. The maintenance-of-membership clause requires union members to maintain their membership during a specific period, such as the duration of the contract.

Financial remuneration—including wages and salaries, shift differentials, overtime rates, holiday pay, cost-of-living adjustment, longevity, and merit increases—receives considerable attention. Nonfinancial remuneration—including insurance, retirement plans, employee services such as free lunches and parking, vacations, holidays, leaves, and educational assistance—also receives considerable attention. The union usually strives to have rewards made on the basis of seniority. Guidelines for discipline, grievance procedures, and professional standards are also negotiated. After acceptance of the contract by the union members through a ratification vote, the contract is signed by employee and employer representatives and becomes binding.

CONTRACT ADMINISTRATION

Implementation of the agreement, the final phase of the unionization process, interprets and enforces the agreement developed during negotiations. When one of the parties involved does not abide by the terms of the contract, a grievance may result. Grievances are most commonly filed against management because management has a more active role than the union in the administration of the contract. The grievance procedure is usually addressed in the contract.

Underlying causes of grievances should be identified and corrected so that future grievances will be prevented. Different types of grievances require different reactions from managers and union leaders. A legitimate grievance results when one party violates the agreement between parties. Managers' ignorance of the agreement and lack of commitment are the major causes. It is not uncommon for first-line managers to function without having read the contract and with the attitude that labor relations are a chore. On the other hand, union stewards are more motivated to understand the agreement and must have an interest in labor relations to obtain

their positions. Consequently, most legitimate grievances are against management. It is advisable to develop training programs to familiarize managers with the contract and to set labor relations objectives as priorities for managers.

Imagined grievances occur when a party incorrectly believes that there has been a violation. Employees sometimes imagine a grievance because they do not understand their rights. The steward should correct the misunderstanding before it becomes a formal grievance.

Political grievances occur for reasons other than the concern itself. Management may want to appear supportive to subordinate managers and stewards to union members, so they do not adequately advise the complainant. A cooperative atmosphere between labor and management is the best way to avoid political grievances.

Harassment grievances are fabricated to distress the other side. They are most commonly used by unions in connection with negotiations. Management usually denies the grievances, forcing the union to drop the grievance or request arbitration. If the contract indicates that both sides share arbitration expenses, harassment grievances are usually dropped.

Organizations should have a grievance procedure even if they are not unionized. This allows employees access to management regarding issues of concern to them and conveys management's intent to be fair. Grievances should be handled quickly through the use of a grievance procedure. Grievances may be handled in a centralized or decentralized manner. In a decentralized process, the immediate supervisor tries to resolve as many problems as possible, and grievances rarely progress further. This encourages a close working relationship between manager and staff associates. Unfortunately, there may be inconsistent decisions because of the number of different people involved in the process. In a centralized grievance procedure, the immediate manager denies the validity of the grievance, and it is handled by the next level of management or by a personnel department. Thus decisions are made consistently among units because of the few people involved in the decision making. Unfortunately, cooperation between the manager and staff associate is not fostered.

Arbitration

Most contracts allow either side to seek arbitration when a grievance is not satisfactorily resolved, but both parties must agree on the arbitrator. The American Arbitration Association and the Federal Mediation and Conciliation Service are primary sources for professional arbitrators. The payment of costs involved is specified in the contract. Commonly, both parties share the costs, but some contracts specify that the loser must pay.

In any case, arbitration is not automatic and must be requested by the dissatisfied party. Both sides select a representative, the grievance is reviewed, fact finding is done, and witnesses are interviewed. Preparation of one's case from the opponent's view encourages one to consider both sides and develop a stronger case. Presenting one's case to a friend who will act as an advocate helps further identify weaknesses in one's presentation and further strengthens the case. Documents should be prepared in triplicate for the hearing so that the arbitrator, opponent, and presenter can each have a copy. Witnesses may be used for the hearing. Their availability should be confirmed. Witnesses should be informed of where and when to attend the hearing and what will be expected of them.

A hearing is similar to courtroom proceedings. The arbitrator makes opening remarks, and the initiating party comments on the purpose of the hearing and outcomes desired. The responding side may respond then or wait until later. Witnesses are presented and cross-examined in an alternating pattern. First, a witness testifies for the initiator, and then one for the responding party testifies and is cross-examined. The initiating party makes closing remarks, followed by the responding party's closing statement, each pointing out evidence to support that side. The arbitrator studies the evidence and makes a decision. The arbitrator may issue a summary judgment shortly after the proceedings or a written decision to both parties within 1 month. The decision of the arbitrator is enforceable in court.

DECERTIFICATION

When employees no longer want to be represented by their present union, they can request a decertification election. Management may also request an election if it is in good faith doubting that the union is representing the majority of employees. The decertification election is similar to the certification process. First, a decertification petition must be signed by at least 30% of the bargaining unit to file a show of interest. In reality, more than 50% and probably closer to 75% need to show interest to guarantee a successful election. The petition is filed with the NLRB by the employer. It can be filed on the expiration date of a contract or ideally during the 30-day period before the 90-day period preceding expiration of the contract.

After receiving the decertification petition, the NLRB distributes a notice about it to the union, the petitioners, and the employer. The employer is asked to submit the following to the NLRB: (1) names and addresses of other interested unions, (2) copies of current and recent contracts covering the employees petitioning for decertification, and (3) names and job classifications of all employees in the bargaining unit.

A preelection hearing may be scheduled if there are questions regarding representation. If neither the union nor the employer requests a hearing, an election date and time are set. The selection of the date is extremely important to the success of the election. Campaigning is limited to 24 hours before the election so that the decertification process momentum is not disrupted by a weekend. Wednesday, Thursday, and Friday are preferable days for the election. A day that will ensure maximal turnout, such as payday, is desirable. The election should be held within 3 weeks of confirmation of the election by the NLRB.

Decertification campaigns are similar to certification efforts. Managers should have various meetings, including individual meetings, small group meetings, and entire unit meetings, to assure personnel that they are in good hands with management and that they will be better off without a union. However, decertification cannot be accomplished just by holding meetings during the campaign. Management needs to have earned the confidence of the employees over time through the use of good management techniques.

The NLRB conducts the election on the specified date. If the union loses the election, management stops negotiating with the union. If not, the next contract is negotiated.

Key terms used in collective bargaining are defined in Box 5-6.

STRIKES

TYPES OF STRIKES

Economic Strikes

Employees attempt to get their employer to meet their demands by withdrawing their services. An employee cannot be fired for participating in an economic strike but can be replaced.

Unfair Labor Strikes

Unfair labor strikes result from an unfair labor practice by an employer or a union.

Sympathy Strikes

Employees of one employer strike in support of another. Workers can refuse to cross picket lines.

Jurisdictional Strikes

In jurisdictional strikes there is a work stoppage over the assignment of work to two or more unions. Employees may strike because the employer assigned a particular job to another union.

Recognition Strikes

A recognition strike is a work stoppage to force an employer to bargain with a particular organization.

BOX 5-6 Key Terms Used in Collective Bargaining

Agency shop: A business where nonmembers are required to join the union as a condition of employment

Arbitration: Procedures for using the services of a third party to settle labor disputes

Arbitrator: The person chosen by agreement of both parties to decide the dispute between them

Authorization cards: Cards the employees sign to authorize representation by a specific union

Bargaining agent: A person or group accepted by an employer and chosen by members of the bargaining unit to represent them in collective bargaining

Bargaining unit: An employee group that the state or National Labor Relations Board recognizes as an appropriate division for collective bargaining

Certification: The official recognition of a labor organization as the exclusive bargaining agent for employees of a specific bargaining unit

Collective bargaining: A legal process used by organized employees to negotiate with an employer about wages and related concerns resulting in an employment contract

Contract violations: Acts that break the terms of a contract

Deadlock: A stall in negotiations when neither party is willing to compromise about an issue

Decertification: The withdrawal of official recognition of a union as the exclusive bargaining agent for a bargaining unit

Grievance: Any complaint by an employer or union concerning an aspect of employment

Grievance procedures: Steps both sides have agreed to follow to settle disputes

Mediation: A process for settling labor disputes where a mediator helps the parties reach their own agreements

Open shop: A business where employees are not required to belong to the bargaining unit

From Foley M, Center for Labor Relations: *Key terms used in collective bargaining*, Washington, DC, American Nurses Association.

Illegal Strikes

The category of illegal strikes comprises violent strikes, boycott or secondary strikes, and wildcat or surprise strikes that are not authorized by the union (Vestal, 1995).

NURSE MANAGERS' ROLE IN COLLECTIVE BARGAINING

Nurse managers should evaluate their management skills and take continuing education courses to improve them. Motivational techniques are particularly important for nurse administrators to possess because they work through others. They must listen carefully to staff concerns and represent staff associates' wishes to top management. Nurse administrators need to know about labor relations.

The director of nursing should not serve as the chief negotiator during collective bargaining because it would put the director in an adversary role. The agency's legal representative is usually the negotiator. During negotiations the director of nursing defines what is best for the nursing care of patients. Once the contract has been negotiated, nurse managers must learn the terms of the contract and have copies of the contract available to them. Problems should be solved through problem-solving techniques as they arise.

ADVANTAGES AND DISADVANTAGES OF COLLECTIVE BARGAINING

There are advantages and disadvantages to collective bargaining. Some equalization of power between administrators and staff associates can be obtained because of the staff associates' strength in numbers. Professionalism can be promoted. Nurses can gain control of practice. Grievance procedures become viable, and staffing for systematic and equitable distribution of work can be established. Unfair treatment of employees can be reduced. The quality of services can be influenced. Economic security can be increased. Unfortunately, an adversary relationship may develop between administration and staff associates, and strikes may not be prevented. Unionization is considered unprofessional by many nurses. Unions can interfere with the management of the organization. Leadership for unions may be difficult to obtain

TABLE **5-1**   Advantages and Disadvantages of Collective Bargaining

ADVANTAGES	DISADVANTAGES
Equalization of power	Adversary relationship
Viable grievance procedures	Strikes may not be prevented
Equitable distribution of work	Leadership may be difficult to obtain
Professionalism promoted	Unprofessional behavior
Nurses control practice	Interference with management

because many professional nurses have little experience in positions of authority. Women tend to view employment as a job instead of a career, minimizing interest in leadership positions, and if the bargaining unit and the professional association are the same, top administrators may have to drop membership in the professional organization, further depleting the leadership (Table 5-1).

Chapter Summary

Chapter 5 covered the following:
Power, Authority, and Politics
    Sources of Power
        Reward
        Coercive power
        Legitimate power
        Referent power
        Expert power
        Information
        Connection
    Sources of Personal Power
    Sources of Interpersonal Power
        Connection power
        Information power
        Group decision-making power
    Sources of Position Power
        Centrality
        Criticality
        Flexibility
        Relevance
        Visibility

On-line Resources

evolve Additional critical thinking activities, worksheets, and case studies are available on-line at http://evolve.elsevier.com/Marriner/guide/

References

ANA House of Delegates conference materials, June 1999.

Block P: *The empowered manager,* rep ed, San Francisco, 1991, Jossey-Bass.

Cleary PJ: *The negotiation handbook*, Armonk, NY, 2001, ME Sharp.

Cohen SS, Mason DJ, Kovner C, et al: Stages of nursing political development: Where we've been and where we ought to go, *Nurs Outlook* 44:259-266, Nov-Dec 1996.

Cummings S: Atilla the Hun versus Atilla the hen: Gender socialization of the American nurse, *Nurs Adm Q* 19(2):19-29, 1995.

Davis CK, Oakley D, Sochalski JA: Leadership for expanding nursing influence on health policy, *JONA* 12:15-21, Jan 1982.

Decker PJ, Sullivan EJ: *Nursing administration,* Norwalk, Conn, 1992, Appleton & Lange.

Dienemann J: *Nursing administration: Strategic perspectives and application,* Norwalk, Conn, 1990, Appleton & Lange.

Fisher R, Brown S: *Getting together*, Boston, 1988, Houghton Mifflin.

Fisher R, Ertel D: *Getting ready to negotiate*, New York, 1995, Penguin Books.

Fisher R, Ury W: *Getting to yes,* ed 2 (rep ed), Boston, 1991, Penguin Books.

Gillies DA: *Nursing management: A systems approach,* Philadelphia, 1994, WB Saunders.

Grohar-Murray ME, DiCroce HR: *Leadership and management in nursing,* Stamford, Conn, 1997, Appleton & Lange.

Hein EC: *Contemporary leadership behavior,* Philadelphia, 1998, Lippincott.

Kalisch BJ, Kalisch PA: *Politics of nursing,* Philadelphia, 1982, Lippincott.

Loveridge CE, Cummings SH: *Nursing management in the new paradigm,* Gaithersburg, Md, 1996, Aspen.

Management Science Associates: *Positive employee relations and union free management,* Independence, Mo, 1997, Management Science Associates.

Marquis BL, Huston CJ: *Leadership roles and management functions in nursing,* ed 3, Philadelphia, 2000, Lippincott.

Marquis BL, Huston CJ: *Management decision making for nurses: 124 case studies,* Philadelphia, 1998, Lippincott-Raven.

Mason DJ, Leavitt JK, Chaffee MW: *Policy & politics in nursing and health care,* ed 4, St Louis, 2002, Mosby.

May R: *Power and innocence,* New York, 1972, WW Norton and Co.

McCrory JL and Ivers W of Steward and Irwin, PC in Indianapolis. Personal communication, 2003.

Mishra AK: Organizational response to crisis: the role of mutual trust and top management teams, doctoral dissertation, Ann Arbor, 1992, University of Michigan.

National Labor Relations Act, 1935.

Negotiating self-taught, Stamford, Conn, 1984, Learning International.

Spreitzer GM: When organizations dare: The dynamics of individual empowerment in the workplace, doctoral dissertation, Ann Arbor, 1992, University of Michigan.

St. Francis Hospital #NLRB 948, 1984.

Steinberg L, D'Orso M: *Winning with integrity: Getting what you're worth without selling your soul*, Villard, NY, 1998, Leigh Steinberg & Michael D'Orso.

Tappen RM: *Nursing leadership and management: Concepts and practice,* Philadelphia, 1995, FA Davis.

Ury, W: *Getting past no: Negotiating with difficult people*, New York, 1991, Bantam Books.

Vestal KW: *Nursing management: Concepts and issues,* ed 2, Philadelphia, 1995, Lippincott.

Vroom VH, Jago AG: Decision making as social process: Normative and descriptive models of leader behavior, *Decision Sciences* 5:743-769, Oct 1974.

Vroom VH, Yetton PG: *Leadership and decision making,* Pittsburgh, 1973, University of Pittsburgh Press.

Whetten DA, Cameron KS: *Developing management skills,* Reading, Mass, 1998, Addison-Wesley.

Yoder-Wise PS: *Leading and managing in nursing ed 3,* St. Louis, 2003, Mosby.

Conflict Management

6

---

*"Build your adversary a golden bridge to retreat
across."* —Sun Tzu

Chapter Overview

Chapter 6 presents sources of conflict, types of conflict, reactions to
conflict, escalation techniques, stages of conflict, approaches to conflict
management, deescalation tactics, mediation, arbitration, and strategies
for managing intrapersonal, interpersonal, group, intergroup, and
organizational conflict. Nominal group technique, role negotiations, and
decision charting are discussed in detail. Sexual harassment and
workplace violence are also addressed.

Chapter Objectives

- List at least five sources of conflict.
- Identify at least five kinds of conflict, and describe them.
- Describe reactions to conflict.
- Identify five approaches to conflict resolution, describe each, and identify appropriate
  times to use each.
- Outline nominal group technique.
- Explain role negotiations.

Major Concepts and Definitions

Conflict clash, fight, battle, struggle
Role ambiguity person does not know what is expected
Role overload person is unable to accomplish what is expected within the allotted time frame
Nominal group technique a group participation method for making decisions
Role negotiations the process of preventing role conflicts, role ambiguities, and role overload

CONFLICT THEORY

Conflict, which is closely related to power and political issues, is inevitable and can be constructive or destructive. It may offer an individual personal gain, provide prestige to the winner, be an incentive for creativity, and serve as a powerful motivator. Indeed, there seems to be an optimal level of conflict or anxiety necessary for effective functioning. Conflict that is managed instead of avoided, ignored, or suppressed can be used effectively. If conflict goes beyond the invigorating stage, it becomes debilitating. Conflict is a warning to management that something is amiss, and it should stimulate a search for new solutions through problem solving, the clarification of objectives, the establishment of group norms, and the determination of group boundaries. However, eliminating conflict is not necessary. If managers learn the sources and types of conflict and how to manage them, they can minimize stress on individuals and the organization and maximize effectiveness (Box 6-1).

SOURCES OF CONFLICT

Cultural differences may contribute to differing attitudes, values, beliefs, and behaviors. Conflict can arise because the individuals involved do not have the same facts. They define the problem differently, have different pieces of information, place more or less importance on various aspects, or have divergent views of their own power and authority. Varying goals and objectives or contrasting procedural strategies for accomplishing mutually acceptable goals produce conflict. Variations in personal value systems or in perceptions of ethical responsibilities can lead to

divergence in choices of both goals and methods, thus producing conflict.

When people work together in a complex organization, there are numerous sources of

---

BOX **6-1** Model for Managing Conflict

Determine the basis of the conflict:
    Intrapersonal
    Interpersonal
    Group
    Intergroup
    Organizational
Analyze the sources of the conflict:
    Cultural differences
    Different facts
    Separate pieces of information
    Different perceptions of the event
    Defining the problem differently
    Divergent views of power and authority
    Role conflicts
    Number of organizational levels
    Degree of association
    Parties dependent on others
    Competition for scarce resources
    Ambiguous jurisdictions
    Need for consensus
    Communication barriers
    Separation in time and space
    Accumulation of unresolved conflict
Consider alternative approaches to conflict
    management:
    Avoiding
    Accommodating
    Compromising
    Collaborating
    Competing
Choose the most appropriate approach.
Implement the conflict management strategy.
Evaluate the results.

conflict. Conflict increases with both the number of organizational levels and the number of specialties. It is greater as the degree of association increases and when some parties depend on others. Competition for scarce resources, ambiguous jurisdictions, and the need for consensus all contribute to conflict. Communication barriers impede understanding, and separations in time and space foster factionalism rather than mutual cooperation. Although standardized policies, rules, and procedures regulate behavior, make relationships more predictable, and decrease the number of arbitrary decisions, they impose added controls over the individual. Men and women who value autonomy are likely to resist such control. Clearly, the sources of conflict are endless, and the number of conflicts increases with the number of unresolved differences.

TYPES OF CONFLICT

Structurally based conflict is either vertical or horizontal. Differences between managers and staff associates (vertical conflict) are often related to inadequate communication, opposing interests, and lack of shared perceptions and attitudes. In vertical situations, managers often attempt to control staff associates' behavior, and the staff associates resist, often causing managers to apply their position power through impersonal bureaucratic rules. Line-staff conflict, which is usually horizontal, is commonly a struggle among domains related to activities, expertise, and authority and is often related to interdepartmental strife.

Interdepartmental differences are related to the degree of interdependence among departments. Interdependence demands collaboration, and the latter provides the occasion for conflict. The need for consensus, the work sequence, and common use of shared facilities or services are areas of interdependence aggravated by differing departmental goals. Both the personalities and the status of the individuals involved affect attitudes such as trust and cooperation, which are just as important as the communication and interaction structures.

There are several types of role conflict (Box 6-2). *Intrasender* conflict originates in the sender who gives conflicting instructions or expects conflicting or mutually exclusive behavioral responses. For example, the same supervisor may demand a higher quality of nursing care, refuse to allow the head nurse to fire incompetent help, and, in an effort to cut costs, refuse to increase an inadequate staff or to permit overtime.

Intersender conflict arises when an individual receives conflicting messages from two or more sources. For example, management may implement an incentive plan to stimulate production and peer pressures may discourage rate busting. In university settings, the dean may expect department chairpersons to function as administrators, and the faculty may expect them to act as their advocates. The matrix organization that imposes project management on a functional structure creates intersender role conflict. Anytime one is responsible to more than one person, one can anticipate intersender role conflict.

Interrole conflict can occur when an individual belongs to more than one group. Simultaneous, multiple roles within the same organization or the conflicting expectations that result from being a member of more than one organization are sources of such conflict. For example, a person may be expected to attend two different committee meetings at the same time. Job expectations can easily interfere with one's family life. The individual has to develop a system of trade-offs to determine how to behave at certain times.

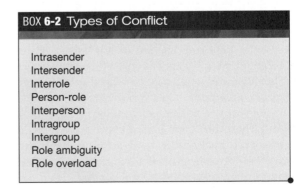

BOX **6-2** Types of Conflict

Intrasender
Intersender
Interrole
Person-role
Interperson
Intragroup
Intergroup
Role ambiguity
Role overload

Person-role conflict is the result of disparity between internal and external roles. An individual has perceived roles and expectations based on one's values and perceptions of oneself. When one's values, needs, or capabilities are incompatible with the role requirement, person-role conflict is created. Behavioral expectations that exceed one's current level of knowledge and skill are also stressful. If the nurse believes that people are important but must process patients through a large clinic in a relatively impersonal manner, the nurse is bound to experience person-role conflict.

Interperson conflict is common among people whose positions require interaction with other persons who fill various roles in the same organization or other organizations. Interperson conflict is usually not personal but rather the result of each person's acting as a protagonist for that person's department. For example, the director of nursing competes with other departmental heads for resources. Occasionally the conflict arising from the nature of the roles involved is complicated by personal animosity.

Intragroup conflict occurs when the group faces a new problem, when new values are imposed on the group from outside, or when one's extragroup role conflicts with one's intragroup role. In an academic setting, pressures to have baccalaureate nursing students prepared by faculty with master's degrees and graduate students prepared by faculty with doctoral degrees produces intragroup conflict. Faculty members are caught in a conflict over their teaching responsibilities, continuation of their own education, and fulfillment of expectations for service and scholarly work. A group facing a new problem may require a change in role relationships that requires role negotiations. When intragroup conflict becomes intense, two new groups may form and give rise to intergroup conflict.

Intergroup conflict is common where two groups have different goals and can achieve their goals only at the other's expense. The conflict may be between groups on the same level or between groups on different levels within an organization. Competition between groups also produces conflict. Resolution may be reached by the dominance of one group over the other, by a compromise that rarely satisfies either group, or by an integration of goals attained when each group recognizes the role of the other group in the system. Intergroup conflict need not be dysfunctional. It can stimulate creativity, innovation, and progress. A conflict-free organization suggests stasis, a situation that offers little challenge for group members.

Role ambiguity, a condition in which individuals do not know what is expected of them, frequently occurs in organizations. Inadequate job descriptions, incomplete explanations of assigned tasks, rapid technological change, and the increasing complexity of organizations contribute to role ambiguity and produce uncertainty and frustration.

If individuals cannot meet the expectations placed on them, they will experience *role overload*. This does not involve a questioning of the legitimacy of the request or of what is expected. Rather, the person is simply unable to accomplish so much within a limited time period. As a result, quality is sacrificed for quantity, the ego is threatened, and frustration develops.

REACTIONS TO CONFLICT

Numerous psychological mechanisms exist for coping with one's own behavioral reactions to conflict, but such stress contributes to somatic reactions, for example, cardiovascular diseases and gastric disorders. Box 6-3 lists some common reactions to conflict.

Sublimation is one of the most constructive psychological mechanisms whereby unacceptable feelings are repressed and channeled into socially acceptable activities. Energy from hostility and anger that would be destructive if expressed directly is diverted with positive results into other activities, such as jogging, tennis, or community service. *Vigorous physical activity* often reduces interpersonal aggression.

People who are displeased with the results of their behavior may *increase their efforts*. Working

BOX **6-3** Reactions to Conflict
Sublimation
Vigorous physical exercise
Increased efforts
Identification
Reinterpreting goals
Substituting goals
Rationalization
Attention getting
Reaction formation
Flight into fantasy
Projection
Displacement
Fixation
Withdrawal
Repression
Conversion

longer and harder is likely to increase productivity. Flight into activity, a defense mechanism whereby a person keeps busy to avoid thinking about problems, provides some temporary relief but does not solve the problems.

Identification is the practice of enhancing one's self-esteem by imitating another's behavior. The values and beliefs of the other person are internalized, and both achievements and suffering are experienced vicariously. This illustrates the adage, "If you can't beat them, join them." An individual may compensate for a real or imagined inadequacy in one area by substituting a high degree of proficiency in another area. For example, one who lacks social skills may excel academically.

Goals may be *reinterpreted* to attain an unmet goal, or the goal may be lowered or another goal *substituted.* A person promoted to vice president with little hope of becoming president may decide that the vice presidency is a satisfactory position. A rejected job applicant may find another job the applicant enjoys more.

Rationalization provides acceptable explanations for undesirable beliefs or behaviors. Managers may find reasons to fire someone they do not like or pad the expense account because "everyone does it."

Attention getting may involve seeking highly visible jobs, engaging in loud or excessive talking, wearing bright or sexy clothing and unusual hair styles, or driving flashy cars. These displays are destructive only if they divert attention from problem solving.

When individuals repress unacceptable behaviors and values and substitute the opposite attitudes and behaviors, they are using a coping mechanism called *reaction formation.* For example, an employee who was denied a merit pay increase may defend the manager and vigorously support the related policies.

Another mechanism people use to cope with stress is *flight into fantasy.* Flight into fantasy allows one to think about something else. For example, the nurse's aide may daydream about being the charge nurse. Although daydreaming, watching television, and going to the movies are constructive forms of relaxation, engaging in excessive fantasy interferes with one's productivity.

People may protect themselves from their undesirable feelings and traits by attributing them to others. This defense mechanism is called *projection.* For example, a student who is unable to answer a test question may claim that the question is unclear. An unsuccessful person who wants to block another's success claims that the colleague is hostile and uncooperative. Projection is a destructive way to meet needs.

Displacement redirects emotions toward ideas, people, or objects other than the source of the emotions. For example, after the director corrects the head nurse, the nurse manager may displace aggression by snapping at the staff. Some individuals reacting to conflict may resort to negativism, picking apart every idea and action and putting everything in the worst light.

Fixation is the maintenance of a certain maladaptive behavior even though it is obvious that it is not effective in this situation. One who depends on this escape mechanism will make the same mistake repeatedly.

Withdrawal removes one from the area of frustration. For example, a staff nurse who is frustrated by hospital working conditions may go into teaching. This mechanism can be constructive if the person withdraws from a dangerous situation.

Repression pushes painful information and memories into the subconscious, but the material is not truly forgotten. An individual may revert to earlier, even childish behavior. When regressing, staff members may transfer their attitudes toward their parents to their manager and expect the manager to act like a parent. Some people may even have temper tantrums. Regression moves one away from the present and is rarely constructive.

An individual may unconsciously convert an emotional conflict into physical symptoms, for example, the common tension headache. Paralysis of an arm to avoid writing a report or losing one's voice to avoid discussing an unpleasant topic is an extreme form of the coping mechanism called *conversion.*

Everyone uses psychological mechanisms. They are our unconscious defenses against impaired self-esteem, anxiety and guilt, and other threatening or uncomfortable feelings. Defense mechanisms serve a purpose. They become harmful only when excessive.

ESCALATION-OF-CONFLICT TACTICS

Competition escalates conflict. One tries to outdo the other and often vice versa. When we feel we are righteous, we often stop listening. Then we lose an opportunity to learn. Labeling, such as calling someone lazy, escalates the conflict. Identifying the behavior and the negative outcomes can assist with problem solving; for example, "You are often late. That means you do not get the change-of-shift report in a timely way, and patients do not get the care they deserve at the beginning of the shift. People have to tell you what you missed, and we all seem to get off to a bad start." Dealing with personalities escalates conflict and is not appropriate. We should separate the person from the problem. Issue expansion includes issues from other times. We should stay focused. Bickering often makes conflict worse unless we identify the

BOX 6-4 Escalation-of-Conflict Tactics

Competition
Righteousness
Stop listening
Labeling
Dealing with personalities
Issue expansion
Bickering
Coalition formation
Threats
Constricting others
Intentional hurt

problem causing the discomfort and take a problem-solving approach. Coalition formation gets other people involved and is a power strategy. Constricting others and making threats escalate conflict. One of the most difficult situations to handle is intentional hurt. That may lead to revenge (Box 6-4).

STAGES OF CONFLICT

Conflict may be divided into four progressive stages (Box 6-5): latent, perceived, felt, and manifest. *Latent conflict* is a phase of anticipation in which antecedent conditions, such as scarcity of resources, predict conflict behavior. When change is required, the manager anticipates differences of opinion about the desirability of the change, how it should be implemented, and how the consequences should be handled.

Perceived conflict, which may or may not be discussed, indicates a cognitive awareness of a

BOX 6-5 Stages of Conflict

Latent—antecedent conditions predict conflict behavior.
Perceived—cognitive awareness of stressful situation exists.
Felt—feelings and attitudes are present and affect the conflict.
Manifest—overt behavior results from three earlier stages.

stressful situation. One's personal perceptions can contribute to either an accurate or inaccurate assessment of the situation and affect the amount of threat and potential loss the individual anticipates. Conflicts can be perceived when antecedent conditions do not exist, such as when individuals have a limited knowledge of the facts or do not know others' opinions and values. For instance, a manager may think there are limited resources or that someone else wants to use the same materials when, in fact, there is plenty for everyone or no one else is interested anyway. Personal perceptions also can help to avoid conflict. A suppression mechanism may be used to ignore conflict that involves low potential loss or is only minimally threatening. An attention-focus mechanism helps the individual select which conditions to change and which to ignore.

Affective states such as stress, tension, anxiety, anger, and hostility are present during the *felt conflict*. Feelings and attitudes may create or avoid conflict. Trust, for example, is a significant factor in the development of a manifest conflict. If the individuals involved possess trusting attitudes, they share information and control and recognize their mutual vulnerability. In the absence of trust, individuals may withhold information so it cannot be used against them or distort communications to their advantage. They may scheme to increase their control over others and strive to decrease others' control over them. Clearly, trusting attitudes may prevent potential conflict, and the lack of them may actually create conflict. Two self-serving individuals are more likely to have manifest conflict than a dominant and submissive pair.

The personalization or depersonalization of the situation affects the evolution of conflict. When the situation is personalized, the individual is threatened or judged negatively. With a depersonalized approach, the behavior rather than the individual is identified as creating the problem. "You are wrong" is personalized, whereas "your views are very different from mine" is depersonalized. Personalized comments increase anxiety; a depersonalized approach is conducive to problem solving.

Manifest conflict is overt behavior resulting from the latent, perceived, and felt conflict. It can be either constructive or destructive to problem solving. Unfortunately, aggression, competition, and other defenses are learned unconsciously, whereas problem solving requires a more deliberate, conscious effort.

"Better bend than break." —Scottish saying

CONFLICT MANAGEMENT

APPROACHES TO MANAGING CONFLICT

Some common approaches to handling conflict are avoiding, accommodating, compromising, collaborating, and competing (Box 6-6). *Avoiding* creates lose-lose situations through unassertive and uncooperative means. The conflict is simply not addressed. This approach may be appropriate when the other party is more powerful, the issue is unimportant, one has no chance of meeting the goals, or the cost of dealing with the conflict is higher than the benefit of the resolution. It may also be used when it is more appropriate for others to solve a problem, when more information is needed, or when one wishes to reduce tension and gain composure. Withdrawing from a conflict does not resolve it, and the individual who retreats frequently harbors a gnawing anger over a situation that drains energy needed for more constructive purposes.

Accommodating is cooperative but unassertive. It is self-sacrificing—the opposite of competing. One neglects one's own needs to meet the goals of the other party. It is appropriate when the

---

BOX 6-6 Approaches to Conflict Resolution

Avoiding—unassertive and uncooperative
Accommodating—cooperative but unassertive
Compromising—assertive and cooperative
Collaborating—assertive and cooperative
Competing—assertive but uncooperative

opponent is right, the opponent is more powerful, or the issue is more important to someone else. It can be used when preserving harmony is important or when collecting social credits is necessary for later, more important issues. By complimenting one's opponent and accentuating points of agreement, one may smooth out an agreement on minor issues, but the real problems still have to be dealt with.

Compromising moderates both assertiveness and cooperation. It addresses a problem more effectively than avoidance but less than collaboration. Compromisers are willing to yield less than accommodaters but more than competitors as they seek expedient, mutually acceptable answers. Because both parties feel that they sacrifice something, they are only partially satisfied, and a lose-lose atmosphere results. Compromising is useful for reaching expedient answers for limited periods when the goals are only moderately important and the parties have equivalent power.

Collaborating is assertive and cooperative. It is a win-win strategy. It contributes to effective problem solving because both parties try to find mutually satisfying solutions. This method integrates insights from different perspectives with the commitment developed through participation and the resolution of hard feelings. Problems are identified, alternatives explored, and ramifications considered until difficulties are resolved. Unfortunately, it may take more time than the results are worth. Generally this is a most effective method of conflict resolution. It should be used for important issues and can be used to find creative solutions to interpersonal problems.

Competing is a power-oriented mode that is assertive but uncooperative. In competition one is aggressive and pursues one's own goals at another's expense. This creates a win-lose situation. Nevertheless, it is appropriate when a quick or unpopular decision is needed, when the person is very knowledgeable about the situation and able to make a sound decision, or when one must protect oneself from other aggressive people. If this strategy is used too often, colleagues may become afraid to admit mistakes and may simply say what they think the aggressor wants to hear. A manager can always fall back on authority and give orders to a subordinate, but because the resolution is forced, it almost certainly will be unsatisfactory (Thomas and Kilmann, 1974, 2002).

A foundation of mutual trust must underlie any attempt to understand alternative views and to actively seek solutions that will allow each party to achieve its goals. This trust creates an atmosphere conducive to successful conflict resolution.

DEESCALATION-OF-CONFLICT TACTICS

Listening is a good way to deescalate conflict. It shows that you care about the person by taking your time to listen to them. The other person may be able to talk through the problem and solve it, particularly if you ask questions that lead her through problem solving, such as the following: What is the problem? What are your options? What will happen if you do that? What do you think is the best way to handle this situation? What are you going to do? Showing tact and concern for others is important. Appealing to deescalation by saying something such as "I don't want to fight about this" can help. Goodwill gestures such as "Let's get a cup of coffee and discuss this" and allowing the airing of feelings are good. Our feelings often dissipate after we talk about how we are feeling. We usually feel better after talking about our feelings. Negative inquiry is an assertive technique of asking for more information and trying to resolve the problem. When we are criticized, we tend to get defensive, which escalates the conflict. Then the other person has to work harder to get us to understand where we went wrong. When we ask for more information, the criticizer may end up defending the accused.

Using metacommunications, one discusses the communication as it is occurring. "I am trying to talk to you, and you are walking away from me." It is important to respond to all levels of communications, the facts and the feelings. "I know that it is my weekend to work, but I am angry that I have to work." Once again, expressing the feelings helps dissipate them. Focusing on the facts helps with reality testing and problem solving. Fractionalization breaks the problem down into more manageable components. Position papers help move people from opposite poles to a more middle-of-the-road stance. People will often follow flat statements with qualifiers. Problem solving is a very effective deescalator. When all else fails, establishment of outside criteria may be used (Box 6-7).

STRATEGIES FOR MANAGEMENT OF CONFLICT

There are three ways of dealing with conflict: the *win-lose, lose-lose,* or *win-win* strategy (Box 6-8). *Win-lose* methods include the use of position power, mental or physical power, failure to respond, majority rule, and railroading a minority position over the majority. *Lose-lose* strategies include compromise, bribes for accomplishing disagreeable tasks, arbitration by a neutral third party, and resorting to the use of general rules instead of considering the merits of individual cases. In win-lose and lose-lose strategies, the parties often personalize the issues by focusing on each other instead of on the problem. Intent on their personal differences, they avoid the more important matter of how to mutually solve their problem. Solutions are emphasized instead of goals and values. Rather than identifying mutual needs, planning activities for resolution,

---

BOX 6-8 Strategies for Conflict Resolution

WIN-LOSE	LOSE-LOSE	WIN-WIN
Position power	Compromise	Consensus
Mental or	Bribes	Problem solving
physical power	Arbitration	Collaborating
Failure to respond	General rules	
Majority rule		
Railroading		
Competing		

---

and solving the problem, the parties involved look at the issue from their own point of view and strive for total victory.

By contrast, *win-win* strategies focus on goals. They emphasize consensus and integrative approaches to decision making. The consensus process demands a focus on the problem (instead of on each other), on the collection of facts, on the acceptance of the useful aspects of conflict, and on the avoidance of averaging and self-oriented behavior. Thus the group decision is often better than the best individual decision.

Problem-solving strategies include identifying both the problem and each party's needs, exploring alternatives, choosing the most acceptable alternative, planning, defining roles, implementing, and evaluating the decision.

MEDIATION

Mediation is a friendly intervention by consent and invitation for settling differences between parties. It is negotiation that involves a third party who is knowledgeable about negotiation procedures and can help the parties do their bargaining. A mediator plays several roles. The mediator serves as a housekeeper who reviews the ground rules and keeps the records. The mediator serves as a ringmaster who chairs the meeting and determines when to recess, when to adjourn, and when to have separate meetings. The mediator helps the parties define the problems, identify the issues, and prioritize multiple issues. The mediator is an educator

---

BOX 6-7 Deescalation-of-Conflict Tactics

Listening
Showing tact and concern for others
Appealing to deescalation
Goodwill gestures
Airing feelings
Negative inquiry
Metacommunications
Responding to all levels of communication
Fractionalization
Position paper
Problem solving
Establishing outside criteria

who facilitates the bargaining process and helps each party consider how to achieve his or her objectives while accommodating the opponent to create a win-win solution. The mediator is a communicator and an innovator. Innovation can come about by making suggestions, but the suggestions should be explored in separate meetings because the mediator should never raise questions in the presence of both sides that could be embarrassing for either side. If one party opposes the suggestion, it can be dropped. The mediator is a problem explorer who helps analyze issues from a variety of viewpoints; a resource expander who links parties to outside resources; and an agent of reality who helps create a reasonable and implementable settlement. The mediator is a leader who takes initiative to advance negotiations forward procedurally and may at times offer suggestions for consideration. The mediator may also serve as a scapegoat and take some responsibility and blame for an unpopular decision (Kheel, 2001; Moore, 1986).

The mediator starts by (1) creating a positive climate and introducing the mediator and parties, (2) commending the parties for their willingness to cooperate in seeking a solution to their problems, (3) defining mediation and the mediator's impartial role, (4) describing the mediation process, (5) defining the parameters of confidentiality, (6) describing the logistics, (7) suggesting behavioral guidelines, (8) answering questions about process, and (9) getting a joint commitment to begin (Mayer, 2000; Moore, 1986).

After bringing the disputants together and creating the effective atmosphere, the mediator clarifies perceptions by helping parties feel heard, hearing each other, and focusing on individual and shared needs. The biggest and most dangerous disputant is to be seated in the deepest and softest chair available. The mediator tries to keep the disputants' eyes on the mediator and the disputants talking to the mediator instead of each other. If the disputants get out of control, the mediator can stand up between them, hold hands out to separate them, and restate the ground rules of listening to one person at a time. The mediator

can hold a hand out at the disputant who is not to be talking while looking at the other party. The mediator starts with a low level of force but can escalate to match the disputants' level. Each disputant is to tell only his or her own views of the situation one problem at a time. The mediator frames and reframes issues, concerns, and suggestions to develop shared positive power and an atmosphere of safety. The mediator helps parties learn from the past and focus on the future to generate options and realistic doable actions. The mediator helps manage communications and emotions and works across cultural, gender, class, and other differences to come to a mutual-benefit agreement. Parties decide who does what by when and set a time for follow-up. To wrap up, the mediator completes all paperwork, writes a written memorandum confirming the understanding, arranges for any necessary follow-up, holds people accountable for their promises, and keeps essential information only (Beer and Stief, 1997; Mayer, 2000; Patterson, Grenny, McMillan, et al, 2002; Potter, 1996; Weeks, 1992).

In order to come to resolution, the parties should be encouraged to share facts because facts are less controversial and more persuasive. Then they should each tell their stories, talking tentatively and encouraging testing. Parties should disentangle impact and intent; describe feelings carefully instead of ventilating; share their story rather than evaluating it; describe feelings without judging, attributing, or blaming; and acknowledge the other person's feelings. Exaggerations such as "always" and "never" should be avoided. Open-ended questions should be asked. Listening transforms conversations and encourages others to listen in return. Parties should share where their conclusions come from and not present them as the truth. The mediator asks parties what they think and feel, helps them solve their own problems while teaching the problem-solving process, and then reviews and sums up (Levine, 1998; Patterson, Grenny, McMillan, et al, 2002; Stone, Patton, and Heen, 2000).

ARBITRATION

Arbitration is a structured method of dispute resolution. The arbitrator does not interact with the parties but renders a binding decision based on a formal presentation of information (Goodman, 1994).

INTRAPERSONAL CONFLICT

Intrapersonal conflict occurs within the person and usually involves a struggle over values, desires, or incompatible activities. The conflict is internalized. One should set personal goals and priorities and do problem solving. Being self-aware and working to resolve the conflict as soon as possible are important for the manager to remain physically and psychologically well. The manager should help associates be self-aware and do problem solving too (Douglas, 1996; Marquis and Huston, 1996; Wywialowski, 1997).

INTERPERSONAL CONFLICT

Interpersonal conflict is inevitable, but the manager can lessen its impact by coaching staff associates in assertive communication and fair fighting. Engaging in a fair fight demands that individuals with a complaint first ask their opponent for a meeting. Once a time and place are agreed on, both parties should determine whether their manager should be present. Moreover, a fair fight demands that both parties know the purpose of the meeting so neither will be caught off guard—each can be prepared. The encounter should begin with a statement of the problem. The manager, if present, should act as a mediator, asking the complainer to explain the perceived problem to the opponent. The opponent then should relate her understanding of how the complainer perceives the problem. After each has spoken, each can clarify any differences over the statement of the problem. Next, the opponent describes her perception of the problem; this description then should be followed by the complainer's repeating her understanding of how the opponent perceives the problem. Again, there is a pause for clarification.

A clear statement of the problem helps shed light on the negative effects of each person's behavior. This feedback process, which requires each party to repeat what the other has just said, forces each to listen carefully. Were it not for such interaction, one might be so busy thinking of what one is going to say next that one fails to hear what is being said. Feedback does not imply parroting, because an understanding of meaning is more important than sheer memorization of words. Differences often begin to disappear when both parties really hear each other for the first time.

By exploring the alternatives to the problem and the ramifications of their options, the parties can identify and request changes in each other's behavior and respond to the other's requests. The discussion should close with an agreement on whether to change and the establishment of the accompanying conditions. A follow-up engagement should be set to discuss the success or failure of the agreement (Bach and Goldberg, 1974).

Helpful strategies for mediating interpersonal conflict include the following (Loveridge and Cummings, 1996):

- Do not blame anyone for the problem.
- Focus on the issues, not the personalities.
- Protect each party's self-respect.
- Facilitate open and complete discussion of the issues.
- Give equal time to each party.
- Encourage the expression of both positive and negative feelings.
- Encourage each party to listen actively and try to understand the other person's point of view.
- Help develop alternative solutions.
- Summarize key points and plans.
- Later follow up on the plans and give positive reinforcement as appropriate.
- Facilitate further problem solving as necessary.

Sexual Harassment

Interpersonal conflict can result from sexual harassment. The employer is vicariously liable for harassment. The only defense the employer will have is an effective antiharassment policy in place. In-service classes about sexual harassment are appropriate.

Awareness of sexual harassment in the workplace was heightened in 1991 during the Senate confirmation hearing for Judge Clarence Thomas's appointment to the U.S. Supreme Court. Thousands of sexual harassment complaints are filed each year in the United States. Women seem more likely to be sexually harassed than men, often by male coworkers. There seems to be a high prevalence of sexual harassment in the hospital setting. Nurses are often harassed by physicians, patients, and coworkers. Harassment may include repeated requests for dates, sexual teasing, sexual jokes, suggestive looks or gestures, actual touching and fondling, or trapping and leaning over a worker. These can lead to low morale, inefficiency, and decreased productivity resulting from embarrassment and anger

related to sexual harassment. Women often do nothing but try to avoid the harasser because of guilt from thinking one must have done something to cause the other's behavior or fear of retaliation.

Sexual harassment is a legal issue that should be confronted immediately. Be assertive and confront the issue. "I want to be very clear that I will not tolerate this sexual harassment. I do not want you telling me dirty jokes, brushing against me, and asking me out with an offer of serving me breakfast in bed." Then listen to the harasser's response, hope for an apology, and accept it, making your position clear. "I accept your apology, but I will follow the sexual harassment policies and report this to my supervisor. I will take action on any further harassment. Sexual harassment is illegal." That way you have made your position clear and implied legal action. File a report. If a situation occurs again, confront

RESEARCH Perspective 6-1

Data from Fiedler A, Hamby E: Sexual harassment in the workplace, *JONA* 30(10):497-503, 2000.

Purpose: The purpose of this study was to examine the perceptions of nurses and nursing administrators of various types of sexual harassment.

Methods: Surveys were sent to a random sample of 423 nurse administrators and 802 registered nurses licensed in Florida. The researchers received 303 usable responses, including 103 nursing administrators and 200 registered nurses. A total of 24 scenarios were given in a scrambled order in the Sexual Harassment Scale. The scale included four subscales: male-female, female-male, male-male, and female-female. There were also demographic questions.

Results/conclusions: Just over one half of the female registered nurses and nursing administrators and almost one third of the

male registered nurses and nursing administrators believed they had been sexually harassed. They were significantly more sensitive to opposite-gender harassment than to same-gender harassment. They were more sensitive to men harassing other men than to women harassing other women. Nursing administrators were significantly more sensitive to sexual harassment than nonadministrative nurses. There were no significant differences between the perceptions of female nursing administrators and male nursing administrators on the total harassment scale. Nurses who had been victims of opposite-gender harassment were more sensitive to all types of harassment. Nurses who had been victims of same-gender harassment showed no increased sensitivity on any of the scales. Nurses do not find all types of sexual harassment equally disturbing.

the behavior immediately and follow the policies of the agency (Douglas, 1996).

Deborah Swiss (1996) discusses resolving the harassment dilemma in *Women Breaking Through: Overcoming the Final 10 Obstacles at Work.* The women interviewed advised other women to trust their instincts. If they feel harassed, they probably are. Then they have to assess their risk/reward situation, decide how to stop the harassment, and decide whether to deal with it informally or to file a formal complaint. Women are advised to choose an option to stop harassment that feels right to them. One may be able to handle the harassment privately by dealing directly with the offending individual or may need to go public. One may write a letter to the harasser, even if it is never sent. That will help organize thoughts for a confrontation. Role playing how to approach the offender with a friend will help build confidence. If one wants to be less direct, one can send a highlighted version of the company's sexual harassment statement to the offender. Copies of the policy can be posted on bulletin boards. One can send a clear, anonymous, generic message, or one may have an intermediary help confront the harasser directly.

It is advisable to record the dates and details of the harassment—noting in particular incidents that can be substantiated by others—if only for one's private files. If harassment continues, one will have historical documentation to take formal action. Otherwise, one may read the account later to find assurance that nothing was done to encourage the harassment and to help relieve self-blame and embarrassment.

If the risk is not too high, a direct approach can be assertive. Allowing the harasser to save face when the harassment has stopped will decrease the likelihood of damage to one's career. If the offender harasses women, makes explicit threats if sexual favors are not granted, or uses physical contact, a formal complaint is appropriate. It is advisable to have contingency plans such as the following: If confronting the harasser does not work, I will discuss the situation with my boss. If my boss is not responsive, I will discuss the situation with the personnel officer or other appropriate official.

RESEARCH Perspective 6-2

Data from Madison J, Minichiello V: Sexual harassment in healthcare: Classification of harassers and rationalizations of sex-based harassment behavior, *JONA* 31(11):534-543, 2001.

Purpose: The purpose of this study was to identify how 16 Australian registered nurses classified gender-based harassers and explained their own behavior and the behavior of the harasser.

Methods: A qualitative research design was used. In-depth interviews of 16 Australian nurses were used to collect data.

Results/conclusions: Subjects identified obvious sexual harasser, sex-based (gender) harasser, unexpected (trusted) harasser, same-gender harasser, and mixed behavior harasser. Rationalizations of actions or inactions of the harassed were expected nurse role behavior, self-flagellation, lack of social skills, misinterpretation or mistake, denial or inaction, professional silence, and assertiveness. Rationalizations of actions or inactions of the harasser were expected patient role behavior, expected male role behavior, mental illness, emotional immaturity, and organizational science. The researchers suggest that health care managers should demonstrate and teach interpersonal strategies that assist the harassed in developing and using assertive confrontational strategies.

Women are encouraged to discuss the harassment with a friend. Otherwise, the harassment may be an emotional drain that causes a decrease in self-confidence.

GROUP CONFLICT

Team development can help prevent and resolve conflict. Planning, goal setting, and rating goals represent the first step in team development. The statement of the core mission of the team is developed by brainstorming and sharing individual mission statements.

The *nominal group technique* is very effective for developing team-performance goals and priorities (Box 6-9). First, individual group members list on separate pieces of paper what they think team-performance goals should be. The group leader helps keep the group problem centered by presenting the question and prevents interruptions of thoughts by asking participants to work silently and independently. This step allows time for thinking, avoids status and conformity pressures, prevents focusing on a particular idea because of a vocal person, and helps avoid choosing among ideas prematurely.

Second, during a round-robin session, each person in turn states one team-performance goal, which is then written on a chalkboard or paper for all to see. It is probable that equalization of participation and sharing of all ideas foster group creativity. By citing one goal, each member is encouraged to participate equally. By the second round, each member has participated and the precedent is set, and thus competition from aggressive or high-status members is minimized.

If all of an individual's listed goals have been cited, that individual passes and other members continue to offer listed goals in turn until all are exhausted. Ideas are not repeated. However, "hitchhiking" may occur. An idea listed by one member may stimulate another member to have an idea not previously listed. That idea can be added to the member's list and cited during the round-robin session.

It is common for many of an individual's ideas about a problem to remain unspoken because of fear of self-disclosure and embarrassment. When one person states several ideas at once, those ideas tend to be associated with that person. However, with the round-robin method, it is difficult to remember who presented what ideas and full disclosure is encouraged.

The written list can be the basis of recorded minutes and serve as a source of information from which the group continues to work. During this step the group leader should see that ideas are recorded as rapidly as possible and in the words used by the contributor. The entire list should be made visible to all group members. Tearing completed sheets from a flip chart and taping them on the walls work well, and they are an early reward in that the group can see the array of ideas generated. The written ideas are more objective and less personal than oral comments because the personality and position of the contributors are separated from the written statement. The group leader should encourage the simple listing of ideas by explaining that a discussion period will follow. Discussion of the ideas, arguments about them, and side conversations while the list is being made should not be allowed.

The third step is a serial discussion for clarification. During this step each listed idea is discussed in order. This provides an opportunity to clarify ideas, state differences of opinion, provide the logic behind ideas, and prevent undue focusing on one idea. The group leader's responsibility is to clarify the purpose of this step and to pace the group. Arguments can be curtailed by stating that both points of view have been

---

BOX **6-9** Nominal Group Technique

Listing ideas on paper
Round-robin session
Serial discussion for clarification
Preliminary vote
Analysis of votes
Discussion of preliminary vote
Revote

noted and then moving on to the next point. It is better not to ask the contributors to clarify their own items, because such a request can put them on the spot. Instead, the group members can be asked what the items mean to them. The contributor can clarify when appropriate. This method helps reduce identification of items with specific individuals.

The preliminary vote on item importance is the fourth step. In the nominal group process individuals make independent judgments, express their judgments mathematically by ranking items, use the mean value of the independent judgments for the group's decision, talk over the results, and revote (Delbecq, Van de Ven, and Gustafson, 1975).

Alternative ways to determine a group decision are consensus, majority rule, and independent listing. When using consensus, group members may distort their judgments to maintain group cohesion, and consequently a regression toward the mean may occur. A showing of hands for majority rule is subject to social pressure, and minority positions do not count. Consequently, it may not truly reflect group preference. Independent listing, however, overcomes status, personality, and conformity pressures but does not indicate degree of importance. For example, an item listing might look like the one shown in Table 6-1. An analysis of the votes in Table 6-1 suggests that items 1, 4, 5, and 6 are considered the most important by frequency. Information about degree of importance can be obtained by having the items ranked. Ranking of the list might look like the one shown in Table 6-2. Using a scale of 5 as most important and 1 as least important, an analysis of the votes reveals that items 6, 4, 1, 5, and 8 are considered most important in descending order from 6 to 8. This method is more likely to reflect the true group preference.

The group leader asks each individual to select a specific number of most important items from the list. Individuals seem most able to accurately list five to nine items. Each member is asked to take that specific number of 3×5 index

TABLE **6-1** Analysis by Frequency

ITEM	VOTES
1	5
2	1
3	2
4	5
5	5
6	5
7	1
8	2

cards, identify that number of items from the list, place the item number in the upper left-hand corner, and write some identifying words in the middle of the card (Figure 6-1). Then the participants are asked to spread out the cards, choose the item they consider most important, and put the high number in the lower right-hand corner of the card and underline it. If five items are being selected, 5 would be the high number. For nine items, 9 would be the high number. That card is turned over, the remaining cards are assessed, and a 1 is put in the lower right-hand corner and underlined for the least important card. That card is turned over, and the next most important item is selected and rated as one less than the highest number: for instance, 8 for nine items or 4 for five items. Then the next-to-the-lowest item is chosen and marked as 2, and so on, until the middle item is left and numbered. This process encourages careful decisions.

When the card ranking is complete, the group leader collects and shuffles the cards and records the votes on the written list of items.

TABLE **6-2** Analysis by Ranking

ITEM	VOTES	TOTALS
1	1-2-5-5-1	14
2	2	2
3	3-2	5
4	4-3-2-4-2	15
5	1-2-1-3-1	8
6	5-5-4-5-4	23
7	1	1
8	3-3	6

```
┌─────────────────────────────────────────────┐
│                                               │
│   6 (item number from original list)          │
│                                               │
│                                               │
│                                               │
│              Setting goals for the unit        │
│                (identifying words)             │
│                                               │
│                                               │
│                                       2        │
│                              (rank order number)│
│                                               │
└─────────────────────────────────────────────┘
```

Figure 6-1 Index card illustrating rank order.

The fifth step is an analysis of the preliminary vote. Inconsistent voting patterns can be examined, and items receiving many or few votes can be discussed. The sixth step, discussion, will probably allow for corrections of misinformation, misunderstandings, and unequal information, thereby offering a more accurate indication of preferences than voting only.

The final step is the revote, which determines the outcome of the process, documents the group judgment, and closes the nominal group process.

Role negotiations—the process of preventing role conflicts, role ambiguities, and role overload—become important once priorities have been set. During this process group members clarify each individual's role on the team and help resolve any disagreements over the team members' roles. Members initially send one written message to each team member indicating that for them to act, they need the other team member to do more, to do less, or to continue her previous performance (Figure 6-2). *To whom* and *from whom* are essential parts of the message. The number of role messages sent to any one individual should be limited to prevent an information overload. The message must clearly state how the sender wants the receiver to behave and how a change will help the sender. Each role message must indicate the need for more, less, or the same of some activity. More than one message

in the "same" category indicates support for the other person.

Receivers respond by indicating what they can or cannot do, explaining why, and offering alternative solutions, for example, "I can't do *x*, but I can do *y*, which should help solve your problem," or "If I do *x*, I would like you to do *y*." Receivers analyze the role messages they receive in the "do more, do less, and do the same" categories according to who sent the message and their response to that message. Do the receivers know what is expected of them? Do different people want them to do more and less of the same activity at the same time? Do the receivers have time to meet all the demands made of them? Role definition helps identify role ambiguity, role conflict, and role overload. After roles are negotiated, a contract (Figure 6-3) is written that defines the problem, identifies what each involved person will do, and sets a date for a follow-up check.

Negotiating involves good communication skills. One can identify needs, ideas, and information by using open-ended probes to clarify. Closed probes can be used to pinpoint specifications and to confirm understanding. One should indicate one's intent ("I support your idea") when one offers ideas of information. It is preferable to present reasons before conclusions, because they seem to be heard better that way, and the speaker is more likely to be considered

ROLE MESSAGE FORM

To:_____
From:_____

In order for me to _____, I need you to do

   Less of:

   Same of:

   More of:

Figure 6-2 Role message form.

ROLE CONTRACT

1. Problem:

2. Person **x** agrees to:

3. Person **y** agrees to:

4. Others agree to:

We agree that a follow-up check will be done by _____.
                                      (date)

                     Signatures

                     _____
                     x

                     _____
                     y

                     _____
                     others

Figure 6-3 Role contract.

reasonable. To build on ideas, one should acknowledge the connection ("Bill's comment made me think of …") and then add value. To criticize constructively, merits should be stated before concerns. One should then ask for ways to retain merits and eliminate concerns. One should confront counterproductive tactics by confirming the behavior and expressing its impact. ("That seemed like a personal attack. Is that what you intended? I feel angry when I am treated that way.") To break an impasse, one can indicate one's desire to continue and then initiate a change of pace. ("Let's go get a cup of coffee and then try to solve this problem.")

To come to an agreement, the purpose of the meeting and a review of the situation should be discussed. Identify the needs and restrictions, examine ideas from both points of view, and determine the best alternative. The discussion can be closed by summarizing the agreement and confirming the next steps (*Negotiating Self-Taught*, 1984).

Decision charting is the next major phase of team development and is concerned with who should be involved in decision making and with the nature of that involvement. To determine who should be involved in decision making, one should assess who has the information necessary to make a sound decision and who is responsible for implementing that decision. The latter needs to understand the decision and be committed to it.

People can be involved in decision making in a variety of ways. Some are directly involved because they have the necessary information and are responsible for implementing the decision. The involvement of some may be limited to input or consultation. Others need to be informed about the decision, and someone must be responsible for managing the overall decision-making process.

A decision chart helps one visualize the decision-making process (Figure 6-4). Decisions to be made are listed down the side of the page, and the involved people are listed across the top in a grid pattern. Placing an *M* in a square indicates who manages the process; *D* indicates who is directly involved; *C* indicates who should be consulted; and *I* indicates who should be informed. Anyone who is expected to implement the decision obviously must be informed (Rubin, Plovnick, and Fry, 1975, 1978).

INTERGROUP CONFLICT

Intergroup conflict is common and can be dysfunctional. As with interpersonal conflict, intergroup resistance may result from low trust, poor communications, and false assumptions. People resist what they perceive as threatening. Intergroup actions may threaten territorial rights and contribute to role overload and conflict. By preventing win-lose situations, emphasizing the organization's goals and effectiveness, rotating personnel among groups to facilitate

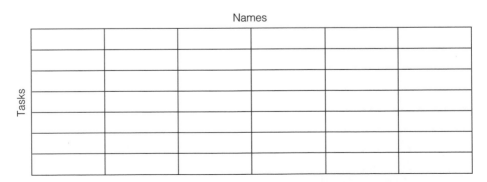

Figure 6-4 Decision chart. *M*, Manages the process; *C*, consulted before the decision; *D*, makes the decision; *I*, informed of the decision.

understanding, and increasing interaction and communication among groups, one can help reduce intergroup conflict.

When a group recognizes its need to solve some intergroup conflict, it must first decide how to begin. A study of the organizational chart will determine who should be involved. Who should represent the group—a person or a committee? Someone who is already friendly with members of the other group? Someone with strong or moderate feelings about the position? What is the group's position, and how much negotiation is acceptable? It helps to emphasize common goals and discuss constraints. The same process used in interpersonal conflict should be used in group conflict situations: setting and rating goals, negotiating roles, and making decisions.

"An open enemy is better than a false friend."
—Greek saying

ORGANIZATIONAL CONFLICT

Organizations in conflict display the collective symptoms of their members. Personnel feel frustration at work. If they do not think their skills are being used, they experience a loss of self-esteem and a sense of powerlessness, both of which lead to withdrawal from the situation instead of an attempt to solve the problems. Group members also engage in backbiting and blame others for the problems. Subgroups commonly form. Members of the organization identify the same task and group maintenance problems but act contrary to the information, thereby increasing their frustrations. However, personnel do not have the same frustrations or exhibit the same dysfunctional behavior outside the organization.

Organizational factors that increase conflict include the number of organizational levels, number of specialties, degree of association, and some parties' dependency on others. The higher the number of levels and specialties, the more opportunities for conflict. More need to associate with others and greater dependency of one on another increase the risk of conflict. Competition for scarce resources, ambiguous jurisdictions, and need for consensus increase conflict. Communication barriers, including separation in time and space and differing values, increase conflict. An accumulation of unresolved conflict increases the challenge for conflict management.

A manager may soothe a party during organizational conflict to facilitate the process and then deal with the underlying problem later. Managers should encourage personnel to confront each other and work their problems out themselves. Appropriate behavior change should be expected and may require sensitivity training, team development, and educational tools. The manager should assess things such as the organizational structure, titles, job descriptions, policies, and procedures as related to the apparent conflict. Responsibility charting can help clarify jurisdictional conflicts. A consultant may be appointed to assess the situation and make recommendations (Marquis and Huston, 1996).

The consultant must analyze the organization's structure, the leadership and authority of the institution, the communication patterns, the amount of intergroup cooperation and competition, the group's norms and goals, the group's problem-solving and decision-making processes, and various individual roles and functions within the group. Organizational research can help provide the information necessary to solve the problem.

After data have been collected and analyzed, the consultant offers feedback. Members of the organization can publicly vote on whether they agree with the consultant's views. A public vote facilitates ownership of ideas. If there is disagreement, the consultant helps the group clarify the reasons for the differences and modifies the statement until it reflects the group's thinking.

The consultant then asks all members to write a few sentences about how they contribute to the situation so that they can recognize their own part in the problem. Individuals are likely to maintain the status quo for fear of serious consequences if they confront the issues.

The consultant shares his or her theory with the group, helps develop an awareness of dysfunctional behavior, helps individuals cope with their feelings, encourages fantasy and reality testing, and coaches group members toward new behaviors.

WORKPLACE VIOLENCE

Unacceptable behavior includes excessive noise, malicious allegations, offensive gestures, general verbal abuse, racial and sexual abuse, drug and alcohol abuse, damage, theft, threats, and violence (Richards, accessed 9/8/02).

A number of factors (U.S. Department of Health and Human Services, July 1996) may increase a worker's risk for workplace assault:

- Contact with the public
- Exchange of money
- Delivery of passengers, goods, or services
- Having a mobile workplace...
- Working with unstable or volatile persons...
- Working alone or in small numbers
- Working late at night or during early-morning hours
- Working in high-crime areas
- Guarding valuable property or possessions
- Working in community-based settings

Health care workers face increased risk in poorly lighted parking areas and where there is a prevalence of handguns or other weapons, drugs, or money. Solo work in remote locations, isolated work with patients during examinations and treatments, low staffing levels during increased activity time such as mealtimes and visiting hours, and unrestricted movement of the public are increasing the presence of drug and alcohol abusers, gang members, trauma patients, and patients and families distraught and frustrated from long waits. Lack of training of staff for recognizing and managing assaultive and hostile behavior also increases risk (U.S. Department of Labor, 1998).

Warning signs of violence include attendance problems, carelessness at work, history of physical violence, performance problems, personality changes, poor hygiene, substance abuse, and social isolation. A sudden change in behavior, clenched jaws or fists, increased movement, increased respirations, pacing, shouting threats, staring or pointing, and use of profanity are signs of impeding physical violence (Gates and Kroeger, 2003). Workplace bullying is also a problem. The following are examples of bullying (U.S. Health and Safety Authority, 2001):

- Purposely undermining someone
- Targeting someone for special negative treatment
- Manipulation of an individual's reputation
- Social exclusion or isolation
- Intimidation
- Physical abuse or threats of abuse
- Aggressive or obscene language
- Jokes that are obviously offensive to one individual by spoken word or e-mail
- Intrusion by pestering, spying, and stalking
- Unreasonable assignments to duties that are obviously unfavorable to one individual
- Reported requests with impossible deadline or impossible tasks

The Department of U.S. Occupational Safety and Health Administration (Gates and Kroeger, 2003) has recommended eight essential components to a violence prevention plan that is recommended for all workplaces to develop and implement. They include (1) management commitment, (2) employee involvement, (3) work site analysis, (4) prevention of hazards, (5) training and education, (6) prompt recognition, control, and monitoring, (7) record keeping, and (8) evaluation.

Management commitment should include the following:

- The endorsement and visible involvement of top management
- Assigned responsibility for the various aspects of the workplace violence prevention program
- Appropriate allocation of authority and resources to responsible parties
- A system of accountability
- A comprehensive program of medical and psychological counseling and debriefing for employees witnessing violent incidents

- Commitment to support and implement appropriate recommendations from the safety and health department

Employee involvement should include the following:

- Understanding and complying with the workplace violence prevention program and other safety measures
- Participation in an employee complaint or suggestion procedure
- Prompt and accurate reporting of violent incidents
- Participation on safety and health committees
- Taking part in a continuing education program

Work site analysis includes the following aspects:

- Record analysis and tracking
- Monitoring trends and analyzing incidents
- Screening surveys
- Workplace security analysis

Engineering controls for hazard prevention include the following:

- Assess new construction plans to eliminate security hazards.
- Install and regularly maintain alarm systems.
- Provide metal detectors.
- Use a closed-circuit video for high-risk areas.
- Place curved mirrors at hallway intersections.
- Enclose nurses' stations, and install deep service counters or bullet-resistant, shatterproof glass.
- Provide employee "safe rooms."
- Establish "time-out" or seclusion areas.
- Provide patient waiting rooms designed to maximize comfort and minimize stress.
- Ensure that counseling or patient care rooms have two exits.
- Limit access to staff counseling rooms and treatment rooms controlled by using locked doors.
- Arrange furniture to prevent entrapment of staff.
- Provide lockable and secure bathrooms for staff members separate from patient-client and visitor bathrooms.
- Lock all unused doors to limit access.

- Install bright, effective lighting indoors and outdoors.
- Replace burned-out lights and broken windows and locks.
- Keep automobiles well maintained and locked.

Administrative and work practice controls include the following:

- State clearly to patients, clients, and employees that violence is not permitted or tolerated.
- Establish liaison with local police and state prosecutors. Report all incidents of violence. Provide physical layouts of facilities to expedite investigations.
- Require employees to report all assaults or threats. Keep logbooks and reports of such incidents.
- Advise and assist employees requesting police assistance when assaulted.
- Provide management support during emergencies.
- Set up a trained response team.
- Use properly trained security officers.
- Ensure adequate and properly trained staff for restraining patients or clients.
- Ensure adequate and qualified staff coverage at all times.
- Institute a sign-in procedure with passes for visitors.
- Establish a list of restricted visitors for patients with a history of violence.
- Supervise the movement of psychiatric clients and patients throughout the facility.
- Control access to facilities other than waiting rooms, particularly drug storage or pharmacy areas.
- Prohibit employees from working alone.
- Establish policies and procedures for secured areas.
- Ascertain the behavioral history of new and transferred patients.
- Treat and/or interview aggressive or agitated patients in relatively open areas.
- Use case management conferences.
- Prepare contingency plans to treat patients who are "acting out."
- Transfer assaultive patients to acute care units.

- Make sure that nurses and/or physicians are not alone when performing intimate physical examinations.
- Discourage employees from wearing jewelry to prevent possible strangulation.
- Periodically survey the facility to remove tools or possessions left by visitors.
- Provide staff with identification badges.
- Discourage employees from carrying keys, pens, or other items that could be used as weapons.
- Provide staff members with security escorts to parking areas.
- Use the buddy system, especially when personal safety may be threatened.
- Develop policies and procedures covering home health care providers.
- Establish a daily work plan.
- Conduct a comprehensive postincident evaluation.

Training should cover topics such as the following:

- The workplace violence prevention policy
- Risk factors that cause or contribute to assaults
- Early recognition of escalating behavior or recognition of warning signs or situations
- Ways of preventing or diffusing volatile situations or aggressive behavior, managing anger, and using medications as chemical restraints
- Information on multicultural diversity to develop sensitivity to racial and ethnic issues and differences
- A standard response action plan for violent situations, including availability of assistance, response systems, and communication procedures
- How to deal with hostile persons
- Progressive behavior control methods and safe methods of restraint application or escape
- The location and operation of safety devices such as alarms systems, along with the required schedules and procedures
- Ways to protect oneself and coworkers, including use of the buddy system

- Policies and procedures for reporting and record keeping
- Policies and procedures for obtaining medical care, counseling, workers' compensation, or legal assistance for a violent episode or injury

Record keeping is essential to the success of a workplace violence prevention program. Good records help determine the severity of the problem, evaluate methods of hazard control, and identify training needs; they include the following:

- U.S. Occupational Safety and Health Administration (OSHA) Log of Injury should be filled out.
- Medical reports of work injury and supervisor's report for each recorded assault should be kept.
- Incidents of abuse, verbal attacks, or aggressive behavior: should be part of an assault incident report.
- Information on patients with a history of past violence, drug abuse, or criminal activity should be on the patient's chart.
- Minutes of safety meetings, records of hazard analysis, and corrective actions recommended are to be documented.
- Records of all training programs, attendees, and qualifications of trainers should be maintained.

An evaluation program should involve the following:

- Establishing a uniform violence reporting system and regular review of reports
- Reviewing reports and minutes from staff meetings on safety and security issues
- Analyzing trends and rates in illnesses/injuries or fatalities caused by violence or workplace violence
- Keeping up-to-date records of administrative and work practice changes to prevent workplace violence and evaluate their effectiveness
- Surveying employees before and after making job or work site changes or installing security measures
- Keeping abreast of new strategies available to deal with violence

- Surveying employees who experience hostile situations about the medical treatment they received again several weeks afterward and then several months later
- Requesting periodic law enforcement or outside consultant review of the work site for recommendations for improving employee safety

These ideas are explained in more detail in *Violence in the Workplace* and *Guidelines for Preventing Workplace Violence for Health Care Service Workers* (U.S. Department of Labor, Occupational Safety and Health Administration, 1996, 1998), and OSHA consultation services are available.

The National Institute for Occupational Safety and Health (NIOSH) is the federal agency responsible for research and recommendations for the prevention of work-related illness and injury. Job stress is harmful physical and emotional responses that occur because the requirements of the job do not match the capabilities, resources, or needs of the worker. It can lead to poor health, injury, and workplace violence.

Interventions could include the following:
- Target source of stress for change.
- Propose and prioritize intervention strategies.
- Communicate planned interventions to employees.
- Implement interventions.

Evaluations of interventions can include the following aspects:
- Conduct both short- and long-term evaluations.
- Measure employee perceptions of job conditions, stress, health, and satisfaction.
- Include objective measures.
- Refine the intervention strategy.

The following can reduce the effects of stressful working conditions:
- Balance between work and family or personal life
- A support network of friends and coworkers
- A relaxed and positive outlook

(NIOSH, accessed 12/6/02):

PREVENTION OF CONFLICT

"The best general is the one who never fights."
—Sun Tzu

Careful development of an organization's structure, strategic and comprehensive planning, management and organizational development, and careful selection and placement of personnel help prevent organizational conflict. The same strategies also prevent intergroup, group, and interpersonal conflict. Although conflict can be reduced, it cannot be totally avoided. Conflict can be constructive or destructive. By capitalizing on the positive aspects, the negative features can seem more bearable.

Chapter Summary

Chapter 6 covered the following:
Conflict Theory
    Sources of Conflict
    Types of Conflict
    Reactions to Conflict
    Escalation-of-Conflict Tactics
    Stages of Conflict
Conflict Management
    Approaches to Managing Conflict
    Deescalation-of-Conflict Tactics
    Strategies for Management of Conflict
    Mediation
    Arbitration
    Intrapersonal Conflict
    Interpersonal Conflict
        Sexual harassment
    Group Conflict
    Intergroup Conflict
    Organizational Conflict
    Workplace Violence
    Prevention of Conflict

On-line Resources

evolve   Additional critical thinking activities, worksheets, and case studies are available on-line at http://evolve.elsevier.com/Marriner/guide/

References

Bach GR, Goldberg H: Creative aggression: The art of assertive living, New York, 1974, Avon Books.

Beer JE, Stief E: The mediator's handbook, Gabriola Island, BC, Canada, 1997, New Society Publishers.

Delbecq AL, Van de Ven AH, Gustafson DH: Group techniques for program planning: A guide to nominal group and Delphi processes, Glenview, Il, 1975, Scott Foresman.

Douglas LM: The effective nurse, ed 5, St Louis, 1996, Mosby.

Gates DM and Kroeger D: *Violence against nurses: the silent epidemic. ISNA Bulletin* 29(1):25-29.

Goodman AH: Basic skills for the new mediator, Rockville, Md, 1994, Solomon Publications.

Kheel TW: The keys to conflict resolution, New York, 2001, Four Walls Eight Windows.

Levine S: Getting to resolution: Turning conflict into collaboration, San Francisco, 1998, Berrett-Koehler.

Loveridge CE, Cummings SH: Nursing management in the new paradigm, Gaithersburg, Md, 1996, Aspen.

Marquis BL, Huston CJ: Leadership roles and management functions in nursing, Philadelphia, 1996, Lippincott.

Mayer B: The dynamics of conflict resolution: A practitioner's guide, San Francisco, 2000, Jossey-Bass.

Moore CW: The mediation process: Practical strategies for resolving conflict, San Francisco, 1986, Jossey-Bass.

National Institue for Occupational Safety and Health: Stress. DHHS (NIOSH) Publication No. 99-101. http://www.cdc.gov.iosh/stresswk.htm. Accessed 12/6/03.

Negotiating self-taught, Stamford, Conn, 1984, Learning International.

Patterson K, Grenny J, McMillan R, et al: Crucial conversations: Tools for talking when stakes are high, New York, 2002, McGraw-Hill.

Potter B: From conflict to cooperation: How to mediate a dispute, Berkeley, Calif, 1996, Ronin Pub, Inc.

Richards J: Management of workplace victims…Violence …/2?action=Attachment.View&Item.Attachment.id=2 &User.context=dmiwMithodHi&Item.drn=19/8/02.

Rubin IM, Plovnick MS, Fry RE: Improving the coordination of care: A program for health team development, Cambridge, Mass, 1975, Ballinger.

Rubin IM, Plovnick MS, Fry RE: Managing human resources in health care organizations: An applied approach, Reston, Va, 1978, Reston.

Stone D, Patton B, Heen S: Difficult conversations: How to discuss what matters most, New York, 2000, Penguin Books.

Swiss DJ: Women breaking through: Overcoming the final 10 obstacles at work, Princeton, NJ, 1996, Peterson's/ Pacesetter Books.

Thomas KW, Kilmann RH: Thomas-Kilmann conflict mode instrument, Sterling Forest, Tuxedo, NY, 1974, 2002, XICOM.

U.S. Department of Labor, Occupational Safety and Health Administration. (1998). Guidelines for preventing workplace violence for health care workers. http://www.osha-slc.gov/SLTC/workplaceviolence/guideline.html. Accessed 12/6/02.

U.S. Department of Health and Human Services. (July 1996). Violence in the workplace: Risk factors and prevention strategies. DHHS (NIOSH) Publication No. 96-100 http//www.cdc.gov/nioshviolcont.htm. Accessed 12/6/02.

U.S. Health and Safety Authority: Prevention of workplace bullying: Dignity in the workplace. http://www.has.ie/safety/bullying/index.htm. Accessed 12/6/02.

Weeks D: The eight essential steps to conflict resolution: Preserving relationships at work, at home, and in the community, New York, 1992, GP Putnam's Sons.

Wywialowski EF: Managing client care, ed 3, St Louis, 2004, Mosby.

7

Theories of Leadership

"Lead, follow, or get out of the way."
—Anonymous

Chapter Overview

Chapter 7 discusses several theories of leadership and the development
of management thought.

Chapter Objectives

- Identify the two dimensions of leadership behavior and at least three activities in each dimension.
- List the three aspects of a situation that structure the leader's role as identified by Fiedler in contingency theory.
- Identify the variable from which Hersey and Blanchard's situational leadership theory predicts the most appropriate leadership style.
- Describe the differences between transactional and transformational leadership.
- Identify at least three of the strategies for taking charge as identified by Bennis and Nanus.
- Outline the five basic practices and two specific behaviors for each practice as identified by Kouzes and Posner in *The Leadership Challenge: How to Get Extraordinary Things Done in Organizations.*
- Identify at least two theorists in each of the following management eras: scientific management, classic organization, human relations, and behavioral science.
- Identify at least five of the concepts stressed in each management era.
- Compare Maslow's, Herzberg's, and McGregor's theories.
- Describe each of Likert's four types of management systems.

> ## Major Concepts and Definitions
>
> **Lead** to show, mark the way, guide the course
> **Transaction** the negotiation of business
> **Transformation** a change in the nature of someone or something
> **Charisma** an inspirational quality that some leaders possess
> **Situational** appropriate to the requirements of different situations
> **Contingency** the uncertainty of an event's occurrence
> **Management** act of planning, organizing, staffing, directing, and controlling
> **Scientific management** focused on the best way to do a task
> **Classic organization** focused on planning, organizing, and controlling of the organization as a whole
> **Human relations** focused on the effect individuals have on the success of the organization
> **Behavioral science** focused on scientific validation

THEORIES OF LEADERSHIP

Theories of leadership are numerous. The following survey covers the alternatives, beginning with the oldest notion and advancing to ideas currently in vogue. By familiarizing themselves with these theories, nurses can select and adapt the most suitable approach for dealing with different situations. As a role model, the nursing leader can reduce the autocratic atmosphere and, hence, some of the role conflicts.

Leaders need to do the right things, are challenged by change, focus on purposes, and have a future time frame. They ask why and use strategies on their journeys to human potential. On the other hand, managers do things right, are challenged by continuity, and focus on structures and procedures in a present time frame. They ask who, what, when, where, and how as they use schedules to get to destinations and evaluate human performance (Table 7-1).

GREAT MAN THEORY

The great man theory argues that a few people are born with the necessary characteristics to be great. Leaders are well rounded and simultaneously display both instrumental and supportive leadership behavior. Instrumental activities include planning, organizing, and controlling the activities of subordinates to accomplish the organization's goals. Obtaining and allocating resources such as people, equipment, materials, funds, and space are particularly important. Supportive leadership is socially oriented and allows for participation and consultation from subordinates for decisions that affect them. People who use both instrumental and supportive leadership behaviors are considered "great men" and supposedly are effective leaders in any situation. Many find this theory unattractive because of its premise that leaders are born and not made, which suggests that leadership cannot be developed.

CHARISMATIC THEORY

People may be leaders because they are charismatic, but relatively little is known about this intangible characteristic. What constitutes charisma? Most agree that it is an inspirational quality possessed by some people that makes others feel better in their presence. The charismatic leader inspires others by obtaining emotional commitment from followers and by arousing strong feelings of loyalty and enthusiasm. Under charismatic leadership one may overcome obstacles not thought possible. However, because charisma is so elusive, some may sense it while others do not.

Gary Yukl (1994) has reported findings from Robert House's, Bernard Bass's, and Jay Conger

TABLE **7-1** Comparison of Leadership and Management

	LEADERSHIP	MANAGEMENT
Motto	Do the right things	Do things right
Challenge	Change	Continuity
Focus	Purposes	Structures and procedures
Time frame	Future	Present
Methods	Strategies	Schedules
Questions	Why?	Who, what, when, where, and how?
Outcomes	Journeys	Destinations
Human	Potential	Performance

From Bennis W, Nanus B: *Leaders: The strategies for taking charge*, New York, 1985, 1997, Harper & Row.

and Rabindra Kanungo's research about charisma. House found that followers of charismatic leaders trust the leader's beliefs; have similar beliefs; exhibit affection for, obedience to, and unquestioning acceptance of the leader; and are emotionally involved in and believe they can contribute to the mission. He found that charismatic leaders have a strong conviction in their own beliefs, high self-confidence, and a need for power. They are likely to set an example by their behavior, communicate high expectations to followers and express confidence in them, and arouse motives for the group's mission.

Conger and Kanungo's (1998) research approached charisma as an attributional phenomenon. They found that charisma is more likely attributed to a leader who advocates a vision discrepant from the status quo, emerges during a crisis, accurately assesses the situation, communicates self-confidence, uses personal power, makes self-sacrifices, and uses unconventional strategies.

Bass proposed that charismatic leaders perceive themselves as having supernatural purpose and destiny and that followers may idolize and worship them as spiritual figures or superhumans. This blind obedience can lead to bad outcomes, such as group suicide. Transformational leaders use charisma for good.

TRAIT THEORY

Until the mid-1940s, the trait theory was the basis for most leadership research. Early work in this area maintained that traits are inherited, but later theories suggested that traits could be obtained through learning and experience. Researchers identified the leadership traits as energy, drive, enthusiasm, ambition, aggressiveness, decisiveness, self-assurance, self-confidence, friendliness, affection, honesty, fairness, loyalty, dependability, technical mastery, and teaching skill. Asking themselves what traits leaders possess, various researchers arrived at different conclusions but identified some common leadership traits:

1. Leaders need to be more intelligent than the group they lead. However, a highly intelligent person may not find leadership responsibilities challenging enough, may prefer to work with abstract ideas and research, and may have difficulty relating to the group.
2. Leaders must possess initiative, the ability to perceive and start courses of action not considered by others.
3. Creativity is an asset. Having originality—the ability to think of new solutions to problems and ideas of new ways to be productive—is helpful.
4. Emotional maturity with integrity—a sense of purpose and direction, persistence, dependability, and objectivity—is another important trait. Mature leaders do what they say they will and are consistent in their actions. They often work long hours, apply themselves intensely, and spread enthusiasm to followers. Energy, drive, and good health are necessary to endure the long hours, overcome obstacles,

and sustain continuous achievement. Self-assurance is self-confidence. It is hoped that leaders perceive themselves as effective problem solvers who can successfully handle the difficulties that confront them.

5. Communication skills are important. The leader needs to understand others and speak and write clearly.

6. Persuasion often is used by leaders to gain the consent of followers. The leader may make suggestions, supply supportive data, ask penetrating questions, make compromises, and request action to persuade others.

7. Leaders need to be perceptive enough to distinguish their allies from their opponents and to place their subordinates in suitable positions.

8. Leaders participate in social activities. They can socialize with all kinds of people and adapt to various groups. Approachable, friendly, and helpful, they gain the confidence and loyalty of others in such a way that makes people willing to cooperate.

The authoritarian leader maintains strong control, does the planning, makes the decisions, and gives the orders. Autocratic leaders tend to be directive, critical, and punitive. They may make decisions that are not in the best interest of the group. They give themselves a higher status than the group members, which reduces open communications and trust. They tend to get good quantity and quality of output but little autonomy, creativity, or self-motivation. This can be appropriate for an emergency situation when the leader knows what to do, but it does not develop people (Table 7-2).

Democratic leaders maintain less control; ask questions and make suggestions rather than issue orders; and get the group involved in planning, problem solving, and decision making. The participation tends to increase motivation and creativity. It works when people have knowledge and skills and work well together over time. It can be cumbersome. It is often less efficient than autocratic control.

Laissez-faire is very permissive, nondirective, passive, and inactive. Members may work independently and possibly at cross purposes because there is no planning or coordination and little cooperation. Chaos is likely to develop unless an informal leader emerges. This style can work with very mature, autonomous workers, but it is more likely to be inefficient and unproductive.

The trait theory expanded knowledge about leadership, but it was not without its flaws. Few if any traits are identified in all trait theory research. They are not mutually exclusive, and there is considerable overlap between categories or definitions of the characteristics. It is not clear which traits are most important, which traits are needed to acquire leadership, and which traits are needed to maintain it. Trait theory does not view personality as an integrated whole, does not deal with subordinates, and avoids environmental influences and situational factors.

Ohio State Leadership Studies researchers compiled a list of about 1800 examples of leadership behavior that factored out two dimensions: consideration and initiating structure. Consideration involves behaving in a friendly and supportive way, looking out for others' welfare, showing

TABLE **7-2** Comparison of Autocratic, Democratic, and Laissez-Faire Leadership

AUTOCRATIC	DEMOCRATIC	LAISSEZ-FAIRE
Strong control	Less control	No control
Gives orders	Offers suggestions	Nondirective
Does decision making	Makes suggestions	Abdicates decision making
Leader does planning	Group does planning	No planning
Directive	Participative	Uninvolved
Fosters dependency	Fosters independence	Fosters chaos

concern, treating others as equals, taking time to listen, consulting others on important matters, being willing to accept suggestions, and doing personal favors.

Initiating structure is the way the leader structures roles to attain the goals. It includes assigning tasks, defining procedures, setting deadlines, maintaining standards, suggesting new approaches, and coordinating activities.

Researchers at the University of Michigan focused on identification of relationships among leader behavior, group process, and group performance. They found that three types of leadership behavior marked the difference between effective and ineffective leaders: (1) task-oriented behavior, (2) relationship-oriented behavior, and (3) participative leadership. Task-oriented behavior includes planning, scheduling, and coordinating activities. Relationship-oriented behavior includes acting friendly and considerate, showing trust and confidence, expressing appreciation, and providing recognition. Participative leadership uses group meetings to enlist associate participation in decision making, improve communications, promote cooperation, and facilitate conflict resolution.

John Maxwell (1999) discusses 21 qualities of a leader as character, charisma, commitment, communication, competence, courage, discernment, focus, generosity, initiative, listening, passion, positive attitude, problem solving, relationships, responsibility, security, self-discipline, servanthood, teachability, and vision in *The 21 Indispensable Qualities of a Leader* (1999). Warren Blank provides self-assessment tools in *The 108 Skills of Natural Born Leaders* (2001).

SITUATIONAL THEORY

Situational theories became popular during the 1950s. These theories suggest that the traits required of a leader differ according to varying situations. Among the variables that determine the effectiveness of leadership style are factors such as the personality of the leader; the performance requirements of both the leader and followers; the attitudes, needs, and expectations of the leader and followers; the degree of interpersonal contact possible; time pressures; physical environment; organizational structure; the nature of the organization; the state of the organization's development; and the influence of the leader outside the group. A person may be a leader in one situation and a follower in another or a leader at one time and a follower at others because the type of leadership needed depends on the situation.

CONTINGENCY THEORY

During the 1960s Fred Fiedler introduced the contingency model of leadership. Refuting the ideal leadership style theory, he argued that a leadership style will be effective or ineffective depending on the situation. He identified three aspects of a situation that structure the leader's role: (1) leader-member relations, (2) task structure, and (3) position power.

Leader-member relations involve the amount of confidence and loyalty the followers have with regard to their leader. Leadership is assessed by a group-atmosphere scale (Box 7-1). Fiedler also used a sociometric index of the least-preferred coworker (LPC) score. Followers were asked to think of everyone with whom they have ever worked and to rate the least-preferred coworker on an eight-point bipolar adjective scale, which includes adjectives such as friendly and cooperative. A high score describes the person in favorable terms, and a low score is a negative rating. Although the LPC scores are difficult to interpret and it is hard to say what they measure, Fiedler suggests that high scorers are relationship oriented and low scorers are mostly task oriented.

Task structure is high if it is easy to define and measure a task. The structure is low if it is difficult to define the task and to measure progress toward its completion. Fiedler used four criteria to determine the degree of task structure: (1) goal clarity: extent to which a goal is understood by followers; (2) extent to which a decision can be verified: knowing who is responsible for what; (3) multiplicity of goal paths: number of

---

BOX 7-1 Group-Atmosphere Scale

Describe the atmosphere of your group by checking the following items:

	8	7	6	5	4	3	2	1	
1. Friendly	:___:___:___:___:___:___:___:___:								Unfriendly
2. Accepting	:___:___:___:___:___:___:___:___:								Rejecting
3. Satisfying	:___:___:___:___:___:___:___:___:								Frustrating
4. Enthusiastic	:___:___:___:___:___:___:___:___:								Unenthusiastic
5. Productive	:___:___:___:___:___:___:___:___:								Nonproductive
6. Warm	:___:___:___:___:___:___:___:___:								Cold
7. Cooperative	:___:___:___:___:___:___:___:___:								Uncooperative
8. Supportive	:___:___:___:___:___:___:___:___:								Hostile
9. Interesting	:___:___:___:___:___:___:___:___:								Boring
10. Successful	:___:___:___:___:___:___:___:___:								Unsuccessful

From Fiedler FE: *A theory of leadership effectiveness*, New York, 1967, McGraw-Hill, p. 269.

---

solutions; and (4) specificity of solution: number of correct answers. Technical nursing, which focuses on procedures, may have a high task structure, but situations involving human relations and value judgments may have numerous solutions with no specific correct answer and consequently have a low task structure.

Position power refers to the authority inherent in a position, the power to use rewards and punishment, and the organization's support of one's decisions. Directors of nursing, managers, and sometimes patient care coordinators have high position power with the right to hire and fire, promote, and adjust salaries. People with low position power may be elected, function in an acting position, or be subject to removal by peers or subordinates. Elected committee chairpersons have low position power. Team leaders and staff nurses usually have low position power. Given the critical conditions, Fiedler argues that one can predict the most productive leadership style (Table 7-3).

If a task is structured but the leader is disliked and therefore needs to be diplomatic, or if the task is ambiguous and the leader is liked and therefore seeks the cooperation of the workers,

---

TABLE **7-3** Summary of Fiedler Investigations of Leadership Group Situation

CONDITION	LEADER-MEMBER RELATIONS	TASK STRUCTURE	POSITION POWER	LEADERSHIP STYLE CORRELATION WITH PRODUCTIVITY
1	Good	Structured	Strong	Directive
2	Good	Structured	Weak	Directive
3	Good	Unstructured	Strong	Directive
4	Good	Unstructured	Weak	Permissive
5	Moderately poor	Structured	Strong	Permissive
6	Moderately poor	Structured	Weak	No data
7	Moderately poor	Unstructured	Strong	No relationship level
8	Moderately poor	Unstructured	Weak	Directive

From Donnelly JH Jr, Gibson JL, Ivancevich JM: *Fundamentals of management functions, behavior, models*, Dallas, 1981, Business Publications, © 1981 by Business Publications, Inc.

the considerate, accepting leadership style probably will be most productive. When a disliked leader faces ambiguous tasks, a directive style is more productive. The most productive leadership style is contingent on the situational variables.

Empirical evidence does not supply conclusive evidence for the contingency model. It is difficult to say what the psychologically distant manager and psychologically closer manager measures are really recording. Correlations were used for predicted direction even when they were not statistically significant. The model is primarily academic in that it has not been used in management development for improving group performance and organizational effectiveness, and Fiedler's complex, three-dimensional contingency model has contributed to leadership theories (Fiedler, 1967; Fiedler and Chemers, 1974; Fiedler, Chemers, and Mahar, 1976).

PATH-GOAL THEORY

House derived the path-goal theory from the expectancy theory. The expectancy theory argues that people act as they do because they expect their behavior to produce satisfactory results. In the path-goal relationship, the leader facilitates task accomplishment by minimizing obstructions to the goals and by rewarding followers for completing their tasks. The leader helps staff associates assess needs, explores alternatives, helps associates make the most beneficial decisions, rewards personnel for task achievement, and provides additional opportunities for satisfying goal accomplishment.

House noted that studies done during the 1950s revealed that leaders who structured activities for staff associates generally had more productive work groups and got higher performance evaluations from superiors. Structure

RESEARCH Perspective 7-1

Data from Newhouse RP, Mills MEC: Enhancing a professional environment in the organized delivery system: Lessons in building trust for the nurse administrator. *Nursing Administration Quarterly* 26(3):67-75, 2002.

PURPOSE: The purpose of this study was to examine the level of system integration if a relationship exists between the level of nursing development and system integration.

METHODS: Contingency theory was used as the theoretical framework. Primary data were collected from nurse administrators in Maryland acute care hospitals in December 1999. A survey of 23 Maryland nurse administrators was conducted utilizing three tools. The Perceived Systemness and Integration Measure was used to measure the level of integration within the system or network. The level of professional practice development was measured utilizing a Likert-scale tool designed by the researchers based on the Transformational Model for Professional Practice in Health Care Organization. A narrative response

questionnaire was included to determine mechanisms in place to promote professional practice and clinical integration.

RESULTS/CONCLUSIONS: The level of system integration was moderate in all domains: functional, physician-system, and culture. Significant correlations were found between transformational leadership and culture and between strategic planning and resource allocation. No significant relationship was found between the level of clinical integration and the development of nursing. Few mechanisms to enhance clinical integration exist across the delivery system. Nurse executives need to promote structure and processes to enhance the development of nursing in integrated systems and networks.

includes planning, organizing, directing, and controlling through activities such as clarifying expectations of staff associates, scheduling work, making assignments, determining procedures, and setting standards. Structured activity can increase motivation by reducing role ambiguity and allowing for externally imposed controls. In contrast, considerate leaders had more satisfied workers. They created an atmosphere of friendliness, warmth, and support by tending to the personal welfare of their subordinates. Leader consideration seems particularly important for routine jobs. People who perform a variety of tasks may find their jobs more satisfying and have less need for social support.

House recognized that individual differences will affect the staff associates' perception of leader behavior. For instance, experienced staff associates may prefer a task-oriented style, whereas less mature, less experienced, and consequently less secure individuals may prefer a considerate leader. Staff associates with a high

need for achievement probably will prefer a task-oriented leader, but people with a high need for affiliation will prefer a considerate leader. The path-goal theory introduced staff associates as a variable (House, 1971).

"Instruction does much, but encouragement does everything." —Johann Wolfgang Von Goethe

SITUATIONAL LEADERSHIP THEORY

The situational leadership theory predicts the most appropriate leadership style from the level of maturity of the followers. Paul Hersey and Kenneth Blanchard illustrate this theory in a four-quadrant model (Figure 7-1). A horizontal continuum registers low emphasis on the accomplishment of tasks on the left side of the model to high emphasis on task behavior on the right side. The vertical continuum depicts low emphasis on interpersonal relationships at the bottom of the model to high emphasis on relationships at

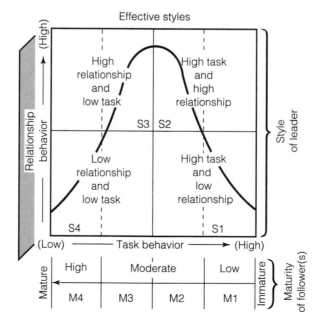

Figure 7-1 Situational leadership theory. (From Hersey P, Blanchard KH: *Management of organizational behavior: Utilizing human resources,* ed 3, Upper Saddle, NJ, 1977, Prentice Hall.)

the top. The lower left quadrant therefore represents a laissez-faire type of leadership style with little concern for production or relationships. The lower right quadrant represents an autocratic leadership style with considerable concern for production but little concern for relationships. The upper right quadrant designates a high concern for both tasks and relationships. The upper left quadrant represents a leadership style that stresses relationships but shows little concern for tasks.

The maturity level of the group or individual is depicted on a continuum from high maturity on the left to low maturity on the right under the four quadrants. The maturity levels are superimposed on the quadrants with dashed lines. The best leadership style for given levels of maturity is shown by a curvilinear line in the four quadrants. To determine the most appropriate leadership style, one must assess the maturity level of the individual or group, plot it on the maturity continuum, and project a line at a right angle from that point until it intersects with the curvilinear line. The quadrant in which the intersection occurs depicts the most appropriate leadership style. With increased maturity less structure and emotional support are needed. In contrast, high-task and low-relationship style is considered best for below-average maturity. The leadership styles in quadrants 2 and 3 are recommended for the average group or individual.

This model is consistent with Chris Argyris's immaturity-maturity continuum, which indicates that as people mature, they progress from a passive to an active state and from dependence to independence. With maturity they pass from a need for structure and little relationship through a decreasing need for structure and increasing need for relationship to little need for either. The progression is not always smooth. Stress may cause members of the group to regress, and leaders must adjust their behavior accordingly. The situational leadership theory therefore emphasizes the importance of the maturity level of the group, and the leader needs to adapt leadership styles accordingly.

TRANSACTIONAL LEADERSHIP

Transactional leadership is an exchange posture that identifies needs of followers and provides rewards to meet those needs in exchange for expected performance. It is a contract for mutual benefits that has contingent rewards. The leader is a caretaker who sets goals for employees, focuses on day-to-day operations, and uses management by exception. It is a competitive, task-focused approach that takes place in a hierarchy.

TRANSFORMATIONAL LEADERSHIP

Transformational leadership promotes employee development, attends to needs and motives of followers, inspires through optimism, influences changes in perception, provides intellectual stimulation, and encourages follower creativity. The leader is a role model who uses individualized consideration, provides a sense of direction, and encourages self-management. Transformational leadership is a cooperative, process-focused networking. Table 7-4 summarizes the key points of several views of transactional and transformational leadership.

Bass (1985) has described transformational leaders in terms of charisma, inspirational leadership, individualized consideration, and intellectual stimulation.

Warren Bennis and Burt Nanus (1985) indicate that leaders do the right things, whereas managers do things right. Leaders focus on effectiveness; managers deal with efficiency. Bennis and Nanus identify four strategies for taking charge: (1) attention through vision, (2) meaning through communication, (3) trust through positioning, and (4) deployment of self. The leader's vision should be clear, attractive, and attainable. Communication through stories, allegories, fables, parables, analogies, and so on helps give meaning to the vision. The leader's position must be clear because associates are more likely to be trusting when they know the leader's view of the organization. Open communications, honesty, and consistency are important to building trust. Leaders are continuous learners and use the organization as a learning

TABLE **7-4** Comparison of Transactional and Transformational Leadership

TRANSACTIONAL	TRANSFORMATIONAL
Hierarchy	Networking
Competitive	Cooperative
Task focus	Process focus
Exchange posture	Promote employee development
Identify needs of followers	Attend to needs and motives of followers
Provide rewards to meet needs	Inspire through optimism
Exchange for expected performance	Influence change in perception
Contract for mutual benefits	Provide intellectual stimulation
Contingent rewards	Encouragement of follower creativity
Caretaker	Role model
Set goals for employees	Individualize consideration
Focus on day-to-day operations	Provide sense of direction
Management by exception	Encouragement of self-management

environment. They deploy themselves as they foster a learning environment.

James Kouzes and Barry Posner (1987, 1990) identify five basic practices and 10 specific behaviors that leadership involves: (1) challenging the process by searching for opportunities and experimenting and taking risks, (2) inspiring a shared vision by envisioning the future and enlisting others, (3) enabling others to act by fostering collaboration and strengthening others, (4) modeling the way by setting an example and planning small wins, and (5) encouraging the heart by recognizing individual contributions and celebrating accomplishments.

Bernard Bass and Bruce Avolio (1993) indicate that transformational leaders change the organization by realigning the organization's culture with the new vision and revision of assumptions, values, and norms. They identify four components that characterize transformational leaders: (1) idealized influence, (2) inspirational motivation, (3) intellectual stimulation, and (4) individualized consideration. They believe that organizations should maintain a base of effective transactional qualities while moving in the direction of transformational qualities.

William Hitt (1993) defines leadership as affecting people so that they will strive willingly toward group goals. He identifies five types of knowledge needed by a leader: (1) knowing oneself, (2) knowing the job, (3) knowing the organization, (4) knowing the business, and (5) knowing the world. He also identifies six core functions of leaders: (1) valuing, (2) visioning, (3) coaching, (4) empowering, (5) team building, and (6) promoting quality. He lists the attributes essential for leadership as identity, independence, authenticity, responsibility, courage, and integrity.

INTEGRATIVE LEADERSHIP MODEL

From a review of leadership theories, obviously there is no one best leadership style. Leaders are rarely totally people oriented or task oriented. Leader, followers, situation—all influence leadership effectiveness. Consequently, an integration of leadership theories seems appropriate. Leaders need to be aware of their own behavior and influence on others, individual differences of followers, group characteristics, motivation, task structures, environmental factors, and situational variables and adjust their leadership style accordingly. Leadership requires adaptive behavior.

DEVELOPMENT OF MANAGEMENT THOUGHT

A familiarity with the development of management thought can be useful to nursing leaders in creating their own management styles. No single management theory is sufficient in itself to guide the nursing leader's every action, but through an eclectic approach, drawing from the best and most applicable theories in each situation, nurse administrators can create individual management styles to meet their particular needs.

SCIENTIFIC MANAGEMENT

Theories of management do not remain static. Since the introduction of the earliest principles of scientific management nearly a century ago, management thought has been marked by constant change.

Taylor

Frederick Taylor (1856-1915) is generally recognized as the father of scientific management. Through the use of stopwatch studies, he applied the principles of observation, measurement, and scientific comparison to determine the most efficient way to accomplish a task. Taylor conducted time-and-motion studies to time workers, analyze their movements, and set work standards. He usually found that the same result could be obtained in less time with fewer or shorter motions. When the most efficient way to complete a task was determined, workers were trained to follow that method. The most productive workers were hired, and even when they were paid an incentive wage, labor costs per unit were reduced.

Taylor, an engineer in steel manufacture, applied his pioneering experience in scientific management to the service of Bethlehem Steel in 1898 and later became an independent business consultant. Identifying the responsibilities of management and separating them from the functions of the workers, Taylor threw aside rule-of-thumb judgments and developed a systematic approach to determine the most efficient means of production. He considered management's function to be planning. Working conditions and methods had to be standardized to maximize production. It was management's responsibility to select and train workers rather than allow them to choose their own jobs and methods and train themselves. An incentive plan whereby workers were paid according to their rates of production was introduced to minimize worker dissent and reduce resistance to improved methods, increase production, and produce higher profits. Taylor's scientific management reduced wasted efforts, set standards for performance, encouraged specialization, and stressed the selection of qualified workers who could be developed for a particular job. His *Shop Management* (1903) and *The Principles of Scientific Management* (1911) spread his ideas throughout Europe and the United States.

Gilbreth

Frank Gilbreth (1868-1924) and Lillian Gilbreth (1878-1972) also did pioneering work in time-and-motion studies. They emphasized the benefits of job simplification and the establishment of work standards, as well as the effects of the incentive wage plans and fatigue on work performance. As an apprentice bricklayer, Frank Gilbreth was instructed differently by each workman on how to lay bricks. To add to his confusion, the men used one set of motions to teach him, another for a slow pace, and still another for a fast pace. Wondering what methods would be most efficient, the young bricklayer started studying the workers' motions. Gilbreth reduced the number of motions required to lay a brick from 18 to 4 by developing a new way to stack bricks; developed an adjustable stand to eliminate excessive stooping, bending, and walking back and forth; and prescribed a mortar consistency that prevented excessive tapping on the brick with a trowel. His system of "speed work" eliminated haste and also increased work output by cutting out unnecessary motions. Workers could be paid higher wages because they accomplished more in a shorter time (Gilbreth, 1909; Gilbreth and Gilbreth, 1919).

The Gilbreths were among the first to use motion-picture films to analyze workers' motions. Because early cameras did not work at a steady speed, Gilbreth developed a micro-chronometer, a clock with a large hand measuring 1/2000 of a minute. The clock was photographed with the task and used to study motion patterns. A small, blinking electric bulb was attached to the worker's hand so speed and direction of movement could be studied. For his study of hand motions, Gilbreth developed 17 classifications for hand movements, such as "find," "select," "grasp," "position," and "rest," which he labeled "therbligs" (Gilbreth spelled backward with the th transposed). The Gilbreths also developed the flow diagram and the process chart to record their observations. The work process was diagrammed to indicate operations, delays, inspection, transportation, and storage, and the process was then studied to shorten, combine, or eliminate steps. The Gilbreths recommended written instructions to prevent misunderstandings and started a merit-rating system for workers (Gilbreth, 1911; Gilbreth and Gilbreth, 1917).

Lillian Gilbreth is known as the first lady of management. Her doctoral dissertation, *The Psychology of Management* (1914), was published with the author listed as L.M. Gilbreth, thus obscuring the fact that she was a woman. It was one of the first contributions toward understanding human factors in industry. Her work on the effects of fatigue complemented her husband's efforts. The Gilbreths and their 12 children are the subjects of the popular book *Cheaper by the Dozen* (1984).

Gantt

Henry Gantt (1861-1919), a disciple of Taylor, also was concerned with problems of efficiency. He contributed to scientific management by refining previous work rather than introducing new concepts. The Gantt chart, a forerunner of the PERT (program evaluation and review technique) chart, depicts the relationship of the work planned or completed on one axis to the amount of time needed or used on the other. Gantt also developed a task and bonus remuneration plan whereby workers received a guaranteed day's wage plus a bonus for production above the standard to stimulate higher performance. Gantt recommended that workers be selected scientifically and provided with detailed instructions for their tasks. He argued for a more humanitarian approach by management, placing emphasis on service rather than profit objectives, recognizing useful nonmonetary incentives such as job security, and encouraging staff development (Gantt, 1916, 1919).

CLASSIC ORGANIZATION

Classic administration-organization thinking began to receive attention in 1930. Deductive rather than inductive, it views the organization as a whole rather than focusing solely on production. Managerial activities are classified as planning, organizing, and controlling. The concepts of scalar levels, span of control, authority, responsibility, accountability, line-staff relationships, decentralization, and departmentalization became prevalent.

Fayol

Henri Fayol (1841-1925), known as the "father of the management process school," was a French industrialist concerned with the management of production shops. Fayol studied the functions of managers and concluded that management is universal. All managers, regardless of the type of organization or their level in the organization, have essentially the same tasks: planning, organizing, issuing orders, coordinating, and controlling.

Fayol derived some general principles of administration from his observations. A believer in the division of work, he argued that specialization increases efficiency. Fayol recommended centralization through the use of a scalar chain or levels of authority, responsibility accompanied by authority, and unity of command and direction so that each employee receives orders from only one superior. He believed that although individual interests should be subordinated to agency interest, workers should be allowed to think through and implement plans and should be adequately remunerated for their services. Fayol encouraged development of group harmony through equal treatment and stability of tenure of personnel. A firm believer in order, he advocated "a place for everything and everything in its place." He also urged that management be taught in the colleges (Fayol, 1925).

Weber

Max Weber (1864-1920), a German sociologist, earned the title of "father of organization theory" by his conceptualization of bureaucracy with emphasis on rules instead of individuals and on competence over favoritism as the most efficient basis for organization. He conceptualized a structure of authority that would facilitate the accomplishment of the organizational objectives. The three bases of authority, according to Weber, are (1) traditional authority, which is accepted because it seems things have always been that way, such as the rule of a king in a monarchy; (2) charisma, typified by Abraham Lincoln and Otto von Bismarck; and (3) rational, legal authority, which is considered rational in formal organizations because the person has demonstrated the knowledge, skill, and ability to fulfill the position. Weber recognized that if subordinates do not believe a person is qualified for the position, they may not accept that person's authority.

Favoring a rational, legal basis for authority, he suggested the avoidance of traditional and charismatic leadership through systematic selection of personnel. Administrators are chosen for their competence; their authority is clearly defined; they are given legal means for exercising their authority; and continuity of administration is provided. In Weber's bureaucracy administrators are appointed, not elected. They are career officials who work for fixed salaries and do not own what they administer. Like other personnel, they are subject to strict rules that are applied impersonally and uniformly. All personnel are selected for competence; the division of labor, authority, and responsibility is clearly defined; and positions are organized into a hierarchy.

Mooney

Working independently of Fayol and Weber, James Mooney (1884-1957) formed similar ideas. Mooney believed management to be the technique of directing people and organization the technique of relating functions. Organization is management's responsibility. Mooney enumerated four universal principles of organization: (1) coordination and synchronization of activities for the accomplishment of a goal can be accomplished in part through (2) functional effects, the performance of one's job description, and (3) scalar process organizes (4) authority into a hierarchy. Consequently, people get their right to command from their position in the organization (Mooney and Reiley, 1931, 1939).

Urwick

Lyndall Urwick (1891-1939) integrated the ideas of Fayol and Mooney with those of Taylor. His conceptual framework blended scientific management and classic organization theory into the beginnings of classic management theory. He described the managerial process as planning, coordinating, and controlling, and he popularized concepts such as the balance of authority with responsibility, span of control, unity of command, use of general and special staffs, the proper use of personnel, delegation, and departmentalization.

HUMAN RELATIONS

"There is something that is much more scarce, something finer far, something rarer than ability. It is the ability to recognize ability." —Anonymous

The human relations movement began in the 1940s with attention focused on the effect individuals have on the success or failure of an organization. Classic organization and management theory concentrates on the physical environment and fails to analyze the human element; human relations theory stresses the social environment. The chief concerns of the human relations movement are individuals, group process, interpersonal relations, leadership, and communication. Instead of concentrating on the organization's structure, managers encourage workers to develop their potential and help them meet their needs for recognition, accomplishment, and sense of belonging.

Barnard

Chester Barnard (1886-1961) studied the functions of the executive while he was a manager for the New Jersey Bell Telephone system.

Barnard saw the manager's responsibilities as defining objectives, acquiring resources, and coordinating activities. Stressing the importance of cooperation between management and labor, he noted that the degree of cooperation depends on nonfinancial inducements, which informal organization can help provide. Formal channels of communication must be known and should be as short as possible. Barnard said authority depends on acceptance by the followers, and he stressed the role of informal organizations for aiding communication, meeting individuals' needs, and maintaining cohesiveness. Because small units are the building blocks for complex organizations, the worker contributes to the large organization, as well as the basic work unit. Barnard's work, which was done at the end of the classic period before human relations were emphasized, influenced the development of a behavioral focus (Barnard, 1938, 1940).

Follett

In the 1920s Mary Follett (1868-1933) stressed the importance of coordinating the psychological and sociological aspects of management. Perceiving the organization as a social system and management as a social process, she considered subordination offensive. Follett distinguished between power with others and power over others and indicated that legitimate power is produced by a circular behavior whereby superiors and subordinates mutually influence one another. The law of the situation dictates that a person does not take orders from another person but from the situation. For instance, nurses will work through their lunch break during an emergency. The problem with this idea is that it is difficult for workers to know the total situation. Follett advocated that managers study the total situation to achieve unity because she believed that control would be obtained through cooperation among all of the elements, people, and materials. Her work was a link between the classic and human relations eras (Follett, 1949).

The Hawthorne Studies

The Hawthorne studies, although criticized for poor research methods, stimulated considerable interest in human problems on the job. Conducted at the Chicago Hawthorne plant of Western Electric by researchers from Harvard University under the direction of the psychologist Elton Mayo (1880-1949) and reported by the sociologist Fritz Rothlesberger, the studies investigated the effects of changes in illumination on productivity. Lighting was changed for the experimental group but remained constant for the control group. As the illumination was increased for the experimental group, the production of both groups increased. When it was decreased for the experimental group, production continued to increase for both groups until the level of illumination reached moonlight, at which point there was a significant decrease in output. The researchers concluded that lighting had little effect on production. The effects of the number and length of work breaks, refreshments, length of workdays and workweeks, temperature, and humidity were observed on five volunteers with little or no effects shown. A group piecework incentive plan was studied. The researchers anticipated that fast workers would pressure slow workers to increase their output. However, they found that group norms were set and workers were pressured not to be rate busters by overproducing or chiselers by underproducing. Workers slacked off when it became apparent that they could meet the rate for the day. Work norms obviously had more influence than wage incentive plans. The Hawthorne studies gave the human relations movement its thrust.

Lewin

In the early 1930s Kurt Lewin (1890-1947), a Jewish psychologist, fled from Germany to the United States, where he revived the study of group dynamics. Lewin maintained that groups have personalities of their own: composites of the members' personalities. He showed that group forces can overcome individual interests. He confirmed the importance of group control over output and coined the terms *life space, space of free movement,* and *field forces* to describe group pressures on individuals.

Lewin advocated democratic supervision. His research indicated that democratic groups in which participants solve their own problems and have the opportunity to consult with the leader are most effective. Autocratic leadership, on the other hand, tends to promote hostility and aggression or apathy and to decrease initiative. Conducting experiments during World War II to change people's eating habits to consumption of more organ meats, he found that only 3% of the women who attended lectures (autocratic method) changed their behavior, but 32% of the women who participated in a discussion after the lecture (democratic method) started eating more organ meats. Lewin was one of the first to apply Gestalt psychology to the study of individual personality (Lewin, 1951).

Moreno

Jacob Moreno (1892-1974) developed sociometry to analyze group behavior. Claiming that people are attracted to, repulsed by, or indifferent toward others, he developed the sociogram to chart pairings and rankings of preferences for others. This process of classification can be used to calculate which workers are capable of harmonious interpersonal relationships. With this knowledge, work groups can be organized with a predicted minimum of disruptive tendencies for maximal efficiency and for promotion of high morale. Moreno also contributed to psychodrama (individual therapy), sociodrama (related to social and cultural roles), and role-playing techniques for the analysis of interpersonal relations.

BEHAVIORAL SCIENCE

During the 1950s advocates of the behavioral sciences became concerned that much scientific, classic, and human relations management theory had been accepted without scientific validation. Behavioral science emphasizes the use of scientific procedures to study the psychological, sociological, and anthropological aspects of human behavior in organizations. Behavioral scientists indicate that management is not strictly a technical process, that it cannot be haphazard, and that it should not be executed through authority. Rather, they stress the importance of maintaining a positive attitude toward people, training managers, fitting supervisory action to the situation, meeting employees' needs, promoting employees' sense of achievement, and obtaining commitment through participation in planning and decision making.

Maslow

Abraham Maslow (1908-1970) initiated the human behavioral school in 1943 with his development of a hierarchy-of-needs theory. He outlined a hierarchical structure for human needs classified into five categories: (1) physiological, (2) safety, (3) belonging, (4) esteem, and (5) self-actualization. The physiological needs are the most important and the most necessary for survival. They include the needs for oxygen, water, food, sleep, sex, and activity. Safety includes freedom from various kinds of danger, threat, and deprivation, such as physical harm, economic distress, ill health, and unnecessary, unexpected occurrences. Belonging needs are composed of affectionate relations with others, acceptance by one's peers, recognition as a group member, and companionship. Esteem comprises self-respect, positive self-evaluation, and regard by others. Self-actualization is composed of self-fulfillment and achievement of one's full capacity. In Maslow's hierarchy physical needs must be met before other needs become prepotent and so on, and the satisfaction of self-actualization needs is possible only after all other needs are met. Once a need is satisfied, it is no longer a motivator and the next need becomes prepotent. As a need begins to be satisfied, it decreases in importance as a motivator in relation to other needs, some of which are never completely satisfied and never completely cease to motivate.

Maslow's work has been very influential in management and has stimulated subsequent research. Although Maslow's outline is correct in general, human needs are more complex than a simple listing would indicate. Because no two people are alike, needs vary in type and intensity from one person to another. People differ in the amount of gratification needed before the next goal becomes prepotent. For example, some people do well with 6 hours of sleep per day, but others need 10 hours to function. Varying degrees of importance may be placed on the needs dependent on cultural and individual differences. One person may desire recognition, whereas a sense of belonging to a group may be more important to someone else. People do tend to attach importance to what they do not have. It is socially more acceptable to request that physical needs be met than that social or psychological goals receive attention. The process of motivation is complicated by the fact that one's needs change. When one accepts a job, the pay, work hours, and geographical location may be prepotent. Soon after, the social needs and need for achievement and recognition may become prepotent. People also meet their needs in different ways. Some people may get recognition for the quantity and quality of work they produce, whereas others may get even more attention through negative behavior such as inferior work and tardiness. There are some situations that seem to defy Maslow's theory. Although most of us will eat if we are hungry, some people fast to achieve higher-level needs. Maslow's work marked the beginning of behavioral science. Much subsequent work has been based on his theory (Maslow, 1970).

Herzberg

Frederick Herzberg (1923-2000) and his colleagues used the critical-incident method in 1959 to interview 200 Pittsburgh-area engineers and accountants about job situations that they had found satisfying or dissatisfying. The stories were analyzed according to content and classified according to the job factors each contained. The researchers found that job factors in situations associated with satisfaction were different from job factors in situations associated with dissatisfaction. The motivators or satisfiers identified were achievement, recognition, work itself, responsibility, advancement, and the potential for growth. These job-content factors (factors in the job) can raise the level of performance and meet the higher-order needs. In Maslow's hierarchy-of-needs model, the hygiene factors or dissatisfiers identified were supervision; company policy; working conditions; interpersonal relations with superiors, peers, and subordinates; status; job security; and effect on one's personal life. These job-context factors (surrounding environmental factors) cannot motivate but can lower performance and cause job dissatisfaction. They meet lower-order needs in Maslow's model.

Herzberg's theory is very controversial and has stimulated considerable research, some of which supports the theory and some of which does not. His work has been the subject of much criticism. He studied only two jobs and used only one measure of job attitude. No validity or reliability data were reported. Statements of critical incidents were subject to memory loss and selective perception. The mere fact that one is more likely to blame others than oneself when asked about an unpleasant experience but is willing to assume the responsibility when something good happens could explain Herzberg's findings. No observations or measurement of job behavior were taken. Wrong categories could be identified, and the highly subjective stories could be misclassified. Herzberg did, however, develop a taxonomy of job situations based on research that has contributed to a better understanding of human motivation. His work complements Maslow's (Herzberg, 1959, 1977). (See Figures 4-2 and 4-3.)

McGregor

Douglas McGregor (1932-) developed the managerial implications of Maslow's theory. He notes that one's style of management depends on one's philosophy of humans and categorizes those assumptions as Theory X and Theory Y. In Theory X the manager's emphasis is on the goal of the organization. The theory assumes that people dislike work and will avoid it; consequently, workers must be directed, controlled, coerced, and threatened so that organizational goals can be met. According to Theory X, most people want to be directed and to avoid responsibility because they have little ambition. They desire security. Managers who accept the assumptions of Theory X will do the thinking and planning with little input from staff associates. They will delegate little, supervise closely, and motivate workers through fear and threats, failing to make use of their potentials.

In Theory Y the emphasis is on the goal of the individual. It is the manager's assumption that people do not inherently dislike work and that work can be a source of satisfaction. Theory Y managers assume that workers have the self-direction and self-control necessary for meeting their objectives and will respond to rewards for the accomplishment of those goals. They believe that under favorable conditions people seek responsibility and display imagination, ingenuity, and creativity. According to Theory Y, human potentials are only partially used. Managers who believe the assumptions of Theory Y will allow participation. They will delegate, give general rather than close supervision, support job enlargement, and use positive incentives such as praise and recognition.

McGregor suggests that when people are unable to satisfy their higher-level needs, they experience personal frustrations resulting in negative behaviors. Some managers have responded to the consequences of the personal frustration with punitive measures without determining the cause. Managers with a human relations orientation have made working conditions pleasant and have provided rewards unrelated to job performance. McGregor believes that both approaches are ineffective and recommends that the work situation be structured so that workers can meet their personal goals while working toward the goals of the organization. He suggests collaboration between the manager and the worker for integration of goals. Table 7-5 shows the relationships among the Maslow, Herzberg, and McGregor theories (McGregor, 1960).

Ouchi, Pascale, and Athos

William Ouchi published Theory Z: *How American Business Can Meet the Japanese Challenge* in 1981. Richard Pascale and Anthony Athos gave a more extensive discussion of *The Art of Japanese Management: Applications for American Executives* in 1981. Ouchi contrasts Japanese organizations with organizations in the United States. The Japanese organizations have "lifetime employment; slow evaluation and promotion; nonspecialized career paths; implicit control mechanisms; collective decision making; collective responsibility; and wholistic concern," whereas the organizations in the United States have "short-term employment; rapid evaluation and promotion; specialized career paths; explicit control mechanisms; individual decision making; individual responsibility; and segmented concern" (pp. 48-49). Pascale and Athos explain that organizations in the United States tend to favor strategy, structure, and systems, whereas the Japanese organizations focus on staff, skills, style, and superordinate goals (Ouchi, 1981; Pascale and Athos, 1981).

TABLE **7-5** Relationships Among the Maslow, Herzberg, and McGregor Theories

MASLOW	HERZBERG	McGREGOR
Physiological needs		
Safety needs	Hygiene	Theory X
Belonging needs	factors	
Esteem needs	Motivators	Theory Y
Self-actualization needs		

Modified from Kelly J: *Organizational behaviour*, rev ed, Homewood, Ill, 1980, Irwin, p. 220. © by Richard D. Irwin.

Argyris

Chris Argyris (1923-), focusing his research on the coexistence of personal and organizational needs, found that individuals give priority to meeting their own needs. He found that the greater the disparity between individual and organizational needs, the more tension, conflict, dissatisfaction, and subversion result. Argyris recommends that leaders help workers achieve self-actualization by implementing a Theory Y philosophy and maintains that this will help one's personality to grow from passivity and dependence to activity and independence. Incongruency between the mature personality and management based on classic principles makes workers subordinate, dependent, and passive, thereby causing psychological failure and job dissatisfaction. Managers can make jobs more meaningful by taking advantage of people's talents and letting them participate in planning, goal setting, and problem solving (Argyris, 1953, 1957, 1964, 1993; Argyris, Putnam, and Smith, 1985; Argyris and Schon, 1978).

Likert

Rensis Likert's (1903-1981) theory of management is based on his work at the University of Michigan's Institute for Social Research. He identified three types of variables in organizations: (1) causal, (2) intervening, and (3) end result. The causal variables include leadership behavior, organizational structure, policies, and controls. Intervening variables are perceptions, attitudes, and motivations. The end-result variables are measures of profits, costs, and productivity. Likert believed that managers may act in ways harmful to the organization because they evaluate end results to the exclusion of intervening variables. Consequently, he developed a Likert scale questionnaire that includes measures of causal and intervening variables. The Likert scale measures several factors related to leadership behavior process, motivation, managerial influence, communication, decision-making processes, goal setting, and staff development.

Likert also identified four types of management systems: (1) exploitative-authoritative, (2) benevolent-authoritative, (3) consultative, and (4) participative group. He associated the first system with the least effective performance. Managers show little confidence in staff associates and ignore their ideas. Consequently, staff associates do not feel free to discuss their jobs with their managers. Responsibility for the organization's goals is at the top; goals are established through orders. What little communication is used is directed downward, is often inaccurate, and is accepted with suspicion. Although managers do not know about their staff associates' problems, they make decisions without input from below. Policing and punishment are used as control functions by top administration. Allowed no input, the workers strongly resist the organization's goals and develop an informal organization of their own.

In the benevolent-authoritative system, the second type of system, the manager is condescending to staff associates. Staff associates' ideas are sometimes sought, but they do not feel very free to discuss their jobs with their manager. Top management and middle management are responsible for setting goals. There is little communication, and it is mostly directed downward after being censored by the manager and is received with some suspicion. Decisions are made at the top with some delegation. Managers do have some knowledge of the staff associates' situation, and staff associates are occasionally consulted for problem solving. Goals are established through orders with some comment invited and moderate resistance received. Rewards and punishment are used as control functions by top administration. There is usually an informal organization resisting the formal one.

In the third system, the consultative system, the manager has substantial confidence in staff associates. Their ideas are usually sought, and they feel free to discuss their work with the manager. Responsibility for setting goals is fairly general. Although there is considerable communication, both upward and downward, it has limited accuracy and is accepted with some caution. Managers are quite familiar with the problems faced by their staff associates. Broad policy is set at the top with delegation; goals are set after discussion; and there is decision making throughout the organization. Control functions are delegated to lower levels, where reward and self-guidance are used. Sometimes an informal organization resists the formal goals.

Participative management, the fourth system, is associated with the most effective performance. Managers have complete confidence in their staff associates. Staff associates' ideas are always sought, and they feel completely free to discuss their jobs with the manager. Goals are set at all levels. There is a great deal of communication—upward, downward, and sideways—that is accurate and received with an open mind. Managers are very well informed about the problems faced by their staff associates, and the decision making is well integrated throughout the organization with full involvement of staff associates. Because goals are established through group action, there is little or no resistance to them. There is not an informal organization resisting the goals of the formal organization, because the goals of both are the same. Control is widely shared through the use of self-guidance and problem solving.

Likert was a strong proponent of participative management and supportive relationships. His linking-pin concept is based on studies about the differences between good and poor managers as measured by their level of productivity. Good managers were found to have more influence on their own managers than did poor managers, and their managerial procedures were better received by their staff associates. Consequently, Likert suggested that managers form groups for supportive relationships and that those groups be linked by overlapping groups of managers. This facilitates three-way communications—upward, downward, and sideways. When middle

managers have the opportunity for interaction with their manager, workers can have input, and there is a chance for the individual's and the organization's goals to become similar (Figure 7-2) (Likert, 1961).

Blake and Mouton

Robert Blake (1918-) and Jane Mouton (1930-) maintain that there are two critical dimensions of leadership: (1) concern for people and (2) concern for production. They depict these on a 9×9 or 81-square managerial grid (Figure 7-3). The two dimensions are independent, so a manager can be high on both, low on both, or high on one and low on the other. The vertical axis represents the manager's concern for people, and the horizontal axis represents concern for production. Each axis is on a 1 to 9 scale, from a minimal concern for people or production to a maximal concern. The five basic styles are located at each corner and in the middle.

The task manager at 9,1 has the highest regard for production and the lowest concern for people. This manager stresses operating efficiency through controls and views people as tools of production. Workers are paid to do what they are told without questioning.

As reflected on the grid, 1,1 management is impoverished. The manager has a lack of concern for both production and people. This style may be found in some managers who feel they have been repeatedly denied promotion or otherwise mistreated and who have consequently compensated through a low level of involvement with their jobs. The organization man management at 5,5 represents a moderate concern for both people and production but not necessarily at the same time. The manager's emphasis shifts. The country club manager, 1,9, is thoughtful and friendly but has little concern for production.

Blake and Mouton consider team management, 9,9, the optimal managerial style. These managers integrate their concern for people and production. Problems are confronted directly,

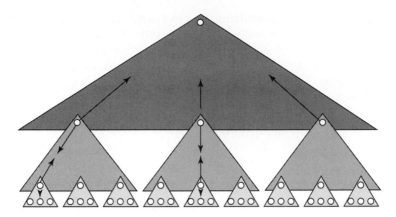

Figure 7-2 Linking-pin concept. Arrows indicate linking-pin function. (From Likert R, Likert JG: *New ways of managing conflict,* New York, 1976, McGraw-Hill.)

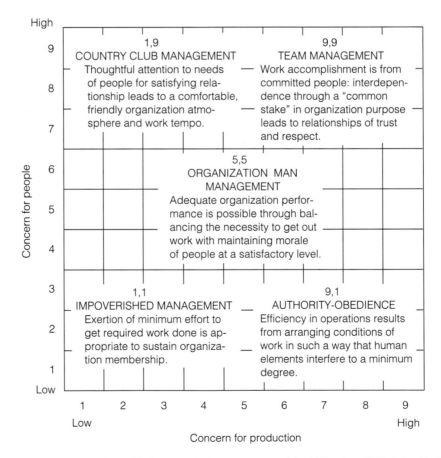

Figure 7-3 Managerial grid. (From Blake RR, Mouton JS: *The new managerial grid,* Houston, 1978, Scientific Methods, Inc.)

and mutual trust, respect, and interdependence are fostered (Blake and Mouton, 1978).

Fiedler

During the 1960s Fred Fiedler (1922-) introduced the contingency model of leadership effectiveness. He identified three important dimensions of a situation for his contingency model: (1) leader-member relations, (2) task structure, and (3) position power. Leader-member relations are related to the amount of confidence and loyalty followers have in their leader. Task structure is related to the number of correct solutions to a problem. Position power depends on the amount of organizational support available to the leader (Fiedler, 1967; Fiedler and Chemers, 1974; Fiedler, Chemers, and Mahar, 1976).

Hersey and Blanchard

Paul Hersey (1930-) and Kenneth Blanchard (1939-) extended the work of Blake, Mouton, and Fiedler by considering the maturity of the followers in more detail. As the maturity of one's followers increases, the leadership style requires less structure and emotional support. Groups with below-average maturity function best under leaders with high task–low relationship orientations. Groups with average maturity function best under leaders with high task–high relationship or high relationship–low task orientations. The most effective leadership style depends on the maturity of the group (Hersey, 1984; Hersey and Blanchard, 1969, 1982; Hersey and Duldt, 1989).

Drucker

In his prolific writings about management, Peter Drucker (1909-) maintains that the only way for management to justify its existence is through economic results. However, he recognizes noneconomic consequences of managerial decisions, such as job satisfaction, as by-products of the focus on economic performance. He identifies three areas of management: (1) managing a business, (2) managing managers, and (3) managing workers. Activity, decision, and relations analyses are recommended to determine the structure and organization needed. Drucker has studied the advantages and disadvantages of decentralization, supports decentralization, and says managers should create markets and products rather than being passive.

Drucker introduced management by objectives as a way to manage managers. Relying on self-control instead of control from above, managers are directed by objectives of performance rather than by their manager. For management by objectives, the manager develops the framework, and the staff associate supplies the goals, which are agreed on by both. The staff associate gives progress reports to the manager. Objectives are developed for every level of management in the hierarchy and each unit in the organization. The manager checks objectives for compatibility with other units and contribution to the objectives at the next level of the hierarchy. Drucker maintains that it is more productive for workers to set their own norms and measure their own performance than for minimal standards to be set.

For managing the worker, Drucker recommends that jobs be designed to fit the worker, that workers be given more control over their jobs, and that the worker be considered the most vital resource in the agency. For decades Drucker has been one of the leading thinkers about the study and practice of management through his landmark articles in *Harvard Business Review* and numerous books. He has stressed the importance of managing for the future. He believes it is pointless to predict the future, that the future has already happened, and that we should identify major events that have occurred and identify the predictable effects, such as demographics including the overpopulation of the world with increasing underpopulation of the developed countries. By the late 1990s he was indicating the importance of managing society's knowledge resources. Selections of management works by Peter F. Drucker are published in *The Essential Drucker: Selections From the Management Works of Peter F. Drucker* (2001). See also Drucker (1964, 1974, 1980, 1985, 1986, 1992, 1995, 1998).

Odiorne

George Odiorne (1920-1992), director of the Bureau of Industrial Relations of the University of Michigan, was previously assistant director of personnel for General Mills, Inc., where he pioneered the installation of a management-by-objectives system. He advocated effective management through personal and agency goals and had written about the executive's responsibilities for implementing a management-by-objectives system. He also recommended training by objectives as an economic strategy for management training (Odiorne, 1965).

Peters

Tom Peters has been provocative during the 1980s and 1990s through seminars and several books. In the book *In Search of Excellence,* he and Robert Waterman (1982) stressed the importance of managing ambiguity and paradox, having a bias for action to get things done, remaining close to the customer to know his or her needs and anticipate wants, fostering autonomy and entrepreneurship, reinforcing shared values by celebrating heroes, getting productivity through people, demonstrating values through direct interventions, keeping to what you know instead of widely diversifying, keeping a simple form and lean staff, and maintaining simultaneous loose-tight properties. In 1985 he and Nancy Austin stressed the importance of having a passion and searching for excellence through team-based innovations in *A Passion for Excellence.* In 1987 he did a handbook for management of revolution, *Thriving on Chaos.* He did a guide to economic excellence, *Liberation Management,* in 1992. *The Tom Peters Seminar* (1994) presented the slides and lecture content from a typical 2-day seminar. In *The Circle of Innovation* (1997) Peters continued to discuss how the obsessed transformational leader lives life out loud and presents current trends.

Kotter

John Kotter has reported his research about topics related to leadership in a number of books, including but not limited to *The General Managers* (1982), *Power and Influence* (1985), *The Leadership Factor* (1988), *A Force for Change* (1990), *Leading Change* (1996), and *The Heart of Change: Real-Life Stories of How People Change Their Organizations* (2002). The research is primarily about traits, management, and transactional issues.

TRANSFORMATIONAL LEADERSHIP

Transformational leadership became popular during the 1980s and 1990s with stress on the need for leadership versus management, the importance of values, and a commitment to service.

Bass

In *Leadership and Performance Beyond Expectations* (1985) Bernard Bass identifies the need for charisma, inspirational leadership, individualized consideration, and intellectual stimulation to have transformational leadership instead of just transactional or a contingent reinforcement leadership. In *Transformational Leadership: Industry, Military, and Educational Impact* (1998) Bass indicates that women are more inclined to transformational leadership than men.

Bennis and Nanus

Warren Bennis has stressed the importance of leading rather than just managing. In *Leaders: The Strategies for Taking Charge* (1985), he and Burt Nanus lead a paradigm shift to transformative leadership. They discuss the need to manage oneself to lead others, attention through vision, meaning through communication, trust through positioning, deployment of self, and empowerment. In his second report based on his study of leadership, *On Becoming a Leader* (1989), Bennis describes how people become leaders, how they lead, and how organizations can encourage or stifle leaders. He and Joan Goldsmith did a workbook on becoming a leader and published it as *Learning to Lead: A Workbook on Becoming a Leader* (1997). In *Organizing Genius* (1997) Bennis tells the stories of seven groups and concludes by describing the characteristics of great groups. In *The Leader's Edge* (1989) Nanus discusses four conceptual skills: (1) farsightedness, (2) mastery of interdependence, (3) anticipatory learning, and (4) high integrity; four roles: (1) direction setter, (2) change agent, (3) spokesperson, and (4) coach; and three action skills: (1) organization design, (2) initiative, and (3) mastery of change.

Kouzes and Posner

In *The Leadership Challenge: How to Get Extra-ordinary Things Done in Organizations,* James Kouzes and Barry Posner (1987, 1990) identify five practices and 10 behaviors to implement those practices: (1) challenging the process by searching for opportunities by (a) confronting and changing the status quo and (b) experimenting and taking risks and learning from mistakes and successes; (2) inspiring a shared vision by (a) envisioning the future through imagining ideal scenarios and (b) enlisting others by attracting people to common purposes; (3) enabling others to act by (a) getting people to work together through collaboration and (b) sharing power and information to strengthen others; (4) modeling the way by (a) leading by example and doing and (b) building commitment to action through small wins; and (5) encouraging the heart by (a) linking rewards with perform-ance and recognizing contributions and (b) cele-brating accomplishments. In *Credibility* (1993) they identify credibility as the cornerstone of leadership and discuss how leaders encourage initiative, risk taking, and productivity through trust in people and by using principles rather than positions to manage conflict. They elaborate on seven essentials of encouragement: (1) setting clear standards, (2) expecting the best, (3) paying attention, (4) personalizing recognition, (5) telling the story, (6) celebrating together, and (7) setting the example in *Encouraging the Heart* (1999).

Tichy

Noel Tichy and Stratford Sherman present *Control Your Destiny or Someone Else Will* (1993) as a three-act play: (1) the awakening, (2) the vision, and (3) revolution as a way of life. Tichy and Mary Anne Devanna think that transformational leaders would control the quality of life inside and outside the workplace. In *The Transformational Leader* (1986, 1997) they too present corporate transformation as a three-act drama: (1) recog-nizing the need for revitalization, (2) creating a new vision, and (3) institutionalizing change. In *The Leadership Engine* (1997) Tichy and Eli Cohen stress the importance of developing leaders at all levels and the necessity of quantum transforma-tion, not just incremental quality improvement. In *The Cycle of Leadership: How Great Leaders Teach Their Companies to Win* (2002) Tichy and Nancy Cardwell indicate good leaders teach and great leaders learn.

Blanchard

Ken Blanchard has written numerous books during the 1980s and 1990s. In *Raving Fans* (1993). Blanchard and Sheldon Bowles identified the three steps to a revolutionary approach to customer service as (1) deciding what you want, (2) discovering what the customer wants, and (3) delivering plus one In *Gung Ho!* (1998) he and Sheldon Bowles report lessons learned by observing the worthwhile work of squirrels, the control of achieving the goal by beavers, and how the geese cheer each other on. In *The Heart of a Leader* (1999), Blanchard has collected many inspirational passages. *High Five: The Magic of Working Together* is a parable by Blanchard, Bowles, Carew, et al (2001) that demonstrates why teams are important and what organiza-tions can do to build successful ones. Blanchard, Lacinak, Tompkins, et al tell how the technique of accentuating the positive used to train killer whales at SeaWorld can also be used on people in organizations in *Whale Done* (2002). Blanchard and S. Truett Cathy discuss the joy of giving time, talent, and treasures in *The Generosity Factor* (2002).

Anderson and Collins

Terry D. Anderson (1998) provides a sophisticated discussion about equipping oneself and coaching others to build the leadership organization in *Transforming Leadership: Equipping Yourself and Coaching Others to Build the Leadership Organization.*

Jim Collins (2001) has developed a model for level 5 leadership to make the leap from *Good to Great: Why Some Companies Make the Leap . . . and Others Don't.*

SERVANT LEADERSHIP
Greenleaf and Others

Robert Greenleaf wrote *Servant Leadership* (1977, 1991). He conceptualized the idea of the servant as leader from Hermann Hesse's *The Journey to the East* (1956), in which the servant who does the menial chores also sustained the party's spirits through his extraordinary presence. When the servant left the group, the group fell into disarray and the journey was abandoned. Servant leadership puts serving first, takes a holistic approach, shares decision making, and builds community. Larry Spears has identified 10 characteristics of the servant-leader by studying Greenleaf's work: (1) listening, (2) empathy, (3) healing, (4) awareness, (5) persuasion, (6) conceptualization, (7) foresight, (8) stewardship, (9) commitment to the growth of people, and (10) building community. Spears has edited the following anthologies about servant leadership: *Reflections on Leadership: How Robert K. Greenleaf's Theory on Servant Leadership Influenced Today's Top Management Thinkers* (1995), *Insights on Leadership: Service, Stewardship, Spirit, and Servant Leadership* (1998), *The Power of Servant Leadership* (1998), and *Focus on Leadership: Servant-Leadership for the 21st Century* (2002).

Max DePree, author of *Leadership is an Art* (1989) and *Leadership Jazz* (1992), and *Leading Without Power: Finding Hope in Serving Community* (1997), has been influenced by Greenleaf. He stresses the importance of connecting one's voice and one's touch. The personal transformation can be related to Parker Palmer's works *The Courage to Teach: Exploring the Inner Landscape of a Teacher's Life* (1998) and *To Know as We Are Known/a Spirituality of Education* (1983). He believes that good teaching comes from the identity and integrity of the teacher, not just from good technique, and that inner work can help create communities of learning.

M. Scott Peck addresses the new psychology of love, traditional values, and spiritual growth in *The Road Less Traveled* (1978). Ann McGee-Cooper, D. Trammel, and B. Lau describe a program to bring joy, energy, and balance back into one's life in *You Don't Have to Go Home From Work Exhausted* (1990, 1992). Peter Vaill believes that executive development is spiritual development and uses a metaphor, *Managing as a Performing Art* (1989), to discuss his ideas.

Peter Block wrote *The Empowered Manager: Positive Political Skills at Work* (1987) but found that the rhetoric about visionary leadership, customer-driven service, and quality improvement addresses only cosmetic changes. Then he wrote *Stewardship: Choosing Service Over Self-Interest* (1993). Stewards hold themselves responsible and accountable. They lead by serving. He discusses how acting on what matters, the relationships, is important in *The Answer to How is Yes: Acting on What Matters* (2000).

Stephen Covey's books *The 7 Habits of Highly Effective People* (1989), *Principle-Centered Leadership* (1990), and *First Things First* (Covey, Merrill, and Merrill, 1994) teach how to managing relationships instead of just managing time around priorities. Joseph Jaworski describes his personal transformation in *Synchronicity: The Inner Path of Leadership* (Jaworski and Flowers, 1996, 1998).

Elizabeth Jeffries describes leadership from the inside out in *The Heart of Leadership: Influencing by Design* (1993). Calvin Miller tells the 10 keys to servant leadership in a religious book, *The Empowered Leader: 10 Keys to Servant Leadership* (1995). Stacy T. Rinehart tells about the paradox of servant leadership in a religious book, *Upside Down: The Paradox of Servant Leadership* (1998). Tom Chappell discusses seven intentions of values-centered leadership in *Managing Upside Down: The Seven Intentions of Values-Centered Leadership* (1999). Russ S. Moxley weaves together spirit and leadership in *Leadership and Spirit: Breathing New Vitality and Energy Into Individuals and Organizations* (2000). Randolph A. Pohlman and Gareth S. Gardiner present value-driven management as a comprehensive philosophy of management in *Value Driven Management: How to Create and Maximize Value Over Time for Organizational Success* (2000). Ann McGee-Cooper and Gary Looper provide a sophisticated discussion of the development of servant-leaders in *The Essentials of Servant-Leadership: Principles in Practice* (2001). Peter G. Northouse discusses transformational leadership with other leadership theories in *Leadership: Theory and Practice,* ed 2 (2001). James A. Autry gives powerful examples of how to build a creative team, develop great morale, and improve bottom-line performance in *The Servant Leader* (2001).

LEARNING ORGANIZATIONS
Senge and Others

Peter Senge discusses five disciplines—(1) systems thinking, (2) personal mastery, (3) mental models, (4) shared vision, and (5) team learning—in his book *The Fifth Discipline: The Art and Practice of the Learning Organization* (1990), and he discusses tools and strategies to build a learning organization in *The Fifth Discipline Fieldbook* (Senge, Kleiner, Roberts, et al, 1994). They address participation as a basis of learning to prevent organizational learning disabilities instead of participation as an entitlement.

Senge's beliefs about systems thinking have been influenced by many people and books. In *Belonging to the Universe* Fritjol Capra, David Steindl-Rast, and Thomas Matus (1991) explain changes from seeing things as structures to seeing them as processes, from linear thinking to systems thinking. For example, a tree is not just a structure. It is a photosynthesis process that unites sun and earth. Margaret Wheatley (1992) observes nature and concludes in *Leadership and the New Science* that everything is a bundle of potentiality and that order emerges from chaos. Wheatley and Myron Keller-Rogers use pictures, poetry, and narrative to look for patterns in nature, learn, and seek meaning. They recommend playfulness in *A Simpler Way* (1996). Now the new science describes the nature of people's lives better than mechanical models.

David Meadows, Dennis Meadows, and Jorgen Randers indicate the global limits have already been exceeded in some areas in *Beyond the Limits* (1992). So it does not make sense to continue toward the same kind of growth. In *The Breakthrough Strategy* (1988) Robert Schaffer recommends a simple and direct approach to small, tangible steps toward strategic breakthroughs, looking for projects that do not take additional resources, and choosing indicators that show results within a few months.

There are a number of books about simulations, use of computer technology, and mapping techniques. In *Improving Performance* Geary Rummler and Allen Brache (1995) address improving process relationships to form a link between individuals and the organization strategy. The book is a practical guide for a holistic view of the organizational skeleton, process levels, and interdependencies. Christopher Meyer indicates that *Fast Cycle Time* (1993) is achieved by aligning the organization to learn faster rather than merely work faster. Sometimes we have to slow down to speed up. In *Creating the Corporate Future: Plan or Be Planned For,* Russell Ackoff (1981) describes interactive planning as a participative systems approach to corporate development.

The Path of Least Resistance (1989) and *Creating* (1991), both by Robert Fritz, provide exercises and ideas for developing personal mastery and creativity. Argyris influenced thought on mental models and has been studying learning in organizations for a long time. He has published *Organizational Learning: A Theory of Action Perspective* (Argyris and Schon, 1978), *Action Science* (Argyris, Putnam, and Smith, 1985), *Knowledge for Action* (1993), and *On Organizational Learning,* ed 2 (1999) among other books. Edgar Schein describes how culture emerges and changes through birth and early growth, midlife, maturity, and possibly destruction in *Organizational Culture and Leadership* (1985, 1997).

In *Creating Shared Vision* Marjorie Parker (1990) tells a story of how a Norwegian aluminum company had each employee sketch his or her personal vision of the organization and link it with other images. The vision statement was a garden mural with each plant having metaphorical meaning.

Team learning is influenced by conversations. *The Abilene Paradox* by Jerry Harvey (1988) is a metaphor of how groups can agree to take action that contradicts individual members' beliefs of what is right and end up where no one wanted to go. *You Just Don't Understand: Women and Men in Conversation* by Deborah Tannen (1990) addresses the differing communication styles of men and women and was the seminal work for *Men Are From Mars, Women Are From Venus* (Gray, 1992). Men tend to be problem solvers, whereas women want to make connections.

Although Henry Sims published *The Thinking Organization: Dynamics of Organizational Social Cognition* in 1986, Senge's *The Fifth Discipline: The Art and Practice of the Learning Organization* (1990) was the path-breaking book on learning organizations. The book is based on science, psychology, and spiritual wisdom. The field book contains success stories, essays, ideas, and exercises for individuals and teams.

Leading the Learning Organization (2000) by Alan T. Belasen is a sophisticated discussion about communication and competencies for managing change. *Building Leaders: How Successful Companies Develop the Next Generation* (1999) by Jay A. Conger and Beth Benjamin is about how to develop the next generation of leaders.

EMOTIONAL INTELLIGENCE
Goleman and Others

Daniel Goleman's *Working With Emotional Intelligence* (1998) applies the concepts from his *Emotional Intelligence* (1995) in the workplace. In his emotional competence framework he identifies self-awareness, self-regulation, and motivation as important to personal competence and empathy and social skills as important to social competence. He stresses the importance of teaching emotional competence and gives guidelines for training, including how to assess the job, assess the individual, deliver assessments with care, gauge readiness, motivate, make change self-directed, focus on clear and manageable goals, prevent relapse, give performance feedback, encourage practice, arrange support, provide models, encourage, reinforce change, and evaluate. Emotional intelligence is more important than intelligence quotient (IQ) or technical expertise for success in organizations. In *Primal Leadership: Realizing the Power of Emotional Intelligence* (2002), Goleman, Boyatzis, and McKee continue to deal with the power of emotional intelligence.

In *Putting Emotional Intelligence to Work: Successful Leadership is More Than IQ*, Ryback (1998) identified the seven core qualities of successful leadership as strategic planning, communication and alignment, team building, continuous learning, dynamic accountability, systemic results, and actualized integrity. Goleman (2001) in *The Emotionally Intelligent Workplace: How to Select for, Measure, and Improve Emotional Intelligence in Individuals, Groups, and Organizations* identified leadership style for objectives and the necessary emotional intelligence competencies as (1) visionary to mobilize others to follow a vision through self-confidence, empathy, change catalyst, and visionary leadership; (2) affiliative to create harmony through empathy, building bonds, and conflict management; (3) democratic to build commitment through participation; (4) coaching to build strengths for the future through developing others, empathy, and emotional self-awareness; (5) coercive for immediate compliance to kick start a turnaround through achievement, drive, initiative, and emotional self-control; and (6) pace setting to perform tasks to a high standard through conscientiousness, achievement drive, and initiative.

In *The Handbook of Emotionally Intelligent Leadership: Inspiring Others to Achieve Results*, Feldman (1999) indicated that leaders need core skills for effective individual contribution plus higher-order skills. He identified the five core skills as (1) knowing yourself (recognizing your emotions, differentiating between emotions, knowing the reason behind the emotion), (2) maintaining control (resisting or delaying an impulse, drive, or temptation to act; controlling aggression, hostility, and irresponsible behavior; managing emotions in a flexible and adaptable way), (3) reading others (being aware of the emotions of others, appreciating the emotions of others, understanding how and why people feel and act as they do), (4) perceiving accurately (accurately assessing a situation, having clear vision, keeping a broad perspective, being objective), and (5) communicating with flexibility (having a full range of emotional expression, being authentic, addressing your needs as well as the needs of others).

Feldman identified the following higher-order skills that leaders need to make an emotional connection with others: (1) take responsibility (act independently and with accountability, own a problem as well as the solution), (2) generate choices (open self to varied possibilities, discover available choices), (3) embrace a vision (commit self to a particular view of the future, use the vision to guide actions), (4) have courage (look at choices, take responsibility, buck standard modes, make tough decisions), and (5) demonstrate resolve (make decisions about what to do with a firm determination, demonstrate to others our commitment to the plan of action.) By the late 1990s attention turned to action management, results-based leadership, and the accountability revolution.

RESULTS-BASED LEADERSHIP
Welch and Others

Under Jack Welch's leadership, GE became a benchmark for excellence. He did it in three stages: destruction, creation, and quality During the 1980s he globalized the company, especially into Europe and Japan. During the late 1980s, he introduced "work out." He had workers tell managers what was wrong and make suggestions for improvements. The goals were to build trust, empower employees, eliminate unnecessary work, and create a boundaryless culture by tearing down the walls between management and workers and between functions such as marketing and production. He started with relatively short-lived change instead of incremental change. To create the boundarylessness, he (1) listened to the people closest to the customers; (2) gave people who did the work a say in how the work could be done better; (3) lowered boundaries among vertical (hierarchical relationships), horizontal (between functions), external (suppliers and customers), and geographic (different countries) structures, realizing that not all the answers were within the company walls; and (4) implemented the best ideas no matter where they originated. He hired "A" leaders who could articulate a vision and rally workers to take responsibility to make the vision a reality. Those "A" leaders had "Four *E's*": energy, edge, energizer, and execution. He did not tolerate managers who used intimidation. He nurtured only those leaders who shared the company's vision and harnessed the power of change. He searched out confident managers who put the customer first. They used learning to build confidence, moved decision making down the hierarchy, and let employees know that their ideas were valued. They used story boards to give attention to the best practices. Welch fired 10% of the least productive workers each year. He recommended simplifying practices and procedures. Limiting the number of approvals needed and the number of pages in forms could do streamlining.

Welch met with his managers on a regular basis in a comfortable place away from e-mail and phones. He did not set a rigid agenda and kept the meetings informal. The group members had ground rules such as (1) members agreed to attend every meeting; (2) substitutes for team members were not allowed; (3) only emergencies were allowed to interrupt the meeting; (4) members were to come to meetings with their assignments completed; (5) they started on time if at least 80% of the team was there: (6) they discussed the best decision model for each decision and agreed to support the decision of the group; (7) they agreed to use data to make decisions; and

(8) they encouraged honest disagreements with respect and could use a facilitator if they needed help resolving conflict. Welch involved as many managers as possible in training and distribution of information to increase knowledge. He paid attention to globalizing the training.

In the mid-1990s, Welch started the product services focus that generated revenues and Six Sigma, an employee-driven quality movement. Quality became an issue for everyone in the organization. The six ingredients in Six Sigma were as follows: (1) a genuine focus on the customers, (2) a data-driven management, (3) a management- and improvement-focused process, (4) a proactive management, (5) boundaryless collaboration, and (6) a drive for perfection with a tolerance for failure. The four-step process included measuring, analyzing, improving, and rigorously controlling each process and trans-action once they had been improved. People learned that strategy cannot be reduced to a formula, and that long-range plans should not be followed blindly. In the late 1990s after watching his employees order Christmas presents online, Welch started the eInitiative and got the company into the e-business movement.

Recurring themes include the following: (1) leaders who live the values are more important than those who make the numbers; (2) command and control are not the best ways to run an organization; (3) ideas should rule over tradition and hierarchy; (4) involving everyone is a key to enhancing productivity; (5) developing a learning community creates a competitive enterprise; and (6) market-leading business can ensure long-term growth (Crainer, 1999; Kramer, 2001; Pande, Neuman, and Cavanaugh, 2002; Slater, 1999, 2000; Welch and Byrne, 2001).

Ulrich, Zenger, and Smallwood (1999, p. 179) outlined how a person can become a results-based leader as follows:

1. Begin with an absolute focus on results.

2. Take complete and personal responsibility for your group's results.

3. Clearly and specifically communicate expectations and targets to the people in your group.

4. Determine what you need to do personally to improve your results.

5. Use results as the litmus test for continuing or implementing leadership practice.

6. Engage in developmental activities and opportunities that will help you produce better results.

7. Know and use every group member's capabilities to the fullest, and provide everyone with appropriate developmental opportunities.

8. Experiment and innovate in every realm under your influence, looking constantly for new ways to improve performance.

9. Measure the right standards, and increase the rigor with which you measure them.

10. Constantly take action; results will not improve without it.

11. Increase the pace or tempo of your group.

12. Seek feedback from others in the organization about ways you and your group can improve your outcomes.

13. Ensure that your subordinates and colleagues perceive that your motivation for being a leader is the achievement of positive results, not personal or political gain.

14. Model the methods and strive for the results you want your group to use and attain.

They present the reasoning behind each proposed action and share ideas about implementation.

Perkins (2000, pp. vii, viii) identifies 10 strategies for leading at the edge as follows:

1. Never lose sight of the ultimate goal, and focus energy on short-term objectives.

2. Set a personal example with visible, memorable symbols and behaviors.

3. Instill optimism and self-confidence, but stay grounded in reality.

4. Take care of yourself: Maintain your stamina, and let go of guilt.

5. Reinforce the team message constantly: "We are one—we live or die together."

6. Minimize status differences, and insist on courtesy and mutual respect.

7. Master conflict—deal with anger in small doses, engage dissidents, and avoid needless power struggles.

8. Find something to celebrate and something to laugh about.

9. Be willing to take the Big Risk.

10. Never give up—there is always another move.

Redwood, Goldwasser, and Street (1999) indicate that the less communication used the more resistance received. Bossidy and Charan (2002) stress the importance of having the right people in the right place, linking strategy and operations, and linking people with both the operations and the strategies.

Buckingham and Coffman (1999) of the Gallup Organization interviewed more than 80,000 managers in more than 400 companies and found the best managers in the world seem to have little in common. However, they did seem to break every rule believed by conventional wisdom, and they turned employees' talent into performance.

Samuel (2001) identified an accountability continuum from entitlement through individual work unit, cross-functional to organizational accountability. With the entitlement attitude, employees get paid to show up regardless of performance. For individual accountability, employees take responsibility for doing their own assignments based on their job descriptions, without concern about the impact on others. They tend to be competitive and tend to give little support to others. Frustration is created from low consistency and high fragmentation. Poor utilization of resources results from little coordination.

Teams are the next stage. People on the team help each other be successful. The team is more important than any individual's success. Coordination is high within the team but not among functional areas. Therefore resources get wasted. Territorialism is high. Teams deal with the behaviors that keep the team from being successful, but decisions are made without considering the impact on the system.

For cross-functional accountability the organizational outcomes determine the composition of the team regardless of the members' functions. Many functions or departments are represented. The team achieves outcomes important to the organization. Resources are shared, and competition is minimal. Organizational accountability exemplifies the "fluid" organization that adapts to situations that arise. This type of organization works with other organizations in collaborative partnerships to improve products and services.

"Two heads are better than one." —Old adage

DIVERSITY AMONG LEADERS

DIVERSITY

Diversity should be defined in a broad and inclusive way to prevent widespread opposition. Employees should understand that everyone's diversity is valued. Diversity can affect individuals' values, perceptions of self and others, and opportunities at work. Primary dimensions include age, ethnicity, gender, mental and physical abilities, race, and sexual orientation. Secondary dimensions include communication style, education, family status, first language, geographical location, income, military experience, organizational role, religion, work experience, and work style. Organizations should value primary and secondary diversity.

At first, organizations focus on expectations, norms, and operating assumptions. As the organization moves up the continuum of diversity implementation, diversity in styles, communications, and problem solving gains greater acceptance. In *Implementing Diversity* Marilyn Loden (1996) identifies five segments of a diversity adoption curve: innovators, change agents, pragmatists, skeptics, and traditionalists. Adoption is speeded up by compatibility, high relative advantage, observability, simplicity, and testability. Adoption is slowed down by complexity, incompatibility, little or no relative advantage, little observability, and little or no testability. The different concerns and needs of all segments of the diversity should be considered in a plan to ensure a rapid and successful adoption.

It seems to be the diversity mind-set that separates effective facilitators from those who merely pay lip service to the need to implement diversity. The valuing diversity mind-set includes valuing that diversity benefits all and is good for individuals as well as the company.

Diversity must be inclusive, requires investment of time and human resources, and requires a long-term culture change. Building support among those who are willing to adopt change while minimizing involvement of resistant people helps minimize backlash. Building a business case of the strategic and financial arguments for valuing diversity will help strengthen the adoption. Although excellent training will not ensure cultural change, inappropriate training can harm diversity efforts. Focusing on the common needs for inclusion, opportunity, and respect can help close the gaps among diverse employee groups. Administrative support is the single most important factor for predicting implementation success.

Segmentation helps adoption occur more quickly with less confusion and less conflict. Innovators generally look for opportunities to create. Change agents are among the first to try out new ideas and are interested in self-learning. Pragmatists are suspicious about the practicality of change and tend to wait rather than move quickly. They want to know that something is "good for the people." Skeptics are predisposed to delay implementation of change. They start considering change when they find themselves out of synch with mainstream values. Traditionalists tend to totally avoid involvement. They need ongoing repetitive endorsements from leaders about the strategic importance and adoption of change as less painful than continued resistance.

The timing and content of training should differ for different segments. Loden identifies best practices across organizations as follows: (1) setting the context for change, (2) providing ongoing communication, (3) focusing on data-driven change, (4) providing awareness and skill-based training, (5) encouraging ongoing learning, (6) multicultural mentoring, (7) providing flexible benefits and scheduling, (8) linking rewards to effective diversity management, and (9) building common ground.

Gender Differences

There are differences in male and female leadership styles. Women tend to be more democratic and participative by sharing power and information, encouraging consultation, and enhancing group members' self-worth. They use their interpersonal skills, charisma, and networking to influence others toward the accomplishment of goals. Men tend to be more direct and autocratic. They use the organization's formal authority structure and their positions as their power base. With the organizational trends from competitive individualism, secrecy, and control toward trust, teamwork, and information sharing, women seem well equipped for leadership beyond the 1990s.

In the classic book *The Managerial Woman*, Margaret Hennig and Anne Jardim (1966, 1977) discuss why women are at a comparative disadvantage to men for advancement in companies; how they are socialized to be a nurse, not a doctor, or a secretary, not a boss; and how "queen bees," women who have made it to the top, do not want to share their power with other women. It and *Games Mother Never Taught You: Corporate Gamesmanship for Women* by Betty Harragan (1977) describe games that still exist, making it difficult for women to advance in business. Harragan elaborates on a football metaphor to explain how women need to act. JoAnn Ashley (1976) speaks specifically to *Hospitals, Paternalism, and the Role of the Nurse*. In *Breaking Into the Boardroom: What Every Woman Needs to Know*. Jinex Melia (1986) indicates that it is women keeping women out of the boardroom.

Melia says that men stab each other in the back for gain, but women do it just to do it.

With the help of Equal Opportunity Employment legislation, women have been able to make an impact in business. Ann Morrison, Randall White, and Ellen Van Velsor (1987) did a 3-year study to determine success or derailment factors in *Breaking the Glass Ceiling: Can Women Reach the Top of America's Largest Corporations?*; the glass ceiling is a transparent barrier that few women have been able to break. They found that men and women did not score differently on most factors measured. The few statistically significant gender differences that emerged were as follows (p. 50):

Executive men are more likely than executive women to feel equal to the demands for time and energy.

Executive men feel more in tune with their surroundings and are more likely than executive women to perceive things as their peers do.

Executive men are more comfortable than executive women in an environment where conformity to intellectual authority is desirable and the criteria for excellence are clearly specified (called "achievement via conformance").

Executive women are more likely than executive men to move in new and original directions.

Executive women are more likely than executive men to behave as individuals and to personalize their experiences.

Many of the 76 executive women said they needed to take risks but be consistently outstanding; be tough but not macho; be ambitious but not expect equal treatment; and take responsibility and follow others' advice (pp. 57-70). The six lessons learned were as follows: (1) learn the ropes, (2) take control of your career, (3) build confidence, (4) rely on others, (5) go for "the bottom line," and (6) integrate life and work (pp. 74-122).

In *On Our Own Terms* Liane Enkelis, Karen Olsen, and Marion Lewenstein (1995) present 14 portraits of women business leaders who have broken the glass ceiling.

To know how women manage differently from men, Sally Helgesen needed to know how men manage. She referred to Henry Mintzberg's 1968 dissertation, which was published in 1973 as *The Nature of Managerial Work.* Mintzberg followed five male executives through their days and found that they worked at a relentless pace without breaks. Their days were filled with interruptions, discontinuity, and fragmentation. They had little time for activities not directly related to their work. They had a preference for live action encounters and maintained a complex network of relationships with people outside the organization. They immersed themselves in their jobs, had little time for reflection, had difficulty sharing information, and identified with the job.

Helgesen (1990) did diary studies on four women, two of whom are entrepreneurs. She found that women worked at a steady pace with small breaks throughout the day. The pace was steady and fast but not frantic. The subjects did not view unscheduled tasks as interruptions. They made time for activities not directly related to their work. They did not sacrifice important family time or restrict their reading to work-related items. They preferred live action but did schedule time to read the mail. They too maintained a complex network of relationships with people outside the organization. They focused on the ecology of leadership, scheduled time to share information, and saw their identities as complex and multifaceted. Men have been socialized to work sun up to sun down, whereas women know their work is never done. Women's work is cyclical and unending. They are process oriented and get pleasure from doing the work instead of getting it done. Women repeatedly used the metaphor of voice. They lead with voice. Helgesen found that the most successful women executives knew they had complex identities with various roles in both public and private life.

In *Everyday Revolutionaries* Helgesen (1998) addresses how the entry of women into the workforce since 1970 has changed how businesses are managed, how families are structured, how communities are organized, how services are conceived and marketed, and how children are raised. Entry of women into the public arena has been occurring at the same time as rapid economic and technological change. The postindustrial economy has been influenced by women who are pioneers in new ways of learning and who improvise their own lives instead of just conform to the needs of large organizations.

Rosabeth Kanter's *Men and Women of the Corporation* (1977, 1993) hypothesized that large numbers of women in the workforce would overcome the problem of sexual discrimination. However, many women are clustered at entry-level and mid-level positions. Not many women have reached the top or broken sexual stereotypes. For *Reach for the Top* Nancy Nichols (1977, 1994) interviewed women who described themselves as transformational. They did interactive leadership by encouraging participation, sharing power and information, enhancing people's self-worth, and getting others excited about their work (pp. 13-23).

Arlie Hochschild and others (1989) interviewed 50 families, including artisans, students, and professionals, in Berkeley, California, in the late 1970s. The results were published in *The Second Shift*, indicating that men who shared the load at home felt just as pressed as their wives. However, the majority of the men did not share the load at home. As women have moved into the economy, there has been a speedup at work and at home. Consequently, women talk of being overly tired, sick, and emotionally drained. Women who do all the work at home and have a job become known as supermoms. Yet the black woman who works to support her family is known as a matriarch instead of a supermom.

In *Backlash: The Undeclared War Against Women*, Susan Faludi (1991) chronicled the resentment of women's accomplishments that is characterized by antagonism and scapegoating. Some angry white men believe that women's growing presence in the workforce is depriving them of well-paying jobs and job security.

America's Competitive Secret: Utilizing Women as a Management Strategy reports the results of Judy Rosener's (1995) telephone interview with executive men across the United States. A content analysis revealed four working relationships: supervising women, working with women as peers, competing with women, and working for women. The major issues of concern for the men were loss of power and control, loss of male identity and self-esteem, and increasing discomfort or sexual static. Women have some of the same career aspirations and receive challenging assignments, but taking time off for family reasons continues to be a problem for them. The men thought that women bring attention to detail, compassion, different perspectives, sensitivity, and a willingness to work hard to the job. Black men felt differently about working with women. They are sympathetic about the underutilization of women in the workforce but also think women have taken jobs away from them. There is a need for corporations to increase gender awareness through specific training, including role playing, videos, case studies, and skill development. The female underutilization is worldwide. The number of Japanese women with career aspirations is quite small, and there is an increase in Japanese women requesting to be assigned abroad. American and British women, especially married women, feel underutilized. Some believe that women are the greatest undeveloped natural resource in the world.

In *Career Strategies for the Working Woman*, Adele Scheele (1994) discusses discovering one's self at work; building relationships with management, clients, and colleagues; and triggering one's ambition. She recommends that one provide bosses with what they need, study leaders in the organization, read profiles and biographies of achievers, develop one's own talents into expertise, make one's self visible, and work in a safe environment by joining professional and civic organizations.

Pamela Gilberd (1996) gives *The Eleven Commandments of Wildly Successful Women* as follows:

1. Create your own definition of success by finding your passion so you can love your work, believing that you deserve success, asking yourself the right questions, expanding your view of the world, knowing your priorities and values, integrating your career and your personal goals, learning how to get back on track, and giving your own definition of success the test of time.

2. Take responsibility for your career by adopting an entrepreneurial attitude, describing what you want, keeping the big picture in mind, using transitions to evaluate your work choices, being willing to change gears, and creating your own solutions.

3. Change your thinking and change your life by using the power of belief to create success, adopting a "why not?" attitude, choosing to deal with your circumstances, remembering the importance of flexibility, stretching your comfort zone, and practicing optimism.

4. When the odds are against you, defy the odds by seeing yourself as a player, taking the first step, refusing to believe conventional wisdom, doing what you know best, getting support when you need it, knowing when you need help and asking for it, and being willing to learn.

5. Fantasize about your future but create your game plan by creating a vision from your dreams, knowing your destination, creating your own luck, making preparation part of planning, and using action plans to make your dreams come true.

6. Get ready, get set, risk by knowing your tolerance for risk, understanding the risk and its consequences, looking at the long term, not being afraid of the imposter syndrome, calling on your past experience, trusting your intuition, having a fall-back plan, and using networking.

7. When someone says "you can't," say "watch me" by addressing your obstacles, keeping your sense of humor, ignoring the nay sayers, following your passion with conviction, and remembering your past successes.

8. Become financially savvy by understanding the big financial picture, taking charge of learning what you need to know, making sure you get paid what you are worth, researching and writing your own business plan, and setting solid financial goals.

9. See mistakes as road signs, not road blocks, by assuming that mistakes are useful teachers, avoiding the really big mistakes, learning to recognize warning signs, and moving on after a mistake.

10. Enjoy your work and your life by defining and enriching your creative side, nurturing your own growth, starting anew when you have outgrown your work, and creating incentives and teamwork.

11. Give back to keep the cycle of success going by sharing what you know to help others succeed, believing that each person makes a difference, learning to be a good mentor, and participating in organizations that further others' success.

In *Seven Secrets of Successful Women*, Donna Brooks and Lynn Brooks (1997) indicate that successful people (1) realize the importance of a mentor/advocate/cheerleader/coach, (2) know how to increase their visibility, (3) know how to develop an effective network, (4) have learned to communicate effectively, (5) know how to balance work and home, (6) know when to take smart risks, and (7) understand the politics of the organization. The second part of the book discusses gender differences at length. In *Success on Our Own Terms* Virginia O'Brien, Virginia O'Brien, and Lynn Martin (1998) say a key to success is finding a culture that matches your values.

Advancing Women in Business—the Catalyst Guide by Catalyst (1998) indicates that efforts to maximize women's talents will probably be successful only if an organization takes a comprehensive, problem-solving approach. Both internal and external benchmarking of women's advancement should be done. Internal research allows companies to establish the current status of women in the organization by reviewing recruitment, retention, and advancement data; develop short- and long-term goals for improvement after the baseline has been determined; and evaluate the effectiveness of the initiatives that were generated from the benchmarking by measuring and reporting the progress toward specific goals.

Racial Differences

William Wilson (1994) identifies three stages of race relations in the United States: (1) plantation economy and racial-caste oppression, (2) industrial expansion, class conflict, and racial oppression, and (3) progressive transition from racial inequalities to class irregularities. Racial diversity is visible and subject to stereotyping, in which the person is viewed as a member of a group and the images others have about that group are ascribed to the person, and prejudice, when predetermined negative attitudes toward people are based on a group identity. Taylor Cox and Ruby Beale (1997) identify numerous ways of *Developing Competency to Manage Diversity*, including providing awareness training; providing opportunities for in-house trainers; creating interorganizational relationships with organizations with different dominant groups; providing some support for on- and off-site dialogue meetings; providing a reading list on diversity; sponsoring cultural diversity celebrations; sponsoring events to facilitate mentor-protege matchups; providing overseas assignments; allowing time for travel or sponsoring travel for career development; providing financial support for college courses about diversity, foreign language courses, and national conferences on diversity; sponsoring cultural social events; creating diversity task forces; sponsoring educational activities and diversity roundtables; integrating cultural diversity issues into staff meetings; and helping employees obtain requested job assignments.

The working environment is often lonely and unfriendly for nontraditional managers.

Sometimes people of color and women have information withheld from them to sabotage them. They may have trouble finding role models and mentors. They may lack organizational savvy, take comfort in working with their own kind, have difficulty balancing career and family, get a backlash from threatened white males, have infighting from the oppressed group, and have to deal with prejudice. Agencies should give management training. Helping new managers get acquainted with key workers so they will feel comfortable dealing with them later is important (Morrison, 1992).

Sexual Orientation Differences

Lesbian, gay, and bisexual development is more invisible than some other minorities. They are less likely to be considered to have mental illness than earlier but still risk loss of employment, housing, and family relationships (Trickett, Watts, and Birman, 1994).

Disabilities

Many disabilities are visible and affect people at different chronological ages with a variety of physical disabilities. The disability culture is built on a kinship based on identification of shared understandings of life experiences (Trickett, Watts, and Birman, 1994).

FOLLOWERSHIP

We need great followers as well as great leaders. Leaders contribute only about 20% to the success of organizations. Followers do the remaining 80%. We spend more time reporting to others than having them report to us. Some leaders have been such good followers that their peers have asked them to take on leadership responsibilities. In *Leadership Is an Art*, DePree (1989) suggests that leadership and followership involve intimacy and personal covenants that people at work make with each other.

Effective followers view themselves as equals of the leaders and work for the common good. Conformist followers believe they must always please the boss, and alienated followers tend to snipe at leaders. Less effective followers have a limited worldview, mainly considering their own needs and rarely considering the pressures the leader has. Excellent followers work cooperatively with leaders rather than as adversaries.

Effective followers do not always agree with the leader but are likely to use the following guidelines: When disagreeing with the leader, discuss the disagreement privately rather than in a public forum. Do not approach the leader during a crisis or deadline. Present the situation as a joint problem, not as the leader's stupid idea. Go to the meeting with potential solutions. Take the leader's point of view into consideration when brainstorming alternatives. Do not go to the leader while angry, because that is likely to escalate conflict.

In *The Power of Followership* Robert Kelley (1992, pp. 177-182) recommends that followers ask themselves the following six questions to choose their battles wisely:

1. What is at stake for the organization?
2. What will happen if you fail to act?
3. Does the leader have both the expertise and the legitimate authority to issue this order?
4. Are human costs and societal values being overlooked?
5. What role are you being asked to play?
6. What is at stake for you personally?

Followers do maintain independent and critical thinking. They are vigilant about unchecked leaders. Kelley also outlines 10 steps to a courageous conscience as follows (pp. 185-197):

1. Be proactive.
2. Gather your facts.
3. Before taking a stand, seek wise counsel.
4. Build your fortitude.
5. Work within the system.
6. Frame your position so it will be heard.
7. Educate others on how your view serves their best interests.
8. Take collective action.
9. If you meet leader resistance, seek higher authority.
10. Have the financial and emotional cushions to exercise other alternatives.

Janice Ellis and Celia Hartley (1995, pp. 22-23) suggest the following to be a good follower:

1. Invest yourself.
2. Clearly identify your responsibilities as a follower.
3. Clearly identify your expectations of the leader.
4. Support your leader and your group.
5. Challenge your leader and your group.
6. Follow channels of communications and responsibilities.

CHARACTER DEVELOPMENT

"Always do right. That will gratify some of the people, and astonish the rest." —Mark Twain

There is an increased focus on character development resulting from a rise in violence; increasing lying, cheating, and stealing; growing disrespect for authority figures; increasing peer cruelty; a rise in prejudice and hate crimes; a deterioration of language; a decline in the work ethic; declining personal and civic responsibility; increasing self-destructive behaviors such as premature sexual activity, substance abuse, and suicide; and the growing ethical illiteracy (Center for the 4th and 5th Rs, http://.cortland.edu/www/c4n5rs/signs_iv.htm, accessed 6/21/01).

There are a variety of approaches to moral and character education. First, some ignore it. Second, some take a value neutral approach and assume that no values or character traits are more valid than others. Third, some assume that moral and character decisions are made rationally and teach a decision-making process. Fourth, some use the approach that changing thinking will lead to changes in behavior and engage students in discussion of moral issues. It is the change in behavior that differentiates values education from character education. Fifth, some teach students a given set of values and accompanying appropriate actions. Sixth, some use the inculcation, values education, analysis, and moral development approaches and have students put their thoughts and feelings into actions through a variety of social actions. This approach involves action learning or service learning. The combination of approaches includes the volition and action aspects of character development that are not present in values education (Educational Psychology Interactive: Moral and Character Development, http://chiron.valdosta.edu/whuitt/col/morchr/morchr.html, accessed 1/7/03).

The Character Education Partnership has identified the following 11 principles of effective character education: (1) character education promotes core ethical values as the basis of good character; (2) character must be comprehensively defined to include thinking, feeling, and behavior; (3) effective character education requires an intentional, proactive, and comprehensive approach that promotes the core values in all phases of school life; (4) the school must be a caring community; (5) to develop character, students need opportunities for moral action; (6) effective character education includes a meaningful and challenging academic curriculum that respects all learners and helps them succeed; (7) character education should strive to develop students' intrinsic motivation; (8) the school staff must become a learning and moral community in which all share responsibility for character education and attempt to adhere to the same core values that guide the education of students; (9) character education requires moral leadership from both staff and students; (10) the school must recruit parents and community members as full partners in the character-building effort; and (11) evaluation of character education should assess the character of the school, the school staff's functioning as character factors, and the extent to which students manifest good character (Character Education Partnership, Eleven Principles of Effective Character Education, http://character.org/principles/index/ cgi, accessed 6/21/01).

Allen Elementary School is an inner-city school in Dayton, Ohio where more than 60% of the students lived in single-parent families and more than 70% of the families received public assistance. The faculty had trouble teaching because of the discipline problems. The faculty started a word of the week program to promote a different value each week. Values promoted included cheerfulness, citizenship, cleanliness, courage, courtesy, helpfulness, honesty, kindness, loyalty, patience, punctuality, respect, responsibility, self-control, self-reliance, sportsmanship, thrift, and tolerance. Students brainstormed examples of the behaviors and had short homeroom discussions about the word of the week. Teachers tried to connect classroom activities to the word. Students were sent to the principal's office for compliments about their exemplary ways. A newsletter was sent to parents with discussion topic and bedtime story suggestions to promote the week's value. Within 2 years, student respect and other behaviors had markedly improved, suspensions dropped, teacher absenteeism decreased, PTA funding increased, and faculty relationships improved through staff development and trust building (Center for the 4th and 5th Rs, Word of the week, http://www.cortland.edu/www/4cn5rs/suxcs 4.htm). Other words that have been associated with character development include accountability, caring, compassion, cooperation, excellence, integrity, perseverance, promise keeping, loyalty, self-discipline, truthfulness, fairness, faith, friendship, justice, and citizenship. Rules and procedures, cooperative learning, teaching for thinking, quality literature, and service learning can help structure a character education program (Character Education Group, Character education and how it works, http://www.character-ducation.com/home2.htm., accessed 1/7/03). These strategies can be adapted to health care organizations. Rules and procedures help clarify expected behaviors. Staff can learn together by brainstorming and discussing virtues periodically. Bennett's (1993) *The Book of Virtues* is a collection of moral stories. Short selections could be selected and discussed. Staff can also be encouraged to do community service through the health care organization's outreach to the community.

IMPLICATIONS FOR NURSING ADMINISTRATION

Surveying the development of management thought, one can see that there has been a trend from autocratic to democratic management and from a focus on efficiency to a greater regard for the well-being of personnel. Although the focus has changed, elements from each era maintain their validity and can be used by the nurse administrator. For example, Taylor's time studies and the Gilbreths' motion studies in the scientific era are illustrations of how the nurse can study complexity of care to predict staffing needs and study efficiency of nursing care. An adaptation of Gantt's chart can be used to visualize the time element of planning and controlling.

Nurse administrators should be aware of their managerial tasks as defined by Fayol: planning, organizing, directing, coordinating, and controlling. His definition of management can help clarify the manager's role, and his principles of management can help direct one's actions. Assistance with the organizing function can be obtained from Weber's conceptualization of bureaucracy and authority and Urwick's popularization of concepts such as balancing authority with responsibility, unity of direction, unity of command, and span of control.

To a large extent the social environment results from organization and management. The work of Barnard, Follett, Mayo, and Lewin during the human relations era should remind the nurse administrator of the importance of developing workers to their potential and meeting their needs for recognition, accomplishment, and sense of belonging. It is hoped that nurse administrators will consider the results of Lewin's research about autocratic and democratic leadership when determining their own style. They can use Moreno's sociometry to study the group behavior of workers.

Much has been learned about management from the behavioral science studies. The nurse can apply Maslow's hierarchy-of-needs theory to the care of individual patients, to functions of individual workers, or to groups of people. The importance of achievement, recognition, responsibility, and advancement as motivators and satisfiers is stressed in Herzberg's two-factor theory. The research of McGregor, Argyris, Likert, Blake, and Mouton supports the benefits of positive attitudes toward people, development of workers, satisfaction of their needs, and commitment through participation. Fiedler indicates that a leadership style may or may not be effective, depending on the situation. Nurse administrators can use his work in assessing their work situation to determine the most effective style or choosing the work situation according to what fits their style best. The leader can also incorporate Drucker's and Odiorne's work on management by objectives for the planning, directing, and controlling phases of the management process. We have much to learn and apply from the transformational leadership, learning organizations, and results-based leadership theorists.

By studying the development of management thought, nurse administrators can define their management role, develop their philosophy of management, learn tools and techniques for implementation of their responsibilities, and gain an increased understanding of how to work with others to accomplish goals.

CHAPTER SUMMARY

Chapter 7 covered the following:
Theories of Leadership
    Great Man Theory
    Charismatic Theory
    Trait Theory
    Situational Theory
    Contingency Theory
    Path-Goal Theory
    Situational Leadership Theory
    Transactional Leadership
    Transformational Leadership
    Integrative Leadership Model
Development of Management Thought
    Scientific Management
        Taylor

Gilbreth
Gantt
Classic Organization
  Fayol
  Weber
  Mooney
  Urwick
Human Relations
  Barnard
  Follett
  The Hawthorne studies
  Lewin
  Moreno
Behavioral Science
  Maslow
  Herzberg
  McGregor
  Ouchi, Pascale, and Athos
  Argyris
  Likert
  Blake and Mouton
  Fiedler
  Hersey and Blanchard
  Drucker
  Odiorne
  Peters
  Kotter
Transformational Leadership
  Bass
  Bennis and Nanus
  Kouzes and Posner
  Tichy
  Blanchard
  Anderson and Collins
Servant Leadership
  Greenleaf and others
Learning Organizations
  Senge and others
Emotional Intelligence
  Goleman and others
Results-Based Leadership
  Welch and others
Diversity Among Leaders
  Diversity
    Gender differences
    Racial differences
    Sexual orientation differences
    Disabilities
Followership
Character Development
Implications for Nursing Administration

On-line Resources

evolve Additional critical thinking activities, worksheets, and case studies are available on-line at http://evolve.elsevier.com/Marriner/guide/

REFERENCES

Ackoff RL: *Creating the corporate future: Plan or be planned for,* New York, 1981, John Wiley & Sons.

Anderson TD: *Transforming leadership: Equipping yourself and coaching others to build the leadership organization*, ed 2, Boca Raton, Fla, 1998, St Lucie Press.

Argyris C: *Executive leadership*, New York, 1953, Harper & Bros.

Argyris C: *Integrating the individual and the organization,* New York, 1964, John Wiley & Sons.

Argyris C: *Knowledge for action,* San Francisco, 1993, Jossey-Bass.

Argyris C: *On organizational learning,* Malden, Mass, 1999, Blackwell Publishers Inc.

Argyris C: *Personality and organization,* New York, 1957, Harper & Bros.

Argyris C, Putnam R, Smith DM: *Action science,* San Francisco, 1985, Jossey-Bass.

Argyris C, Schon DA: *Organizational learning: A theory of action perspective,* Reading, Mass, 1978, Addison-Wesley.

Ashley JA: *Hospitals, paternalism, and the role of the nurse,* New York, 1976, Teachers College Press.

Autry JA: *The servant leader,* New York, 2001, Prima Publishing.

Barnard CI: *The functions of the executive,* Cambridge, Mass, 1938, Harvard University Press.

Barnard CI: *The nature of leadership,* Cambridge, Mass, 1940, Harvard University Press.

Bass BM: *Leadership and performance beyond expectations,* New York, 1985, Free Press.

Bass BM: *Transformational leadership: Industry, military, and educational impact*, Mahwah, NJ, 1998, Lawrence Erlbaum Associates, Publishers.

Bass BM, Avolio BJ: Transformational leadership and organizational culture, *Publ Admin Q* 17:112-121, Spring 1993.

Belasen AT: *Leading the learning organization*, Albany, NY, 2000, State University of New York Press.

Bennett WG: The book of virtues, NY,1993, Simon & Schuster.

Bennis W: On becoming a leader, Reading, Mass, 1989, Addison-Wesley.

Bennis W: Organizing genius, Reading, Mass, 1997, Perseus Books.

Bennis W, Goldsmith J: Learning to lead: A workbook on becoming a leader, Reading, Mass, 1997, Perseus Books.

Bennis W, Nanus B: Leaders: The strategies for taking charge, New York, 1985, 1997, Harper & Row.

Blake RR, Mouton JS: The new managerial grid, Houston, 1978, Gulf.

Blanchard K: The heart of a leader, Tulsa, Okla, 1999, Honors Books.

Blanchard K, Bowles S: Gung ho! New York, 1998, William Morrow and Co.

Blanchard K, Bowles S: Raving fans, New York, 1993, William Morrow and Co.

Blanchard K, Bowles S, Carew D, et al: High five: The magic of working together, New York, 2001, William Morrow and Co.

Blanchard K, Cathy ST: The generosity factor, Grand Rapids, Mich, 2002, Zondervan.

Blanchard K, Lacinak T, Tompkins C, et al: Whale done, New York, 2002, The Free Press.

Blank W: The 108 skills of natural born leaders, New York, 2001, AMACOM.

Block P: The answer to how is yes: Acting on what matters, San Francisco, 2000, Berrett-Koehler.

Block P: The empowered manager: Positive political skills at work, San Francisco, 1987, Jossey-Bass.

Block P: Stewardship: Choosing service over self-interest, San Francisco, 1993, Berrett-Koehler.

Bossidy L, Charan R: Execution: The discipline of getting things done, New York, 2002, Crown Pub.

Brooks DL, Brooks LM: Seven secrets of successful women, New York, 1997, McGraw-Hill.

Buckingham M, Coffman C: First, break all the rules: What the world's greatest managers do differently, New York, 1999, Simon & Schuster.

Capra F, Steindl-Rast D, Madison T: Belonging to the universe, San Francisco, 1991, Harper.

Catalyst: Advancing women in business—The catalyst guide, San Francisco, 1998, Jossey-Bass.

Center for the 4th and 5th Rs, http://cortland.edu/ www/ c4n5rs/signs_iv.htm. Accessed 6/21/01.

Center for the 4th and 5th Rs, Word of the week, http;//www.cortland.edu/www/4cn5rs/suxcs4.htm.

Chappel T: Managing upside down: The seven intentions of values-centered leadership, New York, 1999, William Morrow and Co.

Character Education Group, Character education and how it works, http://www.charactereducation.com/home2.htm. Accessed 1/7/03.

Character Education Partnership, Eleven Principles of Effective Character Education, http://character.org/principles/index/cgi. Accessed 6/21/01.

Collins J: Good to great: Why some companies make the leap...and others don't, New York, 2001, Harper Business.

Conger J, Kanungo R: Charismatic leadership in organizations, Newbury Park, Calif, 1998, Sage.

Conger JA, Benjamin B: Building leaders: How successful companies develop the next generation, San Francisco, 1999, Jossey-Bass.

Covey SR: Principle-centered leadership, New York, 1990, Summit Books.

Covey SR: The 7 habits of highly effective people, New York, 1989, Simon & Schuster.

Covey SR, Merrill AR, Merrill RR: First things first, New York, 1994, Simon & Schuster.

Cox T, Beale RL: Developing competency to manage diversity, San Francisco, 1997, Berrett-Koehler.

Crainer S: Business the Jack Welch way: 10 secrets of the world's greatest turnaround king, New York, 1999, AMACOM.

DePree M: Leadership is an art, New York, 1989, Dell.

DePree M: Leadership jazz, New York, 1992, Doubleday.

DePree M: Leading without power: Finding hope in serving community, Holland, Mich, 1997, Shepherd Foundation.

Donnelly JH Jr, Gibson JL, Ivancevich JM: Fundamentals of management functions, behavior, models, Dallas, 1981, Business Publications.

Drucker P: The frontiers of management, New York, 1986, EP Dutton

Drucker P: Innovation and entrepreneurship: Practice and principles, New York, 1985, Harper & Row.

Drucker P: Managing for results: Economic tasks and risk-taking decisions, New York, 1964, Harper & Row.

Drucker PF: The essential Drucker: Selections from the management works of Peter F. Drucker, New York, 2001, Harper Business.

Drucker PF: Management: Tasks, responsibilities, practices, New York, 1974, Harper & Row.

Drucker PF: Managing for the future: The 1990s and beyond, New York, 1992, Truman Talley Books/Plume.

Drucker PF: Managing in a time of great change, New York, 1995, Truman Talley Books/Dutton.

Drucker PF: Managing in turbulent times, New York, 1980, Harper & Row.

Drucker PF: On the profession of management, Boston, 1998, Harvard Business School.

Educational Psychology Interactive: Moral and Character Development, http://chiron.valdosta.edu/whuitt/col/morchr/morchr.html, accessed 1/7/03.

Ellis JR, Hartley CL: Managing and coordinating nursing care, Philadelphia, 1995, JB Lippincott.

Enkelis L, Olsen K, Lewenstein M: *On our own terms,* San Francisco, 1995, Berrett-Koehler.

Faludi S: *Backlash: The undeclared war against women,* New York, 1991, Anchor Books/Doubleday.

Fayol H: *Administration industrielle et generale,* Paris, 1925, Dunod.

Feldman D: *The handbook of emotional intelligent leadership: Inspiring others to achieve results,* Falls Church, Va, 1999, Leadership Performance Solutions Press.

Fiedler FE: *A theory of leadership effectiveness,* New York, 1967, McGraw-Hill.

Fiedler FE, Chemers MM: *Leadership and effective management,* Glenview, Ill, 1974, Scott, Foresman and Co.

Fiedler FE, Chemers MM, Mahar L: *Improving leadership effectiveness: The leader match concept,* New York, 1976, John Wiley & Sons.

Follett MP: *Freedom and coordination,* London, 1949, Management Publications Trust.

Fritz R: *Creating,* New York, 1991, Fawcett Columbine.

Fritz R: *The path of least resistance,* New York, 1989, Fawcett Columbine.

Gantt HL: *Industrial leadership,* New Haven, Conn, 1916, Yale University Press.

Gantt HL: *Organizing for work,* New York, 1919, Harcourt, Brace and Howe.

Gates DM, Kroeger D: Violence against nurses: The silent epidemic, *JSNA Bulletin* 29(1):25-29, November, December, 2002, January, 2003.

Gilberd P: *The eleven commandments of wildly successful women,* Tappan, NJ, 1996, Macmillan Spectrum.

Gilbreth FB: *Bricklaying system,* New York, 1909, Myron C Clark.

Gilbreth FB: *Motion study,* New York, 1911, D Van Nostrand.

Gilbreth FB, Carey EG, McKay D: *Cheaper by the dozen,* New York, 1984, Bantam Books.

Gilbreth FB, Gilbreth LM: *Applied motion study,* New York, 1917, Sturgis and Walton.

Gilbreth FB, Gilbreth LM: *Fatigue study,* ed 2, New York, 1919, Macmillan.

Gilbreth LM: *The psychology of management,* New York, 1914, Sturgis and Walton.

Goleman D. An EI-based theory of performance. In Cherniss C, Goleman D, editors: *The emotionally intelligent workplace: How to select for, measure, and improve emotional intelligence in individuals, groups, and organizations,* San Francisco, 2001, Jossey-Bass.

Goleman D: *Emotional intelligence,* New York, 1995, Bantam Books.

Goleman D: *Working with emotional intelligence,* New York, 1998, Bantam Books.

Goleman D, Boyatzis R, McKee A: *Primal leadership: Realizing the power of emotional intelligence,* Boston, 2002, Harvard Business School Press.

Gray J: *Men are from Mars, women are from Venus,* New York, 1992, HarperCollins.

Greenleaf RK: *Servant leadership,* New York, 1977, 1991, Paulist Press.

Harragan BL: *Games Mother never taught you: Corporate gamesmanship for women,* New York, 1977, Warner Books.

Harvey JB: *The Abilene paradox,* San Diego, 1988, University Associates.

Helgesen S: *Everyday revolutionaries,* New York, 1998, Doubleday.

Helgesen S: *The female advantage: Women's ways of leadership,* New York, 1990, Bantam Doubleday Dell.

Hennig MM, Jardim A: *The managerial woman,* Garden City, NY, 1966, 1977, Anchor Press/Doubleday.

Hersey P: *The situational leader,* New York, 1984, Warner Books.

Hersey P, Blanchard KH: *Management of organizational behavior: Utilizing human resources,* Paramus, NJ, 1969, 1982, Prentice Hall.

Hersey P, Duldt BW: *Situational leadership in nursing,* Norwalk, Conn, 1989, Appleton & Lange.

Herzberg F: One more time: How do you motivate employees? In Carroll L, Paine R, Miner A, editors: *The management process,* ed 2, New York, 1977, Macmillan.

Herzberg F, Mausner B, Snyderman BB: *The motivation to work,* ed 2, New York, 1959, John Wiley & Sons.

Hesse H: *The journey to the east,* New York, 1956, Noonday Press.

Hitt WD: The model leader: A fully functioning person, *Leadership Organ Development J* 14(7):4-11, 1993.

Hochschild A: *The second shift,* New York, 1989, Viking Penguin.

House RJ: A path-goal theory of leader effectiveness, *Adm Sci Q* 16:321-339, 1971.

Jaworski J, Flowers BS: *Synchronicity: The inner path of leadership,* San Francisco, 1996, 1998, Berrett-Koehler.

Jeffries E: *The heart of leadership: Influencing by design,* Dubuque, Iowa, 1993, Kendall/Hunt Pub Co.

Kanter RM: *Men and women of the corporation,* New York, 1977, 1993, Basic Books.

Kelley R: *The power of followership,* New York, 1992, Doubleday Currency.

Kelly J: *Organizational behaviour,* rev ed, Homewood, Ill, 1980, Irwin.

Kotter JP: *A force for change,* New York, 1990, Free Press.

Kotter JP: *The general managers,* New York, 1982, Free Press.

Kotter JP: *The heart of change: Real-life stories of how people change their organizations,* Boston, 2002, Harvard Business School Press.

Kotter JP: *The leadership factor,* New York, 1988, Free Press.

Kotter JP: *Leading change,* Boston, 1996, Harvard Business School Press.

Kotter JP: *Power and influence,* New York, 1985, Free Press.

Kouzes JM, Posner BZ: *Credibility,* San Francisco, 1993, Jossey-Bass.

Kouzes JM, Posner BZ: *Encouraging the heart,* San Francisco, 1999, Jossey-Bass.

Kouzes JM, Posner BZ: *The leadership challenge: How to get extraordinary things done in organizations,* San Francisco, 1987, 1990, Jossey-Bass.

Krames JA: *The Jack Welch lexicon of leadership,* New York, 2001, McGraw-Hill.

Lewin K: *Field theory in social sciences,* New York, 1951, Harper & Row.

Likert R: *New patterns of management,* New York, 1961, McGraw-Hill.

Likert R, Likert JG: *New ways of managing conflict,* New York, 1976, McGraw-Hill.

Loden M: *Implementing diversity,* Chicago, 1996, Irwin.

Maslow A: *Motivation and personality,* ed 2, New York, 1970, Harper & Row.

Maxwell, JC: The 21 indispensable qualities of a leader: Becoming the person others will want to follow. Nashville, 1999, Thomas Nelson Publishers.

McGee-Cooper A, Looper G: *The essentials of servant-leadership: Principles in practice,* Waltham, Mass, 2001, Pegasus Communications.

McGee-Cooper A, Trammel D, Lau B: *You don't have to go home from work exhausted,* New York, 1990, 1992, Bantam Books.

McGregor D: *The human side of enterprise,* New York, 1960, McGraw-Hill.

Meadows DH, Meadows D, Randers J: *Beyond the limits,* Past Hills, Vt, 1992, Chelsea Green.

Melia J: *Breaking into the boardroom: What every woman needs to know,* New York, 1986, GP Putnam's Sons.

Meyer C: *Fast cycle time,* New York, 1993, Free Press/Macmillan.

Miller C: *The empowered leader: 10 keys to servant leadership,* Nashville, 1995, Broadman & Holman Pub.

Mintzberg H: *The nature of managerial work,* New York, 1973, Harper & Row.

Mooney JD, Reiley AC: *Onward industry!* New York, 1931, Harper & Bros.

Mooney JD, Reiley AC: *The principles of organization,* New York, 1939, Harper & Bros.

Morrison AM: *The new leaders,* San Francisco, 1992, Jossey-Bass.

Morrison AM, White R, Van Velsor E: *Breaking the glass ceiling: Can women reach the top of America's largest corporations?* Reading, Mass, 1987, Addison-Wesley.

Moxley RS: *Leadership and spirit: Breathing new vitality and energy into individuals and organizations,* San Francisco, 2000, Jossey-Bass.

Nanus B: *The leader's edge,* Chicago, 1989, Contemporary Books.

Nichols NA: *Reach for the top,* Boston, 1977, 1994, Harvard College.

Northouse PG: *Leadership: Theory and practice,* ed 2, Thousand Oaks, Calif, 2001, Sage.

O'Brien V, O'Brien V, Martin L: *Success on our own terms,* New York, 1998, John Wiley & Sons.

Odiorne GS: *Management by objectives,* New York, 1965, Pitman.

Ouchi WG: Theory Z: *How American business can meet the Japanese challenge,* New York, 1981, Avon Books.

Palmer PJ: *The courage to teach: Exploring the inner landscape of a teacher's life,* San Francisco, 1998, Jossey-Bass.

Palmer PJ: *To know as we are known/a spirituality of education,* New York, 1983, HarperCollins.

Pande PS, Neuman RP, Cavanaugh, RR: *The six sigma way team fieldbook: An implementation guide for project improvement teams,* New York, 2002, McGraw-Hill.

Parker M: *Creating shared vision,* Oslo, 1990, Norwegian Center for Leadership Development.

Pascale RT, Athos AG: *The art of Japanese management: Applications for American executives,* New York, 1981, Warner Books.

Peck MS: *The road less traveled,* New York, 1978, Simon & Schuster.

Perkins, DNT: *Leading at the edge: Leadership lessons from the extraordinary saga of Shackleton's Antarctic Expedition,* New York, 2000, AMACOM.

Peters T: *The circle of innovation,* New York, 1997, Alfred A Knopf.

Peters T: *Liberation management,* New York, 1992, Fawcett Columbine.

Peters T: *Thriving on chaos,* New York, 1987, Harper & Row.

Peters T: *The Tom Peters Seminar,* New York, 1994, Vintage Books.

Peters T, Austin N: *A passion for excellence,* New York, 1985, Warner Books.

Peters T, Waterman RH: *In search of excellence,* New York, 1982, Harper & Row.

Pohlman RA, Gardiner GS: *Value driven management: How to create and maximize value over time for organizational success,* New York, 2000, AMACOM.

Redwood S, Goldwasser C, Street S: *Action management: Practical strategies for making your corporate transformation a success,* New York, 1999, John Wiley & Sons, Inc.

Rinehart ST: *Upside down: The paradox of servant leadership,* Colorado Springs, Col, 1998, NAVPRESS.

Rosener JB: *America's competitive secret: Utilizing women as a management strategy,* New York, 1995, Oxford University Press.

Rummler G, Brache AP: *Improving performance,* San Francisco, 1995, Jossey-Bass.

Ryback D: *Putting emotional intelligence to work: Successful leadership is more than IQ,* Boston, 1998, Butterworth-Heinemann.

Samuel M: *The accountability revolution: Achieving breakthrough results in half the time,* ed 2, Tempe, Ariz, 2001, Mark Samuel.

Schaffer RH: *The breakthrough strategy,* New York, 1988, Harper Business.

Scheele A: *Career strategies for the working woman,* New York, 1994, Simon & Schuster.

Schein EH: *Organizational culture and leadership,* San Francisco, 1985, 1997, Jossey-Bass.

Senge PM: *The fifth discipline: The art and practice of the learning organization,* New York, 1990, Doubleday.

Senge PM, Kleiner, Roberts, et al: *The fifth discipline fieldbook,* New York, 1994, Doubleday.

Sims HP: *The thinking organization: Dynamics of organizational social cognition,* San Francisco, 1986, Jossey-Bass.

Slater R: *The GE way fieldbook: Jack Welch's battle plan for corporate revolution,* New York, 2000, McGraw-Hill.

Slater R: *Jack Welch and the GE way: Management insights and leadership secrets of the legendary CEO,* New York, 1999, McGraw-Hill.

Spears LC, editor: *Insights on leadership: Service, stewardship, spirit, and servant leadership,* New York, 1998, John Wiley & Sons.

Spears LC, editor: *The power of servant leadership*, San Francisco, 1998, Berrett-Koehler.

Spears LC, editor: *Reflections on leadership: How Robert K. Greenleaf's theory on servant leadership influenced today's top management thinkers,* New York, 1995, John Wiley & Sons.

Spears LC, Lawrence M, editors: *Focus on leadership: Servant leadership for the 21st century,* New York, 2002, John Wiley & Sons Inc.

Tannen D: *You just don't understand: Women and men in conversation,* New York, 1990, Ballantine Books.

Taylor FW: *The principles of scientific management,* New York, 1911, Harper & Bros.

Taylor FW: *Shop management,* New York, 1903, Harper & Bros.

Tichy NM, Cardwell N: *The cycle of leadership: How great leaders teach their companies to win,* New York, 2002, Harper Business.

Tichy NM, Cohen E: *The leadership engine,* New York, 1997, HarperCollins.

Tichy NM, Devanna MA: *The transformational leader,* New York, 1986, 1997, John Wiley & Sons.

Tichy NM, Sherman S: *Control your destiny or someone else will,* New York, 1993, Doubleday.

Trickett EJ, Watts RJ, Birman D: *Human diversity: Perspectives on people in context,* San Francisco, 1994, Jossey-Bass.

Ulrich D, Zenger J, Smallwood N: *Results-based leadership*, Boston, 1999, Harvard Business School Press.

Urwick L: *The elements of administration,* New York, 1944, Harper & Bros.

Vaill PB: *Managing as a performing art,* San Francisco, 1989, Jossey-Bass.

Welch J, Byrne JA: *Jack : Straight from the gut,* New York, 2001, Warner Books.

Wheatley M: *Leadership and the new science,* San Francisco, 1992, Berrett-Koehler.

Wheatley MJ, Keller-Rogers M: *A simpler way*, San Francisco, 1996, Berrett-Koehler.

Wilson WJ: The declining significance of race: Blacks and changing American institutions. In Grusky DB: *Social stratification*, Boulder, Colo, 1994, Westview Press, pp. 520-531.

Yukl GA: *Leadership in organizations,* ed 3, Gaithersburg, Md, 1994, Aspen.

PART TWO

MANAGEMENT

Strategic and Operational Planning

*"The greatest thing in this world is not so much
where we are, but in what direction we are moving."*
—Oliver Wendell Holmes

Chapter Overview

Chapter 8 illustrates the planning process, history of strategic planning,
strategic planning process, vision, values, mission, philosophy, goals,
objectives, strategies, policies, and procedures.

Chapter Objectives

- Identify at least two differences between strategic and operational planning.
- Describe at least five changes in health care delivery systems that should be taken
  into account in strategic planning.
- List at least five benefits of strategic planning.
- Explain the relationships among purpose, philosophy, goals, and objectives.
- Explain the relationship between policy and procedure.

Major Concepts and Definitions

Strategic planning long-range planning usually extending 3 to 5 years into the future
Operational planning short-range planning that deals with day-to-day maintenance activities
Belief conviction that certain things are true
Vision mental image of something not actually visible
Value the worth, usefulness, or importance of something
Mission/purpose an aim to be accomplished; mission statement
Philosophy statement of beliefs and values that directs behavior
Goal the end to be accomplished
Objective something aimed at or striven for; things done to achieve the goal
Policy a governing plan for accomplishing goals and objectives
Procedure chronological sequence of steps within a process
Protocols documents of agreement
Business plan plan for new ventures, such as new products or services

PLANNING PROCESS

There are two major types of organizational planning: long-range, or strategic, planning and short-range, or operational, planning. Strategic planning extends 3 to 5 years into the future. It begins with in-depth analysis of the internal environment's strengths and weaknesses and the external opportunities and threats so that realistic goals can be set for the preferred future. It determines the direction of the organization, allocates resources, assigns responsibilities, and determines time frames. Strategic planning goals are more generic and less specific than operational planning.

Nurse managers are more likely to be involved in the operational planning. Operational planning is done in conjunction with budgeting, usually a few months before the new fiscal year. It develops the departmental maintenance and improvement goals for the coming year.

HISTORY OF STRATEGIC PLANNING

Private business started using strategic planning in the mid-1950s when the demand for products began to level off and decline and substitute products became available from foreign competitors. The health care industry started during the mid-1970s when the federal government established restricted payment regulations.

Third-party payers also developed restrictions, and payment shifted from the federal government to individuals and other payers. This increased price sensitivity and competition. Alternative delivery systems, such as preferred provider arrangements, health maintenance organizations, self-help and wellness programs, and ambulatory services, proliferated. As chief executive officers looked at job redesign to increase productivity while cutting costs, mergers, acquisitions, joint ventures, and informal networking increased.

High-cost technology responded to the competitive environment with greater acuity of care in acute-care settings, tertiary settings, and homes. At the same time the population was aging, increasing numbers of the population were underinsured and uninsured. Quality of life and ethics also became important issues. Consequently, strategic planning became prevalent in health care settings and literature during the 1980s.

During the 1990s trends moved from individual specialist providers to team primary care providers; from reliance on physician care to use of physician extenders; from hospital episodic care to ambulatory care; from institutional care to alternative care; from individual-based treatments to population-based treatments; from curative, uncoordinated care to preventive, integrated care; from acute care to chronic care; from technological orientation to humanistic orientation; from younger population to older population; from content mastery to process mastery; from being governed professionally to being governed managerially; from competitive to cooperative; from cost unaware to cost aware; from fee for service to capitation; from paper health records to computerized health records; and from no data on best practices to emerging data about best practices (Table 8-1).

PURPOSE OF STRATEGIC PLANNING

Strategic planning clarifies beliefs and values: What are the organization's strengths and weaknesses? What are the potential opportunities and threats? Where is the organization going? How is it going to get there? It gives direction to the organization, improves efficiency, weeds out poor or underused programs, eliminates duplication of efforts, concentrates resources on important services, improves communications and coordination of activities, provides a mind-expanding opportunity, allows adaptation to the changing environment, sets realistic and attainable yet challenging goals, and helps ensure goal achievement.

Leaders need vision that is realistic and feasible. Development of a strategic vision involves analysis of the agency's environment, capabilities, and resources; development and articulation of a conceptual image; clarification of values; development of a mission statement; identification of goals and objectives; and identification of strategies for reaching the goals. The strategic vision should be clear, cohesive, consistent, and flexible (Box 8-1).

STRATEGIC PLANNING PROCESS

"Decision makers can turn opportunities into realities." —Anonymous

TABLE **8-1** Trends During the 1990s

MOVING FROM:	MOVING TO:
Individual provider	Team provider
Physician's needs	Payer's/customer's needs
Specialties	Primary care
Reliance on physician care	Use of physician extenders
Hospital episodic care	Ambulatory continuum of care
Institutional care	Alternative care
Individual-based treatment	Population-based treatment
Curative care	Preventive care
Acute care	Chronic care
Technologically oriented	Humanistically oriented
Younger population	Older population
Content mastery	Process mastery
Governed professionally	Governed managerially
Competitive	Cooperative
Cost unaware	Cost aware
Fee for service	Capitation
Paper health record	Computerized health record
No data on best practices	Emerging data on best practices

BOX **8-1** Strategic Planning Process

External assessment
   Opportunities and threats
Internal assessment
   Strengths and weaknesses
Priority strategic issues and programs
Vision
Values
Mission
Philosophy
Goals
   Strategic
      Organization
   Operational
      Division
      Unit
Objectives
Strategies
   Timelines
   Plans
Policies
Procedures
Implementation
Evaluation
   Production/operations
   Finance
   Marketing

It is important that top-level administrators are committed to strategic planning. Otherwise such planning may be viewed as mere busy work. Managers need to be taught the importance of long-range planning and the way to do it.

An external assessment looks at opportunities and threats, whereas an internal assessment checks for strengths and weaknesses. A situation audit, or environmental assessment, analyzes the past, current, and future forces that affect the organization. Expectations of outside interests such as opinion leaders, governmental officials, insurance companies, and consumers are sought. Expectations of inside interests such as physicians, staff, administrators, and patients are collected.

The management team can use a grid to visualize the situation audit. The past, present, and future are represented on the horizontal axis. Criteria for areas such as clients, competition, market share, environment, demographics, economics, laws, politics, technology, resources and facilities, finances, and human resources are represented on the vertical axis.

A SWOT (strengths, weaknesses, opportunities, threats) analysis worksheet is also helpful. Each quadrant of a paper is labeled as one of the four categories, and appropriate factors are listed in each quadrant for a bird's-eye view of the situation audit (Box 8-2). Internal strengths or weaknesses may include management development, qualifications of staff, medical staff expertise, abundance or scarcity of staff, financial situation, cash flow position, marketing efforts, market share, facilities, location, and quality of services.

Opportunities include nurse and physician recruitment, referral patterns, new programs, new markets, diversification, population growth, improved technology, and new facilities.

Threats may be shortage of nurses, decrease in patient satisfaction, decrease in insured patients, increase in accounts receivable, decrease in demand for services, competition, regulations, litigation, legislative changes, unionization, and loss of accreditation.

After the situation audit is done, the management team reviews the philosophy, identifies

---

BOX 8-2 SWOT Analysis

STRENGTHS	WEAKNESSES
Management development	Scarcity of staff
Qualifications of staff	Financial situation
Medical staff expertise	Cash flow position
Facilities	Marketing efforts
Location	Market share
Quality of services	

OPPORTUNITIES	THREATS
Nurse recruitment	Shortage of nurses
Physician recruitment	Decrease in patient satisfaction
Referral patterns	Increase in accounts receivable
New programs	Decrease in demands for services
New markets	Competition
Diversification	Regulations
Population growth	Litigation
Improved technology	Unionization
New facilities	Loss of accreditation

SWOT, Strengths, weaknesses, opportunities, threats.

---

vision and values, writes a purpose or mission statement, identifies organizational goals and objectives, plans strategies to accomplish the objectives, identifies required resources, determines priorities, sets time frames, and determines accountability.

Business plans are plans for new ventures, such as new products or services that meet many of the standards for strategic plans (Box 8-3). They integrate strategic, operational, and financial planning. The cover page notes the name of the company, the business plan and year, and names and phone numbers of the contact person or persons. The executive summary, which is about two pages long, is a brief overview of the entire plan. The table of contents should identify at least each major section of the report. The introduction describes the nature of the organization and identifies philosophy, goals, objectives, and projected outcomes. The market analysis identifies the product, price, place, and promotions for the new product or service. The analysis of the competition describes the competition

BOX **8-3** Business Plan

Cover page
Executive summary
Table of contents
Introduction
　　Description of the business
Analysis of the market
Analysis of the competition
Product or service development
Operational plan
Marketing plan
Organizational plan
Development schedule
Financial plan

BOX **8-4** Planning Tools

Vision
Values
Mission
Philosophy
Goals
Objectives
Policies
Procedures

"Look upon the present as the past of your future." —Anonymous

and identifies the competitive edge. Product development identifies the resources needed and a time frame for the development of the new product or service and presents a quality control plan. The operational plan identifies the desired location and the needed facilities, equipment, and personnel. The marketing plan describes the mission, goals, strategies, staffing, and financial plans for marketing. The organizational plan presents an organizational chart with job descriptions and short resumes. The development schedule identifies tasks and timelines. The financial plan identifies developmental costs and projects income goals and expenditures (Burton and McBride, 1999; Swansburg, 1996).

Top-level managers, such as chief executive officers, presidents, and division heads, do strategic planning for 3 to 5 years. Middle-level managers, such as supervisors and clinical specialists, do intermediate planning for 6 months to 2 years. Lower-level managers, such as managers of nursing units, team leaders, case managers, and primary care nurses, do operational planning of 1 week to 1 year (Douglas, 1996) (Table 8-2).

VISION

Vision is a mental image or the power of imagination to see something that is not actually visible. When doing strategic planning, the vision should be the preferred future (Boxes 8-4 and 8-5).

"Good customer service springs from individuals within the organization. It requires compassion, and the rare ability to understand that only by routinely putting the needs of the customer first can we hope to be first as an organization."
—Unknown

BOX **8-5** Sample Vision

GENERAL HOSPITAL VISION STATEMENT

The vision for General Hospital is to be the preeminent health care provider in the region by doing the following:
Being the premier full-service, integrated health care delivery network that provides a continuum of health services
Creating an environment that exceeds the expectations of our customers
Developing creative solutions to the challenges facing us
Providing economically viable, cost-effective services to our customers
Working in partnership with other leading health care organizations

TABLE **8-2** Levels of Planning

Strategic planning	Top-level management
Intermediate planning	Middle-level management
Operational planning	Lower-level management

VALUES

Value is the worth, usefulness, or importance of something. Leadership, management, and personnel should determine what their values are and keep their plans and actions consistent with their values. A values statement is a planning tool (Box 8-6).

PURPOSE OR MISSION STATEMENT

Organizations exist for a purpose. Clarification of the mission or purpose is a high priority for planning. Most nursing services exist to provide high-quality nursing care to clients. Some also encourage teaching and research. Each specialty area, with its own specific purposes, contributes to the overall purpose of the institution. For example, the purpose of the in-service education department is to orient staff to the job and to provide educational programs to improve the quality of the staff work. The burn unit exists to provide good-quality nursing service to patients with burns.

The mission or purpose influences philosophy, goals, and objectives. For example, if a progressive care unit exists to help patients adjust to their diseases, it should be staffed with professional nurses particularly skilled in teaching and counseling. If, however, the unit's purpose is to cut hospital and patient expenses, it may be a minimal care unit with reduced services given by nonprofessional workers. The relationships

---

BOX **8-6** Sample Values Statement

The guiding values for General Hospital are as follows:
Quality
Compassion
Fairness
Integrity
Innovation
Fiscal responsibility

BOX **8-7** Sample Mission Statement

The mission of General Hospital is to deliver comprehensive health care services to promote physical and mental health; to prevent disease, injury, and disability; and to promote healing of the body, mind, and spirit. Related instruction, public service programs, and research will facilitate high-quality health care.

---

among the mission, philosophy, goals, and objectives should be examined periodically for consistency. Box 8-7 provides an example of a mission statement.

PHILOSOPHY

The philosophy articulates a vision and provides a statement of beliefs and values that direct one's practice. It should be written, included in appropriate documents, and reviewed periodically. If the philosophy is stated in vague, abstract terms that are not easily understood, it is useless. Conflicting philosophies between overlapping units cause confusion and should be avoided. Workers are most likely to interpret the philosophy from the pronouncements and actions of the leaders in the institution. Therefore conformity of action to belief is important.

When developing or reevaluating a philosophy, the manager should consider theory, education, practice, research, and nursing's role in the total organization. Gaye Poteet and Alice Hill (1988) identify three approaches that can be used to incorporate nursing theory into the philosophy. An eclectic approach would select ideas from various nursing theories and incorporate them into the philosophy statements: a theory might be adopted and integrated into the philosophy, or another might be referred to throughout. Attaching an explanation of the theory to the philosophy would also be useful.

Myra Levine and Dorothea Orem focus on nursing therapeutics. Dorothy Johnson and Sister

---

RESEARCH Perspective 8-1

Data from Tuck I, Harris LH, Baliko B: Values expressed in philosophies of nursing services. *JONA* 30(4):180-184, 2000.

Purpose: The purpose of this study was to identify the values that are evident in philosophies of nursing services.

Methods: Ten community hospitals and medical centers within a southeastern state submitted their philosophies of nursing services for content analysis.

Results/conclusions: The most frequently cited value was caring. Professionalism was the second most frequently found value. Individualism was the third reported value. The remaining categories of need fulfillment, culture, well-being or health, and adaptation were distributed selectively across the philosophies.

Callista Roy emphasize the client. Imogene King, Margaret Newman, Ida Orlando, Josephine Patterson, Loretta Zderad, Joyce Travelbee, and Ernestine Wiedebach discuss interaction. Martha Rogers focuses on the environment and inter-actions of human beings (Marriner Tomey and Alligood, 2002).

It is appropriate to comment on skill levels needed, advanced preparation for certain posi-

tions, need for continuing education, provision of educational opportunities for students, and specific practice modalities. Value of applying research findings to practice, supporting research efforts, and nursing's role in the overall organization could also be clarified in the philosophy (Box 8-8).

GOALS AND OBJECTIVES

"Wishing consumes as much energy as planning."
—Anonymous

Goals and objectives state actions for achieving the mission and philosophy. In fact, if the mission or purpose and philosophy are to be more than good intentions, they must be translated into explicit goals. The more quantitative the goal, the more likely its achievement is to receive attention and the less likely it is to be distorted. Goals are central to the whole management process—planning, organizing, staffing, directing, and controlling. Planning defines the goals. The institution is organized and staffed to accomplish the goals. Direction stimulates personnel toward accomplishment of the objectives, and control compares the results with the objectives to evaluate accomplishments.

BOX **8-8** Sample Philosophy

PHILOSOPHY OF GENERAL HOSPITAL

General Hospital is committed to assessing and meeting the physical, emotional, spiritual, environmental, social, and rehabilitative health needs of the citizens in the region. The worth, dignity, and autonomy of individuals (customers, employees, and others) are recognized, as is each individual's right to self-direction and responsibility for one's own life. Individual uniqueness will be considered when assessing needs and delivering quality care. Educational pursuits, research, and public service programs will be used toward innovations and improvement of health care in the region. General Hospital personnel will work in collaboration with customers and in partnership with other organizations to provide cost-effective services.

Goals and objectives may address services rendered, economics, use of resources—people, funds, facilities—innovations, and social responsibilities. Objectives are selective rather than global, are multiple, and cover a wide range of activities. The immediate, short-term, and long-term goals should be balanced, interdependent, and ranked in order of importance. It is common to have more short-term than long-term goals.

Classic theory contends that the board of directors and top administration should determine institutional goals. Behavioral scientists are interested in having workers involved in setting goals and identifying real versus stated goals. Observing the day-by-day decisions and actions can identify the real goals. Service interest, profit motives, governmental regulations, union representation, and personal goals all influence decision making.

It is appropriate for the board of directors and top administrators to set institutional goals and objectives; for the vice president for nursing, directors of nurses, and patient care coordinators to set the goals and objectives for the nursing service; for the staff associates to determine the unit goals and objectives; and for the nurses to determine their goals and objectives with their immediate manager. The overlap created by the vice president's and director's working on institutional and nursing service goals and the patient care coordinator's contributing to nursing service and her unit's goals helps facilitate continuity and compatibility of goals. Participation in the determination of goals and objectives increases commitment, transforming them from stated to real goals. Because goals are dynamic, they change over time. They should be reviewed periodically so that they can be changed in an evolutionary rather than a radical manner. Goals should be specific rather than vague and challenging yet reachable. Necessary support elements should be available (Box 8-9).

Goals help focus attention on what is important and are broader statements than objectives. Objectives are more specific ways to reach the

---

BOX 8-9 Sample Goal and Objectives

GOAL

Develop and implement staff development programs to meet the need for increased knowledge

OBJECTIVE

Develop and implement at least 12 staff development programs by the end of the fiscal year

STRATEGIES

Continue to develop, implement, and evaluate continuing education programs for personnel

Evaluate, revise, and implement the orientation program for new personnel

Develop, implement, and evaluate in-service programs regarding new products

---

goal. It is recommended that objectives be achievable, specific, measurable, and outcome oriented, starting with "to" followed by a verb. Each objective should be about a single result with a target date. Strategies identify how the organization will attain the vision. The development of long- and short-term objectives is appropriate. A form with four columns (one for goals/objectives, one for strategies/actions, one for target dates and person or persons responsible, one for accomplishments) can be a helpful planning tool (Swansburg and Swansburg, 2002; Yoder-Wise, 2003) (Table 8-3).

POLICIES

"Honesty is a question of right and wrong, not a matter of policy." —Anonymous

Policies and procedures are means for accomplishing goals and objectives. Policies explain how goals will be achieved and serve as guides that define the general course and scope of activities permissible for goal accomplishment. They serve as a basis for future decisions and actions, help coordinate plans, control performance, and increase consistency of action by increasing the probability that different managers will make similar decisions when independently facing

TABLE **8-3** Planning Tool

GOALS/OBJECTIVES	STRATEGIES/ACTIONS	TARGET DATES/PERSON(S) RESPONSIBLE	ACCOMPLISHMENTS
1. To develop and implement at least 12 staff development programs by the end of the fiscal year	A. Develop class regarding performance appraisal for middle managers.	January 2005/nurse manager educator	Collect materials first week; write lesson plans second week; develop course teaching tools third week; print course packet fourth week.
	B. Implement performance appraisal class for middle managers.	February 2005/nurse manager educator	Class taught February.
	C. Evaluate class regarding performance appraisal.	February 2005/nurse manager educator	Pass out evaluation form at end of class; tabulate data within week.

similar situations. Consequently, morale is increased when personnel perceive that they are being treated equally. Policies also serve as a means by which authority can be delegated.

Policies should be comprehensive in scope, stable, and flexible so they can be applied to different conditions that are not so diverse that they require separate sets of policies. Consistency is important because inconsistency introduces uncertainty and contributes to feelings of bias, preferential treatment, and unfairness. Fairness is an important characteristic that is attributed to the application of the policy. Policies should be written and understandable.

Policies can be implied or expressed. Implied policies are not directly voiced or written but are established by patterns of decisions. They may have either favorable or unfavorable effects and represent an interpretation of observed behavior. Courteous treatment of clients may be implied versus expressed. The presence or absence of workers who are over 50 or 55 years of age, minority members, women, or pregnant women may lead to an interpretation of implied policies. Sometimes policies are implied simply because no one has ever bothered to state them. At other times they may deliberately be only implied because they are illegal or reflect questionable

ethics. Sometimes implied policy conflicts with expressed policy. These double standards should be prevented.

Expressed policies may be oral or written. Oral policies are more flexible than written ones and can be easily adjusted to changing circumstances. However, they are less desirable than written ones because they may not be known.

The process of writing policies reveals discrepancies and omissions and causes the manager to think critically about the policy, thus contributing to clarity. Once written, they are readily available to all in the same form; their meaning cannot be changed by word of mouth; misunderstandings can be referred to the written words; the chance of misinterpretation is decreased; policy statements can be sent to all affected by them; they can be referred to whoever wishes to check the policy; and they can be used for orientation purposes. Written policies indicate the integrity of the organization's intention and generate confidence in management.

A disadvantage of written policies is the reluctance to revise them when they become outdated. However, even oral policies become obsolete. Managers should review policies periodically, and if that fails, personnel can appeal for a revision.

BOX **8-10** Emergence of Policies

Originated
Appealed
Imposed

Policies can emerge in several ways—originated, appealed, or imposed (Box 8-10). The originated, or internal, policies are usually developed by top management to guide subordinates in their functions. Strategy for originated policy flows from the objectives of the organization as defined by top management and may be broad in scope, allowing staff associates to develop supplemental policies, or well defined with little room for interpretation. All the lower managerial decisions should implement the broader policy defined by top management.

Sometimes policies are generated at the operating and first-line manager levels and imposed upward. The extent to which this happens is influenced by the organizational atmosphere and adequacy of policies generated by top management. At times policies may be formulated simultaneously from both directions.

When staff associates do not know how to solve a problem, disagree with a previous decision, or otherwise want a question reviewed, they appeal to the manager for a decision. As appeals are taken up the hierarchy and decisions are made, precedents known as appealed policy develop and guide future managerial actions.

Policies developed from appeals are likely to be incomplete, uncoordinated, and unclear. Unintended precedents can be set when decisions are made for a given situation without consideration for possible effects on other dimensions of the organization. This aimless formation of policy makes it difficult to know what policies exist. Sometimes managers dislike facing issues until forced to do so and consequently delay policy making until precedents have been set. Appealed policies can be foresighted and consistent, especially when the manager knows that

the decision constitutes policy. Nevertheless, when a number of policies are being appealed, it is time to assess policies for gaps and needs for updating and clarification so originated policies can dominate. One can expect health care agencies to require policies about patient care assignments, noting physicians' orders, administration of medications, patient safety, charting, and infection control.

Imposed, or external, policies are thrust on an organization by external forces, such as government or labor unions. Policies of the organization must conform to local, state, and federal laws. Collective bargaining and union contracts direct labor policies. Professional and social groups—such as the American Nurses Association, the National League for Nursing, and church, school, and charitable organizations—mold policy.

The planning process involves defining, communicating, applying, and maintaining policies. The development of a policy can originate anywhere in an organization and should involve personnel who will be affected by the policy. They have valuable information for sound policy formation and can ensure that the policy will be implemented. Before writing a policy, one must consider whether there are specific, recurring problems, how frequently they occur, whether they are temporary or permanent in nature, and whether a policy statement would clarify thinking and promote efficiency.

When policies are written, the purpose, philosophy, goals, and objectives should serve as guides. Policies should be consistent and help solve or prevent specific problems. Clear, concise statements that establish areas of authority and perhaps include reference to supporting policies minimize exceptions. Managers need sufficient guidance with accompanying freedom for action. It is advisable to have the policy statement reviewed and approved by superiors and the affected managers before the policy is formalized.

Policies are of no use if no one knows of their existence. Oral communication is appropriate to introduce and explain new policies. It is appropriate to send a letter of purpose and a copy of policies to personnel affected by them. The written policies can then be referred to later. Policies should be written in a specific, concise, and complete manner and stored in a policy manual that is easily accessible to all personnel to whom the policies apply. The manual will be well organized if policies are classified, noted in the table of contents, and indexed by topic. Policies should be easily replaceable with revised ones.

Once a policy has been stated and approved, it is applied. Policy formation is a continuous process; the policy is continually reappraised and restated as necessary (Figure 8-1). Continuing surveillance to determine that the policy is understood and applied is important. Periodic analysis and evaluation of existing policies can suggest the need for revision. Personnel should be encouraged to help formulate, review, and revise policies. Boxes 8-11 through 8-15 present sample policies for generating and reviewing nursing policies, procedures, and protocols.

PROCEDURES

Procedures supply a more specific guide to action than policy does. They help achieve a high degree of regularity by enumerating the chronological sequence of steps. Procedures are intradepartmental or interdepartmental and consequently do not affect the entire organization to the extent that policy statements do.

Procedure manuals provide a basis for orientation and staff development and are a ready reference for all personnel. They standardize procedures and equipment and can provide a basis for evaluation. Good procedures can result in time and labor savings. Box 8-16 presents a sample procedure for ambulating a patient with one assistant.

Improvement in operating procedures increases productivity and reduces cost. Waste in performing work can be decreased by applying work simplification that strives to make each part of a procedure productive. First, one decides what work requires simplification by identifying problem areas. Next, the work selected is analyzed carefully and in detail. Charts that depict the components of the work and the work flow are useful for motion or procedural analysis.

A questioning attitude helps determine why work is done, by whom, when, where, and how. What is the purpose of the procedure? Does it need to be done? Can it be eliminated?

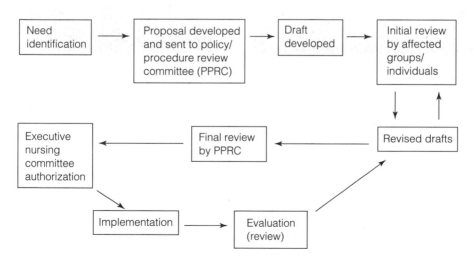

Figure 8-1 Flowchart for policies/procedures/protocols.

BOX 8-11 Process for Generation of Policy/Procedure/Protocol

Issue Date		Policy No.
July 1989	**PROCESS FOR GENERATION OF A NURSING POLICY/PROCEDURE/PROTOCOL**	A/O QA.08
Review Dates		**Subject**
Annually		Quality Assurance

POLICY

Written policies, procedures, and protocols that reflect optimal standards of nursing practice will guide the provision of nursing care.

SCOPE

This policy applies to all of Nursing Services.

PURPOSE

To provide a consistent format for the writing and processing of policies/procedures/protocols (P/P/P); to identify resources for creating, reviewing, and changing P/P/P for Indiana University Hospitals Nursing Services; to eliminate duplication of efforts and ensure current and consistent practice.

PROCESS

1. Any nurse with approval of the unit director or associate director when appropriate may initiate a written P/P/P. A self-study packet is available to assist with this process.
2. A proposal for all new P/P/Ps will be sent to the Nursing Service Policy/Procedure Review Committee (PPRC). (See attached form.) The proposal includes the topic/title, patients affected by the procedure, why it is needed, resource persons who will be used to write or consult, and appropriate signature(s). In some cases a proposal may not be necessary, but the intent to write a P/P/P should be communicated to the PPRC. The committee will then serve as a resource for format, for other resources, and for distribution. Exceptions for the initial proposal might be direction from the Executive Nursing Council or the hospital system.
3. Approval/disapproval to write will then be communicated to the initiating individual(s) by the PPRC after considering the possible overall need, already existent P/P/P, and additional resources. A member of the PPRC will be assigned to each approved proposal to ensure consistency of format. (See attached format guidelines.)

Associated Director of Hospitals for Nursing	Date
Sonna Ehrlich	7/11/89

Used with permission from Indiana Hospitals.

For example, are "closed" and "surgical" beds really necessary, or could "open" beds be used for all purposes? Who does the work? Can someone else do it better, or can it be assigned to someone with less skill? Is there duplication of efforts? Can two or more activities be combined? Will changing the time sequence improve the procedure? Can changing the location reduce transportation? Once these questions have been answered, rearranging, combining, or eliminating components should simplify work. Then the improved methods must be communicated so they can be implemented.

Writing procedures demands a consistent format that considers the definition; purpose; materials needed and how to locate, requisition, and dispose of them; steps in the procedure; expected results; precautions; legal implications; nurse, patient, and physician responsibilities; and appropriate charting. Each step in the procedure leading to the accomplishment of a goal should be necessary and in proper relationship

BOX 8-12 Proposal for Policy/Procedure

PROPOSAL FOR POLICY/PROCEDURE

This form is submitted to the Policy/Procedure Committee of Nursing Services to request a written Policy/Procedure designed to implement policy and maintain policy standards in regard to the following nursing care:

Topic: _____

Patients affected by the policy/procedure: _____

Explanation of the policy/procedure: _____
_____

Problems that arise as a result of not having a written policy/procedure: _____
_____

Resources that you will use to write and document the validity of this policy/procedure: _____

Name _____

Unit director _____

Associate director _____

****

For Use by Policy/Procedure Committee

Date received: _____

Approval for writing of policy/procedure: Yes   No

Contacts within Nursing Services and Medicine that must be made for coordination of the writing of this procedure:
_____

Committee member assigned to supervise project: _____

Guidelines for Procedure Format

Title
Policy statement
Scope
Purpose (optional)
Assessment and planning
   Nursing considerations
   Cautions
   Resources
Implementation
   Sequence of interventions/rationale
   Cautions
Evaluation
Documentation
Authorization signature
Reference:
Written by:
Date of revision(s):
Date of review(s):

Used with permission from Indiana Hospitals.

BOX 8-13 Review Process for Policies/Procedures/Protocols

Issue Date		Policy No.
November 1987	**PROCESS FOR GENERATION OF A NURSING POLICY/PROCEDURE/PROTOCOL**	A/O QA.07
Review Dates		**Subject**
Annually		Quality Assurance

POLICY

All policies, procedures, and protocols (P/P/Ps) will be reviewed annually and revised as necessary.

SCOPE

This policy applies to all Nursing Service policies, procedures, and protocols.

PROCESS

1. Reviews of P/P/Ps will be conducted in quarterly periods (Jan-Mar, Apr-Jun, Jul-Sept, Oct-Dec).
2. Before the beginning of the upcoming quarter, the Policy/Procedure Review Committee (PPRC) will receive notice of which P/P/Ps are due for review. Members of the PPRC will be assigned accountability for the review of specific P/P/Ps.
3. The accountable PPRC member will review the P/P/P and will solicit feedback from appropriate content experts, using the appropriate Policy or Procedure Review Questionnaire. (See attached.)
4. The content experts will complete the Review Questionnaire after obtaining input from most affected groups or individuals. The completed questionnaire and a draft of the revised P/P/P will be returned to the accountable PPRC member by the deadline date indicated.
5. On receipt of the questionnaire and draft, the accountable PPRC member will submit the final draft of the revised P/P/P to the PPRC.
6. Upon approval by the PPRC, the final draft will be submitted to the Executive Nursing Council for authorization and signature.
7. Revised P/P/Ps will then be distributed to all holders of Nursing Service Policy/Procedure Manuals.
8. Requests to review P/P/Ps can be made at any time during the year to the PPRC. (See Figure 8-1.)

Date of Revision(s): 7/89
Date of Review(s): 7/90

Associated Director of Hospitals for Nursing	Date
Sonna Ehrlich	7/21/89

Used with permission from Indiana Hospitals.

to the other steps. Balance between flexibility and stability should be maintained. As with the policy manual, the procedure manual should be easily accessible, well organized with a table of contents, and indexed. Each procedure should be easily replaceable with a revised one. Because there is a tendency to add new procedures instead of revising existing ones, it is important to review and revise the procedure manual periodically.

In reviewing, one should check the effectiveness and workability with personnel to determine whether the procedure has been followed. Procedures should be realistic and written in simple language that is easy to understand. Changes should be dated and provided to all appropriate personnel.

Before spending valuable time writing procedures, one must consider whether a procedure is actually needed. With preservice and on-the-job

BOX **8-14** Procedure Review Questionnaire

PROCEDURE REVIEW QUESTIONNAIRE

Name of Procedure _____

Date of review _____

Reviewer(s) _____

(Name)	(Title)	(Service/Unit)

(Name)	(Title)	(Service/Unit)

(Note: The reviewer may wish to carry out the procedure exactly as written before addressing the questions below.)

Please circle the number that most accurately reflects your response to the following.

Where procedure differs from practice, please note discrepancies on separate sheet of paper. Please write recommended revision on separate sheet of paper and return to _____ by _____.

	Yes	No	Uncertain	Comments
1. Does the procedure accurately reflect all equipment/materials necessary to carry out the procedure				
a) safely?				
b) competently?	1	2	3	
2. Does the procedure reflect equipment used at IUHs?	1	2	3	
3. Is the sequence of steps correct?	1	2	3	
4. Is the sequence of steps complete?	1	2	3	
5. Are the contraindications, if any, clearly identified?	1	2	3	
6. Does the scientific rationale provide a meaningful reason for each intervention?	1	2	3	
7. Does the procedure reflect results of current research and state-of-the-art clinical nursing practice?	1	2	3	
8. Does the procedure reflect current clinical practice at IUHs?	1	2	3	
9. Is the procedure in conflict with any other hospital or Nursing Services' policies/procedures? If so, please list.	1	2	3	

ADDITIONAL COMMENTS:

RECOMMENDED ACTION

_____ The procedure is correct as written. Recommend adoption of procedure.   _____ Discrepancies noted. Recommended revision attached   _____ Recommend procedure not be adopted.

12/84

Used with permission from Indiana Hospitals.

BOX 8-15 Policy Review Form

POLICY REVIEW FORM

Name of policy _____

Date of review _____

Reviewer _____
                    (Name)   (Service)
_____

INSTRUCTIONS: Please circle the number that most accurately reflects your response to the following questions. Please check at the bottom your recommended action.

	Yes	No	Comments
1. Is there a need for the policy?	1	2	
2. Is the policy relevant to this institution and staff?	1	2	
3. Is the policy consistent with Indiana University Hospitals Nursing Services philosophy?	1	2	
4. Is the policy in conflict with any other hospital or nursing policies?	1	2	
5. Does the policy create any inequities between hospital staff or patients?	1	2	
6. Is the policy reasonable (i.e., can compliance be enforced)?	1	2	
7. Is the policy clearly written so that anyone unfamiliar with the subject can understand it?	1	2	
8. Is the information accurate?	1	2	
9. Is the policy complete (i.e., does it include the scope, purpose, and any related information)?	1	2	

ADDITIONAL COMMENTS:

RECOMMENDED ACTION:

_____ No action required   _____ Revision required   _____ Remove from manual
         Approved as written   (Changes attached)   (Justification attached)

Courtesy Indiana Hospitals. Used with permission.

preparation, is there really a need to have on each unit procedures on how to feed a patient and how to make a bed? Goals can be reached in a variety of ways, and consequently nursing students are taught principles rather than procedures. There are textbooks with bedside nursing procedures, and many disposable products with directions are available. It seems most important for the procedure manual to contain information that may vary from institution to institution. Not all parts of the procedure format may be necessary for each procedure. New personnel and float nurses can serve as valuable resources for nursing managers to consult when they are determining what contents are important for the procedure manual.

The planning process is a critical element of management. Nurse administrators must learn it, because it will not happen by accident. Planning is largely conceptual, but its results are clearly visible. The statement of the purpose or mission, philosophy, goals, objectives, policies, and procedures are all consequences of planning. They set the stage for smooth operations.

BOX 8-16 Procedure

PROCEDURE

Ambulating with One Assistant

1. Definition: to walk or move about with help from one person
2. Purpose
   a. Prevent complications of immobility.
   b. Improve balance and muscle tone.
   c. Increase feelings of physical and mental well-being.
   d. Progress from needing assistance to becoming independent in ambulation.
3. Materials needed
   a. Robe or hospital gown to put on backwards to prevent exposure of patient's back
   b. Slippers or shoes that have nonslip soles and fit well
   c. Safety belt if indicated
4. Steps in procedure
   a. Check patient's chart regarding ambulation.
   b. Wash hands.
   c. Explain the procedure and rationale to the patient.
   d. Place the bed in a low position, and help the patient sit on the edge of the bed.
   e. Assess the patient for faintness or dizziness.
      (1) Rationale: Having the patient sit on the edge of the bed before standing to reduce faintness and dizziness will reduce the risk of falling.
   f. Apply safety belt if the patient is unsteady.
      (1) Rationale: The safety belt helps support the patient and decreases the risk of injury.
   g. Help the patient to stand and observe the patient for balance.
   h. Grasp the patient around the waist to stabilize, and grasp the arm near the assistant with the other hand to guide the patient.
   i. Stand by the weaker side except when with cerebrovascular accident patient; then stand on the stronger unaffected side.
      (1) Rationale: Flaccid muscles on the affected side do not provide enough muscle strength for the assistant to grasp and support the patient.
   j. Encourage the patient to look straight ahead and to use good posture.
      (1) Rationale: There is a tendency for the patient to look down, and that may increase vertigo.
   k. Instruct the patient to lift each foot to take a step instead of shuffling.
   l. Remember the patient has to walk back, and pace the distance to the patient's ability.
   m. Chart the activity and the patient's tolerance.

Modified from Smith SF, Duell DJ, Martin BC: *Clinical nursing skills: Basic to advanced skills*, ed 5, Upper Saddle River, NJ, 2000, Prentice Hall Health.

CHAPTER SUMMARY

Chapter 8 covered the following:

Planning Process
    History of Strategic Planning
    Purpose of Strategic Planning
    Strategic Planning Process
Vision
Values
Purpose or Mission Statement

Philosophy
Goals and Objectives
    Policies
    Procedures

On-line Resources

evolve Additional critical thinking activities, worksheets, and case studies are available on-line at http://evolve.elsevier.com/Marriner/guide/

REFERENCES

Burton EJ, McBride WB: *Total business planning: A step-by-step guide with forms,* New York, 1999, John Wiley & Sons.

Douglas LM: *The effective nurse leader and manager,* St Louis, 1996, Mosby.

Marriner Tomey A, Alligood MR: *Nursing theorists and their work,* St Louis, 2002, Mosby.

Poteet GW, Hill AS: Identifying the components of a nursing philosophy, *J Nurs Adm* 18:29-33, Oct 1988.

Smith SF, Duell DJ, Martin BC: *Clinical nursing skills: Basic to advanced skills,* ed 5, Upper Saddle River, NJ, 2000, Prentice Hall Health.

Swansburg RC: *Management and leadership for nurse managers,* ed 2, Boston, 1996, Jones & Bartlett.

Swansburg RC, Swansburg RJ: *Introductory management and leadership for nurses,* ed 3, Boston, 2002, Jones & Bartlett.

Yoder-Wise PS: *Leading and managing in nursing,* ed 3, St Louis, 2003, Mosby.

9

Financial Management, Cost Containment, and Marketing

Chapter Overview

Chapter 9 discusses history of health care financing, budgetary leadership and management, budgets, cost containment, costing out nursing services, personal finances, and marketing.

Chapter Objectives

- Define capitation.
- Identify at least three prerequisites to budgeting.
- Identify at least four types of budgets.
- Differentiate at least three advantages and three disadvantages of budgeting.
- Discuss at least five strategies for cost containment.
- Explain fixed and variable costs as they relate to break-even points.
- Determine at least three factors to consider when costing out nursing services.
- Identify at least five factors that should be considered when making a marketing audit, and ask a question to evaluate each of those factors.
- Describe the four *p*'s of the marketing mix.
- Describe the Boston consulting group's grid of potential growth and profitability possibilities for identifying marketing strategies.
- Identify the four stages in the life cycle of a product.
- Identify at least three ways to do pricing.
- Determine at least four promotion tools.

Major Concepts and Definitions

Accounting a system that accumulates bookkeeping entries into summaries of the financial situation of the agency

Budget a plan for the allocation of resources and a control for ensuring that results comply with the plans

Cost containment to hold back costs within fixed limits

Economics production, distribution, and consumption of wealth

Costing out calculating the cost of specific items

Marketing the analysis, planning, implementation, and control of programs for exchanges of values with target markets to achieve organizational objectives

Exchange resource dependency

Publics distinct groups of people or organizations that have an actual or potential interest in or impact on an organization

Market potential arena for trading resources

Image sum of a person's beliefs, ideas, and impressions about an object or person

Audit identification, collection, and evaluation of information that needs examination to evaluate market relations

Segmentation subsets of the total market

Marketing mix product, price, place, and promotions

Life cycle introduction, growth, maturity, and market decline stages of a product

Break-even calculations direct and indirect costs equal to income

Direct costs specific costs of a program

Indirect costs generalized costs such as maintenance and administration allocated to the program

Variable costs costs that vary in direct proportion to volume

Fixed costs costs unrelated to volume

Semifixed costs costs that are fixed within a range of activity

Semivariable costs costs that are fixed at zero output and increase with volume

HISTORY OF HEALTH CARE FINANCING

During the 1930s most health care was privately financed. Insurance plans increased during the 1950s. During that time cost-based pricing was used. The price of service was based on direct costs (such as salaries, benefits, supplies) and indirect costs or overhead costs (including services such as accounting, administration, housekeeping, medical records, depreciation, interest expenses, repayment of debt, return on investments, bad debts, other uncollectible accounts). The more treatments and services provided, the more income to the health care providers. This retrospective approach increased hospital profits, increased health care costs, and in turn increased insurance rates.

Medicare was developed during the 1960s and brought average pricing to the health care market by establishing the average price it would pay. That led to competitive-based pricing, which forced providers to achieve the marketplace average or lose money.

Health costs have been increasing because of the aging population with chronic diseases and increased health care needs, increased use of expensive technology, new and expensive treatment modalities, litigation, uninsured people, and administrative costs. Previously, third-party payers paid hospitals for services. The employers paid the insurance premiums. The insurance companies paid the bill, and the customers felt little effect. During the 1980s, 1990s, and 2000s, insurance companies raised their premiums dramatically to meet the rising costs, making it difficult for employers to pay the premiums. Consequently customers are required to pay larger portions of the costs as deductibles and are becoming increasingly aware of the high costs of health care and the need to be selective.

A prospective reimbursement system encourages the implementation of cost-effective health care services. The Tax Equity Fiscal Responsibility Act of 1982 added case-mix into Medicare based on diagnostic-related groups (DRGs). A prospective payment system based on 467 DRG categories that provided pretreatment diagnosis billing categories for most U.S. hospitals reimbursed by Medicare was signed into law as HR 1900 (P.L. 98-21) by President Reagan. It used a prospective rather than the traditional retrospective time frame. Reimbursement is by case or costs related to treatment of specific DRGs rather than per diem or total hospital costs divided by patient days. The payment unit is the diagnosis rather than the patient day. Rates are determined from local, regional, and national rural and urban costs instead of the hospital's own costs. There are incentive payments when the length of stay is lower than average and disincentives when costs exceed the standard so that hospitals profit from cost containment. Previously hospitals were reimbursed for costs retrospectively and had little incentive to contain costs. The prospective payment system applies to all Medicare-participating hospitals except long-term care, rehabilitation, children's, and psychiatric care hospitals.

The results of DRGs include a decrease in number of patients in acute care settings caused by early discharge, an increase in the acuteness of illness among hospitalized patients, an increase in the use of ambulatory and home care facilities, and a focus on cost-effectiveness.

Managed care became widespread during the 1980s. Coordination of high-cost health care services became a goal of health care insurance companies. Since 1988 there has been rapid growth of case management or utilization review organizations that monitor the delivery of care and are gatekeepers to providers of care. Clinical pathways use outcome criteria as indicators of quality. Cooperation among health care providers is necessary to reach the expected outcomes in the most efficient manner. By the late 1990s, capitation and global payments were common.

Insurance companies have developed policies to control costs that direct beneficiaries away from providers that have charges above the marketplace average. By 2000 insurance companies were demanding discounted services. Insurance companies were contracting amounts discounted or deducted from patient care revenues that health care providers must write off.

The exclusive provider arrangement provides insurance coverage only for services provided by a contracted professional or institution except in the event of an emergency or while out of a geographical area.

Health maintenance organizations (HMOs) provide comprehensive health care services to enrollees for a fixed periodic payment. Capitation is the fixed rate paid to the provider per member per month for a specified amount of health care services. Actuarial services provide statistical analysis of demographic, financial, and utilization trends to predict health plan premiums or costs. The clients choose their physician from a medical group roster. The primary care physician is a gatekeeper who assesses the patient and determines if referral to a specialist or hospitalization is necessary. The incentive is to keep patients healthy and to reduce physician, diagnostic, and hospital services. Under capitation, the financial risk for provision of care is transferred from the payer to the health care delivery system. Visits to a physician or services are expenses, not revenue to the provider. Hospitals have incentives to lower hospitalizations, decrease the length of stay, and minimize the variance of stays between patients with like diagnosis. Consequently, hospital utilization has dropped drastically, and hospitals have many empty beds. Hospitals may subcontract some services, such as dialysis, to others for less cost. Because hospitals have large fixed costs in physical facilities, the trend of the 1980s and 1990s to give care outside the hospital may be reversed. Hospitals may get involved with services such as home health care and hospice that were provided outside the hospital. Hospital administrators may become health care system managers.

Preferred provider organizations (PPOs) negotiate a special, usually reduced, rate for insurance-plan beneficiaries usually on a fee-for-service basis with incentives of lowered rates for consumers when they use the preferred providers.

Individual provider arrangements (IPAs) allow health care providers to provide medical services in their offices for managed care or prepaid plans. This was one of the first alternative delivery prepaid plans with a set of benefits provided by a group of providers within a specific geographical area. During the 1940s Kaiser Permanente was one of the first employers to provide such a plan.

Now managed competition exists among prepaid providers such as HMOs, PPOs, and IPAs and leads to early discharge of patients; early retirement of the better paid senior nurses; narrow differentials between associate degree (AD), bachelor of science (BS), and master of science (MS) prepared nurses; slower wage growth rates; substitution of registered nurses (RNs) with less trained, more poorly paid unlicensed personnel; substitution of physicians and psychologists with greater use of advanced practice nurses; use of RNs as utilization reviewers; and mergers or resized agencies. In 2000, the federal government introduced Ambulatory Payment Classifications as a new payment system for outpatient services, which changed the basis of payment for outpatient services from a flat fee for individual services to a fixed reimbursement for bundled services.

Supply and demand leads to demand-based pricing. Higher prices are paid for products or services that are in high demand. Reduced demand leads to lower prices. This makes

entrepreneurial activities important both within the organization and to external markets. Entrepreneurs take risks for profits. Strategic planning is needed to determine which activities can be in the most demand and make the most profits. For example, a hospital may provide food service instead of outsourcing that service and open the cafeteria to the public community for profit.

The providers played a major role in setting prices in the cost-based and charge-based systems. They assume increased financial risk in the flat-fee and capitated payment systems. Cost shifting by payers attempting to control their costs and providers trying to pass on unpaid costs from one payer to other payers has caused a great increase in costs to the private sector. Consequently, employers and insurers have become increasingly involved in managing care.

It is appropriate for entrepreneurs to prepare a business plan for their new ventures. They need to identify the new product or service; analyze the competition and identify the competitive edge; identify the resources needed, such as facilities, equipment, and personnel; identify the time frame needed to develop the product or service; and develop a quality control plan. Financial forecasting to predict the future from past and present information should be done along with benefit-to-cost analysis (the number of dollars returned for each dollar invested) and break-even analysis to determine the price. Planning the marketing by determining the purchase cost (price), identifying the product or service (product), determining the market (place), and planning advertising and determining the medium for the least expense (promotions) are important. (See discussion of the four *p*'s of the marketing mix later in this chapter.) Entrepreneurs are leaders (Douglas, 1996; Hein, 1998; Marquis and Huston, 2002; Swansburg, 1997; Zelman, McCue, Millikan, et al, 2003).

BUDGETARY LEADERSHIP AND MANAGEMENT

Budgetary leaders inspire proactive fiscal planning, determine resource needs, guide visioning

RESEARCH Perspective 9-1

Data from Bonace AL: Doccumentation's effect on reimbursement for rapid treatment status patients. *JONA* 30(6):295-297, 2000.

Purpose: The purpose of this study was to determine if a correlation exists between the quality of documentation and reimbursement for patients classified under rapid treatment status.

Methods: A retrospective chart review was conducted in a 465-bed, not-for-profit, tertiary-care medical center located in northwestern Pennsylvania. Charts represented several areas of the institution. The accounts were randomly selected. The data collection instrument was designed using Medical Management Development Associates, Inc. criteria. The known-groups technique was used to construct validity. The director and three outcomes managers, all with master of science degrees in nursing, reviewed the criteria and data collection instrument for accuracy and completeness. The instrument evaluated physician documentation of 16 key criteria and nursing documentation of six key criteria in the medical records. Data were analyzed using descriptive statistics. The Statistical Package for the Social Sciences version 6.0 and DUSTAT 98 were used to perform a chi-square

analysis for the physician and nursing criteria. Data were organized on the basis of 22 key criteria, each of which was considered to be an independent variable.

Results/conclusions: Chi-square analysis showed statistically significant differences in three physician criteria: A physician order that clearly specified admission to rapid treatment status was present in 72% of the charts from the reimbursed group and 91.9% of the non-reimbursed group. Progress notes substantiating the need for rapid treatment status were present in 64% of the charts from the reimbursed group and 94.6% of the nonreimbursed group. Evidence of informed consent to perform invasive procedures, if applicable, was present in none of the charts from the reimbursed group (there were no invasive procedures done) and 24.3% in the nonreimbursed group.

The results of this study did not provide evidence of a clear and direct relationship between the quality of documentation and reimbursement.

---

of justification for resources, negotiate for needed resources, analyze expenses, anticipate, recognize, and creatively deal with budgetary problems, create a financially savvy work environment, involve group members in fiscal planning, and help groups find innovative ways to be more cost effective (Table 9-1). The fiscal manager coordinates fiscal planning, plans the budget, organizes the justification, implements the budget process, determines resource requirements within the constraints, coordinates

expenses and budget control, documents needs to other administrative levels, organizes needed resources, explains budgeting to others, and evaluates technology (Huber, 2000; Marquis and Huston, 2002).

BUDGETS

"Proportion your expenses to what you have not what you expect." —English proverb

TABLE **9-1** Budgetary Leadership and Management

LEADER	MANAGER
Inspires proactive versus reactive fiscal planning	Coordinates fiscal planning to be consistent with organizational goals and objectives
Determines resources/needs	Plans the budget
Guides visioning of justification for resources	Organizes the budget justification
Negotiates for needed resources	Implements the budget process
Locates new sources of resources	Determines resource requirements within constraints
Analyzes expenses	Coordinates expenses and budget control
Anticipates, recognizes, and creatively deals with budgetary problems	Documents needs to other administrative levels.
Creates a financially savvy work environment	Organizes needed resources
Involves group members in fiscal planning	Explains budgeting to others
Helps groups find innovative ways to be more cost-effective	Evaluates technology

Modified from Huber D: Leadership and nursing case management, Philadelphia, 2000, Saunders; Marquis BL, Huston CJ: Leadership roles and management functions in nursing: Theory and application, Philadelphia, 2002, Lippincott.

A budget is a plan for the allocation of resources and a control for ensuring that results comply with the plan. Results are expressed in quantitative terms. Although budgets are usually associated with financial statements, such as revenues and expenses, they also may be nonfinancial statements covering output, materials, and equipment. Budgets help coordinate the efforts of the agency by determining what resources will be used by whom, when, and for what purpose. They are frequently prepared for each organizational unit and for each function within the unit.

Planning is done for a specific period, usually a fiscal year, but may be subdivided into monthly, quarterly, or semiannual periods. The budgeting period is determined by the desired frequency of checks and should complete a normal cycle of activity. Budget periods that coincide with other control devices—such as managerial reports, balance sheets, and profit-and-loss statements—are helpful.

The extent to which accurate forecasts can be made must be considered. If the budget forecasts too far in advance, its usefulness is diminished. On the other hand, factors such as seasonal fluctuations make it impossible to predict long-range needs from short budget periods. Managers therefore necessarily revise budgets as more information becomes available. Top management and the board of directors also may prepare long-term budgets of 3, 5, or more years, but these are not used as direct operating budgets.

PREREQUISITES TO BUDGETING

Some conditions are necessary for the development and implementation of a budgetary program. First, a sound organizational structure with clear lines of authority and responsibility is needed. All employees know their responsibilities and the person to whom they are responsible; they have the authority to do what they are responsible for and are held accountable for their actions. Organization charts and job descriptions are available, and goals and objectives are set for areas of responsibilities. Budgets are then developed to conform to the pattern of authority and responsibility.

Nonmonetary statistical data—such as number of admissions, average length of stay, percentage of occupancy, and number of patient days—are used for planning and control of the budgetary process. Someone must be responsible for collecting and reporting statistical data.

Charts of accounts are designed to be consistent with the organizational plan. Revenues and expenses are reported by responsibility areas, thus providing historical data that are valuable for planning and providing budgetary control for evaluation since performance can be compared with plans. Nurse managers focus their attention on the principle of management by exception by noting what is not going as planned so they can take necessary action.

Managerial support is essential for a budgetary program. Although budgeting is done at the departmental level, it must be valued by top administration. Managers must be willing to devote their time and energy to the budgeting process. They are most likely to do that when they are familiar, through budget education, with the principles of budgeting and its usefulness for planning and controlling.

Formal budgeting policies and procedures should be available in a budget manual, in which objectives of the budgetary program are defined, authority and responsibility for budgeting are clarified, and instructions for budget development are discussed in detail. Samples of standardized forms are available. A calendar of the budgeting activities with the schedule for each stage of the program is presented. Procedures for review, revision, and approval of budgets are discussed in detail.

APPLIED ECONOMICS

Economic goods are goods or services purchased by consumers from suppliers to provide a benefit to the consumer. Goods and services are acquired through exchange, generally of money. *Wealth* is the value of the consumer's resources. *Income* is additional resources gained over time. Consumers do not have the wealth to buy everything they want, so they must make choices about what to purchase.

Utility is the benefit consumers get from the purchase of goods and services. It helps determine how much the consumer is willing to pay. *Marginal utility* is the additional utility gained by consuming one more unit. Marginal utility is not the same for all consumers or for additional units. A person who likes chocolate is more willing to pay for a chocolate candy bar than a person who does not like chocolate but may not be as willing to buy a second or third chocolate bar. People try to maximize their total utility. To do that, a mix of goods should be consumed so that the last unit has the same marginal utility per dollar spent.

Supply and demand influence costs. *Supply* is the amount of goods or services that suppliers are willing to provide at a given price. *Demand* is the amount of goods or services the consumers are willing to buy at that price. For an equilibrium price, the quantity offered and the quantity demanded are the same. As supply goes up and demand goes down, the price is likely to go down. As the supply goes down and the demand goes up, the price is likely to go up.

Elasticity of demand is the degree to which the demand for a good or service decreases in response to a price increase and increases in response to a price decrease. The demand for health care is generally inelastic.

Economies of scale indicate that the cost of providing goods or services falls as quantity increases and fixed costs are shared with the larger volume. Large volumes can eventually lead to decreasing returns to scale as more personnel and supplies are needed.

Incentives encourage action. Managers may use them to encourage good use of scarce resources. Health insurance deductibles are incentives to encourage desirable behavior.

Market efficiency is the optimal allocation and use of goods and services resulting from supply and demand.

Redistribution of resources may be done to improve equality.

Market failure occurs when the free market does not operate efficiently and may result from lack of information, lack of direct patient payment, monopoly, government intervention and government-induced inefficiency, and other externalities.

ACCOUNTING

Accounting is a system that accumulates bookkeeping entries into summaries of the financial situation of an enterprise. The fundamental equation of accounting is as follows:

Assets = Liabilities + Fund balance

Assets are the valuable resources owned by the agency. *Liabilities* are what the agency owes. *Fund balance* is the agency's assets. The *balance sheet* is a financial statement that shows the financial position of the agency and a specific time. The *income statement,* or statement of revenues and expenses, shows the financial results of the agency's activities for a specified period. *Depreciation* is the allocation of a portion of the cost of an asset with a multiyear life over the years the asset will be used. A *journal* is a book or computer file recording the financial events of the agency in chronological order. *Ledgers* are sets of individual accounts to which information from the journal is transferred or posted so that the balance in any account can be determined and reported. *Fund accounting* is an optional accounting system used by not-for-profit agencies to establish a complete, distinct set of accounting records for separate accounts of agency assets. These assets may be restricted and unrestricted funds set aside for specific purposes, such as endowments, renovations, or buildings (Finkler and Kovner, 1999).

Several terms must be understood to interpret financial accounting reports. *Entity* is a definable organizational unit. The accountant considers only *transactions* between one entity and another. Transactions that occur within the entity or do not involve it are not considered. If each department is an entity, performance can be compared between departments. However, if the agency as a whole is the entity, the transfer of resources from one department to another is not taken into account. Accounts deal only with transactions, or definable changes in the financial situation of an entity: income, expenditure, depreciation. *Cost valuation* values goods at their cost minus any depreciation. *Double entry* compares the assets, what is owed to or owned by the entity, with the liabilities, what is owed by the entity to others. Accountants balance total assets with the total liabilities and net worth. The double entry makes it possible to know where the entity stands financially at any given time. *Accrual* allows one to determine the overall assets and liabilities by entering transactions on the accounting records at the time a commitment is made rather than waiting until it is billed or paid. *Matching* is the principle of matching revenues with expenses during a budget period.

There are several standard accounting practices. *Consistency* means that categories of transactions may not be changed during or between reporting periods without noting the changes and providing comparable figures. *Materiality* means that transactions can be combined for accounting purposes unless one transaction has a significant impact by itself. *Conservatism* is the act of understating revenue and overstating expenses to provide a margin of safety. *Industry practices* are specific to industries. Special fund accounts designated by donors and a separate account for charitable care provided are examples of industry practices.

TYPES OF BUDGETS

"To get money is difficult, to keep it more difficult, but to spend it wisely most difficult of all."
—Anonymous

OPERATING, OR REVENUE-AND-EXPENSE, BUDGETS

The operating budget provides an overview of an agency's functions by projecting the planned operations, usually for the upcoming year. The operating table reveals an input-output analysis of expected revenues and expenses. Among the factors that nurse managers might include in their operating budgets are personnel salaries, employee benefits, insurance, medical-surgical supplies, office supplies, rent, heat, light, house-keeping, laundry service, drugs and pharmaceuticals, repairs and maintenance, depreciation, in-service education, travel to professional meetings, educational leaves, books, periodicals, subscriptions, dues and membership fees, legal fees, and recreation, such as Christmas parties and retirement teas.

Both controllable and noncontrollable expenses are projected. The manager determines the number of personnel needed and the level of skills required of each. Wage levels and quality of materials used are other controllable expenses. Indirect expenses, such as rent, lighting, and depreciation of equipment, are noncontrollable. The noncontrollable expenses and the probability of rises in material prices or labor costs during the budgetary period demand that an operating budget include some cushion funds to provide for changes beyond the agency's control.

The operating budget deals primarily with salaries, supplies, and contractual services. Nonfinancial factors, such as time, materials, and space, can be translated into dollar values. Work hours, nurse-patient interaction hours, units of materials, equipment hours, and floor space

also can be assigned dollar values (Swansburg, 1997; Swansburg and Swansburg, 1999). (See Exhibit 9-1.)

PERSONNEL BUDGETS

Personnel budgets estimate the cost of direct labor necessary to meet the agency's objectives. They determine the recruitment, hiring, assignment, layoff, and discharge of personnel. The nurse manager decides on the type of nursing care necessary to meet the nursing needs of the estimated patient population. How many aides, orderlies, licensed practical nurses (LPNs), and RNs are needed during what shifts, in what months, and in what areas? The current staffing patterns, number of unfilled positions, and last year's reports can provide a base for examination and proposals. Patient occupancy and the general complexity of cases affect staffing patterns. Seasonal fluctuations must be considered. Personnel budgets also are affected by personnel policies such as salary related to position and number of days allowed for educational and personal leave. Overtime costs should be compared with the cost of new positions. Employee turnover, recruitment, and orientation costs

Exhibit 9-1 Operating Budget

Medical Unit
December 2004
30 beds

Statistics	Actual	Budget	Variance
Patient days	870	720	(150)
FTEs	79.2	71.4	(7.8)
Revenues			
Inpatient Revenue	$1,287,000	$1,085,700	$201,300
Operating Expenses			
Salaries, Wages, Benefits	$372,780	$246, 450	($126, 330)
Contract Employees	3720	2000	(1720)
Overtime	7712	8640	928
Supplies	17,200	14,700	(2500)
Repairs	1000	1200	200
Travel	650	600	(50)
Continuing Education	1750	2000	250
Total Expenses	404,812	275,590	(129,222)

FTEs, Full-time equivalents.

must be considered (Finkler, 2001; Swansburg, 1997; Swansburg and Swansburg, 1999).

A position is a job for a person no matter how many hours worked. Personnel reports usually describe positions by job categories and the regularly worked hours such as full- or part-time. Vacancy and turnover reports use positions. However, full-time equivalents (FTEs) are more useful for payroll reports. An FTE is a conversion of hours to a standard base of one person working so many hours per day, so many days per week, and so many weeks per year. For example, an FTE for a person working 8 hours per day, 5 days per week, 52 weeks per year is as follows:

Time Frame	Total Hours	8-Hour Shifts
Per week	40	5
Per 2-week payroll period	80	10
Per 4-week payroll period	160	20
Per month	173.33	21.66
Per year	2080	260

The FTEs help interpret payroll reports, identify trends, and compare levels of utilization across time. Productive and nonproductive time should also be considered. Productive worked time includes straight time and overtime. Nonproductive benefit time includes holidays, vacation days, paid sick leave, and other paid nonworked time, such as continuing education hours. The most significant factor influencing paid FTEs is the fluctuation in nonproductive time. Variations in full-time and part-time staff or in professional versus nonprofessional personnel can be determined using FTEs (Finkler, 2001).

CAPITAL EXPENDITURE BUDGETS

Capital expenditure budgets are related to long-range planning. Capital expenditures include physical changes such as replacement or expansion of the plant, major equipment, and inventories. These items are usually major investments and reduce the flexibility in budgeting because it takes a long time to recover the costs. For instance, a patient may be charged per treatment or per day for use of equipment, but it may take many months or even years to recover the cost of the equipment (See Exhibit 9-2).

The hospital administrator usually establishes the ceiling for capital expenses. Under this budget the nurse manager must establish priorities if requests exceed availability of funds. When filling out request forms for capital items, it is advisable to include names of manufacturers and suppliers, trade-in credits, and estimates of purchase, delivery, installation, and maintenance costs. Written justification for each item should be given.

Inventories are helpful in budgeting. (See Exhibit 9-2.) If supplies are checked routinely, use and replacement figures are available for projection of future needs. Central supply services enhance budgetary control, and storage space facilitates inventory maintenance. Stocked supply shelves on each unit with replacement service twice daily can provide a simplified recording system. Disposable equipment and supplies need careful evaluation to determine

Exhibit 9-2 Capital Budget

Capital Budget Request
Calendar Year 2004
Cost Center: Medical Unit

Type	Quantity	Description	Unit Cost	Extended Cost	Priority
Replacement	10	IV pumps	$5000	$50,000	1
Replacement	10	Beds	$6000	$60,000	2

whether they are more economical than nondisposables (Swansburg, 1997). (See Exhibit 9-2.)

There is a 3-year replacement plan for 30 IV pumps and 30 hospital beds (Grohar-Murray and DiCroce, 2003).

CASH BUDGETS

Cash budgets are planned to make adequate funds available as needed and to use any extra funds profitably. They ensure that the agency has enough, but not too much, cash on hand during the budgetary period. This is necessary because income does not always coincide with expenditures. The manager must anticipate fluctuations in resource needs caused by factors such as seasonal variations. If managers have insufficient cash on hand, they will not be able to purchase needed resources. At the other extreme, if too much cash is available, interest or other earnings that money could generate are lost. Budgeting cash requirements may not significantly affect profits, but it does ensure a liquid position and is a sign of prudent management. Using a cash budget, the nurse manager estimates the amount of money to be collected from clients and other sources and allocates that cash to expenditures. If the budget is well planned, it will provide cash as needed and produce interest on excess funds (Box 9-1).

BOX 9-1 Types of Budgets

Operating budget (daily revenues and expenses to operate the health care institution)
    Revenues (income, return on investments and property)
    Expenses (costs)
        Personnel (employed people)
        Supplies (stock, materials—office supplies, pharmaceuticals, medical-surgical supplies)
        Other expenses (spending such as travel, training, dues, rentals, repairs, depreciation)
Capital expenditure budget (capital often defined as something that costs more than $500 and is used more than once)
Cash budget (for money available for immediate use)

FLEXIBLE BUDGETS

Some costs are fixed and do not change with the volume of business. Other costs vary proportionately with changes in volume. Some variable expenses are unpredictable and can be determined only after change has begun: thus the need for flexible budgets to show the effects of changes in volume of business on expense items. Periodic budget reviews help managers compensate for changes. Relationships between the volume of business and variable costs may be predicted by a historical analysis of costs and development of standard costs.

HISTORICAL APPROACH TO BUDGETING

The historical approach is most effective for calculating the relationship between volume of business and variable costs when a company manufactures a few products and each product contributes a relatively stable percentage to the total sales volume. Using the historical approach, the nurse manager may observe that there are more fractures during skiing season. Consequently, more casting materials are used at that time, and there is a need for increased staffing on the orthopedic ward. A supervising community health nurse in a small college town may note that there is less use of family planning services during the summer months and again during December when students leave for vacations. Consequently, there is less need for contraceptive devices and staffing during these months. There may be an increased demand for immunizations just before elementary schools open in the fall. By plotting on a graph the high and low volumes, the nurse manager can predict the expected costs for each level between the extreme volumes. This historical perspective helps determine the amount of supplies to stock and staffing patterns.

STANDARD COST

Standard cost may be developed to predict what labor and supplies should cost. Multiplying the standard cost by the volume predicts the variable cost. Supervising community health nurses can predict the standard number of clinic visits and the number of birth control pills that will be required for each family-planning client who has chosen birth control pills as a method of contraception. Multiplying the number of pills needed by each client by the number of clients using birth control pills, nurse managers can predict the inventory needed and the cost. They also can predict the number of clinic visits needed and plan staffing.

ZERO-BASED BUDGETING

Many budgeting procedures allocate funds to departments on the basis of their previous year's expenditures. Then the department managers decide how the funds will be used. This procedure usually allows for enrichment and enlargement of programs but seldom for decreases in or deletion of programs. Obsolescence is seldom examined, and this leads to increased costs.

With zero-based budgeting, no program is taken for granted. Each program or service must be justified each time funds are requested. Managers decide what will be done, what will not be done, and how much of an activity will be implemented. A decision package is prepared. The package includes a list of the activities that make up a program, the total cost, a description of what level of service can be performed at various levels of funding, and the ramifications of including them in or excluding them from the budget. The manager may identify the activity, state the purpose, list related activities, outline alternative ways of performing activities, and give the cost of the resources needed.

After decision packages are developed, they are ranked in order of decreasing benefits to the agency. They can be divided into high-, medium-, and low-priority categories and reviewed in order of rank for funding. Resources are allocated based on the priority of the decision package. The cost of each package is added to the cost of approved packages until the agreed-on spending level is reached. Lower-ranked packages are then excluded.

A major advantage to zero-based budgeting is that it forces managers to set priorities and justify resources. Unfortunately the process is time consuming (Nowicki, 2001; Swansburg, 1997; Swansburg and Swansburg, 1999).

PERIODIC BUDGETARY REVIEW

Managers should review the budget at periodic intervals, compare actual with projected performances, and make necessary changes. Variance is the difference between the budget and the actual results. It can be a positive profit or a negative loss. A variance analysis investigates the cause. If changes are too frequent or too great, the original budget becomes useless. One way to minimize variance between the annual budget and the revised budget is to anticipate factors such as increased labor costs and the inflationary cost of materials. When discrepancies are found between actual performance and the budget, management must determine the cause of variation to make appropriate adjustments for future plans. A variance may not be reason for changing the budget. It may be a symptom that alerts management to the need for further investigation and explanation. What may demand change is not the budget but the situation (Baker and Baker, 2000; Berkowitz, 1996; Swansburg, 1997).

See Exhibit 9-1 for the variance in an annual budget. The variance analysis (Baker and Baker, 2000; Berkowitz, 1996; Swansburg, 1997) compares the actual results with the preestablished targets. In this case, we can see that the increase in patient days has caused an increase in personnel expenses and supplies. Monthly variance analysis can help manage the budget. Causes or reasons for the variances are considered. There may be seasonal patterns or trends over time. When variance is greater than an established level, the manager may need to investigate the reasons and explain or justify the variance. The level may be a dollar amount or a percentage of the budgeted item. To calculate the variance percentage, divide the dollar variance by the budgeted amount and multiply by 100. For example:

$200 variance for repairs divided by

$1200 budgeted amount equals

0.16666

$0.16666 \times 100 = 16.6666\%$ under the budget for repairs

ADVANTAGES AND DISADVANTAGES

ADVANTAGES AND DISADVANTAGES OF FLEXIBLE BUDGETS

The major advantage of flexible budgets is the study and analysis necessary to prepare one. Fixed and variable costs and their effect on the total cost are analyzed. Unfortunately, flexible budgets are very costly to prepare and very time consuming. It is difficult to predict short-term variations in volume, and it is unlikely that the information can result in savings of variable expenses.

ADVANTAGES OF BUDGETING

Budgets plan for detailed program activities. They help fix accountability by assignment of responsibility and authority. They state goals for all units, offer a standard of performance, and stress the continuous nature of the planning and control process. Budgets encourage managers to make a careful analysis of operations and to base decisions on careful consideration. Consequently, hasty judgments are minimized. Weaknesses in the organization can be revealed and corrective measures taken. Staffing, equipment, and supply needs can be projected and waste minimized. Financial matters can be handled in an orderly fashion, and agency activities can be coordinated and balanced.

DISADVANTAGES OF BUDGETING

Budgets convert all aspects of organizational performance into monetary values for a single comparable unit of measurement. Consequently, only those aspects that are easy to measure may be considered, and equally important factors, such as organizational development and research efforts, may be ignored. Symptoms may be treated as causes. Reasons for the symptoms should be explored; a decrease in revenue from the family-planning clinic may be related to the way people are treated at the clinic, a new competitive service in the neighborhood, or other factors. The budget may become an end in itself instead of the means to an end. Budgetary goals may supersede agency goals and gain autocratic control of the organization. There is a danger of overbudgeting; the budget becomes cumbersome, meaningless, and expensive. Forecasting is required but uncertain because budgetary control is subject to human judgment, interpretation, and evaluation. Skill and experience are required for successful budgetary control. Budget planning is time consuming and expensive.

BUDGETING PROCESS

Identifying financial-planning responsibilities is needed before beginning budget preparation. The governing board, administrator, budget director, steering committee, and department heads are often involved in the budgetary process. The governing board is responsible for the general planning function. It selects the budget steering committee, determines the budgetary objectives, and reviews and approves the master budget. The administrator is responsible for the formulation and execution of the budget by correlating the governing board's goals with the guidelines for budget preparation and supervising the budget preparation. The budget director, who is responsible for the budgeting procedures and reporting, establishes a completion timetable, has forms prepared, and supervises data collection and budget preparation. The budget director serves as the chairperson of the steering committee, which approves the budget before it is submitted to the governing board. Department heads prepare and review goals and objectives and prepare the budgets for their departments.

The first step in the budget process is the establishment of operational goals and policies for the entire agency. The governing board should approve a long-range plan of 3 to 5 years that reflects the community's future health needs and other community health care providers' activities. Because the situation changes over time, flexibility is built into the plan. Then operational goals must be translated into quantifiable management objectives for the organizational units. The department heads use the organizational goals as a framework for the development of departmental goals. A formal plan for budget preparation and review, including assignment of responsibilities and timetables, must be prepared. Historical, financial, and statistical data must be collected monthly so that seasonal fluctuation can be observed. Preparing and coordinating departmental budgets are important. During this phase, units of service, staffing patterns, salary and nonsalary expenses, and revenues are forecasted so that preliminary rate setting can be done. Next, departmental budgets are revised, and the master budget is prepared. At this point, operating, payroll, nonsalary, capital, and cash budgets can be incorporated into the master budget. Then the financial feasibility of the master budget is tested, and the final document is approved and distributed to all involved parties.

During the budget period, there should be periodic performance reporting by responsibility centers.

COST CONTAINMENT

The goal of cost containment is to keep costs within acceptable limits for volume, inflation, and other parameters. It involves cost awareness, monitoring, management, and incentives to prevent, reduce, and control costs.

COST AWARENESS

Cost awareness focuses the employee's attention on costs. It increases organizational awareness of what costs are, the process available for containing them, how they can be managed, and by whom.

Delegating budget planning and control to the unit level increases awareness. Managers should be provided a course about budgeting and be oriented to the agency budgeting process before being assigned the responsibility. They should have a budget manual that contains budget forms, budget calendar, and budget periods.

COST FAIRS

Cost fairs in frequented areas, such as the cafeteria, increase awareness by displaying frequently disappearing items that are labeled with the cost per unit and by posting lists of estimated costs of inventory losses. Staff development programs, unit conferences, and poster contests help increase awareness. Tagging supply items and posting a computer printout of unit charges for supplies and services are revealing. Reviewing a patient's itemized bill during a conference can also be effective.

COST MONITORING

Cost monitoring focuses on how much will be spent where, when, and why. It identifies, reports, and monitors costs. Staffing costs should be identified. Recruitment, turnover, absenteeism, and sick time are analyzed, and inventories are controlled. A central supply exchange chart prevents hoarding of supplies and allows identification of lost items.

COST MANAGEMENT

Cost management focuses on what can be done by whom to contain costs. Programs, plans, objectives, and strategies are important. Responsibility and accountability for the control should be established. A committee can identify long- and short-range plans and strategies. A suggestion box can be used, as can contests for the idea that saves the most money.

Money has been saved by means such as forming a staff pool to maximize flexibility in staffing for census fluctuations, cross-training personnel, closing units for cleaning or remodeling and encouraging staff vacations when census is low, balancing the workload among shifts to minimize peaks and valleys in assigned tasks, reducing shift overlap, charting by exception, tape-recording shift reports, revising forms, improving drug ordering and delivery systems, controlling central supplies, not controlling oral analgesics, modifying food services, allowing volunteers to discharge and transport patients, reducing the amount of time nurses spend in nonnursing functions, and using guest relations personnel, a discharge holding area, outpatient clinics, progressive care, and ambulatory care.

COST INCENTIVES

Cost incentives motivate cost containment and reward desired behavior. Contests for the best money-saving ideas, perfect attendance, and nurse of the month help recognize personnel efforts.

COST AVOIDANCE

Cost avoidance means not buying supplies, technology, or services. Supply and equipment costs should be carefully analyzed. Costs and effectiveness of disposable versus reusable items are compared. The receipt, storage, and delivery of disposables and labor and processing costs of reusable items are part of the analysis. The least expensive and most effective supplies, equipment, and services should be identified, and expensive and less effective items should be avoided.

COST REDUCTION

Cost reduction means spending less for goods and services. The amount of reduction depends on the size of the agency, previous efficiency, skill of managers, and cooperation of employees. Safety programs that reduce the costs of workers' compensation and absenteeism programs that reduce sick time, absenteeism, and turnover reduce costs. Healthy living programs, such as exercise activities, heart-wise foods in the cafeteria, and cease-smoking classes, may help keep workers healthy and thus reduce sick time, absenteeism, and health care costs. Volume buying (getting a cheaper price because of the economies of scale), conservation of supplies, and careful handling of equipment to reduce cost of repairs help reduce costs. Costs can also be reduced through inventory control.

Inventory Control

The manager needs to determine the most economical level of inventory because supplies represent a significant cost factor. The purchasing, order, storage, and costs of long and short stock must all be considered to determine the most economical level of inventory. The purchasing cost is the price paid per item. Cost may be related to the size of the order with cost per item decreasing as the size of the order increases. Purchasing cost equals PD, where P is the cost or price per unit and D is the number of units purchased.

The order costs involve writing specifications, soliciting and analyzing bids, writing orders, receiving the supplies, accounting for the materials, and paying the bills. The order cost may be relatively large the first time an item is purchased or relatively small for routine purchasing processes. The order cost varies with the number of orders placed. The more orders per year, the greater the annual costs will be. Annual order cost equals $(D/Q)O$, where D is the number of units purchased, Q is the order size, and O is the average cost of placing a single order.

The carrying cost is the expense involved with holding inventories. It involves expenses such as storage, insurance, and security. To keep carrying costs down, small orders should be placed frequently; this approach is in direct conflict with keeping the purchasing and order costs low. Carrying cost equals the following:

$$HQ + \frac{IPQ}{2}$$

where H is the cost of storage per item and Q is the order size.

The opportunity cost element is as follows:

$$\frac{IPQ}{2}$$

where *I* represents the highest obtainable rate of return at the current interest rate, *P* is price per unit, and *Q* is the order size.

The short or stock-out costs involved with holding an insufficient amount of inventory must be considered. The manager considers the consequences of running out of stock. Not only is a sale lost, but also client satisfaction may suffer. Although this expense is difficult to measure, it is a real cost.

Total cost is expressed as follows:

$$TC = PD + \frac{DO}{Q} + \left\{ \frac{HQ + IPQ}{2} \right\} + L + S$$

where:

$$TC = \text{Total cost}$$

$$PD = \text{Purchase cost}$$

$$\frac{DO}{Q} = \text{Order cost}$$

$$HQ + \frac{IPQ}{2} = \text{Carrying cost}$$

$$L = \text{Overstocked cost}$$

$$S = \text{Stock-out cost}$$

The economical order quantity is expressed as follows:

$$EOQ = \sqrt{\frac{2DP}{C}}$$

where:

$$EOQ = \text{Economical order quantity}$$

$$D = \text{Usage in units or demand}$$

$$P = \text{Order cost}$$

$$C = \text{Annual cost of carrying one unit in inventory}$$

A large order size is merited when there is a large demand, high order cost, and low carrying cost. However, a small order size is desired when there is little demand for the item, the order cost is small, and the carrying cost is high.

A high inventory turnover is desired. Low inventory turnover may be caused by poor purchasing policies, overstocking, or a decrease in demand for the item. The inventory turnover can be calculated as follows:

$$\text{Inventory turnover} = \frac{\text{Total cost of supplies}}{\text{Inventories}}$$

To determine when to reorder, the manager needs to know the average daily usage and the lead time required to receive the supplies. The manager needs to keep the average daily usage multiplied by the number of days it takes to receive the goods to not run out of stock.

Some managers use the ABC method for maintaining inventories. *A* refers to a small number of items that account for a large percentage of the budget and are carefully monitored; *B* refers to moderate-cost items that receive some monitoring; and *C* refers to a bulk of inexpensive, expendable items such as rubber bands that receive little monitoring.

COST CONTROL

Cost control is effective use of available resources through careful forecasting, planning, budget preparing, reporting, and monitoring. Cost-effectiveness compares costs and identifies the most beneficial outcomes to costs by specifying programs; identifying goals; analyzing alternatives; comparing costs per program, unit of service, and amount of service needed; assessing effect of the outcome; and determining cost outcome and cost-effectiveness. Patient classification systems can be used to predict the appropriate staffing levels. Time management can help control costs. Making meetings worthwhile, reducing repetitious paperwork, improving communication systems, and streamlining the system help save time. Activities to promote retention of personnel, such as a good orientation program, careful placement and mentoring of new personnel, and helping people feel welcome and appreciated, can reduce recruitment, orientation, and development expenses.

Careful selection of supplies and equipment and in-servicing to teach personnel how to use them can save frustration and damage. Proper charging of supplies and use of equipment through things such as bar codes and charge slips could help the health care system recover millions of dollars lost from supplies that were not charged to patients. Delegation of appropriate tasks to unlicensed personnel can save more expensive nurses' time for activities requiring more knowledge and skill. Teaching how to delegate, supervise, and develop teams may help control costs in the long run.

COST-EFFECTIVENESS AND COST-BENEFIT ANALYSIS

Cost-effectiveness is a method of economic evaluation that ranks programs by the cost of achieving the objective. It is measured in non-monetary units, such as fewer readmissions to the hospital or fewer unwed teenage pregnancies. Cost-benefit analysis is a procedure that determines cost of installing and operating a program and converts that into a dollar amount. It also converts all benefits of the program into a dollar amount. A ratio reflects the relationship of costs to benefits. Cost-benefit analysis is measured in monetary units that facilitate a conclusion regarding whether the program savings outweigh the costs. If the benefit/cost ratio is equal to or greater than 1, the investment is considered good. If the ratio is less than 1, it is not advisable to pursue the venture because the number of dollars returned is less than the number invested. It often involves estimating the value of saving a life and adjusting the outcome for quality that is measured as quality-adjusted life-years (QALYs). Each increment of variable costs may not yield a comparable increment in work output. For example, one additional employee decreases the service volume for a time as the work increment of each employee decreases. An additional employee may even cause a decrease in output for the group as communication problems and interpersonal conflict increase. Break-even analysis is used to calculate the break-even point for

Figure 9-1 Variable costs.

each program (Loveridge and Cummings, 1996; Rocchiccioli and Tilbury, 1998; Sullivan and Decker, 1999).

Break-Even Calculations

A *ProForma Income Statement* is a projection of the operations and activities of a business. The ProForma Income and ProForma Cash Flow Statements are used to develop the ProForma Balance Sheet. That reflects the revenue to be generated and cost to be incurred over a period of time. It can be used to help calculate break-even points. Full costs equal all direct costs that can be traced to a source plus indirect costs such as maintenance, administration, and the building that are allocated to the source. Cost finding is an attempt to find the full cost and to allocate indirect costs. Indirect costs allocated may include housekeeping calculated by square feet, utilities by square feet, laboratory by number of tests, and dietary services by number of meals served.

The cost-volume-profit relationships can be visualized on a break-even chart. The manager considers variable, fixed, semifixed, and semi-variable costs when doing a break-even analysis. Variable costs vary in direct proportion to volume (Figure 9-1). Two disposable syringes probably cost twice as much as one. Fixed costs are relatively fixed in total regardless of changes in volume (Figure 9-2). A nurse receives a certain

Figure 9-2 Fixed costs.

Figure 9-3 Semifixed costs.

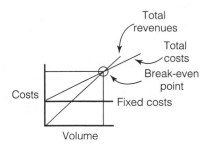

Figure 9-5 Break-even costs.

salary regardless of the number of injections the nurse gives. Sunk costs are fixed costs that cannot be recovered even if the service is not provided. Semifixed costs are fixed within a range of activity (Figure 9-3). One nurse can give just so many injections per shift, and beyond that a second nurse will need to be hired. Semivariable costs are fixed at zero output and increase with volume (Figure 9-4). The break-even point is depicted on a break-even chart where revenues equal expenditures (Figure 9-5). The formula for break-even analysis is as follows:

$$R = FC + VC + P$$

where:

R = Total revenue

FC = Fixed cost

VC = Variable cost

P = Profit

Direct costs are unique to the unit and can be identified with relative certainty. These costs, such as personnel time and supplies, would not occur if the unit was closed.

Indirect costs or overhead costs are from shared resources, such as general administration, housekeeping, information systems, and

maintenance, and are more difficult to calculate than direct costs.

Average cost is the full cost divided by the volume of service units. The average cost decreases as the volume of patients increases because more patients share the fixed costs.

Mixed costs contain both the variable and fixed cost elements.

Marginal costs are the extra costs created by providing care to one more service unit. It is the difference in the total costs before and after adding one more service unit. Decisions about changes should be made on the basis of marginal costs versus average or full costs.

Cost estimation is the prediction of costs. It is a complicated process that involves dividing historical costs into fixed and variable components and adjusting historical costs for inflation to predict future costs.

To adjust cost for *inflation*, the historical cost is multiplied by the current value of the appropriate price index divided by the value of that index when the cost was incurred.

Regression analysis considers costs as the dependent variable and service units as the independent variable. The coefficient of the independent variable represents the variable costs, and the constant term of the regression represents fixed costs.

Contribution margin is the price minus the variable costs per service unit and represents the additional financial benefit for each additional service unit (Baker and Baker, 2000; Finkler, 2001; Finkler and Kovner, 1999; Gapenski, 1999).

Figure 9-4 Semivariable costs.

STRATEGIC COST DECISIONS

Taking a strategic approach to cost containment involves a comprehensive view of costs of the organization without being limited to direct, measurable costs. Albert Einstein said, "Not everything that counts can be counted, and not everything that can be counted counts" (Brinker, 1996, p. D4-1). This approach uses a total cost perspective that includes a broad range of tangible and intangible operating and strategic costs. A cost audit is important in the creation of a cost management strategy. The audit provides an assessment of the organization's cost position, compares it with competitors, and evaluates it for future profitability. This allows an assessment of the organization's current cost management processes.

Some accounting personnel may need to learn about management information needs. Defining what reports are needed is important. Managers and staff need to be supported in cost containment efforts with data that are focused rather than be overwhelmed with data that bury the critical data. Report formats should be clear and simple. Accountants' capabilities should be matched with the needs of management and staff.

Managers need to change their view of cost reductions from a negative exercise to something that can be creative and exciting. Then they should involve employees in the challenging and exciting process. Effective management communication is needed to increase employee awareness for and understanding of cost management. Having more employees involved in the task can create the greatest leverage. Brainstorming can be done with employees at all levels, who can then contribute to cost reduction. Short presentations about what actions are necessary, what employees can do, and rewards for results are key ingredients. Personal talks, videotaped presentations, newsletters, bulletin boards, staff meetings, and the grapevine can be used for communications. Meetings and discussions with employees can help alleviate fears and uncertainties about cost management.

Many ideas do not need simultaneous development and implementation. Factors such as what can be implemented quickly, cheaply, and with the greatest results should be considered. Short-term successes can be celebrated on the way to long-term improvements as management-employee attitudes and relationships change. Cost-reduction successes should be rewarded. Recognition is a reward for most types of agency achievement. It can be formal, such as an employee-of-the-month program or public recognition in the form of a photograph and article in the newsletter or other media, or informal, such as a pat on the back or a simple thank you. Employees may quickly forget positive comments but remember any negative ones, so small token awards such as company pens or other items with the agency logo that may be used to hand out to customers can be used as a physical reminder of the manager's appreciation. Status rewards, such as employee of the month, can be used to create role models and heroes. Money can be rewarded for proposing cost-reducing ideas, usually within a suggestion plan. An effective cost management strategy can take a long time to fully implement. Persistence is a quality of good cost cutters. The long-run commitment to successful cost management strategies helps give the organization the competitive edge.

Cost cutting often involves workforce reduction. Increasing the number of cuts may become increasingly less effective as muscle gets cut with fat. Attrition and early retirement are preferable to layoffs. Unfortunately, negative side effects can offset direct savings. High performers may become insecure and accept other positions, morale and productivity may drop, employees may stop suggesting ways to reduce costs, and absenteeism and grievances are likely to increase. Silent sabotage may occur in the form of increased employee theft; the water cooler gang or company gossip in a public place; huddle and chatter, which is gossip about what happened or might happen, causing hours of nonproductive time; stay-and-quit syndrome, where employees lose their enthusiasm and refuse to go the extra mile; or the deviators, who divert business by not providing good service

(Morin, 1995). Restructuring work relationships, cross-skills utilization, and gaining greater employee involvement may offer significant effects through increased productivity.

Across-the-board cuts may lead to customer complaints, inability to do the work, or lost time because of shortages of parts and maintenance that consequently greatly increase costs. Focused cuts are more useful. Some managers focus on controlling direct expenditures and cut nickel-and-dime items such as free coffee. That can lead to greater losses as employees spend time complaining about the lost privilege instead of getting the work done.

Soft items that lead indirectly to cost reductions are sometimes the first expenditures to be cut. Sometimes it is necessary to spend money to make or save money. Staff development, travel to new experiences, staff meetings on company time, seed money, and maintenance can lead indirectly to cost savings.

Capital- or technology-intensive approaches may lead to cost reductions but may also lead to higher overall costs and can involve painful implementation. Activity-based cost management should be used with caution because a high percentage of the cost in health care organizations is indirect, and the indirect costs are not distributed evenly among units. Activity-based costing software packages translate financial information onto a management tool by aligning costs with the activities and by assigning costs directly to nursing practice. They can help differentiate value-added from non–value-added activities (Cokins, 1996; Storfjell and Jessup, 1996). Developing learning organizations, maximizing employee satisfaction, and simplifying and improving performance measures can be cost management strategies (Brinker, 1996; Ostrenga et al, 1992).

COSTING OUT NURSING SERVICES

The traditional model's equation follows:

$$NT \times (ANHS + BAI + ICA) = TNC \text{ per DRG}$$

where:

NT = Amount of nursing time per intensity level for a DRG

$ANHS$ = Average nursing hourly salary

BAI = Benefits across the institution

ICA = Indirect cost amount

TNC = Total nursing cost

The McCloskey model's equation (Huber, 1996; McCloskey, 1989) follows:

$$NT/NI \times (ANHS + BAI + EC + ICA) = TNC$$

where:

NT = Amount of nursing time

NI = Nursing intervention (instead of intensity level for a DRG)

$ANHS$ = Average nursing hourly salary

BAI = Benefits across the institution

EC = Equipment cost (not in traditional model)

ICA = Indirect cost amount

TNC = Total nursing cost (instead of cost per DRG)

In general, the key problems related to costing out nursing are a lack of comparability of data used, multiple definitions of costs, and neglect of variables that affect nursing care. We need a forum where administrators, researchers, educators, and staff can share ideas about cost-effectiveness. We need models to describe the relationships among cost, quality, and price of nursing functions. We need to continue to compare methods for costing out nursing care and to identify data sets needed to cost out nursing. Levels of care, expected outcomes, and cost of care can be related to pricing of nursing care. Nurses must be concerned about maintaining cost-effective, high-quality health care.

PERSONAL FINANCES

This discussion of personal finances will help you understand broader economic and financial principles by applying them to your personal situation.

ASSESS PERSONAL FINANCES

To assess your personal finances, ask the following:

Assets. How much do you have?
Debts. How much do you owe?
Income. How much do you earn?
Expenditures. How much do you spend?
Savings. Are you saving enough?

evolve   After using Worksheets 9-1 and 9-2 to assess your assets, liabilities, and cash flow, consider making changes in your personal finances by trying to find places to spend less and save more and looking for patterns of spending that could indicate trouble.

"A bank is an institution where you can borrow money if you can present sufficient evidence that you don't need it." —Anonymous

---

MONEY MAKES MONEY

Make sure your money is earning interest whenever possible. You also need cash on hand or assets located where they can be converted into cash. Banks, savings and loans, and credit unions offer a variety of accounts that pay interest and are insured by the federal government, including money-market deposit accounts, savings accounts, and interest-paying checking accounts. Interest rates vary. There may be a fee if your balance falls below a minimum level. There may also be annual fees, monthly maintenance charges, and per-check charges.

FINANCIAL GOALS

evolve   Using Worksheet 9-3, set and prioritize financial goals. Evaluate if your goals are realistic. Achieving your goals depends on the following:

- How soon you want to achieve them
- How much you can save
- How much risk you are willing to take
- What rate of return that risk will bring

There is no risk of losing your money in federally insured savings accounts within the insured limit of $100,000, but savings accounts pay a low interest. Money-market funds and certificates of deposit usually pay a little more than savings accounts with virtually no risk. Bonds pay more interest but have some market risk. When interest rates rise, the market value of stocks rises and the market value of bonds falls. Stocks have brought investors double-digit annual returns over time. Your attitude toward risk will influence which investment you choose. If you cannot meet your goals in the time frame you set, you may need to (1) delay one or more goals, (2) set aside more money for savings, or (3) take more risk in the hope that your savings will grow faster.

INVESTMENT STRATEGIES

The objectives of investment strategies are to preserve capital and to make it grow at a rate faster than inflation. To do that, you need to allocate and diversify your funds. A large portion of your investments and savings should be at low risk. Fewer should be in higher-risk ventures. Spread your risk (Figure 9-6). Box 9-2 lists some low-, medium-, and high-risk investments.

It takes discipline to save money. Savings should be treated as a fixed income, just another bill to pay each month. Payroll deductions can save your money before you get your check, and automatic bank payments can make deposits into mutual funds or savings plans. Planning for

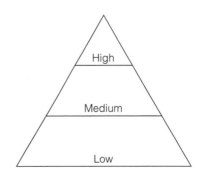

Figure 9-6 Pyramid of risk.

BOX 9-2 Low-, Medium-, High-Risk Investments

LOW-RISK SAVINGS AND INVESTMENTS
Certificates of deposit
Interest-paying checking accounts
Money-market funds
Savings accounts
Savings bonds
Treasury bills and bonds

MEDIUM-RISK INVESTMENTS
Growth and income mutual funds
High-quality bond mutual funds
High-quality municipal and corporate bonds
Income mutual funds
Income stocks
Long-term growth stocks
Long-term growth stock mutual funds
Rental real estate
Tax-deferred annuities
Utility stocks

HIGH-RISK INVESTMENTS
Aggressive growth stock mutual funds
Collectibles
Emerging technology company stocks
Gold and other precious metals
High-yield bonds
High-yield mutual funds
Mutual funds investing in emerging technology firms
Oil and gas partnerships
Stocks of small companies listed in the over-the-counter market

---

college and retirement requires big savings plans. Assets can be protected through insurance—health, disability, auto, home, and life.

It is important to get good financial advice. A lawyer can help with estate planning and wills. A tax adviser can help minimize taxes on various financial transactions. A stockbroker and an independent insurance agent can make valuable recommendations (Swansburg, 1997).

MARKETING

Marketing is the analysis, planning, implementation, and control of carefully formulated programs designed to bring about voluntary exchanges of values with target markets for the purpose of achieving organizational objectives. It relies heavily on designing the organization's offering in terms of the target markets' needs and desires and on using effective pricing, communication, and distribution to inform, motivate, and service the markets" (Kotler 1982, pb).

SOCIAL MARKETING

Social marketing is a fast-growing segment of nonprofit marketing in this age of rapid population growth and economic, social, and environmental problems. Firms should consider consumer short-run wants and long-run welfare and make decisions that are best for consumers and society in the long run. Social marketing applies generic marketing to change social behavior of a target audience or to the well-being of society in general. For example, health care agencies market antismoking campaigns, nutrition education, exercise programs, immunizations, cancer detection, healthy hearts, safe sexual practices, and occupational safety. Marketing can be aimed at one-time or continuing behavior, high or low involvement, and individual or group behavior. Continuing, high-involvement behavior of groups is the most difficult to change. Social marketing may try to influence nonexistent or negative demand and may target relatively nonliterate audiences. It often deals with hard-to-research, sensitive issues or relatively invisible benefits while waiting for long-term change. If one is lucky, sustaining the new behavior becomes an issue. All companies have four basic social responsibilities: (1) economic—to be profitable, (2) legal—to obey the law and do what is legally correct, (3) ethical—to do what is right, just, and fair, and (4) philanthropical—to be a good citizen and contribute resources to improve the quality of life in the community (Andreasen and Kotler, 2002; Kotler and Armstrong, 1996; Kotler and Roberto, 1989; Pride and Ferrell, 1997; Yoder-Wise, 2002).

TRENDS IN MARKETING

Technology has caused changes in marketing. Before the industrial revolution peddlers carried products to the door. They took large pots and pans to communities with many children and smaller pots to retirement communities. Technology can now be used for a large-scale, individualized approach to large markets. The industrial revolution mass-produced products, created a faceless society, and led to marketing designed from economic sciences and consumer models that were based on rational behavior. Target groups were defined for marketing when people wanted the same things.

With cultures that value self-fulfillment and enjoyment of life more than being part of a group, consumption pressure aimed at the masses may not work. The new pattern has people wanting different things with less loyalty to brands. As people want goods and services tailored to them, individual ordering emerges along with the mass markets. A modular product range can give customers a large choice while requiring the production of only a limited number of variants. There may be just a few colors, styles, and sizes, but that gives numerous possibilities of combinations. This creates an abundance of diversity that people can search out with the media to put all kinds of options together, thus creating a fast, interactive means that is available 24 hours per day. Today's health care customers are educated, confident, assertive,

and busy. They want convenience, mastery, quality, and lower costs (Herzlinger, 1999) (Table 9-2).

People do not easily change their habits, so electronics do not supersede everything but offer additional possibilities as people mail what they faxed or copy and distribute what they e-mailed. Agencies formerly used generic, thematic, one-sided bombardment advertising based on market research, generic models, and reported behaviors (which may not be actual behaviors) to manage target groups. Agencies are now more likely to use dialogue to listen and react to actual behaviors by using media and marketing databases to manage personal client relationships (Postma, 1999).

POPCORN AND MARIGOLD'S CULTURAL TRENDS

Leaders need to consider trends to create long-term competitive advantages. Faith Popcorn and Lys Marigold (1996) identify the following 16 trends.

SOS (save our society) is a renewed social conscience with respect to ethics, education, and the environment. People are joining groups to promote social responsibility. Marketers can encourage their agencies to do socially responsible marketing.

Being alive is a desire for more years of quality living. People are increasingly taking more responsibility for their own health because

TABLE **9-2** Trends in Marketing

FROM:	TO:
Masses	Individual
Generic	Specific
Limited choice	Abundance
Print	Electronic
Passive	Interactive
Plenty of time	Fast, faster, fastest
9 AM–5 PM	24-hour service
Agency calls out to market	Agency listens and reacts
One-sided bombardment	Dialogue
Market research	Marketing databases
Generic models	Marketing databases
Generic, thematic advertising	Media
Reported behaviors	Actual behaviors
Management of target groups	Management of personal client relationships

they know lifestyles of eating the wrong foods, smoking, drinking, abusing drugs, breathing bad air, and having unsafe sex can kill them. It is time to market healthier products and services.

Down aging is feeling and acting younger than one is. People buy adult toys, dress young, take adventure vacations, and get plastic surgery. Senior citizens can make good volunteers for social causes.

Cashing out is men and women questioning the price they pay for high-powered jobs and choosing a simpler way of life.

Cocooning is the stay-at-home trend where one is protected from the harsh, unpredictable outside world. With technology one can shop, bank, be entertained, and get an education right from home.

Anchoring is the trend to seek out our spiritual roots and take comfort from the past to secure the future. As people return to church, that may be a good place for social programs.

Clanning is the tendency to join groups with similar beliefs where one can be validated by consensus.

99 Lives is juggling many roles and responsibilities. People resort to fax, car phones, and fast food restaurants to cope. Cluster marketing or one-stop shopping such as a launderette with a copy machine, fax, and exercise bike may meet several needs. **Multi-tasking**

Egonomics is the desire for personalized service. High tech needs to be high touch.

Small indulgences allow people to find an emotional fix by rewarding themselves with affordable luxuries in response to stress. Some may eat ice cream on the weekend to reward themselves for eating well all week or take a weekend trip when unable to afford a luxury vacation. Marketers should note ways people feel deprived and watch for small indulgences that give an emotional lift.

Fantasy adventure is an emotional escape from daily tensions through risk-free adventures such as fantasy parks, food, and travel.

Female think is a trend toward more familial caring and sharing from the goal-oriented, hierarchical model.

Mancipation allows men to be individuals instead of strictly business.

Vigilante consumers are those who demand quality products and services. Agencies should focus on customer-centered, high-quality products and services.

Icon toppling is the questioning and sometimes rejection of our monuments of business and government.

Pleasure revenge is a counterreaction to following rules and regulations without the desirable results. It is the pursuit of pleasure through indulgences such as smoking, drinking, overeating fatty foods, and not exercising (Kotler and Armstrong, 1996; Popcorn and Marigold, 1996).

LEADERSHIP AND MANAGEMENT OF STRATEGIC PLANNING FOR MARKETING

Top-level administrators define the agency mission, which is a statement of the purpose, and set goals and objectives, which will be detailed in each unit. An analysis of strengths, weaknesses, opportunities, and threats is desirable. Administrators also design the agency portfolio, which is the collection of products and services the agency provides (Box 9-3). Market opportunities can be explored using a market expansion grid (Box 9-4).

BOX 9-3 Leadership and Management of Strategic Planning for Marketing

CORPORATE-LEVEL LEADERSHIP
Define agency mission.
Set agency goals and objectives.
Design agency portfolio.

MARKETING UNIT MANAGEMENT
Develop marketing plans from the strategic plan.
Implement the plans.
Evaluate results.
Take corrective actions.

BOX 9-4 Market Expansion Grid

	EXISTING PRODUCTS	**NEW PRODUCTS**
Existing markets	1. Market penetration	3. Product development
New markets	2. Market development	4. Diversification

Agencies have the following market opportunities: (1) market penetration when using existing products in existing markets, (2) market development by taking existing products into new markets, (3) product development by taking new products into existing markets, and (4) diversification by taking new products to new markets.

The marketing unit managers are responsible for developing marketing plans from the agency strategic plan, implementing the plans, evaluating the results, and taking corrective actions (Kotler and Armstrong, 1996; Pride and Ferrell, 1997).

MARKET RESEARCH

Market research is the research process applied to marketing. It involves the following: (1) defining the problem and research questions, (2) designing the research project, (3) collecting data, (4) analyzing data, and (5) interpreting and reporting the findings. It should furnish unbiased information to help avoid the false assumptions and misunderstanding that can lead to poor marketing (Box 9-5).

The first step is to define the problem and state the research questions. The problem may be failure to reach a goal. The research questions may identify the information needed to solve the problem. Refining an indefinite problem into a precise, researchable statement is challenging.

The research project should be designed to be reliable and valid. Reliability is repeatability. Validity is measuring what one intends to measure. The hypothesis is an informed guess about the problem and is tested. An exploratory study has a tentative hypothesis that needs to be made more specific. A descriptive study is intended to

give an accurate portrayal of the characteristics of the situation and may use statistics and predictive tools. Causal studies assume that one variable causes another and tests that the independent variable causes a change in the dependent variable.

Primary and secondary data may be collected. Primary data are collected directly from the subjects. Secondary data are reports and other information from internal or external sources

---

BOX 9-5 Marketing Research

Defining problem and research questions
Designing the research project
  Reliability
  Validity
  Hypothesis
  Exploratory studies
  Descriptive studies
  Causal studies
Collecting data
  Primary data
  Secondary data
  Survey methods
    Interviews
      Mail
      Telephone
      E-mail
      Personal interviews
      On-site computer
    Questionnaires
    Observations
Sampling
  Random
  Stratified
  Area
  Quota
Analyzing data
Interpreting and reporting findings

that may be used to study the problem. There are several ways to collect data. Mail surveys are questionnaires sent to subjects. They are appropriate when subjects are scattered over a large geographical area and the funds are limited. The interviewer records telephone surveys. Computer-assisted telephone interviewing can be done with the interviewer typing the answers to the questions into the computer during the interview. Telephone interviews have better response rates than mail surveys because it takes less effort to answer by telephone, but they are limited to people with telephones. E-mail surveys are an alternative to both mailed and telephone surveys but are limited to people with e-mail. Personal interviews may be in-home, door-to-door interviews, focus interviews with several people at one time, or interviews of people in public places. On-site computer interviewing can be done in public places by putting the questionnaire on the computer, teaching the subjects how to answer the questions on the computer, and letting them self-pace themselves through the questionnaire. For observations researchers observe overt behavior and record it along with notes about the physical conditions and events.

Sampling is the selection of subjects from the total population. The population is all subjects of interest to the researcher. A sample is a limited number of subjects from the population, who can be selected in a number of ways. Random sampling is usually considered the best method of sampling and gives all subjects an equal opportunity to be in the sample. Stratified sampling divides the population into groups and does a probability sample of each group. Area sampling selects subjects from a specific area. Quota samples are not probability samples because not everyone has an equal chance to be in the sample. Variables are unique, such as who wears eyeglasses or has had a specific procedure done. Controls are usually limited to two or three variables, such as age, gender, and education to facilitate representativeness of categories of respondents.

Data are analyzed, often using statistical interpretation, and then interpreted and reported. The report is usually prepared as a formal written document but may also involve verbal presentations (Kotler and Armstrong, 1996; Pride and Ferrell, 1997).

MARKETING CONCEPTS
Exchange

Marketing is based on resource dependency or exchange. Organizations offer satisfactions such as goods, services, or benefits to markets that in return provide needed resources such as goods, services, time, money, or energy (Box 9-6). Exchange involves four conditions: (1) there are at least two parties, (2) each party offers something that the other considers valuable, (3) each party is capable of communication and delivery, and (4) each party is free to accept or reject the offer (Pride and Ferrell, 1997).

Publics

A public is a group of people or organizations that has an actual or a potential interest or impact on an organization. Input publics supply resources and constraints and consist of suppliers, donors, and regulatory publics. The organization's internal publics, such as the board of directors, management, staff, and volunteers, to accomplish the organization's mission, then manage those inputs. Intermediary publics are used to promote and distribute goods and services to consumers. The consuming publics, such as patients, clients, and students, consume the output of the organization. Reciprocal publics

---

BOX 9-6 Exchange Model

Seller has something of value, such as products, services, and ideas, for the buyer.
Buyer has something of value, such as money, credit, services, and products, for the seller.

Data from Pride WM, Ferrell OC: *Marketing: Concepts and strategies*, Boston, 1997, Houghton Mifflin.

are interested in the agency, and the agency is interested in them. Patients are an example. Sought publics are desired by the agency but are not necessarily interested in the agency. For instance, wealthy people who are potential donors could be a sought public. Unwelcome publics are interested in the agency, but the agency is not interested in them. One unwelcome public consists of emergency room patients for nonemergency care. Publics are related to each other, as well as to the agency, and they influence each other's attitudes and behaviors. Publics are groups that have actual or potential interests in or impact on the agency.

Market

A market is a potential arena for the trading of resources. It is a group of people or organizations that have resources that they want to exchange, or might be willing to exchange, for distinct benefits. A market is composed of actual or potential buyers and is a place where people negotiate to transfer goods or services. The health care agency goes to the labor market to obtain employees, to the professional market to obtain physicians, and to the financial market to obtain capital.

Image

An image is the sum of impressions, beliefs, and ideas that a person has of something. Publics with a positive image of an organization will be drawn to it, whereas those with a negative image will avoid or disparage it.

There are two opposite theories about image formation. Object-determined theory maintains that people perceive the reality of the object. They experience the object and process the sensory data in a similar way despite different backgrounds. Therefore when people see a building in a beautiful setting, they perceive it as a beautiful hospital. Person-determined theory maintains that people have different degrees of contact with an object; they selectively perceive different aspects of the object, and through individual ways of processing the sensory data, they experience selective distortion. In this case some

people may perceive the hospital as beautiful and others may not.

Image is a function of deeds and communications. Good deeds about which others are not told and talk without action are not enough. A strong, favorable image develops from satisfied publics that tell others their opinions.

Buyer Decision Process

Both individuals and organizations follow similar processes when making buying decisions. First, the problem or need is identified. Second, specifications needed to solve the problem are identified, and then there is a search for products, services, or ideas to meet the need. Alternatives are evaluated, a purchase decision is made, and then the product, service, or idea is reevaluated on performance (Kotler and Armstrong, 1996; Pride and Ferrell, 1997) (Figure 9-7).

MARKETING PROCESS

Marketing involves informing the market of services provided and fitting services to the market needs. It has evolved through different philosophies (Box 9-7).

Mass marketing occurs when the seller mass-produces, distributes, and promotes one product or service to all customers. *Product-variety marketing* exists when the seller provides variety to the customers by having two or more products with different features. *Target marketing* involves the seller's identifying market segments, selecting specific target markets, and then developing products or services and marketing mixes specific to each target market (Box 9-8).

The marketing process involves several steps.

Market Segmentation

An audit can be used to identify the bases for segmenting the market and to develop profiles of the segments. Marketing involves informing the market of services provided and fitting services to market needs. It is a complex process that generally includes the audit, market segmentation, marketing mix, implementation, and evaluation and control.

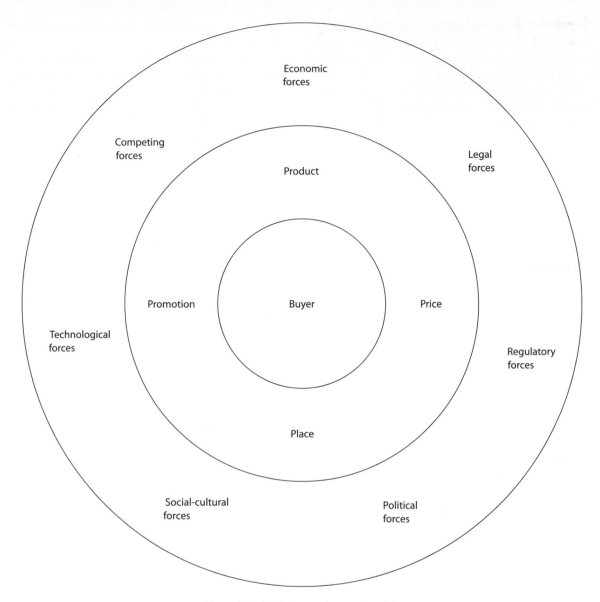

Figure 9-7 Marketing environment model.

The marketing audit involves identification, collection, and evaluation of information that needs to be examined to evaluate market relations. Identifying the market and market segments is required. How large is the area to be served? Is it rural, urban, or both? How many potential customers are there? What are their

BOX **9-7** Philosophies of Marketing

Mass marketing
Product-variety marketing
Target marketing

BOX **9-8** Marketing Process

Market segmentation
　Identify bases for segmenting the market
　Develop profiles of segments
Market targeting
　Develop measures of segment attractiveness
　Select the target segment(s)
Market positioning
　Develop positioning for each target segment
　Develop marketing mix for each target segment
Implement
Evaluate and control

Data from Kotler P, Armstrong G: *Principles of marketing*, ed 7, Upper Saddle River, NJ, 1996, Prentice Hall.

ages, occupations, income levels, and interests? How many are aware of the organization's services? Are there seasonal differences? How satisfied are the clients with the services offered now?

The *organization* should be assessed. What is the mission of the organization? What are its philosophy, goals, objectives, and priorities? What are the services provided? What are the strengths and weaknesses? How do its services compare with those of others? What conditions of the industry affect the organization? What internal and external controls affect it?

As *services* are further analyzed, one should note distinctive superiorities. What services are heavily used? Why? What services are underused? Why? Are there voids? If so, can they be filled? How can needed materials, supplies, and personnel be obtained? Who pays for the services?

Who are the *competitors?* How many are there? Are their numbers increasing or decreasing? Who are the principal competitors? What areas do they serve? How do their size and strength compare? How do their charges compare?

What is the profile of present and future *clients* for the services? Are client profiles different between services? What is the frequency of client usage of the services?

What are the perceptions of the *nursing market?* What are the internal perceptions of nurse recruitment? Focus groups can be formed to discuss reasons why nurses decided to work at the institution, the positive and negative aspects of the job, and ways working conditions can be improved. Interviews with directors of nursing education programs can be used to learn how the institution is perceived, where graduates of that school are going and why, and how personnel at the health care agency can influence those decisions.

What is the organization's pricing philosophy? How are *prices* determined? How do the staff, clients, and competitors view prices?

In what *location* is the service provided? How accessible is it to clients? How far will clients have to travel to obtain the service? Will personnel travel to provide a service? If so, how far? Will the agency charge for travel expenses?

What is the purpose of *promotion?* Is it reaching the intended publics? Is it effective? What media are being used? What media reach whom?

Many *assessment* tools can be used to collect data for the audit. Questionnaires administered by mail, telephone, or interview; in-depth interviews; and observations are common. A consumer panel can be used to discuss relevant issues. A mediator helps keep a representative group of consumers discussing a specific topic in focus groups. Nominal groups aim at generating consensus about a particular issue. Records can be reviewed, and scientific research designs can be planned and implemented to collect data.

A *sampling plan* is important. Who will be surveyed? What will the sample size be? Large samples are more reliable than small samples. How will the sample be chosen? A random sample is the most reliable.

Statistical techniques, such as frequency distributions, means, standard deviations, regression analysis, correlation analysis, factor analysis, discriminate analysis, and cluster analysis, can be useful. Statistical techniques are technical; therefore statistical consultation is often advisable.

Profiles can be developed based on demographical, geographical, psychographical, and product-related variables. Demographical variables can include age, gender, education, income, occupation, race, ethnicity, religion, family size, and family life cycle. Geographical variables include country, region, urban, suburban, rural, city size, county size, state size, climate, and market density. Psychographical variables include personality, social class, lifestyle, benefits sought, readiness state (unaware, aware, informed, interested, desirous, intending to buy), rate of adoption (innovator, early adopter, early majority adopter, late majority adopter, laggard), user status (nonuser, ex-user, potential user, first-time user, regular user), user rate (light, medium, or heavy user), loyalty status (none, medium, strong, absolute), and attitude toward the product (enthusiastic, positive, indifferent, negative, hostile). Product-related variables include benefit expectations, price sensitivity, brand loyalty, and volume usage (Kotler and Armstrong, 1996; Pride and Ferrell, 1997).

Market Targeting

Targeting involves developing measures of segment attractiveness and selecting the target segment or segments to enter. Segmentation identifies subsets of the total market that have similar characteristics (Box 9-9).

There are three major marketing strategies related to segments:
- Differentiated marketing aims directly and differentially at several specific segments.
- Concentrated marketing aims at a specific segment.
- Undifferentiated marketing ignores segments and deals with all as one market.

BOX 9-9 Target Segment Selection Process

Identify targeting strategy.
Determine segmentation variables to use.
Develop market segment profiles.
Evaluate market segments.
Select target market segments.

Data from Pride WM, Ferrell OC: *Marketing: Concepts and strategies*, Boston, 1997, Houghton Mifflin.

Market Positioning

The product position is the way customers describe the important attributes of the product or service. Leaders need to choose and implement a positioning strategy for a competitive advantage, which often involves offering a greater value for a lower price or justifying the higher price for more benefits. The difference promoted should be important, superior, distinctive, affordable, and profitable. The difference should be communicated and made visible to the buyer.

Marketing Mix

A marketing mix is developed for each target segment. It involves the four p's: product, price, place, and promotions (Box 9-10).

Product is something provided for consumption to satisfy a need or want. The inventory of services and analysis of costs, benefits, and target markets indicate which products are overused, underused, and cost-effective and which are perceived as strong or weak. This information should be used to determine the appropriate product mix.

A product line is composed of similar services that are clustered to manage process, quality, costs, and marketing more efficiently. Product line analysis is a method of analyzing products in terms of inputs and outputs and is built on total cost accounting principles. Because determination of actual cost per case is important, all costs for an admission are tracked. All hospital fixed overhead costs are allocated to patients and product lines. All costs from admission to discharge are determined and compared with the reimbursement per case. Length of stay by product line is important. When the patient's

---

BOX 9-10 Marketing Mix

Product
Price
Place
Promotions

length of stay is too long, the total cost may surpass the reimbursement per case even if the daily expense is reasonable.

Product line analysis shows the relationship of inputs to outputs, gives profit and loss information for a product line, attaches all costs to a product line, increases personnel's cost awareness, facilitates planning, promotes efficiency, encourages better review and control of resources, and promotes better decision making.

A Boston consulting group developed a classification system of potential growth and profitability to identify marketing strategies for products (Figure 9-8). They created a grid with growth potential measured on the vertical axis and profitability along the horizontal axis. Low growth potential and profitability are represented at the lower left corner; the factor

becomes higher toward the top and the right of the grid. Products with low profitability and low growth potential are labeled *dogs*. They drain the organization and should be divested if possible. Products in the upper left quadrant have low profitability and high growth potential. They are labeled *question marks*. Aggressive marketing to increase volume and therefore profitability is possible but risky. *Cash cows*, with high profitability but low growth potential, are in the lower right quadrant. That product may be maintained to use the profits to finance other ventures or to cover other losses. In the upper right quadrant are the *rising stars*, which have both high profitability and high growth potential. Promotional money should be put here to increase volume and profitability. After increasing growth, rising stars typically become cash cows.

Figure 9-8 Boston consulting firm's grid.

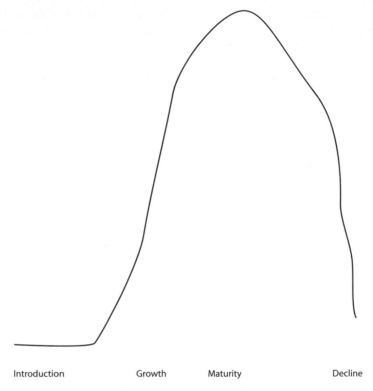

| Introduction | Growth | Maturity | Decline |

Figure 9-9 Product life cycle.

Products have life cycles. The stages of the life cycle are as follows (Figure 9-9):

The introduction stage is the beginning of a new product when the customer's response to the product and its growth potential are relatively unknown.

The growth stage occurs when the number of customers and the size of the market increase.

The maturity stage is the peak market of the product. Competition enters the market to obtain a share. Marketing strategies during the maturity stage are designed to get and keep the agency's share of the market.

The last stage is the market decline stage, when the market decreases because of new ideas, products, technology, or changes in customer needs (Berkowitz, 1996).

Question marks occur during the introductory stage, when the future is risky but there is high growth potential. Rising stars form the growth stage, when profitability and growth potential are high. Cash cows are seen during the maturity stage, when there is high profitability but low growth potential. Dogs occur during the decline stage, with the decreasing growth and profitability.

A fad is a fashion that peaks early and declines rapidly (Figure 9-10, *A*). A fashion is a currently popular style (Figure 9-10, *B*). Style is a basic mode of expression that is distinctive (Figure 9-10, *C*). For example, clothes may be casual or formal; art may be abstract or realistic. A style may last for decades, coming in and out of vogue with periods of renewed interest (Kotler and Armstrong, 1996; Kotler et al, 1999).

Price is another major consideration. Because physicians rather than patients usually determine the services used and health care bills are usually paid by third-party payers, nondollar

Figure 9-10 A, Fads. **B**, Fashions. **C**, Styles.

costs such as time and convenience must be considered. Minimization of nondollar costs should benefit the health care agency and the consumer.

There are several pricing goals:

- *Profit-maximizing pricing* tries to set the maximum price that the demand for the product or service will bear.
- *Market-share pricing* sacrifices short-term profits for long-term market domination and attempts to identify the price that maximizes the agency's share of the market.
- *Market-skimming pricing* places a high price and high profitability on a product or service when it is in high demand with no competition.
- *Current-revenue pricing* tries to maximize the current revenue.
- *Target-profit pricing* attains a satisfactory profit.
- *Promotional, loss-leader pricing* sets the price lower than the cost or competition to introduce customers to the new product or service. Profits are regained when the customers purchase other products.
- *Prestige pricing* sets unusually high prices to convey the image of quality or prestige.

Pricing factors include cost of product, demand for product, and competition. When considering the *cost of products or services,* one can use *mark-up pricing* by adding a certain percentage to the cost, *cost-plus pricing* by adding a fixed amount to the cost, and *target pricing* by setting the price so it yields a specific profit at a particular demand level. When considering the *demand* for the product or service, one can use *perceived-value pricing* by setting the price according to the customer's perception of the value of the product or service or *price-discrimination pricing* by varying the price from one customer or place to another. There

might be a sliding pay scale according to the patient's income. One hospital in a corporation might charge more or less than others because of the clients' income in general or the facility's location in a rich or poor neighborhood. When considering *competition, going-rate pricing* uses the collective wisdom of the marketplace. In *sealed-bid pricing* the lowest bid gets the business.

Place involves the physical location, appearance of the location, its accessibility and availability, resource utilization, the expertise and courtesy of staff, referral mechanisms, and distribution. The goal is to provide the service to the consumer with efficient distribution and minimal inconvenience.

Marketing promotion informs potential consumers of the existence and availability of products and services and persuades them of the benefits to them. Tailoring services to consumer desires is important. Marketing promotion leads to awareness, understanding, interest, decision, utilization, satisfaction, reutilization, and recommendation.

Promotion tools include the following: (1) advertising, which is any paid form of promotion; (2) personal selling, which is an oral presentation by a seller to a buyer; (3) sales promotions, which are short-term incentives for purchasing products or services; and (4) publicity, which is promotion that is not paid for by the agency. *Advertising* includes ads in newspapers, magazines, and journals, direct mail, fliers, billboard advertising, telephone directories, radio, and television. Printed materials can be used—for instance, calendars, matches, pens, telephone stickers, newsletters, and booklets about topics such as diet, exercise, poison control, and first aid. *Personal selling* includes fund-raising, lobbying, and sales calls such as presentations to community groups about health promotion, chemical dependency, weight control, exercise, birth control, and child care. *Sales promotions* include introductory offers, free samples, coupons, discounts, incentives, free lectures, and special credit cards. The best form of *publicity* is the word of mouth of satisfied customers. Other types are public service announcements, public relations campaigns, speakers' bureaus, interviews, health fairs, and screening programs.

Promotion has been revolutionized by technology. Personal computers and multimedia applications are readily available and make graphics, moving pictures, and sound possible. Multimedia notebooks are portable compact computers that are so small they can be taken anywhere they are needed and used without a connecting lead. They are very convenient for traveling representatives. A personal digital assistant (PDA) is fitted with an optic that allows one to write and draw on an electronic slate rather than type on a keyboard. Television facilitates visual communications. Teletex is a popular form of interactivity that allows choices to be made numerically by a standard remote control. People can get information about things such as the weather, traffic updates, airport arrivals, and stock indices. Then interests expressed by the choices can simultaneously be marketed by teletex. Travel arrangements can be booked when interest is expressed in a travel program. Direct-response television is interactive by using a commercial to get customers to call a specific number. Most calls are made within 10 minutes of the advertisement. TV videotex is an electronic information service that allows one to choose a teletex page from a menu. One needs to dial a telephone number to get access to a specific page that lists a variety of services. Near video on demand allows customers to view films as they "go by" on a regular basis. The customer pays for what is viewed. The investment costs for near video on demand are considerably less than video on demand, which is equivalent to a video shop at home (Postma, 1999).

Computers can make databases easily accessible and retrievable. They can then be used for marketing decisions. Electronic bulletin boards are computer network systems that link many computers by phone lines or satellite. They allow marketers to interact with data sources and clients almost instantaneously. Bulletin boards can permit customers to exchange ideas for problem solving, learn from each other, and give the agency new insights into marketing products and services. The Internet is a collection of computers connected by phone lines that enables people to communicate around the world through e-mail, news groups, chat rooms, and more. It links companies with customers around the world by computer networks. Although the Internet has been in existence for a few decades, the World Wide Web was not developed until 1992. It organizes information available on the Internet into interconnected pages that may include text, graphics, sound, and video. Software packages that facilitate navigating the Web have made the Web a multimedia communication tool (Pride and Ferrell, 1997). Fax machines, sales-automation software, personal newspapers, videoconferencing, cable television, and the Internet have revolutionized marketing (Kotler, 1999; Kotler and Kotler, 1999).

IMPLEMENTATION

Implementation can be done incrementally or as an entire package. Designing and implementing a marketing program are expensive projects and require personnel with expertise in marketing. Outside consultants can be hired when qualified people are not available within the organization. Dealing with local political conflicts, reaching communities that are out of touch with their own real demands, and sorting real demands from surface expectations are challenging tasks.

Domestic marketing focuses on the market in the country of origin. Although there may not be an international marketing plan, sometimes international distributors or foreign companies purchase products or services, creating limited exporting. International marketing includes plans for marketing among countries. Global marketing involves strategies for marketing around the world (Box 9-11).

Dealing with international and global markets is even more challenging than domestic marketing. There are different political climates; different histories; cultural differences; different business customs; different laws, legal systems, and regulations; different technological forces;

BOX 9-11 Levels of Global Marketing

Domestic marketing
Limited exporting
International marketing
Global marketing

Data from Pride WM, Ferrell OC: *Marketing: Concepts and strategies*, Boston, 1997, Houghton Mifflin.

---

different stages of economic development; different economic forces; and different local geography. Rather than dealing with one set of market conditions, marketers must address differences for each country and for each market within each country (Cateora and Graham, 1999; Pride and Ferrell, 1997).

Evaluation and Control

The last phase of the marketing process is evaluation and control. It involves identifying goals and objectives, measuring planned and actual results, determining reason for variance between planned and actual results, correcting action based on causal analysis, and revising goals. Evaluation can be done more or less often—daily through weekly, monthly, yearly, or on a more extended basis—to determine whether implementation is accomplishing desired results.

Health Care Marketing and Ethics

Historically, many professionals have argued that marketing health care could sacrifice quality for volume, could shift decision-making power to the public that was not qualified to make the decisions, would lower standards of professions, could be harmful to professional image, and was thus unethical. Now many professional groups are marketing to increase awareness of services without sacrificing standards. Some say marketing has increased sensitivity to client needs. Others recommend marketing to recruit nurses. The American Marketing Association's Academy for Health Services Marketing has developed professional ethics for health care marketing. They include respecting the primacy

of the client's welfare and confidentiality of the relationships; providing communications to inform, not to deceive; being competitive and making fair comparisons; and being vigilant in the application of the standards. Marketing public relations has helped marketing campaigns be successful (Harris, 1998; Sullivan and Decker, 1999).

Chapter Summary

Chapter 9 covered the following:
History of Health Care Financing
Budgetary Leadership and Management
Budgets
Prerequisites to Budgeting
Applied Economics
Accounting
Types of Budgets
    Operating, or Revenue-and-Expense,
        Budgets
    Personnel Budgets
    Capital Expenditure Budgets
    Cash Budgets
    Flexible Budgets
    Historical Approach to Budgeting
    Standard Cost
Zero-Based Budgeting
Periodic Budgetary Review
Advantages and Disadvantages
    Advantages and Disadvantages of Flexible
        Budgets
    Advantages of Budgeting
    Disadvantages of Budgeting
Budgeting Process
Cost Containment
    Cost Awareness
    Cost Fairs
    Cost Monitoring
    Cost Management
    Cost Incentives
    Cost Avoidance
    Cost Reduction
        Inventory control
    Cost Control
Cost-Effectiveness and Cost-Benefit Analysis

On-line Resources

evolve   Additional critical thinking activities, worksheets, and case studies are available on-line at http://evolve.elsevier.com/Marriner/guide/

References

Andreasen A, Kotler P: *Strategic marketing for nonprofit organizations*, Upper Saddle River, NJ, 2002, Prentice Hall.

Baker JJ, Baker RW: *Health care finance: Basic tools for nonfinancial managers*, Gaithersburg, Md, 2000, Aspen.

Berkowitz EN: *Essentials of health care marketing*, Gaithersburg, Md, 1996, Aspen.

Brinker BJ: *Performance measurement: Emerging practices in cost management*, Boston, 1996, Warren, Gorham & Lamont.

Cateora PR, Graham JL: *International marketing*, Boston, 1999, Irwin/McGraw-Hill.

Cokins G: *Activity-based cost management: Making it work*, Chicago, 1996, Irwin.

Douglas LM: *The effective nurse: Leader and manager*, ed 5, St Louis, 1996, Mosby.

Finkler SA: *Budgeting concepts for nurse managers*, ed 3, Philadelphia, 2001, WB Saunders.

Finkler SA, Kovner CT: *Financial management for nurse managers and executives*, ed 2, Philadelphia, 1999, WB Saunders.

Gapenski LC: *Healthcare finance: An introduction to accounting and financial management*, Chicago, 1999, Health Administration Press.

Grohar-Murray ME, DiCroce HR: *Leadership and management in nursing*, ed 3, Upper Saddle River, NJ, 2003, Prentice Hall.

Harris TL: *Value-added public relations: The secret weapon of integrated marketing*, Chicago, 1998, NCT/Contemporary Publishing Group.

Hein EC: *Contemporary leadership behavior: Selected readings*, ed 5, Philadelphia, 1998, Lippincott.

Herzlinger RE: *Market-driven health care: Who wins, who loses in the transformation of America's largest service industry*, Reading, Mass, 1999, Perseus Books.

Huber D: *Leadership and nursing care management*, Philadelphia, 1996, WB Saunders.

Kotler P: *Kotler on marketing: How to create, win and dominate markets*, New York, 1999, Free Press.

Kotler P: *Marketing for nonprofit organizations*. Englewood Cliffs, NJ, 1982, Prentice-Hall.

Kotler P, Armstrong G: *Principles of marketing*, ed 7, Upper Saddle River, NJ, 1996, Prentice Hall.

Kotler P, Kotler P: *Marketing management: Analysis, planning, implementation, and control*, Upper Saddle River, NJ, 1999, Prentice Hall.

Kotler P, Roberto EL: *Social marketing: Strategies for changing public behavior*, New York, 1989, Free Press.

Kotler P et al: *Marketing management: An Asian perspective*, Singapore, 1999, Prentice Hall.

Loveridge CE, Cummings SH: *Nursing management in the new paradigm*, Gaithersburg, Md, 1996, Aspen.

Marquis BL, Huston CJ: *Leadership roles and management functions in nursing: Theory and application*, Philadelphia, 2002, Lippincott.

McCloskey JC: Implications of costing out nursing for reimbursement, *Nurs Manage* 20(1):245-253, 1989.

Morin WJ: *Silent sabotage: Rescuing our careers, our companies, and our lives from the creeping paralysis of anger and bitterness*, New York, 1995, American Management Association.

Nowicki M: *The financial management of hospitals and healthcare organizations,* ed 2, Chicago, 2001, Health Administration Press.

Ostrenga MR et al: *The Ernst & Young guide to total cost management,* New York, 1992, John Wiley & Sons.

Popcorn F, Marigold L: *Clicking: 16 Trends to future fit your life, your work, and your business,* New York, 1996, Harper Collins.

Postma P: *The new marketing era: Marketing to the imagination in a technology-driven world,* New York, 1999, McGraw-Hill.

Pride WM, Ferrell OC: *Marketing: Concepts and strategies,* Boston, 1997, Houghton Mifflin.

Rocchiccioli JT, Tilbury MS: *Clinical leadership in nursing,* Philadelphia, 1998, WB Saunders.

Storfjell JL, Jessup S: Bridging the gap between finance and clinical operations with activity-based cost management, *JONA* 26:12-17, Dec 1996.

Sullivan EJ, Decker PJ: *Nursing administration: A micro/macro approach for effective nurse executives,* Norwalk, Conn, 1999, Appleton & Lange.

Swansburg RC: *Budgeting and financial management for nurse managers,* Boston, 1997, Jones & Bartlett.

Swansburg RC, Swansburg RJ: *Introductory management and leadership for nurses: An interactive text,* Boston, 1999, Jones & Bartlett.

Yoder-Wise PS: *Leading and managing in nursing,* ed 2, St Louis, 2002, Mosby.

Zelman WN, McCue MJ, Millikan AR, et al: *Financial management of health care organizations,* Great Britain, 2003, Blackwell.

10

Organizational Concepts and Structures

Chapter Overview

Chapter 10 outlines factors affecting organizational structures,
organizational concepts, and types of organizational structures, including
health care networks.

Chapter Objectives

- Describe the relationships among span of management, flat or tall structures,
  and decentralization or centralization.
- Describe ways a manager can facilitate adjustments to mergers and
  acquisitions.
- Differentiate between line and staff authority.
- Identify at least three principles of organization.
- Describe disadvantages of the bureaucratic structure.
- Identify at least three adhocracy organizational models.
- Describe the corporate model.

Major Concepts and Definitions

Organizational chart a drawing that shows how the parts of an organization are linked
Span of management the number and diversity of people who report to a manager
Centralize to concentrate power or authority
Decentralize to distribute power and authority among more places
Merger the combination of two or more companies into one company
Line authority the formal chain of command
Staff authority advisory or service oriented in nature
Organization consolidated group of elements; systematized whole
Structure formation or pattern of arrangement
Hierarchy a group of persons arranged by rank, grade, or class
Bureaucracy administration through departments and subdivisions managed by officials
following an inflexible routine
Adaptive able to change to make suitable to new or changed circumstances
Matrix the formation of cells in the organizational structure
Corporation a group

FACTORS AFFECTING ORGANIZATIONAL STRUCTURES

"Chaos results when the world changes faster than people." —Anonymous

Organizational structures are affected by the economic, political, social, and technological pressures in society and follow changes in vertical and horizontal integration, geographical dispersion, and unit volume. The structure delimits responsibilities, communication channels, and the decision-making environment. The organizational structure should facilitate the vision, values, mission, philosophy, goals, objectives, strategies, policies, and procedures.

Organizational structures are changing from simple, hierarchical structures with formal channels of communication, functional fiefdoms, and division of labor with division and simplification of work to complex, flat organizations with cross-functional teams, free access to information, and no boundaries that empower employees and enrich work through multiple tasks (Martin, 1995; Swansburg and Swansburg, 2002) (Table 10-1).

It used to be that only experts could perform complex tasks, information was located in one place, and decision making was centralized with

TABLE **10-1** Trends Affecting Organizational Structures

FROM:	TO:
Hierarchical management	Flat organizations with cross-functional teams
Formal channels of communication	Free access to information
Functional fiefdoms	Organization without boundaries
Division of labor	Empowerment of employees
Division and simplification of work	Enrichment of work through multiple tasks and expanded knowledge
Simple	Complex.

TABLE **10-2** Technological Influences

OLD WAYS	NEW WAYS
Information was in only one place.	Information is simultaneously in many places.
Only experts could perform complex tasks	Generalists can do expert tasks.
The organization was centralized or decentralized.	The organization is simultaneously centralized and decentralized.
Managers made the decisions.	Everyone makes decisions.
Field personnel needed offices.	Field personnel can work anywhere.
Best contact was a personal contact.	Best contact is an effective contact by any of numerous modes.
Field personnel had to find out where things were.	Things tell where they are.
Plans got revised periodically.	Plans get revised instantaneously.

Modified from Wall DK, Proyect MM: *Critical pathway implementation guide: A methodology for managing critical pathways*, Chicago, 1997, Precept Press.

managers. Plans got revised periodically. Field personnel needed an office and had to find out where things were. The best contact was a personal contact. Now generalists can do expert tasks, everyone makes decisions, and the organization is simultaneously centralized and decentralized. Information is simultaneously in many places, and plans can be revised instantaneously. Field workers can work anywhere and can make effective contacts through numerous means. Things tell where they are (Table 10-2).

Leaders evaluate the organizational structure, encourage employees to follow the chain of command, counsel employees who do not follow the chain of command, model responsibility and accountability, help staff see how their roles fit into the structure, encourage upward communications, facilitate the informal group, explain the organizational culture, and support advisory personnel. Managers are knowledgeable about the structure, maintain and clarify unity of command, establish a span of control, provide organizational charts, follow the chain of command, use the informal organization, are knowledgeable about the culture, and use advisory personnel (Table 10-3).

Managed care; consolidations of health plans, hospitals, and physicians; physician and hospital integration; vertical integration with disease management; and horizontal integration for coordination of care respond to trends in health care. There has been an increase in primary care,

TABLE **10-3** Leadership and Management Regarding Organizational Structure

LEADER	MANAGER
Evaluates the organizational structure	Is knowledgeable about the structure
Encourages employees to follow the chain of command	Maintains unity of command
Counsels employees who do not use the chain of command	Clarifies unity of command
Models responsibility and accountability	Establishes a span of control
Helps staff see how their roles fit into the structure	Provides organizational charts
Encourages upward communications	Follows the chain of command
Facilitates the informal group	Uses the informal organization
Explains the organizational culture	Is knowledgeable about the culture
Supports advisory personnel	Uses advisory personnel

Modified from Marquis BL, Huston CJ: *Leadership roles and management functions in nursing: Theory and application*, ed 2, Philadelphia, 2000, Lippincott.

outpatient services, self-care of chronic diseases, uninsured population, and use of Medicare by the aging population. There are new drugs, therapies, medical technology, and information systems. Electronic medical records and databases are becoming available. Telehealth is increasing, as are e-mails between patients and their physicians. Costs are shifting away from managed care and insurance to physicians, hospitals, and the consumer (Coddington, Fischer, Moore, et al, 2000; Institute for the Future, 2000).

ORGANIZATIONAL CHARTS

An organizational chart is a drawing that shows how the parts of an organization are linked. It depicts the formal organizational relationships, areas of responsibility, persons to whom one is accountable, and channels of communication.

Managers should consider actual working relationships when drawing an organizational chart. The formal organization may not be functioning as outlined on an older chart. Rather, an alternate structure may have emerged that operates very effectively. It is essential, then, that the manager knows what is happening in actual practice. The process of drawing the chart demands a review of current practices, discovery of relationships not previously examined, and clarification of vague associations.

The organizational chart may be used for outlining administrative control, for policy making and planning (including organizational change) to evaluate strengths and weaknesses of the current structure, and for showing relationships with other departments and agencies. It can also be used to orient new personnel or to present the agency's structural design to others. The visual diagram of a chart is a more effective means of communicating the agency's organizational structure than is a written description.

Organizational charts are not used by all managers. Autocratic managers who wish to control and manipulate others may feel that their power would be diminished if staff associates understood the working environment. Adaptive structures are more difficult to chart because they are more fluid and subject to change.

Charts become outdated as changes are made. On charts the informal structure has not been diagrammed, the formal structure may be difficult to define, and duties and responsibilities are not described. Charts may foster rigidity in relationships and communications. People may be sensitive about their relative status in the organization and may not want their positions revealed. It can be expensive to develop, disseminate, and store the charts.

Vertical charts, depicting the chief executive at the top with formal lines of authority down the hierarchy, are most common, but other modifications are available (Figures 10-1 and 10-2). A left-to-right, or horizontal, chart depicts the chief executive at the left with lower echelons to the right (Figure 10-3). It follows the normal reading habit, shows relative length of formal lines of authority, helps simplify the lines of authority and responsibility, and can reveal problems within the structure. A concentric, or circular, chart shows the chief executive in the center with successive echelons in concentric

Figure 10-1 Line-staff relationships.

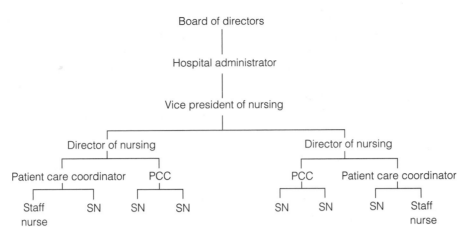

Figure 10-2 Vertical chart.

circles (Figure 10-4). It helps depict the outward flow of formal authority from the top executive and supposedly reduces status implications.

The informal structure can be superimposed on the formal structure or charted through the use of sociograms. Sociograms analyze data on the choice of, communication among, and interaction among members of a small group. Personnel may be asked with whom they prefer to work, or their interactions may be observed

Figure 10-3 Left-to-right chart.

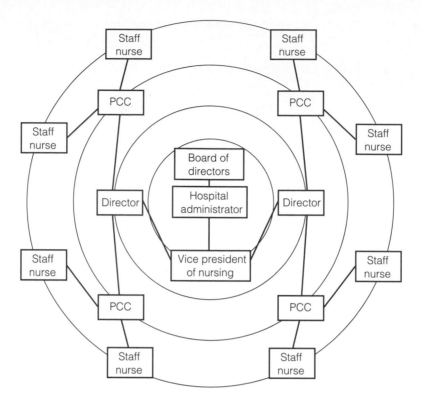

Figure 10-4 Circular chart.

and charted. The person with the most relationships is often the leader. Members of the primary group are those most accepted by other group members. Managers should use this information to increase production, because work groups based on sociograms are generally more productive than those arbitrarily designed.

Advantages of organizational charts are that they can contribute to sound organizational structures, map lines of decision-making authority, show formal lines of communication, and help employees understand their assignments, especially in relation to others (Box 10-1). Unfortunately, organizational charts can become obsolete quickly, show only formal relationships, do not show informal communications, may show how things are supposed to be rather than how they are, and may contribute to confusion about authority and status (Marquis and Huston, 1998, 2000).

CHAIN OF COMMAND

"A person remains wise as long as he seeks wisdom. The minute he thinks he has found it he becomes a fool." —Anonymous

The chain of command is the formal line of authority and communications. In hierarchies authority and communications flow from the top down and authority and responsibility are aligned. In the newer structures the chain of command is flatter, with communications flowing in all directions, and authority and responsibility delegated to the lowest operational level possible (Marquis and Huston, 1998, 2000; Swansburg and Swansburg, 2002).

CENTRALITY

Centrality indicates the location of a position in an organization where frequent communication

BOX **10-1** Advantages and Disadvantages of Organizational Charts

ADVANTAGES

Contributes to sound organizational structure
Maps lines of decision-making authority
Shows formal lines of communication
Shows how people fit into the organization

Helps employees understand their assignments

DISADVANTAGES

Becomes obsolete quickly
Shows only formal relationships
Does not show informal communications
May show how things are supposed to be rather than how they are
May help confuse authority and status

occurs. It is determined by organizational distance. Employees with small organizational distance are able to receive more information than those more peripherally located. Middle managers tend to have a broad view of the organization because of the centrality for receiving upward, downward, and horizontal communications (Marquis and Huston, 1998, 2000).

UNITY OF COMMAND

Unity of command is represented by the vertical solid line between positions on an organizational chart. It indicates one person has one boss. This is still supported in some structures, as with primary nursing. However, health care professionals are getting increasingly involved with matrix organizations, where they answer to more than one person (Marquis and Huston, 1998, 2000; Swansburg and Swansburg, 2002).

AUTHORITY

Authority is the official power to act. It is the power to direct the work of others (Marquis and Huston, 1998, 2000).

RESPONSIBILITY

Responsibility is a duty or an assignment. A person needs the authority necessary to accomplish the assignment (Marquis and Huston, 1998, 2000).

ACCOUNTABILITY

Accountability is a moral responsibility. A manager may delegate responsibility but always remains accountable (Marquis and Huston, 1998, 2000).

SPAN OF MANAGEMENT

Span of management has been of concern since biblical times. Exodus 18:13-26 is an account of how Moses had to deal with the problem of leading the Israelites out of Egypt. His father-in-law, Jethro, observed Moses counseling people all day long, while others had to wait long periods of time to tell Moses their problems. Jethro suggested that he delegate authority by selecting rulers of thousands, hundreds, fifties, and tens who would teach the people laws and leave Moses free to deal only with the exceptions.

Initial work with span of management was quantitative and attempted to devise formulas for determining the most desirable number of people reporting to a manager. General Hamilton, a British officer in World War I, concluded that managers at the lower levels could direct more people than those at higher levels. He thought an effective span of control was three to six others, especially at upper levels. Henri Fayol, a French industrialist and early writer about scientific management, used a similar philosophy to develop a hierarchy.

Hamilton's principle has been elaborated on by A.V. Graicunas, a Lithuanian management consultant whose mathematical analysis of potential relationships illustrates the complex social processes between managers and their staff associates and among the staff; the complexity especially increases with each additional staff associate. Graicunas demonstrated that as the number of staff associates responsible to a manager increases arithmetically, the number of potential interactions increases geometrically. The geometrical interactions can be classified as direct single relationships, direct group relationships, and cross relationships. If a manager has two staff associates, x and y, the manager may have two direct single relationships, one with x and one with y. The manager may speak to either in the presence of the other, forming two group relationships. Two cross relationships exist between x and y and between y and x. Consequently, there are six possible interactions between one manager and two staff associates—two direct, two group, and two cross. If a third staff associate is added, one direct relationship, seven group relationships, and four cross relationships are added, making 18 potential interactions.

Graicunas's formula is as follows:

$$R = n\left(\frac{2^n}{2} + n - 1\right)$$

R equals all types of relationships, and *n* equals the number of subordinates. The results are presented in Table 10-4.

Graicunas's formula calculates the number of potential relationships. It does not deal with the actual frequency or the importance of the various relationships. In reality, the number of relationships with which a manager must deal is probably not so great. One might question whether the relationship in which the manager speaks to x in y's presence is different from speaking to y in x's presence. Graicunas considers them different psychological situations. It is unlikely that people will engage in all the relationships that are theoretically possible. Nevertheless, Graicunas's formula illustrates how complex a situation can become as additional staff associates report to a manager.

The optimal span of management depends on many considerations that affect the time requirements for management. Managers' competence and qualifications and those of their staffs affect their time requirements. Some managers, because of their education and personal qualities, can

TABLE **10-4** Variables Number of Associates and Resulting Number of Potential Relationships

NUMBER OF ASSOCIATES	NUMBER OF RELATIONSHIPS
1	1
2	6
3	18
4	44
5	100
6	222
7	490
8	1080
9	2376
10	5210
11	11,374
12	24,708
13	53,404
14	114,872
18	2,359,602

work with more people than others. The better prepared staff associates are for their jobs, the less time managers must devote to teaching, clarifying responsibilities, and correcting mistakes.

Rapidly changing technology, procedures, and policies increase training problems and the need for problem solving. Availability of expert advice and services to managers can free their time and widen their span of management. However, a larger personal staff does not necessarily allow a broadening of the span of control because of the supervision required for those assistants. It may be more economical to increase the responsibilities of lower-level management. The greater the clarity of delegated authority, the less time it will take for managers to explain responsibilities and tasks. There will be less need for them to make decisions staff associates can make. If staff associates' tasks are not clearly defined, are unaccompanied by the necessary authority, or are beyond their competence, there will be an increase in time required for supervision.

Much of a manager's time is spent explaining plans, giving instructions, and receiving information about problems and progress. Clear and concise communications transmit information quickly and accurately. Much communication can be written. However, some situations cannot be handled with planning documents, policy statements, written reports, memoranda, or other written communications. These require personal contact. Some situations that could be handled by written communications may be better handled by personal contact. These might include delicate situations and instances where attitudes are involved. Personal contacts require considerable time.

If plans are clear, staff associates will know what is expected of them without frequently checking with the manager. If staff associates do their own planning, they will need more supervision. However, clear policies to guide their planning will reduce demands on the manager. Clear and complete policy statements can also simplify managers' decision making and allow expansion of their span of management. Deciding every problem individually requires more time than making policy decisions that anticipate problems.

The demands on the staff associate vary according to the complexity of functions. Standardization reduces time requirements because people know what is expected. Routine work requires less time than innovative work. But we can expect that as the degree of difficulty for performing a task satisfactorily increases, so does the demand on the manager. As the variability of functions increases, the manager must consider more factors and interrelationships; this takes more time. Interdependent functions require more management time than independent functions because of the increased need for coordination. The greater the geographical separation of personnel reporting to the manager, the more limiting the span of control. The greater the nonmanagerial responsibilities, the less time the manager has for management. Managers in flat organizational structures have a broader range of management than those in tall structures, and lower-level managers have a broader range than top management.

LEVELS OF MANAGEMENT

Top-level managers generally make decisions with the help of few guidelines or structures, coordinate internal and external influences, and view the organization as a whole. They include the chief executive officer (CEO), the organization's highest ranking individual, and the top-level nurse manager. The titles vary but could include president, vice-president, or director. Middle-level managers conduct day-to-day operations with some involvement with long-term planning and policy making. Those titles also vary but could include supervisor, unit manager, or head nurse. First-level managers are concerned with a specific unit's work flow. They deal with immediate day-to-day operations problems. Those titles vary and may include case manager, nurse practice coordinator, primary care nurse, team leader, or charge nurse (Marquis and Huston, 1998, 2000; Rocchiccioli and Tilbury, 1998). The trend is to expand the span of top-level management to multiple organizations, of middle-level managers to multiple units, and of lower-level managers to cases across agencies.

FLAT VERSUS TALL STRUCTURES

The flat structure is developed along horizontal dimensions according to the number of organizational functions that are identified separately. There are few levels of management. The tall structure is developed along vertical dimensions by use of the scalar process to define relationships between levels in an organization. Because there are advantages and disadvantages to both the flat and tall structures, it is best to maintain a reasonable balance of dimensions. Changes within the organization bring imbalance over time, so the organizational structure should be reviewed periodically.

The flat structure shortens the administrative distance between top and bottom levels in the organization, thereby minimizing distortions through shorter lines of communication. Communications are direct, simple, fast, and clearly apparent to employees. Another advantage of the flat structure is that large groups have a greater variety of skills available and are capable of solving a greater variety of problems. This structure is believed to contribute to high employee morale and help develop capable, self-confident staff. It lends itself to a democratic approach and general management, which are preferred by many people. This minimal social stratification is consistent with an egalitarian political and social philosophy, which is currently popular.

However, a flat structure may be impractical in large organizations. Large groups have more difficulty reaching a consensus and require more coordination. The flat structure places tremendous pressure on each manager because of the large amount of authority and responsibility and the high penalties for failures. Overburdened managers may not have the time to select, evaluate, and teach subordinates or the energy to think and plan. They may have difficulty making and communicating decisions. Socializing with

staff associates may reduce their authority (Yoder-Wise, 2003).

Tall structures lend themselves to authoritarianism, which is most effective in situations requiring rapid changes and precise coordination. In a tall structure messages from managers are given more attention than those from peers and consequently pass through levels quickly. The narrow range of management allows staff to evaluate decisions frequently. With small groups decision making takes less time, and there is more opportunity for members to participate and to understand the goals. Such interaction facilitates group cohesiveness.

Levels are expensive because of the large number of executives needed with high salaries. Each additional level makes communication more cumbersome. The more levels that communications pass through, the greater the distortion. Therefore a tall structure reduces the

---

RESEARCH Perspective 10-1

Data from Adams CE, Michel Y, DeFrates D, et al: Effect of locale on health status and direct care time of rural versus urban home health patients.
JONA 31(5):244-251, 2001.

Purpose: The purpose of this study was to determine if health status differed between rural versus urban home health patients and to identify if locale was a significant predictor of home direct care time.

Methods: The investigation was a secondary analysis that focused on comparing outcomes and resource utilization in home health patients. Data were collected in four Medicare-certified home health agencies retrospectively on a convenience sample of 2788 patient episodes of care. Patient health status was measured using items from the Outcome Assessment and Information Set obtained from itinerary records. Direct care time was the time clinicians spent in the home.

Results/conclusions: Significantly more urban than rural patients were female. Urban patients were significantly older by an average of 2 years. Significantly more urban than rural patients had an inpatient discharge within the last 14 days, a good rehabilitation prognosis, and a good overall prognosis. When the home health care episode ended, significantly more urban than rural patients remained in the home. On the average, rural patients received more registered nurse direct care time than urban patients. Living in a rural location increased total direct care time by an average of 150 minutes. Urban patients were healthier than rural patients.

understanding between higher and lower levels and increases impersonality.

DECENTRALIZATION VERSUS CENTRALIZATION

Decentralization is the degree to which decision making is diffused throughout the organization. It is relative, for the degree of decentralization is larger when more important decisions affecting more functions are made at lower levels with less supervision. There are several factors to consider when determining the optimal degree of decentralization for an organization. People in top management need a positive attitude toward decentralization, and they need competent personnel to whom they can delegate authority. The latter need access to the information necessary for decision making.

The number of people who need to interact to solve a problem should be considered. In general, the larger the organization, the greater the number of complex decisions that must be made, and that can overburden top management and delay decision making. Smaller, decentralized units reduce the number of decisions made by each manager and increase the time available to devote to each problem. Agencies tend to be more centralized during their early, formative years. If the agency gradually expands from within, it is more likely to remain centralized. An organization that grows rapidly through acquisitions is more likely to be decentralized; thus decentralization is more common in organizations with geographical dispersion of operations. Some functions lend themselves more readily to decentralization than do others; production, marketing, personnel, and some purchasing may be readily decentralized. In contrast, finances, accounting, data processing of statistics, and purchase of capital equipment are likely to remain centralized.

The profit center concept has developed from decentralization and has been popular since World War II. It is particularly characteristic of large organizations with multiple product lines. The organization is divided into manageable units called profit centers that are self-contained and have their own management and staff. Each unit competes with others for profits; this arrangement motivates managers to make decisions that will maximize profits. The manager has considerable freedom for making operational decisions. The profit center concept helps give meaning to decentralization by placing the responsibility for profit making on a number of managers instead of just top management.

The advantages of decentralization seem to outweigh the disadvantages. Decentralization increases morale and promotes interpersonal relationships. When people have a voice in governance, they feel more important and are more willing to contribute. This increased motivation provides a feeling of individuality and freedom that in turn encourages creativity and commits the individual to making the system successful. Decentralization fosters informality and democracy in management and brings decision making closer to the action. Thus decisions may be more effective because people who know the situation and have to implement the decision are the ones who make it. Because managers do not have to wait for the approval of their superiors, flexibility is increased, and reaction time is decreased. Fewer people have to exchange information; consequently, communications are swift and effective. Coordination improves, especially for services, production with sales, and costs with income. Products or operations that are minor to the total production receive more adequate attention. Plans can be tried on an experimental basis in one unit, modified, and proven before used in other units. Risks of losses of personnel or facilities are dispersed.

Decentralization helps determine accountability. It makes weak management visible through semiindependent and often competitive divisions. Operating on the premise that people learn by doing, decentralization develops managers by allowing them to manage. A management pool can be developed that thereby eases the problem of succession. There is usually less conflict between top management and divisions. Decentralization releases top management from the burden of daily administration, freeing them for long-range planning, goal and policy development, and systems integration.

Nevertheless, several problems can also result from decentralization. An organization may not be large enough to merit decentralization, or it may be difficult to divide the organization into self-contained operating units. Top administrators may not desire decentralization. They may feel it would decrease their status, or they may question the abilities of the people to whom they would delegate. They may feel that most people prefer to be dependent on others and do not want decision-making responsibility. An increased awareness of division consciousness and a decrease in company consciousness may develop. Divisions may become individualized and competitive to the extent that they sacrifice the overall objectives for short-range profitability and work against the best interests of the whole organization. Because of conflicts among divisions, it may be difficult to obtain a majority vote, and compromises may result. If the majority vote is delayed, it may come too late to be effective.

Decentralization involves increased costs. It requires more managers and larger staffs. Managers may be underused. Divisions may not adequately use the specialists housed at headquarters. Functions are likely to be duplicated between divisions and headquarters. Because decentralization develops managers, there are novice managers in the system who will make mistakes. Division managers may not inform top management of their problems. There are problems with control and nonuniform policies. Some restrictions on autonomy remain. Even with decentralization, people in top management remain responsible for long-range objectives and goals, broad policies, selection of key executives, and approval of major capital expenditures.

Departmentalization

Departmentalization results from span of management, division of work, and need for cooperation. Its primary purpose is to subdivide the organizational structure so that managers can specialize within limited ranges of activity. Organization of the agency influences group behavior and the effectiveness of the group. The objectives of the agency can be met most easily if the group is properly organized. Two common types of departmentalization are input and output. The input, or process, orientation includes function, time, and simple numbers as bases for departmentalization, whereas the output, or goal, orientation includes product, territory, and client divisions.

The input, or process-oriented, structure emphasizes specialization of skills. It reinforces professional skills by uniting people with similar expertise in the same department. For example, the focus may be on cardiac nursing, respiratory nursing, or transplant nursing, depending on the departmentalization. It is possible for professionals to advance within their field of expertise instead of advancing through the administrative hierarchy. Unfortunately, the process-oriented structure emphasizes professional skills over organizational goals. Conflicts increase as communication and cooperation decrease. Input organization provides less favorable training for general administrators than does a goal-oriented structure.

Departmentalization by function groups activities according to similarity of skills or a group of tasks necessary to accomplish a goal. Logical, simple, and commonly used, it facilitates specialization that contributes to economic operations. It groups functions that can be performed by the same specialists with the same type of equipment and facilities. Less demand for one product may be counteracted by a greater demand for another product. Consequently, staff, equipment, and facilities will have optimal utilization. The combination of administrative activities also is economical. One manager is responsible for all related activities; therefore coordination is improved because it is more easily achieved. The agency benefits from a few people with outstanding abilities, for only top management is able to coordinate the major functions.

For example, the hospital may be organized by medical, surgical, and pediatric units.

Functional departmentalization also has its disadvantages. As the size of the agency increases, centralization may become excessive, making effective control more difficult. The necessary additional organizational levels may slow communications and delay decision making. It becomes more difficult to measure performance. Functional departmentalization does not provide good training for general managers. They become expert in their particular function, have little opportunity to learn about other functions, and may emphasize their previous function while deemphasizing others when they become general managers.

Time factors are another basis for organization. Acute-care settings require coverage 24 hours per day, 7 days per week, whereas preventive services may require coverage for only 8 to 12 hours per day for 5 or 6 days per week at the most.

Grouping by numbers divides undifferentiated labor into manageable units. A certain number of workers are assigned to each manager. This method is common in underdeveloped countries but is disappearing in industrialized areas.

The output, or goal, structure emphasizes service to the client. It collects all the work for a project under one manager and reduces dependence on other units for needed resources. This allows considerable autonomy, and the client, workers, and goals are readily identified. Systems and procedures are highly standardized. Family planning, pregnancy counseling, and school health are examples of services available from some health departments.

Unfortunately, these units may stress their own goals while deemphasizing agency goals. Duplication of equipment and services may develop. Equipment may not be fully utilized, or smaller-scale equipment may be less effective. The grouping of various skills into one unit can reduce the expertise as professional reinforcement is weakened.

A product or group of closely related products may be the basis of organization for autonomous departments. Emphasis is on the product instead of the process. Improvement, expansion, and diversification of the product are possible because one manager is responsible for all activities affecting that specific product. In a large agency this could result in small, flexible units where functional groupings would be too complex. This method identifies profit responsibilities for specific products. Organization on the basis of products has become increasingly popular. It is common for schools of nursing to organize according to the "products" produced—medical nurses, surgical nurses, obstetrical nurses, pediatric nurses, psychiatric nurses, and community health nurses.

Departmentalization by territories is particularly useful for physically dispersed activities where branches provide similar services at each location. This method serves the local clients with greatest efficiency. Managers consider local circumstances that might be overlooked by a central manager. It uses local people who are familiar with local conditions. It reduces delivery time and may reduce transportation costs related to raw materials and finished products. It is particularly useful for production and sales and when perishability is a problem. However, financial management works best if centralized.

Departmentalization by client makes sense when service is important and the welfare of the client is of primary interest. For example, a clinic may have obstetrical, pediatric, and adolescent clinics. Clinics may be open nights and weekends for working people. Schools of nursing may offer night classes for working students. This better uses facilities and is more satisfactory to the client. However, pressure for special consideration and treatment of specific groups may exist, and coordination problems may increase (Galbraith, 1995; Galbraith, Downey, and Kates, 2002).

Clusters

Clusters are two or three clinically similar units that share resources such as staff, equipment, and educational materials. Clustering fosters collaboration and consultation among nurses, decreases the isolation of decentralization, and enhances professional marketability by expanding knowledge and skills.

Units forming cluster work groups should develop written agreements describing how the cluster will work, emphasize sharing resources, and arrange for personnel to meet each other through in-services and social events. New staff should know that clustering is an expectation and should be oriented to the cluster units. Staff should be oriented to cluster units before being shared and during nonstressful times. Cross training facilitates cost-effective, safe, and satisfying nursing services (Ouellette, Martin, Holmes, et al, 1989).

LINE-STAFF RELATIONSHIPS
Line Authority

Line organization is the oldest type of structure. It is a chain of command or a manager–staff associate or leader-follower relationship. The manager delegates authority to a staff associate, who in turn delegates authority to the staff. This progression is the basis for the term *line authority.* The command relationship is a direct line between manager and staff associate and is depicted by a solid line on organizational charts (see Figure 10-1). The line positions are related to the direct achievement of organizational objectives. This arrangement fosters quick decision making because managers are given complete charge of their areas and at most would need to consult only with their immediate managers. Buck passing is reduced, and authority relationships are clearly understood. The manager has the right to give orders, demand accountability, and discipline violators.

Staff Authority

Staff support line-authority relationships and are advisory or service oriented in nature. Staff authority is depicted by a dashed line on an organizational chart. They handle details, locate required data, and offer counsel on managerial problems. Staff function through influence, for they do not have authority to accept, use, modify, or reject plans. They make the line more effective, but organizations can function without staff authority.

The two major categories of staff authority are personal and specialist. The personal category includes the assistant and general staff. The specialist staff is composed of advisory, service, control, and functional personnel.

Assistant Staff

A personal staff member may be called an assistant, a staff assistant, or an administrative assistant and is responsible to one line manager. The assistant's chief purpose is to extend the line manager's capacity for completing a large amount of work by doing the more routine tasks that the manager would otherwise have to perform. The duties vary widely from one manager to another but might include activities such as mail answering, data collection for decision making, consolidation of information from various reports, preparation of documents, development of budgets, interpreting plans to others, and substitution for the manager at various meetings and functions.

Personal staff members have no specific functions. Their duties vary with the assignments. They do not act on their own behalf but rather as personal representatives of a manager. The only specific authority they have comes from a manager on a limited basis, usually for a specific job over a brief time span. With delegated authority, the personal staff member can give instructions in the manager's name and make decisions that affect the organization. It is important for assistants and the people with whom they work to know the extent of their influence. Misuses of and misunderstanding about the assistant are all too common. Some feel that the assistant is unnecessary and that the duties should be delegated to other line managers. When the assistant takes over tasks that belong to others, misunderstanding and poor cooperation result. Some assistants give the impression that they are the manager instead of just acting for one.

General Staff

The general staff is composed of top administrators. The top administrator makes the decision after receiving input from these key people who together have the necessary expertise to make sound decisions for the agency. This is a coordinated group performing to maximize results. They serve in an advisory capacity by collecting and sharing information and are functional through their supervisory activities. The military has used this concept extensively, but it is relatively uncommon in business. Rotating general staff members to various areas and levels within the organization fosters an understanding of line problems.

Advisory Staff

Advisory staff counsel line managers. They study problems, collect and analyze data, offer alternatives, and prepare plans. Their work may be accepted, rejected, or modified by the line manager. Although ideas are heard, they are not always implemented. This puts staff on the defensive, because they must sell their ideas. It is important that they counsel rather than suggest or confirm just what the line manager wants. Chances of an idea's being approved are increased when staff have discussed proposed recommendations with line managers who will be affected by the decision and have received their approval before presenting the plan to the top administrator. Careful evaluation of the plan is important. The better prepared the advice is, the more likely the staff will be heard and their suggestions implemented. If they work in seclusion, secretly preparing reports without listening to or discussing them with line managers, they are likely to get a suspicious and negative reception from others.

Service Staff

Service staff are not advisory. They perform a centralized service that has been separated from the line to prevent duplication and to allow more economical performance and good control. This includes dietary and laundry services in a hospital. Line managers rely on staff to get the job done. They do not do it themselves.

Control Staff

Control staff also do not advise. They control by restraining line authority. They have direct or indirect control over certain line performance. They control directly by acting as an agent for a line manager or indirectly through procedural compliance and interpretation of policies and reports. Quality control personnel and the affirmative action officers are members of the control staff.

Functional Staff

Functional authority exists when a specialist is given decision-making authority for specific activities outside the formal chain of command. This authority may be delegated to line, staff, or service managers and may be exercised over line, staff, and service personnel. Functional staff have limited line authority with power to determine standards in their areas of specialization and to enforce them. This authority is usually of an impersonal nature in the form of schedules, inspection reports, and written orders. It breaks the scalar chain and violates the principle that personnel should only be accountable to one superior. Although done in the interest of convenience and efficiency, it should be restricted, because it can damage line authority, destroy departmentalization, and create confusion.

LINE-STAFF CONFLICT

Conflict is likely to arise in any situation where two or more people must interact to get results. Line-staff conflicts occur when there is a lack of understanding of the roles and functions of others and when their lines of responsibility, accountability, and authority are not clear. Line and staff have different responsibilities and goals. Line is generalized, whereas staff is specialized. Line managers are likely to be pragmatists who have received their positions through competent service. They may not have much formal education but pride themselves on

RESEARCH Perspective 10-2

Data from Travis SS, McAuley WJ: Private pay clients in adult day services. *Nursing Economic$* 12(1):23-28, 2000.

Purpose: The purpose of this study was to learn more about factors that differentiated between private and public payer status for a large, statewide group of current users of adult day care services.

Methods: Data were collected for all 3992 participants in Maryland's adult care programs as of December 1993 and showed that the majority of the clients were supported by publicly supported welfare funding sources. Chi-square tests of association with payer status revealed that every comparison resulted in statistically significant association with payer status.

Results/conclusions: Private pay clients were more likely than publicly supported clients to be older and white and less likely to be in the most dependent category of activities of daily living impairment. However, diminished cognitive functioning was evident. Private pay clients were more likely to have short-term and long-term memory loss. Differences were evident in both the care requirements and social support circumstances of the two groups. Private pay clients were less likely to require special treatments or to require manual or mechanical lifting. Private pay clients were more likely than publicly supported clients to be living with a spouse or an adult child at the time of admission to adult day care. The private payers were also almost twice as likely as their public payer counterparts to be self or family referrals to day services. Adult day care seems like a viable option for private pay patients.

common sense. Staff managers probably consider themselves experts by virtue of their extensive formal education or experience in their areas of competence or both. In addition to their differences in responsibilities and backgrounds, they also have different loyalties. Line managers identify with their work group; staff managers are inclined to be loyal to their professional colleagues and the company as a whole.

Line managers may complain that staff personal are impractical and too academic. Specialists sometimes are not aware of the total picture. Offered from a specialized, narrow viewpoint, their advice is impractical because it ignores the ramifications of a given situation. Staff personnel may be viewed as outside interference who do not understand line or technical problems. Consultation causes delay. Line managers may accuse staff personnel of not keeping them informed in an effort to keep them off balance and to claim credit for good ideas that turn out well, while blaming the line managers for failures. Line managers may believe that staff personal lack responsibility or assume too much authority and run the show.

On the other hand, staff managers complain that line personal ignore them, resist staff assistance, or do not use them properly. Line managers may make decisions in specialized situations without consulting staff personal or may seek their consultation too late. Line managers are often viewed as cautious, conservative, and resistant to new ideas. They want to do things as they have always done them. Staff personnel may feel that line managers do not give them enough authority in their area of expertise and may be concerned about the way line managers implement staff managers' ideas and plans.

IMPROVING LINE-STAFF RELATIONSHIPS

Certain conditions can be created to foster the integration of line-staff efforts. It is helpful if both line managers and staff members have participated in determining objectives and plans and their implementation. Participation increases everyone's awareness of the overall goals to be accomplished. Each should be briefed on the roles and functions of other team members. The lines of responsibility, accountability, and authority should be clearly established and publicized. A team-effort atmosphere is more likely to prevail in structures that allow line and staff members to interact with open communications and that have a problem-solving focus.

ORGANIZATIONAL STRUCTURE

ORGANIZATIONAL REDESIGN, RESTRUCTURING, AND REENGINEERING

To maintain market position by reducing the cost of health care, jobs are being redesigned, organizations are being restructured, and systems are being reengineered. Redesign focuses on individual jobs in one setting although it may be occurring in several areas simultaneously or consecutively. The distribution of activities, excess specialization, role overlap, and waste are examined to redesign each job to appropriate tasks and appropriate qualifications to be efficient and effective. It is also intended to facilitate motivation, higher-quality work, greater job satisfaction, less absenteeism, and lower turnover. Unfortunately downsizing and restructuring efforts such as differentiated practice and shared governance often lead to resistance, job dissatisfaction, and little motivation. People may not desire growth or changes in their jobs. Some fear the increased productivity and sense job insecurity. There may not be clarity about what is to be accomplished. Consequently, restructuring organizations and reengineering systems are important.

Restructuring and reengineering deal with the entire organization's structure to improve its functioning and productivity. Restructuring changes the structure of the organization. It naturally follows organizational affiliations, mergers, consolidations, and integrations. Downsizing or right sizing by cutting the number of positions is also restructuring requiring redesign.

Reengineering examines the process of health care delivery to improve it. Although it is collaborative, patient centered, and data driven, it usually involves the entire organization and makes changes affecting the organization and its members. It is complex and often radical. Common practices have been path development, coordination among departments, case management, implementation of patient-focused care, and development of multiskilled workers.

The role of the nurse manager through redesigning, restructuring, and reengineering involves team building, coaching, mentoring, initiating change, reducing costs, and improving quality of care (Sullivan and Decker, 2001).

FORMAL

Although planning is the key to effective management, the organizational structure furnishes the formal framework in which the management process takes place. The organizational structure should provide an effective work system, a network of communications, and identity to individuals and the organization and should consequently foster job satisfaction. Agencies contain both informal and formal structures.

INFORMAL

The informal organization comprises personal and social relationships that do not appear on the organizational chart. This might include a group that usually takes breaks together, works together on a particular unit, or takes a class together. Informal organization is based on personal relationships rather than on respect for positional authority. It helps members meet personal objectives and provides social satisfaction. People who have little formal status may gain recognition through the informal structure. Informal authority is not commanded through organizational assignment. It comes from the follower's natural respect for a colleague's knowledge and abilities.

Informal structure provides social control of behavior. The control can be either internal or external. If pressure is intended to make a member conform to group expectations, it is internal. Kidding a member about her dirty shoelaces is an example. On the other hand, an attempt to control the behavior of someone outside the social group, such as the manager, is external control.

The informal structure also has its own channels of communication, which may disseminate information more broadly and rapidly than the formal communication system. Unfortunately, the "grapevine" may contain rumors that are not authentic. The best way to correct an invalid rumor is for managers to provide accurate information. It is better that they not state that they are correcting the rumor, for in doing so they may strengthen it, and the facts that they give may be seen primarily as a subterfuge to refute the rumor.

The informal organizational structure is important to management. The manager should be aware of its existence, study its operating techniques, prevent antagonism, and use it to meet the agency's objectives.

PRINCIPLES OF ORGANIZATION

Certain principles of organization help maximize the efficiency of the bureaucratic structure. The organization should have clear lines of authority running from the highest executive to the employee who has the least responsibility and no authority over others. There should be unity of command, with each person having only one boss. All employees should know to whom they report and who reports to them. The authority and responsibility of every individual should be clearly defined in writing. This reduces role ambiguity. Employees should know what is expected of them and what their limitations are. This prevents gaps among responsibilities, avoids overlapping of authority, and helps determine the proper point for decisions. Although many people do not think it is necessary to have their responsibilities in writing, it can be revealing to have them write what they believe their functions are and to note the duplicated efforts and jurisdictional disputes. When someone leaves an agency, it is not uncommon for no one to know exactly what that person did. Under such circumstances it can be difficult to justify replacement and to offer a meaningful orientation.

A clear definition of roles is necessary for effective delegation, but it does not guarantee it. Role clarity allows employees to know what is expected of them, to whom they report, and to whom they should go for help. In contrast, role ambiguity leads to anxiety, frustration, dissatisfaction, negative attitudes, and decreased productivity. Job descriptions increase productivity and satisfaction; however, they should not be so exact that innovation is discouraged.

Patient care coordinators should delegate responsibility to the lowest level within the organization where there is enough competence and information for effective performance and appropriate decision making. Ordinarily, increased delegation and general rather than close supervision increase effective performance, production, and employee satisfaction.

The employee should be given formal authority commensurate with the responsibility delegated. It is not uncommon for managers to delegate authority and then undermine it by making decisions that were supposedly delegated. For example, if patient care coordinators are responsible for the quality of care given on their wards, they should not have to accept members on their team who have been hired by the director without consulting them. In turn, patient care coordinators should not tell patients that they can have a bath at a certain time without consulting the person assigned to give that bath. Preferably the nurse's aide and the patient will determine when various routines can be performed in accordance with the physician's orders and the manager's rationale.

The delegation of responsibility should be accompanied by accountability. Most effective control systems are probably those that provide feedback directly to the accountable person; this seems to increase motivation and provide direction. When feedback from a manager is given as performance evaluation rather than guidance, it tends to be nonfunctional and only infrequently contributes to improved performance. The delegation of functions with accompanying responsibility and accountability is particularly difficult for managers because they remain responsible for the actions of their staff associates. They are as responsible as their staff associates for their associates' performance. Consequently, the span-of-control principle becomes important.

There is a limit to the amount of coordination that can be achieved by one person, and it depends on several factors. One can coordinate more similar positions than dissimilar positions. The more the positions are interdependent, the more coordination is involved. A decreased span of control is required as the complexity of the staff associate's tasks increases. The stability of the agency should also be considered. If the agency has been functioning in a similar manner for a long time, the problems that arise have probably been solved before, and coordination is less difficult than in a changing situation where many new problems arise. The span of control is not likely to be uniform throughout an organization. Top-level managers of positions that are interdependent and dissimilar will probably have a smaller range of control than lower-level managers who are coordinating people doing similar tasks in a confined area. The span of control should not be so wide that managers do not have time to deal with the human relations aspects, such as giving workers individual attention, communicating information about the agency's policies, and listening to suggestions, grievances, and problems. On the other hand, they need a span of control large enough to keep them busy so they will not interfere with the delegated responsibilities of others.

Three types of divisions are commonly used to define span of control: (1) function or process, (2) product or service, and (3) region. Function is associated with specialization. Specialization may apply both to individuals and to departments or divisions. For example, one nurse may pass medications and give treatments, another may just start IV (intravenous) lines, and the nurse's aides may give the baths and change linens. There may be a surgical nursing division with departments for specific types of surgery. It is preferable that if a person is accountable for more than one type of responsibility, they be similar. Efficiency is maximized if employees perform predominantly the tasks they do best and for which their proficiency will consequently continue to increase; they may, however, become bored. It is not uncommon to find individuals within an organization who are assigned several unrelated tasks. Although that may work for some people in given situations, it is not considered good organization, and their replacements are not likely to be successful. It is more viable to hire personnel to fill the organizational structure than to change the structure to fit personnel.

Having individuals perform the same or similar tasks and having divisions with specific functions can help expand the range of control. Similarly, having departments that provide specific services, such as cardiac intensive care, or produce certain products can influence the structure. Organization by geographical location becomes increasingly viable when operations are scattered. Many agencies use a combination of these methods. For instance, a school of nursing may be organized according to campuses (regional division); according to undergraduate, graduate, and continuing education (product division); or according to inpatient, outpatient, medical-surgical, maternal-child, or some other service division; or it may assign individual faculty members to teach according to specialization (functional division).

The organizational structure should be flexible enough to permit expansion and contraction in response to changing conditions, without disrupting the basic design. It should also be kept as simple as possible, because additional levels of authority complicate communications and excessive use of committees may impede progress (Galbraith, 1995).

The formal organizational structure is defined by executive decision determined by planning. It can be diagrammed to show the relationships among people and their positions. It describes positions, task responsibilities, and relationships. The two basic forms of formal organizational structure are the hierarchical, or bureaucratic, model and the adaptive, or organic, model.

BUREAUCRATIC STRUCTURE

A hierarchy or bureaucracy is an organizational design to facilitate large-scale administration by coordinating the work of many personnel. It is associated with subdivision, specialization, technical qualifications, rules and standards, impersonality, and technical efficiency. Figure 10-5 illustrates a typical bureaucratic hierarchy in which the managers are responsible to the director of nursing. The director in turn must answer to the hospital administrator, who is accountable to the board of directors. Managers also have authority over their staff associates, who are accountable to their managers (Yoder-Wise, 2003).

Dual Management

Dual management separates technical and administrative responsibilities. It has one hierarchy in which technical professionals make technical decisions and control technical matters and another hierarchy in which management makes decisions about issues such as personnel and budget. This dual hierarchy gives equal status to managers and technical professionals. It provides a set of titles and job descriptions for each hierarchy.

Advantages of the Bureaucratic Structure

The bureaucracy is suited for work requiring large numbers of moderately educated people who perform routine tasks. Orientation is easy because workers do few procedures in a narrowly circumscribed job description. Orders can be transmitted quickly.

Disadvantages of the Bureaucratic Structure

There are disadvantages to the bureaucratic model. It may be detrimental to healthy personality patterns by predisposing people to the authoritarian leadership style, increasing insistence on the right of authority and status, and fostering a pathological need for control. If managers do not have the technical competence of their staff associates, they may feel insecure and fear their associates. Autocratic behavior may become a defense mechanism through the use of power and fear strategies over staff members and the enforcement of norms through arbitrary or rigid rules. The use of reward and punishment

Figure 10-5 Bureaucratic hierarchy.

to get desired behavior may alienate personnel. Self-serving behavior patterns may develop because of competition for the advancement of individual interests. A certain aloofness can result from the specialization that leads to impersonality. Personnel also may develop a ritualistic attachment to routine, develop monotony and alienation, become attached to subgoals, and show resistance to change.

LINE AND STAFF STRUCTURE

A line and staff organization develops when a simple line structure is altered to provide support to line authorities. The line functions are command and control. The staff functions are separate from the chain of command, involve specialization, and are supportive to line authorities. Staff do what the executives are too busy to do. It is the function of staff to serve the line organization and to submerge personal interests to champion the executives' long-range objectives. Staff can manage policies and procedures, in-service and continuing education, or quality improvement (see Figure 10-1).

Advantages of line and staff structures are that the executive can delegate tasks that the executive does not have the skill or time to do to functional experts. Disadvantages are that executives may get the credit for staff recommendations. Staff may increase their influence by usurping the authority of the executive by making decisions without consulting the executive. The executive may ignore the staff's recommendations.

FUNCTIONALIZED LINE AND STAFF STRUCTURE

Staff have some authority over line executives. The staff expert responsible for a specific management function, such as staffing, staff development, or quality improvement, has authority to command line executives to implement staff plans.

The advantage is that this can increase staff morale. Unfortunately, when the line organization's chain of command is broken, conflict, confusion, and poor communications can result.

ADHOCRACY ORGANIZATIONAL MODELS

Adhocracy, or organic, models are newer organizational frameworks that are more free form, open, flexible, and fluid than older bureaucratic models. Boundaries separating internal and external relationships are more easily penetrated. Temporary affiliations such as consultantships are used.

The underlying assumptions, aims, and structures of adaptive frameworks differ from those of the bureaucratic model. They have resulted from behavioral research to facilitate job satisfaction and creativity, as well as efficiency. They give greater recognition to the informal structure and encourage the group to improve its own norms. Adaptive models recognize realities and are designed to meet them. They are less likely to use organizational charts, because the relationships are flexible. Job descriptions are also less meaningful. The models are ambiguous and consequently require being staffed by independent, self-reliant people who have a high tolerance for ambiguity. They lend themselves to participative management. Motivation is derived from system needs, task-related factors, and peer pressure rather than from supervision. Rewards are based on individual and group results rather than subjective evaluations from managers. Adhocracy comes from an ad hoc committee. Adhocracy structures are loosely structured project organizations.

Task Forces

Task forces are sometimes used for special projects. The task force has a mission, a leader, and a projected completion date. To be most successful, the project should be short range. There must be a pool from which to select talent, and task force members should be readily reabsorbed by the organization. Personnel are relieved of their usual tasks and given a temporary assignment, usually to investigate, analyze, research, and plan. They are less often used for decisions and actions. The task force allows personnel with special qualifications to combine their expertise and concentrate on a project in a manner that would not be possible while performing their usual duties. Structural flexibility is accomplished by adding members when their potential contribution is high and removing them when their specific talents are no longer required. It can be an efficient problem-solving method and can offer training opportunities for managers. It can unleash creative energies and introduce innovations.

On the other hand, it can be disruptive to the organization. Key personnel may be away from their jobs for unknown lengths of time. As members experience different qualities of supervision by moving from one team to another, they may become more critical of the less capable manager. Assignment to a task force may make employees consider themselves better than their peers. They may feel independent and detached from their usual work groups. It is not uncommon for personnel to be promoted and removed from their original departments after the task force responsibilities are completed. Reabsorbing the task force member back into the organization is sometimes difficult, and that realization is almost certain to increase the employee's anxiety; or what began as a short-range, problem-solving task force may become an unwanted permanent arrangement.

Project Management

Project organizational design is used for large, long-range projects where a number of project groups are developed and administered through the various phases of their existence. This method is useful for one-time projects when the task is unfamiliar and complex; when considerable planning, coordination, high-risk research, and development are involved; and when there is a long lead time between planning and production.

There are several types of project units. The general, or functional, management type is the most common. Project activities are done within functional groups that are managed by department heads. The general manager coordinates the activities. With this type of arrangement there is no strong central project authority, and consequently decisions are likely to be made to the advantage of the strongest functional group rather than in the best interests of the project. Lead time and decision-making time are increased because the coordination and approval of all functional groups are required.

Aggregate management has appointed managers who have their own staff and full authority over their projects. All people involved with a project report directly to the manager, giving the manager a high degree of control over each project. This allows rapid reaction time and reduces lead time. Project management is highly regarded by outside sources, and the people involved tend to be loyal to the project because it is their only job at the time.

There are also disadvantages to aggregate management. The people involved are interested in the technology to do the project, but they do not develop the technology, nor do they develop the essential functional organizations. There tends to be little technical interchange between projects and inefficient use of production elements. Because they are managing just one project each, managers cannot keep all production elements in use at all times. With this management method, production elements are not shared with other projects, and there is consequently duplication of functional activities among projects. There is also a lack of career continuity. Anxiety may increase toward the completion of a project, because project personnel do not know where they will be assigned next. It is difficult to balance workloads as projects begin and reach completion. Aggregate management is not often used.

The matrix organization combines concepts from both functional and aggregate organizations. It departmentalizes functions and shares authority among functional heads and project managers. The project manager uses people assigned to functional areas to complete the project while they are still assigned to the functional area. Thus the worker has two bosses. Reaction time is quite rapid. Matrix organization seems well received by outside contacts. It does not slow down the development of technology. It facilitates the interchange of technology between projects and provides career continuity because personnel remain in their functional areas. However, conflicts can arise between project and functional managers. Workers have two bosses, and accountability becomes diffuse (Yoder-Wise, 2003).

In still another design the project manager may monitor the project but serve only in an advisory capacity to the general manager. The project director controls through influence. The director of the project has responsibility without authority. The workers once again report to one boss, the general manager.

Project management offers several advantages. It visualizes projects and focuses on results. It produces good control over the project, shorter development time, improved quality, and lower program costs. This yields higher profit margins and good customer relations. Project management facilitates coordination among functional areas and good mission orientation for people working on the project. It can help elevate morale and develop managers.

There are also numerous disadvantages to project management. It requires changes in patterns of interaction and disrupts the established patterns of hierarchy, span of management, unity of control, resource allocation, departmentalization, priorities, and incentives. Work groups are disrupted, and interfunctional groups develop. Duplication is common. Interdepartmental consensus is used and tends to increase fears of invasion from other departments.

Confusion may arise from authority's ambiguity as new patterns for control develop. Power is one's ability to affect the behavior of others. Authority is power derived from one's position. Influence may be power without authority. Sometimes project managers use authority; at other times they have to use influence. Personnel may report to more than one person with varying patterns of authority. Multiple levels of management are more likely to be problems for project management than functional management. Authority's ambiguity frequently frustrates personnel.

Project managers tend to depend on functional managers for resources. This dependence can create a conflict over those resources. Hence the project may deplete the functional department of premium professional talent, and the competition for talent may disrupt the stability of the organization and interfere with long-range interests by disrupting traditional business. Some professionals complain that incentives for higher-level ego needs are not met. Project personnel are more likely to be anxious about the loss of their jobs, frustrated by make-work assignments between projects, and confused by a lack of role definitions. They are concerned about setbacks in their careers and upset by the apparent lack of concern about their personal development. Conflicts of allegiance result and undermine loyalty to the organization. Shifting personnel can disrupt their training. What is learned may not be transferred from one project to another. Long-range planning suffers when people are more concerned with their temporary projects.

Several factors contribute to the failure of project management. The most common factors include an initially unsound basis for the project, poor selection of the project manager, lack of agency support, use of inappropriate management techniques, poor role and task definitions, and no projected termination date.

Precautions can be taken to prevent failure. Planning is always essential. The project should be well conceived with its scope outlined and the end results described. Well-qualified managers should be selected and their roles defined. It is helpful if their executive rank ensures responsiveness from others. They need the authority to control funds, budgeting, and scheduling for the project; to select subcontractors; and to be able to select, add, or eliminate staff as necessary. They should participate in major managerial activities, especially in policymaking and other decisions related to their projects.

Because functional managers may not wish to take directions from a lesser executive who is suddenly a project manager, top management might select people from high positions of responsibility, assign them impressive titles, support their dealings with functional managers, and have them report to a manager on the same or higher level than the functional managers.

One of the first responsibilities of the project manager is to staff the project. Sometimes several projects compete for the same talent. Functional managers may not be willing to release the requested personnel, or the person may not want to transfer. People may be hesitant to transfer because (1) there is a division of responsibilities between functional and project organizations, (2) the job is less desirable, or (3) they fear unemployment at the end of the project. Management can offer salary increases as incentives. Promotional opportunities may arise from the additional management structure required for the project. Special efforts should be made to relocate people as they are phased out of the project, thus maintaining security. All these measures, however, are expensive.

Next, the project manager sets time controls. The manager determines what tasks are required from each department to complete the project and what their proper sequence is. Each department itemizes what it needs to know from other departments and then commits itself to an estimate of the time required to do its part. An overall schedule can be developed by use of critical-path scheduling. It should be checked frequently to compare actual progress against the projected deadlines. This network can be the focal point of project implementation. Managers develop information links that serve the project and help them prepare to replan jobs as project dynamics change.

The project manager also needs to determine cost controls. The most sound decisions can be made by dividing the comprehensive cost summary into work packages. Then technical decision makers can offer commitment reports, and the project manager can act on the approximate cost data. After reviewing the detailed estimated costs and current expenses, the manager can switch staff from less productive duties to duties that will reduce costs.

To maintain quality control, the manager defines the project objectives in quality standards, describes performance criteria, and monitors individual and project progress against the standards. It is helpful to reward responsibility and performance and to try to accommodate staff members' personal goals while working toward the objectives of the project.

Matrix

Matrix organizational designs try to combine the advantages of project and functional structures. The functional line organization provides support for the project line organization. In a functional organization the functional manager has the authority to determine and rate goals, select personnel, determine pay and promotions, make personnel assignments, and evaluate personnel and the project. Managers are responsible to their superiors but work independently. In a matrix organization the functional manager shares those responsibilities with the project manager, because management by project objectives is important to the matrix organization. Initially, the functional manager may experience a sense of loss in status, authority, and control. Therefore it is important for managers to be able to persuade others by using their personal qualities and knowledge of the program (Figure 10-6). The functional and project managers need each other's cooperation for approvals and sign-offs. The intent in the matrix organization is to have the decision making as far down in the organizational structure as possible. This encourages group consensus. Most decisions are made at the middle-management level, thus freeing top administration for long-range planning. Matrix organizations are more decentralized with fewer levels of decision making and less rigid adherence to formal rules than line and staff or functionalized structures (see Figure 10-6).

The matrix organization increases the amount of contact among individuals, and its complexity makes conflict inevitable. Increased communications are essential. Recognizing and dealing with differences are necessary, because collaborative behavior is needed. Team building between

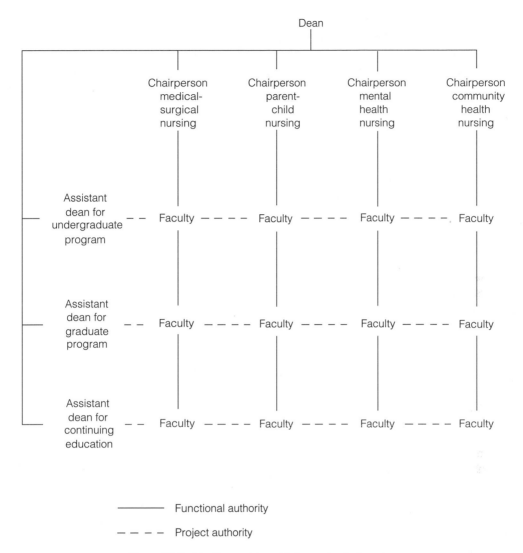

Figure 10-6 Adaptive model; matrix for a school of nursing.

departments is encouraged, and consultants are used as connections between parts. Managers need human relations training. Organizational charts showing task responsibilities and levels of responsibility may reduce conflict.

Matrix organizations foster flexibility in dealing with change and uncertainty. They enable managers to balance conflicting objectives by maximizing technical excellence through efficient use of resources. By moving decision making down in the organization, opportunities are provided for personal development and motivation. Commitment is improved, and top management is freed for long-range planning.

Because people are more familiar with bureaucratic structures, there is considerable need to orient personnel to the matrix structure and philosophy. Rigid lines of authority, inflexible boundaries separating jobs and divisions, unambiguous resource allocation to divisions, and specific loyalties that exist in bureaucracies are not appropriate in dynamic organizations with overlapping and sometimes contradictory interests and goals. But because of multiple and often ambiguous roles, some personnel may get frustrated and feel insecure. Matrix structures are increasingly common in health care systems. Because of the generalized education and time spent with patients, nurses are well qualified to coordinate the clinical and nonclinical care for patients. That may involve integrating care from nutritionist, occupational therapist, pharmacist, physician, physiotherapist, and social worker (Galbraith, Downey, and Kates, 2002) (Box 10-2).

Collegial Management

Collegial management restricts monocratic authority by maintaining a division and balance of power among the top management group through collective responsibility. It is most commonly used in Germany and Holland but is also used in Austria, Switzerland, and France. Consequently, it is also referred to as European-style management. The directors usually represent functional areas of the organization. They may or may not have a chairperson. If so, the chairperson may be the first among equals and merely speak for the directors, may coordinate the others, or may be recognized as the general manager or chief executive. The directors may have vice-directors.

The decision-making process varies from one country to another, but in every case it is the board that makes policy decisions. Essentially, the directors need to persuade each other. Although chairpersons may not have strong decision-making powers, they do have strong veto powers.

Collegial management has several strengths. It limits autocratic leadership, breeds democratic management, and ensures representation of each functional area. Because of their collective responsibility, directors are better informed about the other functional areas; this broadens the approach to problem solving. Collegial management prevents precipitous decisions, encourages long-range planning, and fosters objective appraisal of the functions. Camaraderie is possible.

Collegial management also has limitations. The need for consensus can slow decision making. Consensus based on compromise may be an inferior solution. Logrolling results when directors give reciprocal support to programs that are not viable. Collegial management requires

---

BOX 10-2 Advantages and Disadvantages of Matrix

ADVANTAGES	DISADVANTAGES
Manages dual demands	Dual authority—1 line, 1 project
Good for complex work	Complicated
Focuses on products and functions	May be viewed as confusing
Good for uncertain environment	Complex structure
Good for nonroutine technologies	Need well-educated personnel
High interdependence between functions	Complex communications
Collaborative management	Advanced interpersonal relationship skills needed
Flexible, efficient use of scarce resources	Group and teamwork skills needed
Adaptive	Role conflicts
Innovative	Role ambiguity
Decisions close to operations	Requires frequent meetings
Fluidity	Time consuming
Improved interpersonal skills and conflict management leading to achievement and job satisfaction	Special learning required in conflict management and interpersonal relationships

Data from Sullivan and Decker, 2001; Grohar-Murray and DiCroce, 2003; Nader and Tushman, 1997; Swansburg and Swansburg, 2002; Yoder-Wise, 2003.

considerable, expensive executive time for what may be relatively minor matters or what may be others' functional affairs; this results in a diffusion of responsibility. The management process may even cease at times, especially when policies and programs are to be determined. Differences of opinions may smolder and lead to rudeness and cold wars. Communications are more likely to be vertical than horizontal. Consequently, coordination is a problem. The encouragement of group action may stifle a strong creative director. Because of the inherent problems in collegial management, some organizations are moving toward committee management with an executive to coordinate policy.

Shared Governance

Shared governance was one of the more radical changes during the 1980s. It is an accountability-based governance system for professionals that empowered individuals within the decision-making system and increased nurses' authority and control over their nursing practice. Group professional communications took on an equalitarian structure when joint practice committees were developed to assume power and accountability for decision making. A major resistance has come from nurse managers who were reluctant to change their roles from autocratic decision makers to coaches, consultants, teachers, collaborators, and facilitators of shared decision making. A typical model of shared governance is a committee structure in which representative staff nurses belong to nursing committees that are assigned specific management or clinical functions. The committees are typically composed of a staff nurse or administrative chair appointed by an administrator and representatives of staff and administration. The nursing committee chairs and nursing administrators compose the nursing council or cabinet that makes the final decisions on recommendations from the committees.

Participatory Management

Participatory management is the foundation for shared governance. However, it allows participation only in decision making over which someone else has the power to make the final decisions. For this model, representative staff nurses are members of forums or committees for designated issues. Managers are also members. Recommendations go to an executive committee, which has staff representation, as well as manager membership. The nurse executive retains the decision-making authority and may or may not agree with committee recommendations.

Self-Governance

Self-governance goes beyond participatory management and shared governance to structures that allow nursing staff to govern themselves. These professional practice models place autonomy, authority, and control for services to clients with the professionals providing the care. Representative staff nurses are members of councils with authority for specified functions. The council chairs make up the management committee charged to make the final operational decisions for the organization. Bylaws are developed to specify the authority, responsibility, communication channels, and coordination of the self-governance structure. The councils have the authority to make decisions and are responsible for the results. It is important to clarify what decisions councils will make, what shared decisions will be made by staff and managers, and what decisions will be the responsibility of administration. Councils typically have functional accountability for practice, governance, nursing professional development, peer behavior, and governance with a coordinating council (Marquis and Huston, 2000; Yoder-Wise, 2003).

Systems

Systems design is an adaptive organizational model. It has been facilitated by the use of computers. The systems approach can be applied to bureaucracies that are considered closed systems or to adaptive models viewed as open systems. The design develops from the flow of work and information. It considers relationships, time, and decision points.

Mixed Model

A mixed model may be the most viable. Bureaucratic design can work very well for routine functions. Adaptive designs may be more useful for research and development. However, the success of any organizational design largely depends on the manager's skills.

Corporate Model

A corporation is any group of people who act as one body. Corporations are required to register their articles of incorporation, which specify the purposes and functions of the organization. Corporations may be private or public and proprietary (for-profit) or not-for-profit. A public corporation is subject to government regulations, may issue and trade stock, and is expected to return a profit to the owners of the stock. Most individual investor-owned hospitals are operated for a profit but are privately owned, not public, corporations. However, many hospital management firms are publicly held corporations that manage both for-profit and not-for-profit individual hospitals. Most private corporations are smaller than public corporations.

Corporate growth leads to mergers, buyouts, and other business transactions to increase the value of the business. Large multihospital corporations have emerged within the health care arena. Nurses have opportunities for leadership and management positions in the corporations and may operate their own corporations.

The physician's share of the health care dollar has increased in the newer delivery systems as the hospital's share has decreased and services have moved out of the hospital. The services still tend to be illness based, medically dominated, interventive, and expensive. Decentralization using holding companies with multiple subcorporate entities that provide a range of services is the trend. This trend has created a need to restructure nursing.

For nursing service to be a corporate entity it must be able to sustain its own activities without dependence on other units. Nursing practice must be clearly defined and its contribution to profitability clearly identified. The holding company's mission and purposes must be reflected in the philosophy, purpose, and objectives of the nursing service corporate entity. The relationship to the marketplace and plans to meet market demands should be outlined. Remuneration of nurses should reflect the value of their work in the marketplace.

As nursing becomes increasingly decentralized and incorporated, it is increasingly important to create a network instead of preserving a pyramid. A coordinating council may centralize the activities of individual councils for practice, education, research, and quality assurance. It is an opportunity for the chairpersons of the individual councils to meet together to discuss issues, coordinate councils, and make decisions that affect the entire corporate nursing entity.

The corporate nursing staff should meet at least once per year to (1) review, revise as necessary, and approve as appropriate the nursing staff bylaws; (2) review, discuss, and revise as appropriate the nursing organization's long- and short-range planning process, goals, and objectives; (3) debate issues of concern and vote on them as appropriate; (4) review, discuss, and approve the coordinating council's activities; (5) provide opportunities for informal networking; and (6) provide education sessions.

Interorganizational Relationships

Health care organizations have been forming relationships with one another to survive the increased competition for resources. Horizontal integration occurs when the organizations provide the same or similar services, such as dietary and laundry services. One provides the dietary services to the other while that other provides the laundry services for both organizations. Vertical integration is an arrangement among dissimilar but related organizations to provide a continuum of services. It could include an affiliation of a health maintenance organization with a pharmacy, hospital, home care, and a long-term care facility. Vertical integrations can improve coordination of services, quality, efficiency, and cost-effectiveness (Sullivan and Decker, 2001).

Continuum of Multiorganizational Arrangements

Rakich, Longest, and Darr (1992) depict a continuum of multiorganizational arrangements:

1. Informal affiliations are joint undertakings without written agreements.
2. Formal affiliations occur when two or more organizations formalize undertaking limited activities.
3. Shared or cooperative services have common management, such as joint purchasing or shared laundry facilities for two or more organizations.
4. Consortia and alliances have limited voluntary associations for specific purposes, such as management information systems and labor relations.
5. Management contracts occur when one organization supplies the senior management for the other.
6. Umbrella organizations are new corporations that span but do not replace the existing organizations.
7. Mergers occur when one organization maintains its name and identity while another is dissolved and absorbed.
8. Consolidation occurs when two or more organizations dissolve and are unified into a new legal organization. The management contracts, umbrella corporations, mergers, and consolidations are multiorganizational systems.

Mergers

A merger essentially means that one organization will join its assets with another. Economics are forcing health care organizations to seek mergers, cut staff, and emphasize cost-effectiveness over patient care and service quality. There are some multiinstitutional relationships for sharing assets such as a central laundry service, a purchasing department, or a home health agency. However, mergers usually restructure the relationship of one health care organization with another. These activities can stir many feelings among personnel.

It is appropriate for the nurse manager to assess attitudes toward the merger through a questionnaire, personal interviews, or focus groups. Only personnel who are supportive of the merger should be assigned to leadership positions to accommodate it. Managers need to keep staff informed about the changes. Open communications can help minimize pluralistic views about the merger. Staff may need assistance to understand the new organization culture, and managers can help them understand the unique qualities of the merging agency. Managers should periodically assess how personnel are responding to the merger, identify problems, and do problem solving.

Health Care Networks

Health maintenance organizations (HMOs) are associations of health care professionals and facilities that provide a health care package for a fixed sum of money that was paid in advance for a specific period of time. The HMO contracts with health care professionals and facilities to provide the care. The client cannot usually seek care outside the contract. Primary care physicians see the client first and decide if a specialist is needed. Consequently, patients are not guaranteed the right to see a specialist for consultation or care unless the primary care physician gatekeeper approves.

Preferred provider organizations (PPOs) are groups of health care professionals and hospitals that contract with an employer, insurance company, or other third-party payer to provide health care to a group. The services are not fixed or prepaid and allow more customer choice than an HMO. Consequently, PPOs are more expensive, and customers pay an even greater percentage of fees for services rendered outside those provided by the PPO.

Individual practice associations (IPAs) provide insurance coverage, health care services rates, and bill a fee for services.

Physician hospital organizations (PHOs) allow a hospital and the medical staff to have joint managed care contracts. They vary in terms of administration, credentialing, governance, managed care contracting, and structure. The impetus is usually from the hospital, which incorporates a not-for-profit organization with a hospital and a physician board. Medicare fraud, abuse issues, nonprofit status, and balance of power among hospitals and physicians are issues driving the legal and political perspectives to manage risks and provide what the health care market is demanding. The management skills and infrastructure are critical to the survival of PHOs that will have to develop networks to provide a broader service spectrum to remain competitive. An external focus and customer orientation will be important to success. Care management, risk management, information management, and relationship management are all important components of PHOs to help provide cost-effective care in a timely manner (First Health Associates Consulting Team website, accessed June 5, 1999).

Management service organizations (MSOs) provide medical practice management, physician recruitment, information systems, billing and collection systems, quality monitoring, and other services (Pelinet Internet Services, Pelican Coast Publishers website, 1997).

DISEASE MANAGEMENT

Disease management is a type of product or service offered by some large pharmaceutical companies to get into healthcare services. It involves bundling use of prescription drugs with physicians and allied professionals and large databases to treat many people with specific diseases.

DEMAND MANAGEMENT

Demand management focuses on customer expectations. Demand forecasting uses trends and anticipates shifts in demand. That helps improve revenue and decrease inventory-carrying costs. Research methods are used to acquire, process, and deploy the voice of the customers. (Shillito 2001). Technology can be used to identify the mass market, the target market, the customer, and even to one-on-one marketing (Sharp 2003). Spector (2001) explains lessons learned from Nordstrom, the number one customer service company, about providing customers with choices, creating an inviting place, hiring nice people, selling the relationship, empowering employees to take ownership, being innovative, promoting competition, and committing 100 percent to customer service. Timm (2001) explains the importance of the one-to-one customer future and exceeding customer expectations. That involves dealing with customer turnoffs and dissatisfactions, encouraging positive attitudes, and using behaviors that win customer loyalty like friendly written messages, telephone, e-mail, and web site techniques.

By the early 2000s, private case management companies had become common. Directories, buying guides, market research, statistical reports, databases, and mailing lists for managed care and health care organizations were available. Case managers had access to over 100,000 providers of homecare, rehabilitation, long-term care, addiction, behavioral and psychiatric care, and clinical specialties.

Mergers occur when one organization purchases another of approximately the same size. Acquisitions occur when one organization is considerably larger than the other. Both are used to acquire complementary services or products that are connected by common clients and technologies. By increasing the size, they increase organizational power and leverage through products or services, market access, distribution networks, capital access, economies of scale, technology, people, diversification, name and reputation, and management resources. They gain financial benefits by eliminating employees who have responsibilities that overlap both entities. This makes employees nervous, strains organizational cultures, and often brings out the worst of behaviors. Nurse managers need to resolve their own negative feelings and help employees understand and adjust to the changes (Figures 10-7 and 10-8).

Figure 10-7 Merger collaborative organizational structure. (Modified from Nadler DA, Gerstein MS, Shaw RB, et al: *Organizational architecture: Designs for changing organizations*, San Francisco, 1992, Jossey-Bass, p. 94.)

CONTINUUM OF CARE

Historically the United States has had a two-tiered system for delivering health care: inpatient hospitalization and outpatient treatment. Treatment was often costly. The increasing need for cost containment and developing flexible benefit programs led to a continuum of care. That allowed

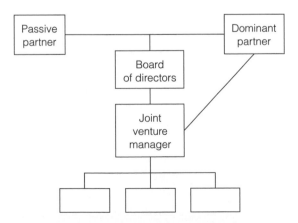

Figure 10-8 Acquisition instrumental organizational structure. (Modified from Nadler DA, Gerstein MS, Shaw RB, et al: *Organizational architecture: Designs for changing organizations*, San Francisco, 1992, Jossey-Bass, p. 96.)

payers to ensure that patients could be directed to the cost-efficient and clinically appropriate services. Expanding services covered by benefit plans lowered costs, and those additional services enhanced patients' treatments and improved patient outcomes. Some of the common treatment settings on a continuum of care include but are not limited to:

Prevention and early intervention services that put screening in primary care offices and nonclinical settings such as schools and work places.

Outpatient offices or clinics are where the patient may be seen by one or more clinicians and may be treated individually or as part of a family or group.

Employee-assistance programs are worksite programs that assist with the identification and resolution of job performance associated with personal concerns that interfere with productivity.

Intensive outpatient programs may include individual or group treatments of at least three times a week.

Intensive case management coordinates financial, legal, and medical services needed to live successfully at home.

Home-based treatment involves a person or team-making home visits to provide intensive treatment to a person or family.

Family support services are services to support and train families to care for a person at home.

Partial hospitalization/day treatment services are structured day programs that may involve an individual, group, or family.

Therapeutic foster home is care by foster parents who provide a therapeutic environment and supervised care.

Group homes are residential homes that provide a therapeutic family-type environment. They may serve as a step-down from a more intensive level of care.

Rehabilitation services address functional problems and deficits that interfere with the person's ability to live in the community. They may include evaluation, treatment, consultation, educational or vocational placement, family or caregive support, and training.

Residential treatment centers are where intensive and comprehensive treatment is provided by a multi-disciplinary team on a 24-hour-a-day basis.

Assisted living is for people who cannot live independently. Food preparation, laundry, cleaning, etc., may be provided.

Respite care is to give caregivers some temporary relief either on a planned basis or in an emergency.

Hospice care may be at home or in an inpatient setting once the patient has agreed to palliative care only.

Day treatment programs provide intensive treatment usually for 5 days a week.

Partial hospitalization or day hospitals provide treatment services during the day, but patients go home each evening.

Crisis residential programs provide short-term of usually less than 15 days crisis intervention and individualized treatment with 24-hours-a-day supervision.

Personal emergency response system is an electronic communication system that can summon emergency assistance 24-hours a day. It automatically dials for help by activating a remote button typically worn around the neck.

Emergency or crisis services are for emergencies and include emergency rooms and mobile crises teams.

Acute inpatient hospital-based treatment includes medically directed interdisciplinary treatment including 24-hour professional nursing care.

Residential treatment facility provides intensive and comprehensive treatment on a long-term basis.

Hospital treatment provides comprehensive treatment based on the patient's needs.

Consumer programs provide support and structure through social centers, club houses, day programs, drop-in centers, and self-help groups like AA, NA, and Al-Anon.

Integrated Health Care Systems

The objective of integrated health care systems is to keep people healthy and treat them in the lowest cost setting when necessary, thus making primary care and managed care pivotal (Figure 10-9). Efforts are toward improving health care outcomes at reduced health care costs while ensuring patient satisfaction. This requires inventing and managing new health care systems. There is a trend toward a reduction in the numbers of managers and the levels of management, retention and training of workers with multiple skills, data-based decision making, and continuous quality improvement. Hospitals are joining together and linking health promotion, clinics, ambulatory care, acute care, home care, and long-term care into integrated health care (Grohar-Murray and DiCroce, 2003). A moderate rate of integration seems desirable. In cases where the parent moves in quickly and tries to integrate in a fast and intense way by imposing its own policies and procedures, the management of the acquired agency often leaves, followed by the technical staff; therefore the parent loses the leverage that was to be gained from the acquisition. If the integration occurs too slowly, people get highly stressed, not knowing what is going to happen to them. This brings out undesirable behaviors, and the best people may accept other positions.

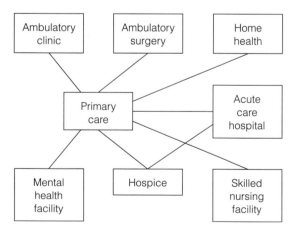

Figure 10-9 Integrated health care system. (Modified from Grohar-Murray ME, DiCroce HR: *Leadership and management in nursing*, Stamford, Conn, 1997, Appleton & Lange, p. 144.)

When there is not integration, the parent may adopt a hands-off approach and let the acquiree operate its separate holdings. With the possible exceptions of limited financial controls and reviews of productivity at the board level, the acquiree remains autonomous. In coupled integrations, some of the activities or functions of the acquired agency are integrated with the parent, whereas others are left independent and separate. In loosely coupled acquisitions, a minimum of activities are integrated. Most are left separate and independent. The acquiree functions largely as an independent entity. Moderately coupled integrations have an increasing amount of integration. Operationally integrated organizations still can be identified as entities, but the key procedures and operations are tightly linked to the parent organization. With complete integration, the organizations are consolidated or merged into one (Box 10-3).

Assessment Phase

During the assessment phase the organization should assess its strategic plan, its ability to handle the operating requirements for a joint venture, and its readiness to manage change. Is the joint venture an appropriate strategic action to address the problem, or are there less complicated alternatives? Is the problem temporary, not meriting a joint venture, or is it a long-term problem that could best be addressed by integration?

All partners should agree to the long-term goals and compatibility. Convergent objectives are those commonly shared and are probably the primary reason the joint venture is being considered. Compatible objectives are those held by each organization that are unique to it and are compatible with other objectives. Objectives in potential conflicts require the most careful assessment. They may be differences in management style, strategies, or whatever presents a potential threat to the viability of the venture. It is better to articulate the potential problems and address them before the joint venture than to be surprised by them later (Box 10-4).

The internal operating and management requirements for the joint venture should be carefully considered. Partners will need to be cooperative and flexible while sharing responsibilities. It can be difficult for some managers to give up power and control. People are likely to resist change. Having a specific plan for the implementation of the change can help manage the change. Is the organization ready to manage change? Is there a deliberate plan of action to minimize disruption during the implementation of change? Is there understanding of the relationship of this venture to the strategic plan? Is there an understanding of the opportunities being sought? Does the other organization provide the resources, skills, or other attributes that are needed? Is the other organization financially sound, trustworthy, and respected? Are the management styles and cultures compatible? Are the people cooperative, flexible, skilled in conflict resolution, and experienced in joint ventures? Are people willing to make a commitment, learn,

---

BOX 10-3 Degrees of Integration

NONE
Separate holding
Loosely coupled

MODERATE
Coupled
Operationally integrated

COMPLETE
Consolidated

Modified from Nadler DA, Gerstein MS, Shaw RB, et al: *Organizational architecture: Designs for changing organizations*, San Francisco, 1992, Jossey-Bass.

BOX 10-4 Phases of a Joint Venture

Phase 1: Assessment
Phase 2: Planning and design
Phase 3: Implementation
Phase 4: Development

Modified from Nadler DA, Gerstein MS, Shaw RB, et al: *Organizational architecture: Designs for changing organizations*, San Francisco, 1992, Jossey-Bass.

and make comparable contributions? Do people understand the joint venture's business?

Planning and Design Phase

After agreeing to integrate, partners need to plan and design the joint venture. The main work in the second phase is to plan the structure, staffing, management style, and support systems. How involved is each partner with the operations? Who makes what decisions? Who reports what to whom? How will the venture be staffed? How do the organizations relate to each other? Chances for success increase when one partner primarily manages the joint venture. The joint venture general manager needs autonomy to act quickly to achieve the responsiveness required to be successful. When both partners are heavily involved in the operations, it slows down decision making. They need compatible styles and orientations, common understanding of the joint venture's necessities, and skills at conflict management and human relationships. Achieving the necessary relationship takes considerable commitment, time, and effort to make it work. The managers need to be able to handle a lot of ambiguity and uncertainty. A participative style that solicits input from all partners tends to get more commitment to plans than an autocratic style. The venture manager should be positioned as the leader for the venture and as the person who is in control. The venture manager and staff need to establish an independent identity and allegiance to the venture. People from both partner organizations in a collaborative structure may staff the venture. In general, however, staff should not be employed from the passive partner organization, because that can create allegiance problems and managerial interference from the passive partner. Staff should be qualified to do the required tasks, should be viewed as competent, and should be respected. A compensatory reward system should be consistent with the performance criteria and expectations of the venture.

Implementation Phase

The implementation focuses on a successful start-up and implementation of the venture.

It deals with the organization's culture and major organizational change that typically involves issues of power, anxiety, and control. During change, individuals and groups often compete for power. Change threatens the balance of formal and informal power. As uncertainty increases, so does the political behavior of people wanting to protect their position and gain power. Competition for control emerges. If the venture is expected to be successful, managers may compete for positions and promise appointments to their staff based on networks rather than job requirements. If failure is anticipated, managers may protect themselves, thus keeping commitment, energy, and resources from the venture and contributing to a self-fulfilling prophecy for failure. During organizational change, people are usually concerned about what will happen to them, become anxious, and experience stress. The redistribution of people, material, tasks, and systems during the change usually results in some loss of managerial control and a deterioration of performance. Managers can help shape the political dynamics associated with change by supporting the change and by getting the support of key power groups. Providing anchors to anxious people can help stabilize the organization. Managers can give assurances about what is not going to change, warn people in advance of what changes will occur and the need for the change, and send consistent messages.

Development Phase

Then people in the venture need to be developed. It is important that they have identity with the venture and independence from the partner organizations. The venture should be seen as distinct from the partner organizations. Building allegiance to the venture and severing formal ties to the partner organizations are necessary. People must not think they can just return to the parent organization if the going gets rough. They need commitment to the venture. The strategic plan can help people assess where they fit into future options.

People need to be developed to deal with the characteristics of future organizations. We can expect that organizations will be networks that cooperate with each other to survive in a competitive market. Organizational forms will be fluid and transitory with fuzzy boundaries. Social and technical systems will be used to create high-performance work systems. Teams will be the norm at all levels and will have relative autonomy. Norms and values will dominate over rules and direct supervision and will facilitate the cohesion necessary to achieve coordination and direction. There will be an emphasis on system-level learning and preparing people to understand the broad strategic issues and the specific tasks to accomplish the strategic plan (Nadler, Gerstein, Shaw, et al, 1992). John Cotter (1995) reminds us of Pareto's law, which says that 20% of the factors in most situations account for about 80% of what happens and advises us to pay attention to the 20% of the factors shaping the future that really matter and to give attention to the 20% of the personnel who will make 80% of what happens happen.

"Worse than a quitter is a person who is afraid to begin." —Anonymous

Chapter Summary

Chapter 10 covered the following:
Factors Affecting Organizational Structures
Organizational Charts
    Chain of Command
    Centrality
    Unity of Command
    Authority
    Responsibility
    Accountability
    Span of Management
    Levels of Management
    Flat Versus Tall Structures
    Decentralization Versus Centralization
        Departmentalization
        Clusters

Line-Staff Relationships
    Line authority
    Staff authority
    Assistant staff
    General staff
    Advisory staff
    Service staff
    Control staff
    Functional staff
Line-Staff Conflict
Improving Line-Staff Relationships
Organizational Structure
    Organizational Redesign, Restructuring, and Reengineering
    Formal
    Informal
    Principles of Organization
    Bureaucratic Structure
        Dual management
        Advantages of the bureaucratic structure
        Disadvantages of the bureaucratic structure
    Line and Staff Structure
    Functionalized Line and Staff Structure
    Adhocracy Organizational Models
        Task forces
        Project management
        Matrix
        Collegial management
        Shared governance
        Participatory management
        Self-governance
        Systems
        Mixed model
        Corporate model
        Interorganizational relationships
        Continuum of multiorganizational arrangements
        Mergers
        Health care networks
    Disease Management
    Demand Management
    Continuum of Care
        Integrated health care systems
        Assessment phase

Planning and design phase
Implementation phase
Development phase

On-line Resources

evolve Additional critical thinking activities, worksheets, and case studies are available on-line at http://evolve.elsevier.com/Marriner/guide/

References

Coddington DC, Fischer EA, Moore KD, et al: *Beyond managed care: How consumers and technology are changing the future of health care*, San Francisco, 2000, Jossey-Bass.

Cotter JJ: *The 20% solution: Using rapid redesign to create tomorrow's organizations today*, New York, 1995, John Wiley & Sons.

First Health Associates Consulting Team: *Positioning your PHO to meet changing market demands* (http://www.fha-inc.com/v1.3positioningyourpho.htm), accessed June 5, 1999.

Galbraith JR, Designing organizations: An executive briefing on strategy, structure, and process. San Francisco, 1995, Jossey-Bass.

Galbraith J, Downey D, Kates A: *Designing dynamic organizations*, New York, 2002, American Management Association.

Grohar-Murray ME, DiCroce HR: *Leadership and management in nursing*, ed 3, Stamford, Conn, 2003, Appleton & Lange.

Institute for the Future: *Health and health care 2010*, San Francisco, 2000, Jossey-Bass.

Marquis BL, Huston CJ: *Leadership roles and management functions in nursing: Theory and application*, ed 2, Philadelphia, 2000, Lippincott.

Marquis BL, Huston CJ: *Management decision making for nurses: 124 case studies*, Philadelphia, 1998, Lippincott.

Martin J: *The great transition: Using the seven disciplines of enterprise engineering to align people, technology, and strategy*, New York, 1995, AMACOM.

Nadler DA, Gerstein MS, Shaw RB, et al: *Organizational architecture: Designs for changing organizations*, San Francisco, 1992, Jossey-Bass.

Nadler DA, Tushman ML: *Competing by design: The power of organizational architecture*, New York, 1997, Oxford University Press.

Ouellette JN, Martin LL, Holmes RB, et al: Clustering: Decentralization and resource sharing, *Nurs Manage* 20:31-35, June 1989.

Pelinet Internet Services, Pelican Coast Publishers: *HMO* (http://www.medicalsocieties.org/hmo.htm), 1997, accessed June 5, 1999.

Rakich JS, Longest BB, Darr K: *Managing health services organizations*, ed 3, Baltimore, 1992, Health Professions Press.

Rocchiccioli JT, Tilbury MS: *Clinical leadership in nursing*, Philadelphia, 1998, WB Saunders.

Sharp DE: *Customer relationship management systems handbook*, Boca Raton, 2003, Auerbach Publications.

Shillito ML: *Acquiring, processing, and deploying voice of the customer*, Boca Raton, 2001, St. Lucie Press.

Spector R: *Lessons from the Nordstrom way: #1 customer service company*, New York, 2001, John Wiley & Sons, Inc.

Sullivan EJ, Decker PJ: *Effective leadership and management in nursing*, Upper Saddle River, NJ, 2001, Prentice Hall.

Swansburg RC, Swansburg RJ: *Introduction to management and leadership for nurses*, Boston, 2002, Jones and Bartlett.

Timm PR: *Customer service: Career success through customer satisfaction*, Upper Saddle River, NJ, 2001, Prentice Hall.

Wall DK, Proyect MM: *Critical pathway implementation guide: A methodology for managing critical pathways*, Chicago, 1997, Precept Press.

Yoder-Wise PS: *Leading and managing in nursing*, ed 2, St Louis, 2003, Mosby.

11

Organizational Culture and Change

Chapter Overview

Chapter 11 explains individual and organizational culture, diversity, process of change, cultural change, behavioral aspects of organizational change, resistance to change, oscillation, and strategies for change.

Chapter Objectives

- Describe the interrelationship of values, attitudes, perception, personality, and roles.
- Identify four factors in organizational culture.
- Explain how managers can use heroes.
- Describe a cultural network.
- Identify at least two rituals.
- Define three strategies for effecting change.
- Define at least three types of change.
- Describe the five tracks that must be carefully planned to facilitate complex organizational change.
- Identify the three developmental stages of an organization and discuss what occurs in each stage.

Major Concepts and Definitions

Values basic convictions and beliefs about what is desirable or important

Attitudes mental states of readiness

Perceptions consciousness, awareness

Personality a relatively stable set of characteristics and temperaments

Roles expected behaviors in given situations

Myers-Briggs Type Indicator a method of self-examination of one's strengths and weaknesses and how one differs from others

Assumptions suppositions, presumptions, something taken for granted

Symbols objects or acts that represent another thing

Language choice of words and sounds used to express thoughts and feelings

Behaviors actions or mannerisms

Organizational culture customary way of thinking and behaving that is shared by members of an organization

Hero a person honored for outstanding qualities

Cultural network primary informal means of communication in the organization

Rituals day-to-day routines

Change to become different

Change agent one who helps bring about change

Organizational development stages of birth, youth, and maturity of organizations

CULTURE OF INDIVIDUALS

Perception is a psychological process that makes sense out of what one sees, hears, smells, tastes, or feels. One's previous experiences and personal value system affect it; thus people may perceive the same situation differently. There are also differences in ability to process data, to remember facts, and to explore alternatives.

VALUES

Values represent basic convictions about what is right, good, or desirable; as a result, they help an individual decide which mode of conduct is preferable to others. Value systems list an individual's values in order of their relative importance and provide the foundation of attitudes, perceptions, personality, and roles. These values cloud objectivity and rationality by containing interpretations of what is right and wrong and implications that certain behaviors or outcomes are preferred over others. They are relatively stable and enduring and generally influence decisions and behaviors.

ATTITUDES

Attitudes are mental states of readiness that are organized through experience and exert specific influences on a person's response to the people, objects, and situations to which they are related. Attitudes, like values, are learned from parents, teachers, and peers, but attitudes are less stable than values. They influence decisions and behavior and are close to the core of personality.

In the late 1950s Leon Festinger proposed the theory of cognitive dissonance to explain the linkage between attitudes and behavior. Cognitive dissonance means a perceived inconsistency or incompatibility between attitudes and behavior. Festinger maintained that this inconsistency is uncomfortable and that people will try to reduce the dissonance and consequently the discomfort. People seek a stable state with a minimum of dissonance. For example, if someone thinks she is being paid more than she is worth, she is likely to work harder, but if she thinks she is underpaid, she may slow down and do less (Festinger, 1957).

PERCEPTIONS

Perception involves receiving, organizing, and interpreting stimuli. The perceptions then influence behavior and form attitudes. People select various cues that influence their perceptions and consequently often misperceive another person, group, or object.

Selective perception means that people select information that supports their viewpoints. Knowing oneself increases the accuracy of perception of others. People tend to identify their own characteristics in others. Consequently, people who accept themselves are more likely to view others favorably.

A stereotype is a judgment made about people on the basis of their gender or ethnic background that can contribute to selective perception.

A self-fulfilling prophecy occurs when people expect certain behavior, use selective perception to see it, and treat others as if it were so. For example, if a nurse manager thinks certain ethnic groups are lazy and irresponsible, she may not assign them challenging tasks. That could lead to boredom and demotivation, which reinforce the stereotype, creating a self-fulfilling prophecy.

COGNITIVE STYLES

People gather and process information differently. The Myers-Briggs Type Indicator shows that people gather information through sensing and intuiting and process or evaluate the information through thinking and feeling. Sensing focuses on detail or specific attributes rather than on the relationships among factors. Intuiting emphasizes commonalities and generalizations in relationships among factors. Thinking systematically evaluates information, whereas feeling gives an internal sense of what to do.

RESEARCH Perspective 11-1

Data from Dunham-Taylor J: Nurse executive transformational leadership found in participative organizations. *JONA* 30(5):241-250, 2000

Purpose: This study explored transformational leadership, stage of power, and organizational climate.

Methods: Three hundred ninety six randomly selected hospital nurse executives and staff reporting to them (1115) rated the nurse executives' leadership style, staff extra effort, staff satisfaction, and work group effectiveness using Bass and Avoio's Multifactor Leadership Questionnaire. Executives' bosses (360) rated executive work group effectiveness. Executives completed Haberg's Personal Power Profile and ranked their organizational climate using Likert's Profile of Organizational Characteristics.

Results/conclusions: Nurse executives used transformational leadership fairly often, achieved fairly satisfied staff levels, were very effective according to bosses, were most likely at stage 3 (power by achievement) or stage 4 (power by reflection), and rated their hospital as a Likert system 3 (consultative organization). Staff satisfaction and work group effectiveness decreased as nurse executives were more transactional. Higher transformational scores tended to occur with higher educational degrees and within more participative organizations.

ATTITUDES TOWARD CHANGE

"A wise man changes his mind, a fool never."
—Anonymous

Tolerance of ambiguity and locus of control influence people's attitudes toward change. Environments are increasingly chaotic, complex, temporary, and overloaded with information. The ability to process information is affected by one's *attitude toward change. Tolerance of ambiguity* refers to how a person is threatened by unpredictability or has difficulty coping with complex situations. People who have a tolerance for ambiguity and complexity are more adaptive. Tolerance of ambiguity involves at least three factors: novelty, complexity, and insolubility. *Novelty* is a tolerance of new and unfamiliar information and situations. *Complexity* is tolerance of multiple unrelated pieces. *Insolubility* is tolerance for situations that are difficult to solve because of unavailable information and unidentified alternative solutions.

There are internal and external *loci of control.* An *internal locus of control* means the person feels responsible for the success or failure of a situation. An *external locus of control* means the person feels that someone or something else has caused the results. A person who has an internal locus of control is more adaptable than one with an external locus of control.

INTERPERSONAL NEEDS

Interpersonal orientations are not actual behaviors but rather are the tendencies to behave in certain ways. They are influenced by one's basic needs related to relationships with others. People need people and tend to seek compatible relationships with others in social situations. There are at least three basic needs: inclusion, control, and affection. *Inclusion* involves introversion, extroversion, joining and including others, and wanting to be included by others. *Control* is the need to balance influence and power in relationships. There are differences in the need to control others or be controlled by

others. People also have a need for *affection,* which is the need for intimacy and the desire for close personal relationships with others (Whetten and Cameron, 1998).

PERSONALITY

Personality is a relatively stable set of characteristics, temperaments, and tendencies that is significantly formed by inheritance and by social, cultural, and environmental factors.

ROLES

Role theory is a collection of concepts, definitions, and hypotheses that predict how actors will perform in certain roles and under what circumstances given behaviors can be expected. Roles are acts or behaviors expected of a person who occupies a given social position. Positions are locations in social systems, such as nurse or teacher. People who occupy a position collectively share common behaviors. Specific behaviors associated with positions constitute roles. Positions and roles have counterparts or counterroles such as nurse-client, teacher-student, or leader-follower.

Positions may be ascribed or achieved. A person has little or no control over ascribed positions such as age, gender, or birth order in the family. Some degree of control is possible for achieved positions, such as marital status, occupation, and social status.

Role structure involves individuals, behaviors, and positions. The individual (or actor, ego, referent, or self) has a set of attributes that can be described from a variety of viewpoints. An interactionist would look at the interaction of roles, the psychiatrist at personality, and the structuralist at position tasks. Behaviors are actions taken by the role enactor. These acts are learned and influenced by norms. They are often voluntary and goal directed. Prescription refers to what should be done by a person in a certain position. Positions often require specific skills, intelligence, or temperament and may be held based on one's age, gender, and education. Positions often imply titles, such as nurse or teacher. People in positions are exchangeable, but the positions are not.

Role socialization is a process of acquiring specific roles and involves role expectations, role learning, and role enactment. Role expectations are beliefs held by others about the specific behaviors inherent in specific positions; they may be general or specific, formal or informal, and extensive or narrow in scope. Some expectations are very clear, whereas others are not. General expectations allow more latitude in the implementation of the role than do specific ones. For example, nurses should be kind and gentle in general. More specifically, nurses use two-way communications skills. Some formal expectations are written, such as codes of ethics and behavioral objectives, whereas informal expectations are communicated indirectly. Expectations for age and gender are extensive in scope in that they transcend other roles. Expectations that apply in only a few positions are narrow in scope. Thus only nurses working in cardiac intensive care units are expected to read and interpret electrocardiograms, and only nurse managers are expected to write a budget.

Role learning involves locating oneself accurately in the social structure. It begins at infancy and early childhood as one prepares to assume adult responsibilities. It involves the development of basic skills such as language, interpersonal competence, and role taking. Role taking is the ability of the person to act out perceptions of how she and others would behave in certain positions. Playing nurse is an example of learning role taking.

Role enactment refers to behaviors and is related to the number of positions one holds, the intensity of involvement in those positions, and the preemptiveness of them. One holds multiple positions at any one time, a situation that sometimes causes conflict and difficulty with role enactment. One may not have enough time to implement each role effectively, and there can be conflicts between various role expectations. A professional nurse who takes a course will have less time for child care. Intensity of involvement

is the degree of effort exerted to enact a role. It may vary from noninvolvement to engrossing involvement. For example, a nurse may merely pay for membership in an organization or may become an officer and serve on several committees. Preemptiveness is the amount of time a person spends enacting one role as compared with others.

Role stress or role dissonance is the difference between role enactment and role expectations. The greater the difference, the greater the stress. Role ambiguity results from a lack of clear role expectations. Role shock arises from discrepancies between anticipated and encountered roles. Role conflict is a consequence of contradictory or mutually exclusive roles.

MYERS-BRIGGS TYPE INDICATOR

The Myers-Briggs Type Indicator is a useful method for performing self-examinations to understand one's strengths and weaknesses and how one differs from others. Isabel Briggs-Myers (1995) has identified four dimensions of psychological type: attitude toward life, perception function, judgment function, and orientation to the outer world. Each of the four dimensions has two categories, thus forming 16 different types, as shown in Table 11-1.

Introverts like to work alone, think before they act, do not like interruptions, like quiet for concentration, may work on a project for a long time, are interested in ideas, are careful with details, may have difficulty remembering names and faces, and may have trouble communicating.

TABLE **11-1** Myers-Briggs Type Indicator

DIMENSIONS	CONTRASTING CATEGORIES	
Attitude toward life	Introversion	Extroversion
Perception	Sensing	Intuiting
Judgment	Thinking	Feeling
Orientation to outer world	Judging	Perceiving

Extroverts like to be around people, communicate freely, may act without thinking, like variety and action, and may become impatient with slow jobs.

Sensing types tend to be good at detail work, are not usually inspired, rarely make errors of fact, are patient with routine details, enjoy using skills they know, like established ways of doing things, and work steadily step by step to an end.

Intuiting types like solving new problems, enjoy learning new skills, follow their inspirations, and work in bursts of energy to reach conclusions quickly.

Thinking types value logic, organize ideas into logical sequences, tend to be brief and businesslike, and may seem impersonal.

Feeling types value sentiment, tend to be friendly and agreeable, may undervalue thinking, and are likely to ramble. They are usually stronger in social skills than in executive ability.

Judging types like to plan their work and follow the plan, make decisions quickly, and get things done.

Perceiving types are curious, may start too many projects, and may have trouble finishing them or coming to a conclusion.

Leaders should know their own styles and those of people with whom they work. When leaders are aware of their own limitations, they can consult opposite types to compensate. By knowing their associates' strengths and weaknesses, they can maximize the strengths, minimize the weaknesses, and develop strong teams (Barr and Barr, 1989; Briggs-Myers and Myers, 1995).

DIVERSITY

"It's OK to be different." —Anonymous

Diversity is a state of difference and having variety. There is strength in diversity. At the center of diversity is one's personality. Other internal factors include age, gender, race, ethnicity, physical ability, and sexual orientation. External factors include education, work experience, income,

religion, marital status, parental status, personal habits, recreational habits, geographical location or living environment, and appearance. Organizational factors include work content field; functional level classification or job roles; division, department, or work environment; seniority; management status; work location; and union affiliation. Respect for diversity comes from finding and acknowledging that good comes from these differences. Multiculturalism refers to maintaining several different cultures. Cross culturalism refers to mediating between cultures. Transculturalism means bridging significant differences in cultural practice.

Cultural differences are common in several areas, including the following:

Values and norms. People in the United States may value individual orientation, independence, and direct confrontation of conflict, whereas other cultures may prefer a group orientation, conformity, and harmony.

Beliefs and attitudes. People in the United States may value egalitarianism, gender equity, and individual control over their own destiny and challenge authority, whereas other cultures may be more hierarchical, respect authority, accept different roles for men and women, and think individuals should accept their destiny.

Mental processes and learning style. People in the United States may be linear, logical, and sequential with a problem-solving approach, whereas other cultures may be lateral, holistic, simultaneous, and accepting of life difficulties.

Sense of self and space. The culture in the United States may be informal and use handshakes, whereas other cultures may be more formal and use hugs and bows, as well as handshakes.

Relationships with family and friends. People in the United States may focus on the nuclear family, value youth, and value responsibility for self, whereas other cultures may focus on the extended family, respect age, and feel loyalty and responsibility to the family.

Time and time consciousness. People in the United States may value promptness and be linear and exact with regard to time consciousness, whereas other cultures may use time to enjoy relationships and may be elastic and relatively time conscious.

Communication and language. People in the United States may use explicit, direct communications with an emphasis on the content, whereas other cultures may use implicit, indirect communications that emphasize contextual meaning found around words.

Food and eating habits. People in the United States may view eating as a necessity and use fast food, whereas other cultures may view dining as a religious and social experience.

Dress and appearance. People in the United States may dress for success and accept a wide range of dress codes, whereas other cultures may see dress as a sign of position and prestige. They may follow religious rules.

Work habits and practices. People in the United States may emphasize tasks, intrinsically value work, and reward workers based on individual achievement, whereas other cultures may put an emphasis on relationships, believe that work is a necessity of life, and reward seniority and relationships.

Cultural imposition is a situation where one culture forces values and beliefs onto another culture or subculture.

Cultural imperialism is a situation of having control over other countries and is often characterized by struggles over control of raw materials and world markets.

Ethnocentrism is believing that one's race, culture, or values are superior to those of others. It is the lowest level of *intercultural sensitivity.* There are several stages in the development of intercultural sensitivity. *Denial of differences* is the inability to construe cultural differences. Isolation in homogeneous groups does not allow for noticing and interpreting cultural differences. Separation allows for some awareness of cultural differences but often yields undifferentiated broad categories such as "Asian" or "black." These are only broad categories for different cultures with a relatively benign effect based on ignorance. *Defense against difference* is the recognition of cultural differences accompanied by a negative evaluation of variations from the dominant culture. The greater the variation, the more negative the evaluation. This may be characterized by dualistic thinking of us and them accompanied by overt negative stereotyping and attempts to convert to the dominant culture. *Minimization of difference* is the recognition and acceptance of superficial cultural differences, such as eating customs. It is assumed that all human beings are essentially the same. There is an emphasis on the similarity of people and basic values. *Acceptance of difference* is recognition and appreciation of cultural differences in both behaviors and values. It emphasizes acquisition of knowledge about cultures, including an increased awareness of one's own culture. *Adaptation to difference* includes a shifting frame of reference to understand and be understood across cultural boundaries, empathy, and communication skills that enable intercultural communication. One is able to consciously shift perspective into an alternative cultural worldview and act in culturally appropriate ways. *Integration of difference* is the internalization of bicultural frames of reference. It is the acceptance of an identity that is not based entirely in one culture (Gardenswartz and Rowe, 1995; Loden, Rosener, and Rosener, 1991; Stewart and Bennett, 1991).

MANAGEMENT OF CULTURAL DIVERSITY

The leader or manager needs to help staff with cultural diversity through awareness building, discrimination control, and prejudice reduction. The organizational mission and goal statements should address diversity. People who want to deal with diversity issues should be supported and open communications encouraged. Development and implementation of a culture audit including focus groups, interviews, and questionnaires help describe the culture. Homogeneous groups who are provided a safe problem-solving environment can make recommendations for solving problems. Long-term contact among culturally and ethnically diverse people can increase awareness. Working with diverse groups may require more time and effort because of the conflict management needed before a mature group emerges. The importance of cultural diversity should be apparent in the organizational philosophy and goals. Orientation programs, seminars, role playing, skill building, and workshops can be used to facilitate intercultural sensitivity. Informal networks for coaching, tutoring, mentoring, and role modeling can help develop people. Leaders should be role models for integration of differences. People should be aware that foreign or minority staff may not consider themselves of lesser status than the majority and that some of the majority may have felt they were part of an oppressed group at some time. People with different lifestyles should not be treated as if they need interventions because they may be happy with their choices. Emotional outbursts may not be anger but may be a communication style. Managers should take time to get to know the staff and help give them a perception of dignity and value. Managers should recognize and value diversity.

All managers should participate in discrimination control. Discrimination is the mistreatment of people based on irrelevant factors, such as race, gender, age, or handicap. Active recruitment, selection, retention, and promotion of women and minorities; monitoring their progress; affirmative action committees to monitor fairness of policies and the implementation of them; and advisory groups representing minorities can help control discrimination. Managers and staff can attend in-service sessions about the appropriate actions to take when aware of discriminatory behavior. Open discussions between representatives of conflicting groups may help minimize discrimination and should focus on the strengths each group brings to the situation to help reach the organizational goals. Clearly written policies

and equal support and resources of career development for all employees can help reduce the risk of reverse discrimination, which occurs when a person of a particular ethnic group is chosen over someone else who has better credentials. People need to be aware that physical features do not always denote a specific race or ethnic group. Jamaicans and Puerto Ricans are not African blacks, and Hispanics may have Asian features. Managers should implement standards of performance and ensure fairness.

Prejudice reduction is more difficult than awareness building or discrimination control. Prejudice is an internal, abstract perception. Organizations can attempt to control the manifestations of prejudice. People who observe and report prejudice can help reduce it. Discouraging racial and gender comments usually decreases the number of racial and gender comments made (Rocchiccioli and Tilbury, 1998; Yoder-Wise, 2002).

ORGANIZATIONAL CULTURE

Organizational culture is the customary way of thinking and behaving that is shared by all members of the organization and must be learned and adopted by newcomers before they can be accepted into the agency. Culture is learned, shared, and transmitted. It is a combination of assumptions, values, symbols, language, and behaviors that manifest the organization's norms and values. Objective aspects exist outside the minds of members of the organization and include artifacts such as pictures of leaders, monuments, stories, ceremonies, and rituals. Subjective aspects are related to assumptions and mind-sets such as shared assumptions, values, meanings, and understandings of how things will be done.

Values are the basic beliefs of the organization. Agencies with strong cultures have a complex system of values that are discussed openly by managers and are accepted by members. They establish the standards for achievement in the organization. They are the essence of the organization's philosophy; they provide a sense of direction, guide daily behavior, serve as an informal control system, help set priorities, and plan strategies.

Heroes personify the organizational culture's values. They show that success is attainable, set a standard for performance, preserve what is special in the organization, motivate employees, serve as role models, and symbolize the organization to the outside world (Shani and Lau, 2000).

The cultural network is the primary informal means of communication within the organization that carries the corporate values and heroic mythology. Managers should use this network to understand what is going on and to get things done (Deal and Kennedy, 2000) (Box 11-1).

Artifacts, or articles made by human work, include a range of verbal and physical symbols, such as stories, myths, verbal or visual forms of humor, rituals, ceremonies, analogies, and metaphors. Gestures are a nonverbal form of communication. Gossip is talk or rumors about others. Jargon is specialized vocabulary or idioms specific to a way of work. A joke is a funny anecdote. Slang is a specialized vocabulary of idioms outside the standard language. A signal is given by a gesture. A slogan is a catchword or motto.

Stories may describe conflicts, heroes, or traditions. Legend is the story of a saint or some wonderful event. Myths are fictitious, traditional stories with a historical basis used to explain something. A saga is a long story of adventure or heroic deeds. Songs are poetry or verse that is sung. Verbal forms of humor could be jokes, whereas visual forms could be cartoons posted on bulletin boards.

Rituals are the day-to-day routines that show employees how they are to behave. Policies and procedures clarify routines. Inductions, promotions, planning retreats, and retirements are rituals that reinforce the values. Ceremonies are extravagant rituals that give visible evidence of the agency's values. Ceremonies keep the values, beliefs, and heroes visible.

Analogies speak to similarities between things that are otherwise unlike or that bear a partial resemblance. For example, the organization is like a battlefield. Metaphors are figures of speech in which one thing is likened to another and spoken of as if it were the other thing. Organizations can be spoken of as follows: (1) anthropology (a family, big daddy, the prodigal son), (2) mechanistic (an assembly line, a factory, a well-oiled machine), (3) television (sitcom, soap opera), (4) military (battles, battle zone, captain, enemies, troops), (5) sports (quarterback, stars, teams), and (6) zoo (chicken, sly fox) (Shani and Lau, 2000; Sullivan and Decker, 2001; Swansburg and Swansburg, 2002). In *Images of Organizations*, Morgan (1997) uses machine, organismic, brain, culture, political, and psychic prison metaphors to describe organizations.

TYPES OF CULTURES

William Schneider (1999) has identified four core cultures with a leadership and management focus. The *control culture* is authoritative, conservative, impersonal, tough minded, realistic, systematic, task driven, objective, and prescriptive. The *collaborative culture* is adaptive, collegial, democratic, informal, participative, personal, relational, supportive, and trusting; the leader functions as a coach, integrator, team builder,

---

BOX **11-1** Cultural Forms

LANGUAGE
Gestures
Gossip
Humor
Jargon
Jokes
Metaphors
Myths
Proverbs
Rituals
Rumors
Taboos
Signals
Slang
Slogans
Signs
Songs

NARRATIVES
Legends
Myths
Sagas
Stories

PRACTICES
Ceremonies
Rituals
Taboos

SYMBOLS
Objects
Performances
Settings

R**ESEARCH** Perspective 11-2

Data from Ingersoll GI, Kirsch JC, Merk SE, et al: Relationship of organizational culture and readiness for change to employee commitment to the organization. *JONA* 30(1):11-20, 2000.

Purpose: The purpose of this study was to determine the relationship among organizational culture, organizational commitment, and organizational readiness in a sample of employees participating in a hospital redesign process.

Methods: Employees of an organization undergoing patient-focused redesign were surveyed after a 6-month period of preparation and before the initiation of the new care delivery model.

Results/conclusions: Organizational readiness was the strongest predictor of employee commitment to the organization. Constructive culture also was predictive, but less so than readiness for change. Findings suggest that when change is seen as a positive characteristic of the environment, employees are more likely to commit to the work of the institution.

and trust builder. The *competence culture* is challenging, efficient, emotionless, formal, impersonal, intense, objective, rational, and task driven; the leader is an assertive, visionary standard setter who recruits the most competent people and then stretches them. The *cultivation culture* is attentive, emotional, enabling, humanistic, nurturing, people driven, personal, promotive, and relaxed; the leader is a catalyst, cultivator, empowerer, inspirer, promoter, and steward.

Robert Cooke and Denise Rousseau (1987) have identified three culture types: (1) positive, (2) passive-defensive, and (3) aggressive-defensive. In a positive culture members are proactive and interactive to meet their satisfaction needs. That culture is based on humanism, affiliation norms, achievement, and self-actualization. In passive-defensive and aggressive-defensive cultures people protect their security and status in reactive, guarded ways. Passive-defensive culture is based on conventional, approval, dependent, and avoidance norms. Aggressive-defensive culture is based on power, oppositional, competitive, and perfectionistic norms. Leaders need to diffuse negativism in oppositional norms and

act as role models for desirable behaviors, encouraging a cultural transition to more positive norms.

INTEGRATED OR DIFFERENTIATED FRAMES OF REFERENCE

Organizations may have action, content, and symbolic consistency. *Action consistency* occurs when content themes are consistent with the formal and informal practices and the artifacts. *Content consistency* is congruence among content themes. *Symbolic consistency* happens when there is congruence among artifacts and informal and formal practices. Integration means that an organization has a single culture with a high level of consistency and consensus. Highly integrated cultures can be repressive and nonadaptive. Differentiation recognizes and allows for variation of cultures within the organization, such as subcultures (Sullivan and Decker, 2001).

Subcultures

Subcultures have the same elements that cultures have, including distinct patterns of shared ideologies and sets of cultural forms. They are collective, dynamic, emotionally charged, historically based, and inherently symbolic. The degree of distinctiveness of subcultures varies. Some resemble the dominant culture in which they are embedded, and others deviate greatly from it. The more unique the subculture, the more it encourages members to weaken their commitment to the dominant culture and violate significant aspects of it. Organizations are usually multicultural, having multiple subcultures within them. Frequency of interactions provides the basis of subcultures. Subcultures require long periods of close association to develop distinctive ideologies. It is shared experiences that stimulate that collective sense making. Shared personal characteristics, such as age, education, ethnicity, occupational training, and social class, also facilitate sense making because people do not need to displace their old beliefs and values very much when they find a common ground with each other. Cohesion is also important to subcultures and is facilitated by small groups; agreement of group goals; tasks requiring interdependence; similar characteristics of members, such as interests and values; physical isolation from others; threats from the outside; and performance success, failure, or crisis. When groups are cohesive, the members are attracted to each other, spend time together, and consequently influence each other. Subcultures tend to form strong norms that govern the behavior of members.

Social cohesiveness is not the same as a subculture. When neighbors respond to a natural disaster, they have social cohesiveness for a while; but when the circumstances that brought them together end, so do the mutual influence and strong emotional bonds. Subcultures are more enduring than social cohesiveness. People's occupations are the most pervasive source of subcultures in an organization. An occupation consists of a set of tasks, and members of the occupation claim exclusive rights to perform and control those tasks. Members of the occupation identify themselves with other members of that occupation and come to share beliefs, norms, and values in a variety of ways. Language, myths,

rituals, songs, and taboos help members vent their emotions and learn ways to frame their activities so they are not overwhelmed. Members then form favorable self-images and social identities from their work that then become part of their presentation of self. Members of occupations may live near one another, spend time together, encourage their children to enter the same profession, and link families through marriage. The subculture then becomes prone to ethnocentrism.

Countercultures

Countercultures develop to oppose the dominant culture. Mergers, rebellious innovators, chronically discontented employees, and illegal or other deviant behaviors encourage the formation of countercultures (Trice and Beyer, 1993).

Leaders help shape the culture by identifying and projecting a vision, demonstrating a philosophy, modeling values, setting policies, creating systems, and supporting a reward system. Leaders must ensure congruity between strategic plans and decision-making processes. They need to identify the actual norms, establish desired norms, identify and close culture gaps, and sustain culture changes. Leaders help others understand and make sense of events and cope with change, instability, and unexpected events. Leaders need to help members of the organization adapt to the dynamic life cycle of the organization. Open and collaborative interaction among leaders and followers is important (Table 11-2).

MANAGEMENT OF CHANGE

FORCES THAT INFLUENCE CHANGE

There are internal and external forces that influence change. Internal forces originate from inside operations that may result from external changes and include changing priorities, need for increased productivity, need for cost containment, staffing pattern changes, shifts in philosophy, work process changes, and need for quality of work life. External forces include health care economics, technology, restructuring, diversity, and changing demographics (Martin, 1995).

TABLE **11-2** Trends: Paradigm Shifts Effecting Change

FROM:	TO:
Automatism	Holism
Fragmentation	Integration
Emphasis on separate parts	Emphasis on relationships
Determinate	Indeterminate
Control	Trust
Certainty/predictability	Uncertainty/ambiguity/rapid change
Reductive	Emergent
Isolated/controlled	Contextual/self-organizing
Parts defining the whole	Whole being greater than the sum of the parts
Top-down management	Bottom-up leadership
Hierarchy	Nonhierarchical networks
Reactive	Imaginative/experimental
Power from top	Power from interacting centers
Competition	Cooperation
Single viewpoint	Many viewpoints
Knowing	Discovering
Quality of work	Quality of life

Data from Zohar D: *Rewiring the corporate brain: Using the new science to rethink how we structure and lead organizations*, San Francisco, 1997, Berrett-Koehler.

Leaders are visionary role models who focus on the future. Managers process the changes and understand the future directions (Table 11-3).

STRATEGIES FOR EFFECTING CHANGE

Whether working with individuals, groups, or systems, the nurse manager is sure to be involved with management of change. Several strategies for managing change have been identified.

Empirical-Rational Strategies

Empirical-rational strategies are based on the assumption that people are rational and behave according to rational self-interest. It follows then that people should be willing to adopt a change if it is justified and if the people are shown how they can benefit from the change.

Nurse managers who use empirical-rational strategies are likely to want the appropriate persons for specific positions. Desirous of having people perform jobs for which they are well qualified, nurse managers give considerable attention to recruitment and selection of personnel. Staff development through independent study, in-service education, continuing education, and formal degree programs is encouraged.

TABLE **11-3** Leadership and Management for Change

LEADER	MANAGER
Is visionary in identifying needed change	Assesses the driving and restraining forces
Is a role model	Identifies and implements strategies
Is sensitive to timing initiatives	Seeks subordinates' input
Is creative in identifying solutions	Supports and rewards individual efforts
Focuses on the future	Understands future directions

Data from Carr DK, Johansson HJ: *Best practices in reengineering: What works and what doesn't in the reengineering process*, New York, 1995, McGraw-Hill; Marquis BL, Huston CJ: *Leadership roles and management functions in nursing: Theory and application*, ed 2, Philadelphia, 2000, Lippincott.

Systems analysis, operations research, and implementation of research findings are consistent with the empirical-rational philosophy, as is long-range futuristic planning.

Normative-Reeducative Strategies

Normative-reeducative strategies are based on the assumption that people act according to their commitment to sociocultural norms. The intelligence and rationality of people are not denied, but attitudes and values are also considered. The manager pays attention to changes in values, attitudes, skills, and relationships in addition to providing information.

Believing that the basic unit of the social organization is composed of individuals, the manager fosters the development of staff members through means such as personal counseling, training groups, small groups, and experiential learning because people need to participate in their own reeducation. Organizational development programs are fostered, and it is typical to collect data about the organization, give data feedback and analysis to appropriate people, plan ways to improve the system, and train managers and internal change agents. The relationships of internal change agents with other personnel can be a major tool in reeducating others.

Power-Coercive Strategies

Power-coercive strategies involve compliance of less powerful people to the leadership, plans, and directions of more powerful individuals. These strategies do not deny the intelligence and rationality of people or the importance of their values and attitudes, but rather they acknowledge the need to use sources of power to bring about change. Use of strikes, sit-ins, negotiations, conflict confrontation, and administration decisions and rulings are power-coercive strategies (Bennis, Benne, and Chin, 1969).

PROCESS OF CHANGE

Lewin's framework for the three phases of change is unfreezing, moving, and refreezing (Figure 11-1). *Unfreezing* is the development through problem awareness of a need for change. Even if a problem has been identified, people must believe there can be an improvement before they are willing to change. Coercion and the induction of guilt and anxiety have been used for unfreezing. Removal of people from the source of their old attitudes to a new environment, punishment and humiliation for undesirable attitudes, and rewards for desirable attitudes effect change.

Stress may cause dissatisfaction with the status quo and become a motivating factor for change. Points of stress and strain should be assessed. Change may begin at a point of stress but ordinarily should not be started at the point of greatest stress. It is most appropriate for it to start with a policymaking body that considers both formal and informal structures. The effectiveness of the change may depend on the amount of involvement in fact finding and problem solving of all personnel.

Moving is working toward change by identifying the problem or the need for change, exploring the alternatives, defining goals and objectives, planning how to accomplish the goals, and implementing the plan for change.

Refreezing is the integration of the change into one's personality and the consequent stabilization of change. Frequently personnel return to old behaviors after change efforts cease. Related changes in neighboring systems, momentum to perpetuate the change, and structural

Figure 11-1 Process of change.

alterations that support the procedural changes are stabilizing factors (Ashkanasy, Wilderom, and Peterson, 2000).

TYPES OF CHANGE

The variables of mutual goal setting, the power ratio between the change agent and the client system, and the deliberativeness of change are differentiating factors in the change process.

Coercive Change

Nonmutual goal setting, imbalanced power ratio, and one-sided deliberativeness characterize coercive change.

Emulative Change

In emulative change, transition is fostered through identification with and imitation of power figures.

Indoctrination

Indoctrination uses mutual goal setting, has an imbalanced power ratio, and is deliberative. Subordinates are instructed in the beliefs of the power sources.

Interactional Change

Mutual goal setting, fairly equal power, but no deliberativeness characterize interactional change.

Parties may be unconsciously committed to changing one another.

Natural Change

Natural changes include accidents and acts of God. They involve no goal setting or deliberativeness.

Socialization Change

Social change is directly related to interactional change. An individual conforms to the needs of a social group. When there is greater deliberativeness on the power side, change becomes indoctrination.

Technocratic Change

Collecting and interpreting data bring about change. A technocrat merely reports the findings of the analysis to bring about change.

Planned Change

Planned change involves mutual goal setting, an equal power ratio, and deliberativeness (Table 11-4).

Ronald Lippitt, Jeanne Watson, and Bruce Westley (1958) have identified seven phases of planned change. First, the client must feel a need for change. The manager, as the change agent, can stimulate an awareness of the need for change, help the client become aware of the

TABLE **11-4** Comparison of Planned Change Theories

LEWIN	LIPPITT	HAVELOCK	ROGERS
1. Unfreezing	1. Diagnosing the problem	1. Building a relationship	1. Awareness
	2. Assessing motivation and capacity for change	2. Diagnosing the problem	2. Interest
	3. Assessing change agent's motivation and resources	3. Acquiring the relevant resources	3. Evaluation
2. Moving	4. Selecting progressive change objective	4. Choosing the solution	4. Trial
	5. Choosing the appropriate role for the change agent	5. Gaining acceptance	
3. Refreezing	6. Maintaining change	6. Stabilization and self-renewal	5. Adoption
	7. Terminating the helping relationship		

Data from Bennis, Benne, and Chin, 1969; Havelock, 1973; Lippitt, Watson, and Westley, 1958; Rocchiccioli and Tilbury, 1998; Rogers, 1995; Swansburg, 1996; Swansburg and Swansburg, 2002; Yoder-Wise, 2003.

problems, and indicate that a more desirable state of affairs is possible. The change agent assesses the client's motivation and capacity for change and the change agent's motivation and resources. Thus unfreezing occurs.

Next, the helping relationship must be established, and the moving process begun. Managers, as change agents, must identify with clients' problems while remaining neutral so that they can remain objective. The change agent needs to be viewed as an understandable and approachable expert. The success or failure of most planned action will depend largely on the quality and workability of the relationship between the change agent and the client. The problem must be identified and clarified. Collecting and analyzing data can facilitate this process. Alternative possibilities for change should be examined. Goals and objectives are planned. The client's emotional and material resources are examined. Strategies for change are determined. The success of planned change is evaluated by the implementation of the plans. It is the active work of modification that completes the moving process.

The refreezing process occurs during the sixth phase—generalization and stabilization. All too often clients slip back to their old ways after change efforts cease. The spread of change to neighboring systems and to subparts of the same system aids the stabilization process. Change momentum, positive evaluation of the change, rewards for the change, and related procedural and structural changes increase the stabilization. The helping relationship ends, or a different type of continuing relationship is established. Dependency is the major factor determining when the relationship will end (Lippitt, Watson, and Westley, 1958).

Lippitt's seven phases, Ronald Havelock's six, and Everett Rogers' five can all be clustered in Kurt Lewin's three, as illustrated in Table 11-4. In addition, Margaret Wheatley (1996, 2001) discusses chaos theory. Organizations are self-organizing and self-renewing open systems that have chaotic, randomly appearing patterns. Wheatley points out that order emerges from chaos. She encourages leading in nonlinear ways, emphasizing the relationships of the parts in forming the whole. Vision, information, and relationships are particularly important. Edward Deevy (1995) speaks to the importance of resilience and hardiness to the survival of organizations. Daryl Conner (1993, 1998) has identified five personal characteristics of resilient behavior as follows: positive, focused, flexible, organized, and proactive. Peter Senge (1990) has addressed learning organizations that stress flexibility and responsiveness. He believes that what makes the difference between learning organizations and traditional organizations is mastery of the five disciplines of a learning organization: (1) systems thinking, (2) personal mastery, (3) mental models, (4) building shared vision, and (5) team learning. Senge, Kleiner, Roberts, et al present strategies and tools for building a learning organization in *The Fifth Discipline Fieldbook* (1999) and discuss sustaining momentum in The Dance of Change (1999).

ROLE OF THE MANAGER AS CHANGE AGENT

As a change agent, the manager identifies the problem, assesses the client's motivations and capacities for change, determines alternatives, explores ramifications of those alternatives, assesses resources, determines appropriate helping roles, establishes and maintains a helping relationship, recognizes the phases of the change process and guides the client through them, and chooses and implements techniques for planned change (Grohar-Murray and DiCroce, 2003; Lippitt, Watson, and Westley, 1958; Swansburg, 1996). Havelock (1973) indicates that change agents facilitate planned change by being a catalyst, solution giver, process helper, and resource linker. Harry Woodward, Steve Bucholz, and Karen Hess (1987) indicate change agents clarify, share, and engage commitment. They clarify by listening, focusing, and restating. They share by signaling the shift from listening to talking, explaining the purpose, overviewing the change, linking the change to the workers' concerns, and netting it out by specifying how their concerns will or will not be met. They engage for commitment by asking for understanding, asking for ideas, suggesting ideas, and agreeing on action steps.

FORCE-FIELD ANALYSIS

Lewin's force-field analysis provides a framework for problem solving and planned change. Status quo is maintained when driving forces equal the restraining forces (Figure 11-2), and change will occur when the relative strength of opposing forces changes. Consequently, when planning change, the manager should identify the restraining and driving forces and assess their strengths.

Driving forces may include pressure from the manager, desire to please the manager, perception that the change will improve one's self-image, and belief that the change will improve the situation. Restraining forces include conformity to norms, morals, and ethics; desire for security; perception of economic threat or threat to one's prestige and homeostasis; and regulatory mechanisms for keeping the situation fairly constant.

Once the driving and restraining forces have been identified, the manager determines their relative strengths. Which are the major factors toward or resisting change? Which are important or moderately important? Which have little effect for or against change? These might be listed in columns under "driving" and "restraining" and ranked (Box 11-2).

To help visualize these forces, the manager can draw a diagram as shown in Figure 11-3, write in key words to identify the forces, and draw arrows toward the status quo line to represent

the strength of the forces. The longer the line, the stronger the force.

Next, the manager plans strategies for reducing the restraining forces and strengthening the driving forces. Managers may do some experiential learning exercises to facilitate the change of group norms, explain each person's role in the change with emphasis on security, and provide some status symbols to reduce the threat to people's prestige. They should also help the workers identify how the change will improve their situation. Steps should be taken to improve self-images. For instance, people may be taught new tasks to prepare themselves for the change, to reduce the threat to their prestige and their fear of making fools of themselves when doing something new, and to improve their self-images. If managers perceive that the workers want to please them, they may inform the workers that they desire the change and give positive reinforcement for it. Keeping the goals in mind, the manager should assess the results of implementing the strategies and revise plans as necessary.

CULTURAL CHANGE IN ORGANIZATIONS

In an adaptive culture members of an organization support each other's efforts to identify and solve problems. The members believe they can manage the problems; have confidence and enthusiasm; and are receptive to change. In a dysfunctional culture members continue behaviors that have worked in the past but are no longer effective. Culture rut occurs when members do not adapt to change and continue to function out of habit even when success is not forthcoming. Culture shock happens when the members realize that the organization is

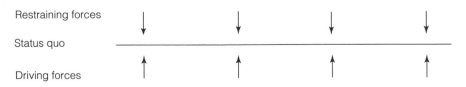

Figure 11-2 Status quo.

BOX **11-2** Driving and Restraining Forces

DRIVING FORCES			RESTRAINING FORCES	
Rank	**Factor**		**Rank**	**Factor**
1	Pressure from manager		4	Conformity
4	Please manager		4	Security
2	Improve self-image		2	Economic threat
2	Improve situation		3	Threat to prestige

Scale
1 = Little strength
2 = Moderate strength
3 = Important strength
4 = Major strength

Modified from Lippitt R, Watson J, Westley B: *The dynamics of planned change*, New York, 1958, Harcourt, Brace & World, p. 126.

out of touch with its setting, mission, and assumptions.

Ralph Kilmann (1991) has identified five stages of organizational planned change: (1) initiate the integrated program for cultural change, (2) diagnose the problems, (3) schedule the tracks, (4) implement the tracks, and (5) evaluate the results (Box 11-3).

The five tracks are as follows: (1) culture, (2) management skills, (3) team building, (4) strategy structure, and (5) reward system (Box 11-4). They require implementation in that order to be most successful. The culture track helps explain organizational differences in decision making and actions, much as personality explains differences in individuals. The culture track reveals the norms of the organization. It exposes the old

culture and helps create a new culture. Without an adaptive culture it can be impossible to make improvements, so removing the cultural barriers has to be accomplished before proceeding to another track.

First, one needs to clarify the actual norms. For instance, one could ask members to list current dos and don'ts. The members can then list what they want the norms to be and identify the culture gaps. Culture gaps are often related to the following: (1) task support—norms related to helping others, information sharing, and concern for efficiency; (2) task innovation—norms related to performing new activities, trying different approaches, and being creative; (3) social relationship—norms about mixing business with pleasure and socializing with coworkers; and

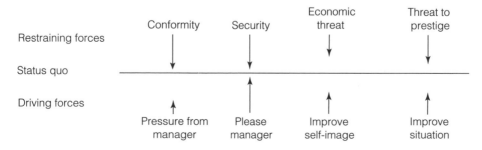

Figure 11-3 Strength of driving and restraining forces.

BOX 11-3 Five Stages of Organizational Planned Change

Initiate the integrated program of cultural change.
Diagnose the problems.
Schedule the tracks.
Implement the tracks.
Evaluate the results.

BOX 11-5 Culture Gaps

Task support norms
Task innovation norms
Social relationship norms
Personal freedom norms

---

(4) personal freedom—norms for pleasing oneself, using self-expression, and exercising discretion (Box 11-5). Culture gaps are generally largest at lower levels in the organization.

Closing the culture gaps then becomes an issue. If the managers and associates decide that changes should occur, they can. Adaptive cultures have internal control. Control is a social reality but not necessarily an objective one. To establish desired norms, members can be asked to list norms they think would lead to organizational success. Then work groups need to develop a sanctioning system to monitor and enforce the new norms. Work groups should decide what will be done if a member violates a new norm or performs the desired behavior. The open sanctioning system is probably more equitable than the old unconscious sanctions.

Now it becomes important to sustain the cultural change. If the new culture is not supported by the remaining four tracks, it is likely that the culture will revert to the dysfunctional ways. The management skills and team-building tracks develop leadership to support the adaptive culture. The strategy-structure track will document the new systems, and the reward system track will support the new norms.

In the management skills track, managers are taught the five steps of problem management: (1) sensing problems, (2) defining problems, (3) deriving solutions, (4) implementing solutions, and (5) evaluating outcomes (Box 11-6). Next, managers examine their personality types. Because one's personality type determines how one will assimilate information and make decisions, managers should be aware of their style and the styles of associates so they can compensate for their natural inclinations and acknowledged limitations and develop strong work teams.

Managers also need to learn assumptional analysis: how to surface, classify by amount of certainty and importance, and synthesize assumptions. Outdated assumptions can lead to the wrong strategy-structure and reward systems. In a climate of trust and openness, associates should be able to examine previously unstated assumptions so they are not held back by faulty assumptions.

The team-building track activates the new culture and skills through the entire organization. Team building involves the following: (1) reuniting the work group, (2) identifying work group problems, (3) identifying solutions and developing action plans, (4) implementing the plans, and (5) evaluating and monitoring the outcomes (Box 11-7). Interteam building is also

---

BOX 11-4 Five Tracks for Cultural Change

Culture
Management skills
Team building
Strategy structure
Reward system

BOX 11-6 Management Skills Track

Sensing problems
Defining problems
Deriving solutions
Implementing solutions
Evaluating outcomes

BOX **11-7** Team Building

Reuniting the work groups
Identifying work group problems
Identifying solutions and developing plans
Implementing the plans
Evaluating and monitoring the outcomes

BOX **11-9** Developmental Stages of an Organization

Birth—creation and survival as a viable system
Youth—stability, reputation, pride
Maturity—uniqueness, adaptability, contribution to society

included in this track. Everyone in the organization needs to learn how to cope with difficult people, understand her own personality style, and appreciate the styles of others.

In the strategy-structure track, strategy sets the direction and structure organizes the goals, tasks, people, and other resources to accomplish the plans. This involves operationalizing strategy, designing subunits, and implementing structure (Box 11-8). The reward system track ensures that associates are rewarded for doing the right things for the right reasons.

ORGANIZATIONAL DEVELOPMENT

Organizations progress through developmental stages—birth, youth, and maturity (Box 11-9). The creation of a new organization and its survival as a viable system are primary concerns during the birth stage. Gaining stability and developing a reputation and pride are the focuses of the youth stage. The maturity stage involves achieving both uniqueness and adaptability and contributing to society.

As organizations are born and grow, they pass through increasingly complex stages of life. They must develop internally and generate new control processes to fit the amount of turbulence and complexity in the environment. At each stage the

BOX **11-8** Strategy Structure Track

Operationalizing strategy
Designing subunits
Implementing structure

environment can become more unknown, unsettled, and difficult. A crisis develops in each stage. Changing its organizational and decision-making structures is needed to fit this new complexity. The new organization copes by developing job descriptions, programs, policies, and procedures. However, as the organization grows and becomes more complex, these policies do not cover the exceptions. As a result, the organization develops a set of hierarchical positions to make judgments about the exceptions to the existing job descriptions and policies. As the organization becomes larger and more complex, the managers in the hierarchy become overloaded. They do not have time to deal with all the exceptions and cannot make sense out of the situation.

Consequently, in the third stage accomplishing orderliness by developing broader goals is required. However, as the organization becomes increasingly complex, conflicts arise among factions, and the organization regresses to hierarchical referral again.

A decentralized system of departments reduces the interconnections among divisions and reduces the number of communications necessary to make decisions; but as the revolutionary cycle continues, conflict among decentralized departments develops.

In the last stage, a vertical information system is developed so that standardized accounting and statistical reporting systems from each department are consolidated at the top, and then resources are allocated among departments. Because all the complex information in turbulent systems cannot be reduced to numbers, human contacts made among department members become a major coping mechanism. Liaisons, teams, committees, task forces, and integrator roles are used.

BEHAVIORAL ASPECTS OF ORGANIZATIONAL CHANGE

Many people are unaware of the factors that initiate change or influence its direction. Even when known, some forces are beyond their control. Some factors that effect change in an agency stem from society, such as new knowledge and technology, new social requirements, changing client needs and demands, and increased competition. Even when known in advance and anticipated, they cannot be controlled by an agency.

The efficiency of an organizational structure is hard to measure, and the factors contributing to success or failure may be impossible to isolate. Organizational structure may not be the problem. A few ineffective people can disrupt an otherwise sound structure, and good people can make a bad structure work. High labor costs, inadequate equipment, ineffective advertising, changing client needs, and increased competition may contribute to inadequate profits.

Some symptoms reflect inefficiencies within the organization and indicate a need for change. If slow and erroneous decision making is a problem, one may question the qualifications of the person making decisions, the level at which responsibility is placed, and access to necessary information. Poor communications, a dearth of innovation, and failure in functional areas are other symptoms indicating a need for change. Diagnosis of the problem is extremely important for planned change. Minor adjustments rather than major reorganizations may correct some problems. However, even a small change in one part of an organization can cause a chain reaction throughout the agency. This domino effect creates problems with coordination and control and brings about a need for comprehensive planning.

RESEARCH Perspective 11-3

Data from Seago JA: Registered nurses, unlicensed assistive personnel, and organizational culture in hospitals. *JONA* 30(5):278-285, 2000.

Purpose: The purpose of this study was to investigate the thinking and behavioral styles that are used to measure the concept of organizational culture among registered nurses and unlicensed assistive personnel in acute care hospitals.

Methods: The Organizational Culture Inventory was used to survey five tertiary-care hospitals on the west coast of the United States. The design was cross-sectional and analytical. A convenience sample was recruited from staff members working at least 20 hours per week in the adult medical-surgical and specialty-nursing units. Analysis included descriptive statistics and multiple regression.

Results/conclusions: Position was a predictor of a number of thinking and behavior styles. Gender was not a predictor of any of the thinking and behavior styles, and neither was the interaction of position by gender. Ethnicity (white versus people of color) was a predictor of several of the thinking and behavior styles. Staff members of color, regardless of position, scored higher on the thinking and behavioral styles of approval, avoidance, and competitiveness. Unlicensed assistive personnel, regardless of ethnicity, score higher than registered nurses on the thinking and behavioral styles of dependence and opposition.

Change disrupts equilibrium. Equilibrium can be maintained only when opposing forces are equal. Production may be maintained when the forces fostering production, such as pressure of the manager to produce, desire for favorable attention from the manager to foster one's own gain, and desire to earn more through the incentive plan, equal the forces limiting production, such as the informal group's standard against rate busting, resistance to training, and the feeling that the job and product are not important. However, when the forces in one direction or the other change in relation to each other, a new grouping forms and change is inevitable.

Changes involve endings, transitions, and beginnings. People grieve when they lose something, when they are threatened with the loss of something, and when they never had and never will have something (Jeffreys, 1995). With change, people go through the grieving process, which Elisabeth Kubler-Ross (1997) has identified as denial, anger, bargaining, depression, and then acceptance. Three stages of loss and mourning are (1) protest, (2) despair, and (3) reorganization. If people do not work through acceptance and reorganization, they may have disengagement (withdrawal), disidentification (sadness and worry), disorientation (confusion), or disenchantment (anger). Disengaged workers may quit and leave or quit and stay, or retire in place. They tend to not ask questions, not seek information, not discuss, and do only the basic requirements; and they may be hard to find. With disidentification, people have lost their self-identity and are vulnerable, like a lobster that has cast off its shell so it can grow. They may sulk, reminisce, dwell on the past, continue to do the old job, and resist new tasks. With disorientation, people have lost sight of where they fit in the organization. They do not know the priorities, do the wrong things, get very detail oriented, and get others to ask questions. The disenchanted people know that what is gone is gone and may become angry and negative. They may talk in a raised tone of voice or refuse to talk, show self-pity, walk out, sabotage, and back stab. Disenchantment can lead to personal problems and destructive behavior (Belasco, 1990; Kanter, 1985, 1989; Marquis and Huston, 1998, 2000; Woodward and Woodward, 1994).

RESISTANCE TO CHANGE

"There comes a moment when you have to stop revving up the car and shove it into gear."
—David Mahoney

Caution should be used when making organizational changes. Changes are disturbing to those affected, and resistance often develops. Giving the structure a chance to work may be better than changing it. Although changing the organizational structure may appear easy on paper, it is quite complicated in reality. It affects the attitudes and effectiveness of personnel whose prestige and status are threatened. Resistance to change is a common phenomenon whether it is initiated by positive stimuli, such as growth or promotion of an employee, or negative forces, such as poor management. Personnel develop vested interests, preferences, habits, and rigidities that attract them to the existing structure. People tend to consider the effects of the change on their personal lives, status, and future more than on the welfare of the agency. Change introduces the risk of error, fear of failure when trying something new, resistance to admission of weakness, fear of losing a current satisfaction, or a fatalistic expectation based on previous unsuccessful attempts to change. Change is most threatening in the presence of insecurity. Even logical, needed changes produce resistance (Maurer, 1996).

Causes of resistance to change include the following: threatened self-interest; embarrassment; insecurity; habits; complacency; inaccurate perceptions; perceived loss of power, rewards, or relationships; objective disagreement; psychological reactions; low tolerance for change; the change's going against the current trends; and the system's having been stable for a long time (Grohar-Murray and DiCroce, 2003; Swansburg and Swansburg, 2002).

Robert Fritz (1996, 1999) explains that organizations either oscillate or advance. If they oscillate, success is neutralized. If they advance, success is possible. Successes breed further success, but with oscillation, success is short term. Because oscillation occurs over a long period and the organization is moving in the desired direction some of that time, oscillation can be hard to observe.

A conflict of interest causes oscillation between tension and resolution. For example, there is tension in a desire for change, which leads to the resolution in change effort; but that creates tension in a desire for continuity, which leads to change avoidance. That further leads to tension in a desire for change, which leads to change effort, which causes tension in a desire for continuity, which leads to change avoidance. Organizations often oscillate between centralized and decentralized decision making, expansion and limitation, growth and stability, investment and cost cutting, and long-term and short-term benefits (Figure 11-4).

Problem-solving approaches identify a problem and take action to solve the problem, which lessens the intensity of the problem, which leads to less action and then to reintensifying the problem. That is oscillation because as problems are solved, the motivation for change is reduced. Problem solving focuses on how to eliminate an unwanted situation instead of envisioning the desired situation. Successful organizations often use a continuous quality improvement approach

within structural tension. Personnel are clear about the desired outcomes and work on improving processes. Then success is measured against standards that reflect improvement toward the vision.

Organizations advance when there is structural tension. That requires structural understanding, leadership, and organizational learning. If the structure remains unchanged, behavior will revert to previous organizational behavior. A change in structure facilitates change in organizational behavior. The structural change is hierarchical because the organization's purpose gives direction to the strategies that are steps to move the organization from the current state to the desired vision. Progression creates a cycle that leads to results that are evaluated. That leads to adjustments and refinements, which lead to new actions or continuous quality improvement and increased capacity over time because it keeps renewing structural tension. Organizations without vision cannot create structural tension and will oscillate instead of advance. Values that dominate in an organization will displace competing lesser values, thus reducing oscillation. Leadership is a critical factor in clarifying the vision. Leaders need to be clear about the vision and the present reality to create the necessary structural tension. They make decisions about competing interests based on values. When leadership is weak, workers support their own interests, which leads to conflicts

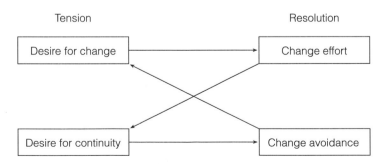

Figure 11-4 Oscillation. (Modified from Fritz R: *Corporate tides: The inescapable laws of organizational structure*, San Francisco, 1996, Berrett-Koehler.)

and oscillation. Leaders need to create fair situations and reward people for their merits and the accomplishments of the team. Organizations renew themselves by learning, which is best motivated when it serves a desired outcome. Training that is directly related to the organization's vision and values is a powerful instrument for change toward expanding capacity.

Gradual changes made in progressive phases are usually less disturbing than radical, sweeping, unpredicted changes. Changes in the structure resulting from sharply defined events that have already been planned—such as changes in size, scope, or objectives—are easier to execute than shifts in personnel, which involve infinitely complex human relations. Careful planning, appropriate timing of communications, adequate feedback, and employee confidence in management can reduce resistance to change.

Informing personnel of the reasons for change can further reduce resistance, especially when the advantages of the change are stressed. Personnel can be involved by requests for their input, including feelings, suggestions, and talents; their negative, as well as positive, feelings should be respected. Communicating honestly about the changes, giving specific feedback, asking what assistance is needed to help them cope, and recognizing their contributions to the implementation of the changes can further minimize resistance.

TYPES OF ORGANIZATIONAL CHANGE

Organizational structure usually grows vertically, then horizontally, and from a functional type to a divisional type. Initially there is vertical growth, but as the amount of work and its complexity increase, horizontal growth develops. Usually organizations develop from a functional type, which is departmentalized by major functions, to one divided by product or territory.

PLANNING FOR CHANGE

Plans for change begin with an evaluation of the existing organization. An organizational audit provides a detailed analysis of the organization, reveals the extent to which goals are accomplished, and examines the use of personnel and the growth of individuals. One begins an organizational audit by collecting and reviewing all available written material about the organization, including statement of the mission or purpose, scope of the agency, goals and objectives, organizational chart, job descriptions, annual reports, performance appraisals, and qualifications needed and not needed by personnel in their present positions. The planner notes whether the reviewed materials are consistent, looks for gaps and overlapping of functioning, and determines if all activities contribute to the major goals of the agency.

Departmentalization, span of management, and balance and emphasis are analyzed. Authority relationships are studied. Leadership patterns, delegation, decentralization, use of committees, and provision of controls are considered. The agency may be compared with what is visualized as an ideal agency or with competitors to identify areas of need and to propose recommended changes. Personnel may be surveyed to identify areas needing improvement. The quantitative approach may be used where ratios are appropriate, such as figuring range of management. Then various organizational patterns are designed, and position breakdown using existing personnel is developed. Personnel who are needed but not presently available and people who are available but not qualified or needed are identified.

A job description and requirements are necessary for each position. Each person's qualifications can be compared with the job requirements. Notations are made of job requirements for which skills are not possessed. Those qualities that can be developed on the job within reasonable time limits should be separated from required skills that cannot be acquired. Unused abilities should be related to requirements of other jobs for which the individual may be better qualified.

Smith (1997) identified the following seven levels of change:

1. Effectiveness: doing the right things . . .
2. Efficiency: doing things right . . .
3. Improving: doing the right things better . . .
4. Cutting: doing away with things . . .
5. Copying: doing things other people are doing . . .
6. Different: doing things no one else is doing . . .
7. Impossible: doing things that can't be done . . .

In *Good to Great,* Collins (2001) indicated that leaders need to get the right people on the bus and the wrong people off the bus and decide where to drive it. Harper (2001) identified seven levels of commitment:

1. Covert resisters: people who resist the change behind the scenes
2. Overt resisters: those who openly resist the change
3. Skeptics: people who need to be convinced of the need for the change
4. Observers: those who watch and withhold judgment about the need or merit of the change
5. Participants: people who accept the change and go through the necessary options
6. Committed: those who embrace the change
7. Champions: those who are the initiators of the change

Who Moved My Cheese? (Johnson, 1998) is a parable about the importance of anticipating change, monitoring it, and changing quickly because the sooner we let go the sooner we can enjoy the change. *Fish Tales* by Lundin, Christensen, and Paul and *Fun Works: Creating Places Where People Love to Work* by Yerkes (2001) stress the importance of creating work places where people can have fun and love work.

Changes in personnel are normal, but they are accelerated during organizational changes. Unless managers are to become obsolete, they must change with the times. Some quickly increase their managerial knowledge and skills. Unfortunately, others are inflexible, overly conservative, and negative. Executive obsolescence is increasingly common with the rapid changes in our society. Managers who previously performed competently may be overwhelmed with increasingly complex duties, or they may have been promoted during an emergency to a position for which they were inadequately prepared.

What can a person do about an unqualified incumbent? In developing a strategy, one should consider the ramifications of the action on the individual and on the group. The strategy should depend on the particular circumstances. An incompetent staff associate may be counseled toward satisfactory performance. Weaknesses should be identified and means to overcome them defined. On-the-job training, in-service education, college courses, and independent study may be explored. A contract may be written between the employer and the incompetent subordinate, specifying what skills are to be developed to what level of achievement and in what time frame.

Incompetent executives may be transferred to positions for which they are more qualified. They may be moved from line to staff authority. The change is most attractive when the advisory staff position is at a higher organizational level than the present line position, carries prestige, and maintains the current salary. Executives may be told there is a problem in the new area that they are to solve. This method fosters high morale and loyalty. It removes incompetence from line authority when damage could be done but uses the executive's knowledge and skills to solve specific problems. This is an expensive method.

Termination is the most extreme way to handle incompetence. It is either direct or indirect. In the direct method employees are informed that their work does not meet the minimal criteria and they are expected to leave the agency. The indirect method may involve giving incompetent employees nothing to do, withholding information from them, leaving their names off memoranda, excluding them from conferences, and generally making them so miserable they will voluntarily resign.

New managers may be hired, particularly when new positions become available during reorganization. They often bring new ideas, objectivity, and enthusiasm to the job. Recruitment is important for development of an executive pool. The best managers do not need to hunt for jobs. The jobs hunt for them. The agency should let its need be known and seek good managers aggressively. Similar agencies may be a resource for managers with new ideas and different approaches. Graduates may be recruited from university programs. Recruiting through advertisements in professional journals and through employment agencies is useful for locating potential managers and well-qualified staff.

Promotions within the agency provide incentives and supply the executive pool. However, some personnel may not be interested in managerial work, and competent, satisfied employees may lack managerial potential.

After the revised organization is decided, developing operational procedures to expedite changes is required. These procedures define activities that are necessary for specific work and identify changes needed. The revised operational procedures should be inclusive, show all details, and ensure coordinated change. Work flow should be maintained and standards upheld. Special activities are likely to be needed during a transitional period. The revised operational procedures should be perceived as carefully thought-out, planned changes and not just as stopgap actions.

STRATEGIES FOR ORGANIZATIONAL CHANGE

"... the very speed of change introduces a new element into management . . . already nervous in an unfamiliar environment, to make more and more decisions at a faster and faster pace."
—Toffler

Visions of what the organization can become, instead of what it is or has been, allow for organizational change. To this end, managers need to create an open atmosphere where questions can be asked. Welcoming criticism instead of forbidding it helps personnel be adequately self-critical. Denying problems has serious consequences. A good recruitment plan is needed for hiring competent, highly motivated personnel. Career development programs should be provided. All employees need to feel that what they achieve is important to the agency and that needed change for the continuing vitality of the organization overrides their vested interests.

David Coleman and Raman Khanna (1995) have identified the issues in managing change as awareness, knowledge, trial, evaluation, and acceptance.

Michael McMaster (1996) has identified the phases of the transformation process as follows:

Awakening. There is an awareness that something is wanted or needed.
Formulation. The iterative process of dialogue facilitates movement from proposals to possibilities.
Experimentation. Isolated experiments and pilot projects test the propositions.
Integration. Isolated projects are added to other parts.
Development. Continuous improvements are implemented.
Mastery. Teaching and learning lead to understanding and excellence.

John Kotter (1996, 2002) outlines an eight-stage process for leading change as follows: (1) establishing a sense of urgency, (2) creating and guiding teams, (3) developing a vision and strategy, (4) communicating the change vision, (5) empowering employees for broad-based action, (6) generating short-term wins, (7) consolidating gains and producing more change, and (8) anchoring new approaches in the culture. He discusses how not doing those things are reasons transformation efforts fail in James Champy and Nitin Nohria's book *Fast Forward: The Best Ideas on Managing Business Change* (1996).

David Carr and Henry Johansson (1995) outline 16 best practices in reengineering as follows:

Recognize and articulate an "extremely compelling" need to change. …

Start with and maintain executive-level support. . . .

Understand the organization's "readiness to change." …

Communicate effectively to create buy-in. Then communicate more. …

Create top-notch teams. …

Use a structured framework. …

Use consultants effectively. …

Link goals to corporate strategy. …

Listen to the "voice of the customer." …

Select the right processes for reengineering. …

Maintain focus: Don't try to reengineer too many processes. …

Maintain teams as the key vehicle for change. …

Quickly come to an as-is understanding of the processes to be reengineered. …

Choose and use the right metrics. …

Understand the risks and develop contingency plans. …

Have plans for continuous improvement. …

David Nadler and M. Nadler (1998) have identified 12 steps in three categories to deal with power, anxiety, and control as follows:

A. Need to shape the political dynamics of change

  Build the support of key power groups

  Use leader behavior to generate support

  Use symbols and language deliberately

  Define points of stability

B. Need to motivate change

  Create dissatisfaction with the current state

Build participation in planning and implementing change

Reward behavior in support of change

Provide people time and opportunity to disengage from the old

C. Need to manage the transition

  Develop and communicate a clear image of the future state

  Use multiple leverage points

  Develop transition management structures

  Collect and analyze feedback

Others speak to the importance of persuasive communications, participation, education, support, role modeling, new structural arrangements, extrinsic rewards, and moving slowly (Grohar-Murray and DiCroce, 2003; Nadler, Shaw, Walton, et al, 1995; Nevis, Lancourt, and Vassallo, 1996; Smith, 1996).

Timothy Galpin (1996) clarifies that resistance may be because people do not know, are not able, or are not willing. When they are not knowing, the leader should communicate the what, why, how, when, who, and where. When they are not able, the leader educates and trains in new skills and management techniques. When they are not willing, the leader sets goals, measures, provides coaching and feedback, rewards, and recognizes.

"If everything seems under control, you're just not going fast enough." —Mario Andretti

Chapter Summary

Chapter 11 covered the following:
Culture of Individuals
  Values
  Attitudes
  Perceptions
  Cognitive Styles

On-line Resources

evolve Additional critical thinking activities, worksheets, and case studies are available on-line at http://evolve.elsevier.com/Marriner/guide/

References

Ashkanasy NM, Wilderom CPM, Peterson MF, editors: *Handbook of organizational culture & climate,* Thousand Oaks, Calif, 2000, Sage.

Barr L, Barr N: *The leadership equation: Leadership, management, and the Myers-Briggs,* Austin, Tex, 1989, Eakin Press.

Belasco JA: *Teaching the elephant to dance: Empowering change in your organization,* New York, 1990, Crown.

Bennis WG, Benne KD, Chin R: *The planning of change,* Fort Worth, Tex, 1969, Holt, Rinehart, & Winston.

Briggs-Myers I : *Gifts differing: Understanding personality type,* Palo Alto, Calif, 1995, S Davies-Black Pub.

Champy J, Nohria N: *Fast forward: The best ideas on managing business change,* Boston, 1996, Harvard Business Review.

Coleman D, Khanna R: *Groupware: Technologies and applications,* Upper Saddle River, NJ, 1995, Prentice Hall.

Collins J: *Good to great,* New York, 2001, Harper Collins.

Conner DR: *Leading at the edge of chaos: How to create the nimble organization,* New York, 1998, John Wiley & Sons.

Conner DR: *Managing at the speed of change,* New York, 1993, Villard.

Cooke R, Rousseau D: Behavioral norms and expectations: A quantitative approach to the assessment of organizational culture, *Group Organ Stud* 13:245-273, 1987.

Deal TE, Kennedy AA: *Corporate cultures: The rites and rituals of corporate life,* Cambridge, Mass, 2000, Persens Pub.

Deevy E: *Creating the resilient organization,* Englewood Cliffs, NJ, 1995, Prentice Hall.

Festinger L: *A theory of cognitive dissonance,* Stanford, Calif, 1957, Stanford University Press.

Fritz R: *Corporate tides: The inescapable laws of organizational structure,* San Francisco, 1996, Berrett-Koehler.

Fritz R: *The path of least resistance for managers: Designing organizations to succeed,* San Francisco, 1999, Berrett-Koehler.

Galpin TJ: *The human side of change: A practical guide to organization redesign,* San Francisco, 1996, Jossey-Bass.

Gardenswartz L, Rowe A: *Diverse teams at work: Capitalizing on the power of diversity,* Burr Ridge, Ill, 1995, Irwin Professional.

Grohar-Murray ME, DiCroce HR: *Leadership and management in nursing,* Stamford, Conn, 2003, Appleton & Lange.

Harper SC: *The forward-focused organization: Visionary thinking and breakthrough leadership to create your company's future,* New York, 2001, American Management Association.

Havelock RG: *The change agent's guide to innovation in education,* Englewood Cliffs, NJ, 1973, Educational Technology Publications.

Jeffreys JS: *Coping with workplace change: Dealing with loss and grief,* Menlo Park, Calif, 1995, Crisp Publications.

Johnson S: *Who moved my cheese?* New York, 1998, GP Putnam's Sons.

Kanter RM: *The change masters,* New York, 1985, Simon & Schuster.

Kanter RM: *When giants learn to dance,* New York, 1989, Simon & Schuster.

Kilmann RH: *Managing beyond the quick fix,* San Francisco, 1991, Jossey-Bass.

Kotter JP: *The heart of change,* Boston, 2002, Harvard Business School Press.

Kotter JP: *Leading change,* Boston, 1996, Harvard Business School Press.

Kubler-Ross E: *On death and dying,* New York, 1997, Simon & Schuster.

Lippitt R, Watson J, Westley B: *The dynamics of planned change,* New York, 1958, Harcourt, Brace & World.

Loden M, Rosener JB, Rosener J: *Workforce America! Managing employee diversity as a vital resource,* Burr Ridge, Ill, 1991, Irwin Professional.

Lundin SC, Christensen J, Paul H: *Fishtales.* New York, 2000, Hyperion.

Marquis BL, Huston CJ: *Leadership roles and management functions in nursing: Theory and application,* ed 2, Philadelphia, 2000, Lippincott.

Marquis BL, Huston CJ: *Management decision making for nurses: 124 case studies,* Philadelphia, 1998, Lippincott.

Martin J: *The great transition: Using the seven disciplines of enterprise engineering to align people, technology, and strategy,* New York, 1995, American Management Association.

Maurer R: *Beyond the wall of resistance,* Austin, Tex, 1996, Bard Books.

McMaster MD: *The intelligence advantage: Organizing for complexity,* Boston, 1996, Butterworth-Heinemann.

Morgan G: *Images of organizations,* ed 2, Thousand Oaks, Calif, 1997, Sage Publications.

Nadler DA, Nadler MB: *Champions of change: How CEOs and their companies are mastering the skills of radical change,* San Francisco, 1998, Jossey-Bass.

Nadler DA, Shaw RB, Walton AE, et al: *Discontinuous change: Leading organizational transformation,* San Francisco, 1995, Jossey-Bass.

Nevis EC, Lancourt J, Vassallo HG: *Intentional revolutions: A seven-point strategy for transforming organizations,* San Francisco, 1996, Jossey-Bass.

Rocchiccioli JT, Tilbury MS: *Clinical leadership in nursing,* Philadelphia, 1998, WB Saunders.

Rogers EM: *Diffusion of innovations,* ed 4, New York, 1995, Free Press.

Schneider WE: *The reengineering alternative: A plan for making your current culture work,* New York, 1999, McGraw Hill Trade.

Senge PM: *The fifth discipline,* New York, 1990, Doubleday,

Senge PM, Kleiner A, Roberts C, et al: *The dance of change: The challenge of sustaining momentum in learning organizations,* New York, 1999, Currency Doubleday.

Senge PM, Kleiner A, Roberts C, et al: *The fifth discipline fieldbook,* New York, 1994, Currency Doubleday.

Shani AB, Lau JB: *Behavior in organizations: An experiential approach,* Boston, 2000, Irwin McGraw Hill.

Smith DK: *Taking charge of change: 10 principles for managing people and performance,* Reading, Mass, 1996, Addison-Wesley.

Smith R: *The 7 levels of change: Create, innovate and motivate with the secrets of the world's largest corporations,* Arlington, Tex, 1997, Summit Publishing Group.

Stewart EC, Bennett MJ: *American cultural patterns: A cross-cultural perspective,* Yarmouth, Me, 1991, Intercultural Press.

Sullivan EJ, Decker PJ: *Effective leadership and management in nursing,* Upper Saddle River, NJ, 2001, Prentice Hall.

Swansburg RC: *Management and leadership for nurse managers,* ed 2, Boston, 1996, Jones and Bartlett.

Swansburg RC, Swansburg RJ: *Introductory management and leadership for nurses: An interactive text,* Boston, 2002, Jones and Bartlett.

Trice HM, Beyer JM: *The cultures of work organizations,* Englewood Cliffs, NJ, 1993, Prentice Hall.

Wheatley MJ: *Leadership and the new science,* San Francisco, 2001, Berrett-Koehler.

Wheatley MJ, Kellner-Rogers M: *A simpler way,* San Francisco, 1996, Berrett-Koehler.

Whetten DA, Cameron KS: *Developing management skills,* ed 4, Reading, Mass, 1998, Addison-Wesley.

Woodward H, Bucholz S, Hess K: *Aftershock: Helping people through corporate change,* New York, 1987, John Wiley & Sons.

Woodward H, Woodward MB: *Navigating through change,* Burr Ridge, Ill, 1994, Richard D Irwin.

Yerkes L: *Fun works: Creating places where people love to work,* San Francisco, 2001, Berrett-Koehler.

Yoder-Wise PS: *Leading and managing in nursing,* ed 2, St Louis, 2002, Mosby.

12

Selection and Development of Personnel

Chapter Overview

Chapter 12 discusses the nursing shortage, leadership and management for recruitment and development of personnel, screening of staff, equal opportunity and affirmative action, multicultural workforce, cultural diversity, sexual preference and gender, generational differences, Americans With Disabilities Act, job analysis, orientation, staff development, career planning, career mapping, group process, and team development.

Chapter Objectives

- Explain why retention measures are at least as important as recruitment efforts.
- Identify three activities related to selection of personnel.
- Define affirmative action.
- Discuss at least four cultural phenomena and their influence on the interviewing process.
- Describe features of job descriptions.
- Differentiate advantages and disadvantages of career ladders.
- Discuss the importance of orientation.
- List at least six ways to accomplish staff development.
- Describe career mapping as a part of career development.
- Diagram four stages of group, or team, process and the major activity in each stage.
- Compare groups and teams.

Major Concepts and Definitions

Personnel persons employed in an agency or department

Recruitment the process of enlisting personnel for employment

Retention capacity to retain employees once they are hired

Affirmative action actions taken to remedy past discriminatory practices

Cultural diversity communication, space, social organization, time, environmental control, and biological variations among cultures

Orientation familiarization with and adaptation to an environment

Job analysis the study of a position to determine what knowledge, skills, aptitudes, and personal characteristics are needed to perform certain responsibilities

Job evaluation process of measuring the remunerative worth of a job in relationship to other positions

Job design specifies what the job requires, job methods, and the relationship among the organizational, social, and personal needs of the worker

Job rotation a horizontal job enlargement technique

Job enrichment vertical approach to job design that uses more abilities and skills of personnel

Job descriptions specifications that are the requirements for the job

Career ladder vertical clinical advancement

Staff development education of the employees

Preceptor teacher or instructor

Mentor a wise and faithful counselor

Career mapping strategic plan for one's career

Group process how the group functions

SELECTION OF PERSONNEL

Leaders predict and plan for the future. They serve as role models, promote the image of the organization, identify and recruit well-qualified people, and assign the new personnel for success for them and the organization. Managers share responsibility for recruitment and retention of well-qualified people. They help establish criteria for selection of personnel and structure interviews to increase validity and reliability of recruitment. They apply their knowledge of legal requirements for hiring and make placement decisions based on employee strengths and the organization's needs (Box 12-1).

DEALING WITH THE NURSING SHORTAGE

Nurses are the main source of care for patients during the most vulnerable times in their lives, making the shortage of nurses a serious problem. Hospitals are the delivery system's most complicated setting of care and the greatest consumer of resources. However, the shortage of nurses is also a grave concern for long-term care organizations and home health agencies. An aging baby boom population with increasing numbers of chronic conditions, higher acuity of care, more complexity of care, and demands for care that exceed capacity are issues. The nursing workforce is also aging at a rate of more than twice that of other workforces in the United States. This nursing shortage impacts patient safety; diminishes hospitals' capacity to treat patients; and contributes to emergency department overcrowding, diversion of emergency patients to other facilities, reduced number of staffed beds, cancellation of elective surgeries, and discontinuation of services.

BOX **12-1** Recruitment Leadership and Management

LEADERSHIP	MANAGEMENT
Predicts the future	Shares responsibility for recruitment and retention of staff
Plans for the future	Structures interview process
Role models for recruitment	Increases validity and reliability of recruitment
Uses interview process to promote image of the organization	Helps establish criteria for selection
Identifies and recruits well-qualified people	Applies knowledge of legal requirements for hiring
Assigns new personnel for success	Makes placement decisions based on employee strengths and organizational needs

Modified from Marquis BL, Huston CJ: *Leadership roles and management functions in nursing: Theory and application*, Philadelphia, 2000, Lippincott.

Conversely, when nursing levels are optimized, there is a positive effect on quality, outcomes, and costs with fewer adverse events; fewer complications such as catheter-related infections, nosocomial infections, decubitus ulcers, and complaints in general; shorter length of stay; lower mortality; more satisfaction of patients, physicians, and staff; and less turnover of staff. The Joint Commission on Accreditation of Healthcare Organizations (JCAHO) in their publication *Health Care at the Crossroads: Strategies for Addressing the Evolving Nursing Crisis* advocates (1) creating cultures of retention in organizations, (2) bolstering the nursing educational infrastructure, and (3) establishing financial incentives for investing in nursing.

To develop a culture of retention the commission recommends providing management training; delegating authority to nurse executives and managers and to staff nurses for patient care resource deployment decisions; recognizing and rewarding hospitals that adopt basic characteristics of "magnet" hospitals (high nurse/patient ratios; nurse autonomy; control over practice setting; nurse participation in organizational policy decisions; good nurse-physician relationships; strong nursing leadership); setting staffing levels based on competency and skill mix appropriate to the patient mix and acuity; measuring, analyzing, and improving staffing effectiveness; adopting zero tolerance policies for abusive behaviors; minimizing paperwork; limiting the

use of mandatory overtime to emergency situations; diversifying the workforce to improve patient care for patients of all backgrounds; adopting information, ergonomic, and other technologies to improve work flow; and adopting fair and competitive compensation and benefit packages.

Nurses have left hospital nursing to work for managed care organizations, insurance companies, pharmaceutical firms, health care technology vendors, medical device vendors, consulting firms, and so on. Many seek regular hours, no nights, no weekends, and no mandatory overtime. However, some nurses like to get overtime with advanced notice. Some states and the federal government have started limiting mandatory overtime. Johnson and Johnson launched a campaign to use advertising to raise the image of nursing and to provide scholarships for students and faculty. Some hospitals use sign-on bonuses to lure nurses away from other hospitals. However, sign-on bonuses do not create employee loyalty. They encourage job hopping to get higher levels of income. There has also been recruitment of foreign nurses that leads to a brain drain and nursing shortage in those countries. Temporary staffing agencies and traveling nurses allow people to earn more money and choose their own hours. That can cause dissatisfaction in the regular staff who are making less and have little control over their work schedules. Although well educated and experienced, temporary nurses may not be familiar with the hospital's policies and practices. Attracting people into nursing seems to be the best option. Some hospitals are targeting high school students for recruitment. Others are considering how to use otherwise retired nurses.

To bolster the nursing education infrastructure, the commission recommends funding nurse faculty positions and student scholarships for all levels of nursing education; increasing federal funding for nursing education; providing fast-track and low-cost opportunities for nurses to get higher levels of education; establishing standardized postgraduate nurse residency programs and funding to support the programs; emphasizing team training in undergraduate and postgraduate nursing education programs; enhancing hospital budgets for nursing orientation, in-service, and continuing education; and creating nursing career ladders that reflect educational levels.

Unfortunately, during the 1990s hospital restructuring, hospital educational budgets to support orientation, in-service, and continuing education were cut. New nurses are receiving less orientation than in the past. Although new drugs, procedures, and technologies have accelerated, there is less in-service education. Nursing residency programs tend to be home grown and vary in length, structure, and content.

Computer-based training, distance education, and simulation programs may require less time and resources than traditional methods. They can be used to select content priorities.

To establish financial incentives for investing in nursing, the commission recommended making new federal monies available to invest in nursing services; requiring demonstrated achievement of criteria and goals to continue receiving federal monies; basing new reimbursement incentives on evidence-based, nursing-sensitive indicators; and aligning private payer and federal reimbursement incentives to reward effective nurse staffing. By connecting quality of nursing service, patient safety, and clinical outcomes to funding, nursing should move from the cost side to the asset side of the balance sheet. That would recognize and reward good nursing care (Joint Commission on Accreditation of Healthcare Organizations, accessed 7/23/03).

RECRUITMENT AND RETENTION

"If a man proceeds confidently in the direction of his dreams and endeavors to live the life he has imagined, he will meet with success unexpected in common hours." —Henry David Thoreau

The acquisition of qualified people in any agency is critical for the establishment, maintenance, and growth of the organization. Therefore active recruitment is important, and the attraction of qualified applicants is the first step in selection of personnel. Modes for active recruitment include employee recommendations and word of mouth; advertisements in local newspapers, nursing organization bulletins, and nursing journals; recruitment literature, such as fliers and newsletters; posters; career days; job fairs; contacts with schools' graduating classes; placement services; open houses; nursing conventions; and frequent, low-cost, credit-carrying continuing education courses for outsiders, as well as employees (Box 12-2).

Word of mouth can be very effective, but it can also lead to the hiring of friends and relatives of the current workforce; this practice may foster

---

BOX 12-2 Modes for Recruitment

Employee recommendations
Word of mouth
Advertisements
Fliers
Newsletters
Bulletins
Posters
Career days
Job fairs
Placement services
Open houses
Nursing conventions

nepotism and violate equal opportunity employment requirements. The use of advertisements in professional journals, in newspapers, and on radio and television; employment agencies; and contacts with schools' graduating classes offers the prospective employer a broader field for selection and more opportunities to hire from minority groups. Hiring minority group members may require active recruitment to meet public policy.

Each institution should have someone who is responsible for recruitment. Recruiters should know nursing qualifications and the needs of the institution. They should be able to represent the institution with candor and enthusiasm. It is important that the recruiter relate well to people. Referrals from employees should be sought and in-house applicants encouraged; however, favoritism should not be shown. To aid in the selection of the best candidate for the job, an adequate budget should be provided for necessary advertisements, and these advertisements should depict an institution that cares about employees and patients. That image should also be reflected at open houses, during conventions, and at high school and college career days.

The content of advertising is more important than the form. The recruiter should determine the needs and desires of potential applicants and demonstrate how the institution will meet those needs. New graduates are likely to be interested in thorough orientation, in-service education, staff development, and intern programs. Some nurses will be interested in tuition reimbursement and release time to work on educational degrees. Single people will be more interested in health benefits than married people whose spouses have family coverage. Older nurses will be increasingly interested in retirement plans. Refresher courses, chartered buses for people who live in suburban areas, child care programs, part-time work, and flexible personnel policies may appeal to inactive nurses. The nurse recruiter needs to assess nurses' interests and show how the institution can address their concerns.

The recruiter should respond to inquiries immediately. Records of inquiries noting the origin (how the job applicant learned of the opening) and disposition (hired or not and length of tenure) should be compiled and evaluated. The most productive recruitment method should be maximized. Out-of-town or out-of-state applicants should be assisted with information about the community and housing.

The major sources of personnel are persons seeking their first jobs, dissatisfied employees, and unemployed individuals. These classifications are important, for the categories indicate types of information the nursing manager should obtain, and they influence the selection process. Recent graduates or nurses who have not practiced since graduation may have a limited idea of job opportunities. Their choice of a first job may be strongly influenced by their education, achievement level, geographical preference, salary, mate's occupation, and peer pressure. They are likely to take several jobs before settling down. This variety of jobs, along with growing family responsibilities and maturity, helps develop the nurse's capabilities.

The dissatisfied employees are often not actively seeking other employment but are likely to be receptive to news of openings and job offers. If nursing managers attribute the dissatisfaction to the misuse of the person's talents and abilities, they may explore how to employ that person more effectively within their own agency. Job dissatisfaction is not uncommon, since every job has disadvantages. Agencies that require special job skills should expect applications from nurses who are looking for a better job with fewer disadvantages.

Hiring an unemployed worker who has been released from a previous job because of an infraction or a quarrel with the previous employer demands careful assessment. The nursing manager may wish to hire nurses who were fired because they refused to falsify records or perform a task for which they were not adequately prepared. They would not want to hire a nurse who was terminated because of high absenteeism and irresponsibility, unless the nurse could adequately explain the situation and assure the nursing manager that the problem has been resolved. For instance, the prospective employee might have been caring for a dying child at that time or having a marital crisis that has since ended in divorce.

It is unlikely that nurse applicants have been laid off from previous jobs because of slack times. If so, the nursing manager should consider the chances of the nurses' returning to their old jobs when the slack has ended. Seniority and other vested interests may influence nurses' desires to return to their previous positions.

Because of the costs of recruiting, selecting, and training employees, the decreased quality of care while orienting new workers, and the emotional drain of turnover on continuing employees, serious attention should be given to retention efforts. Exit interviews, particularly anonymous questionnaires, can help identify the reasons people resign. Posttermination questions mailed to the homes of former employees 1 or 2 months after their resignation may obtain more accurate information than does the exit interview. After a period of time has elapsed, a person may be less emotional and more objective with some distance from the job and may feel more anonymous with less fear of retaliation. In addition, attitude surveys can be used with current employees to identify sources of dissatisfaction and concern. Focus groups can be used to identify and solve problems. Once stressors are identified, strategies to reduce them can be planned. It is important to meet personnel's psychosocial needs for advancement, responsibility, achievement, and recognition. Nurses want input into decision making and control over their own lives.

SCREENING OF POTENTIAL STAFF

Investment in well-qualified nurses can produce a high rate of return; and errors, whether they be failure to hire a promising nurse or hiring someone who fails to achieve the organization's expectations, can be expensive mistakes. In general there are three underlying philosophies in the screening process:

1. The manager should screen out applicants who do not fit the agency's image. Although this practice is common among some corporations, it is not a standard procedure for selecting health care personnel.
2. The manager should try to fit the job to a promising applicant. Examples include part-time positions, split-shift hours, and opportunities for handicapped people.
3. Usually the manager should try to fit the applicant to the job. This philosophy assumes that both the person and the position are unique.

The essential and desirable qualities for the applicant can be identified. Each of the search and screen committee members can list what she thinks are essential and desirable qualities for an applicant for a specific job; the committee members can then discuss the qualities and come to consensus. Next, a qualification assessment form can be developed listing the essential and desirable qualities with yes, ?, and no columns for if the applicant has the quality or not and with a column for comments.

Application Forms and Resumes

Once the applicants have been attracted, they should submit biographical data. The application form is a quick way to collect demographical information. Data in the personal history— educational background, work experience, and other pertinent information—can be used to do the following:

- Determine whether the applicant meets minimal hiring requirements, such as minimal educational level or minimal job experience
- Furnish background data useful in planning the selection interview
- Obtain names of references who may be contacted for additional information about the applicant's work experience and general character

- Collect information for personnel administration, that is, Social Security number, number of dependents, and so forth

Letters of Reference

Letters of recommendation may be requested from references listed on the application form, previous employers, or both. However, these letters may be inaccurate and misleading because the people writing may not have had sufficient exposure to the nurses to become familiar with their capabilities, or they may not have even known the nurse. Because of rapid turnover of nursing personnel, it is possible that few current staff members worked with the previous employee, and the current manager, who joined the agency after the applicant had resigned, may have to write the letter of reference based on an inadequate personnel file. The applicant may not know the current whereabouts of previous managers. To prevent these problems, employees could ask that a letter of reference be sent to a placement bureau at the time of termination, but this measure does not necessarily solve the problem. They have no assurance that the letter writers can express themselves well or are even willing to be accurate.

The preceding discussion indicates that letters of reference should be used cautiously. More emphasis should be placed on comments made by previous employers and coworkers, because they tend to give more critical evaluations than do subordinates and personal acquaintances. Most emphasis should be placed on characteristics consistently cited and on the general tone of the letters.

Interview

A preemployment interview to predict job success should be conducted with the most qualified applicants. Information obtained from the application form and letters of reference should be taken into consideration during the interview. The purposes of the interview are to obtain information, to give information, and to determine if the applicant meets the requirements for the position. The interviewer judges the applicant's dependability, willingness to assume responsibility for the job, willingness and ability to work with others, interest in the job, adaptability, consistency of goals with available opportunities, and conformance of manners and appearance to job requirements. The interviewer answers questions, explains policies and procedures, and helps acquaint the applicant with the position. Finally, the interviewer must predict whether the applicant's overall performance will be satisfactory. The value of the interview is determined by the interviewer's ability to evaluate applicants and to predict accurately their future success.

The interview has definite purposes and should avoid social chitchat, although a brief warm-up period may help put the interviewee at ease. One of the main purposes is to learn about the prospective employee. Therefore it behooves the interviewer to concentrate on listening, as well as to provide necessary information and answer questions from the applicant. Managers should avoid giving clues about what pleases or displeases them, should not be argumentative, and should try to avoid premature judgment. They should also beware of the halo effect: judgment based on appearances. Although individuals wear clothing that reflects their personality, they are likely to select clothes for the interview that project the image they wish to convey.

It is advisable to train managers in the art of interviewing. Training might include methods of establishing rapport with an interviewee, interviewing techniques, therapeutic communication, and predicting applicant job performance. It is helpful to construct an interview recording form designed for the needs of the agency or for a specific position. Use of the job description to define and specify job dimensions on the form increases interviewer reliability. A personal profile of what the person hired should be, including education, experience, abilities, aptitudes, and interests, is helpful. Standardization of the interview promotes nondiscriminatory hiring practices and is particularly important when more than one person does the interviewing.

The heading of the form contains the date, name of the applicant, position desired, and the interviewer's name. The body categorizes traits required for the position. This allows the interviewer to assess applicants more systematically. One area might be work history. Does the applicants' work history indicate that they have the ability to learn and understand the requirements of the job for which they are applying? More specifically, is there any evidence of lack of ability? Have they had past experience in performing the same or similar tasks? Are they familiar with the equipment and procedures? Have they had special project or task force assignments? Have they had job progression? Education is another area to be evaluated. Have applicants had adequate formal education? Is there evidence of on-the-job training? Have they participated in continuing education or in self-initiated skill development by reading books and journals and watching related television specials? Are they active in professional organizations?

Certainly applicants' dependability demands assessment. Is it likely that they will have a good attendance record and maintain good work habits? Or is there evidence of poor work habits or work performance? What do past attendance and safety records indicate? Of equal concern is applicants' sense of responsibility. Will they seek assistance when needed and take initiative when appropriate to get the job done? Will they see jobs through to the end? Is there evidence of past independent thought and action, or do they tend to blame others for problems? Finally, are they capable of assuming leadership when required?

Are applicants cooperative and able to get along with others and work well as team members, or do they prefer to work alone? Is there evidence of success or friction with managers, peers, and staff associates? Are they open to criticism, or do they react excessively? Are applicants involved in the community? Have they been open and candid during the interview?

Job interest, poise, manners, appearance, and aspirations are other areas to investigate.

The interviewer greets the applicant, introduces herself to the applicant, and makes brief comments about the agency and the position available. The interviewer confirms the position for which the person is applying and explains the plan for the interview. Information on the application is discussed, and clarification is sought if necessary. The applicant's qualifications are discussed, preferably using the structured interview format. If the applicant appears qualified, the agency and position can be discussed in more detail, and subsequent hiring procedures can be explained before the interview is terminated.

During the interview the interviewer explains the purpose and plan of the interview. This helps create a positive climate. The interviewer learns the most by listening rather than talking and can encourage the job candidate to talk freely by asking open-ended questions. These are nondirective questions that help reveal feelings and attitudes. Examples of nondirective questions are as follows: What qualifies you for this job? What aspects of your last job appealed to you? How were your relations with your peers?

Closed-ended questions are directive and can often be answered "yes" or "no." They solicit less information than open-ended questions but are appropriate for objective and factual information. The following are examples of closed-ended questions: Who was your last employer? How long did you work for that agency? Did you get along with your coworkers? Do you think you are qualified for this job?

The funnel technique incorporates both open-ended and closed-ended questions. When using the funnel technique, the interviewer starts with an open-ended question, such as "What subjects did you like most in school?" This gets objective information and sets a nonthreatening tone. The scope of the discussion is then funneled by asking a self-appraisal question, such as "Why do you think you liked those courses in particular?" This elicits subjective information. The interviewer closes the discussion of a particular subject by asking direct questions to clarify the self-appraisal. A direct question might be, "What classes did you take for your nursing electives?"

A grid of topics to explore and the funnel technique can help the interviewer sequence questions in a logical order and decide what kind of questions to ask. Initially it may be helpful to fill in the topics and potential questions. The questions may be modified during the interview (Table 12-1).

After obtaining information from the candidate, it is appropriate for the interviewer to share information about the job, policies, the agency, and how the interviewee will be informed of the decision. The applicant is given an opportunity to ask questions. The interviewer closes the interview by telling the applicant when and how she can expect to hear the decision. For example, the interviewer can say, "I will be interviewing a few more applicants this week. You can expect to hear from me by the first of next week" or "You should receive a letter regarding our decision within 2 weeks."

The facts collected during the interview are used as the basis for assumptions or inferences. They should be checked throughout the interview as new information is collected. It is possible to make both positive and negative assumptions from the same information. For example, if an applicant did not work for 3 months between jobs, the negative assumption could be that the person was escaping, undirected, or lazy. A positive inference could be that the applicant was clarifying goals and fulfilling personal objectives. Inferences are often more reflective of the person making them than of the applicant, thus making it particularly important to test interpretations.

Women, men, minority applicants, and persons with disabilities should be treated in the same professional manner. The same general questions and the same standards should be required for all applicants. One should follow a structured interview plan to help achieve fairness in interviewing and should treat all applicants with fairness, equality, and consistency.

Interviewers can talk about applicants' qualifications, abilities, experiences, education, and interests; the duties and responsibilities of the job; where the job is located; travel, equipment, and facilities available; and the organization's missions, programs, and achievements. These are acceptable, but one may not ask about lineage, national origin, race, gender, age, marital status, number or age of children, former addresses, religious affiliations, or handicaps. Although one may ask about academic and

TABLE **12-1**   Topics and Questions to Be Explored During an Employment Interview

TOPICS TO EXPLORE	OPEN-ENDED QUESTIONS	SELF-APPRAISAL QUESTIONS	DIRECT QUESTIONS
Education	Why did you choose to go to that school?	What courses were most useful to you, and how were they useful?	What courses did you take as electives?
Prior employment	Where have you worked?	What did you like best about your job? What did you like least about your last job?	How long did you work there? What was your title? On what service areas did you work?
Life experiences	What life experiences have you had that help qualify you for this job?	How will raising your own children help you in this job?	How long have you spoken Spanish? How frequently do you use sign language?
Professional	What are your professional goals?	How do you plan to accomplish your goals?	What do you plan to be doing 5 years from now?

professional education, schools attended, and ability to read, write, and speak a foreign language, the interviewer may not ask about the racial or religious affiliation of the schools, the date of the schooling, or one's native language. One may ask about professional organizations but not all memberships. A photograph may not be required before employment. The name and address of a person to contact in case of an emergency may be solicited but not the name and address of a relative. Inquiries about relatives who work in the agency or name and address of parents if the applicant is a minor are acceptable. Inquiry into actual convictions that relate to job performance can be asked but not questions relating to arrests.

Discriminatory behavior is improper even when it is not intended, and appearance is as important as reality. Questions not related to the job have been used in a discriminatory way and should be avoided. Because improper significance might be given to questions regarding marriage plans or family matters, one should not inquire about marital status or nonmarital arrangements; what the significant other does or earns; how the significant other feels about the applicant's work life, travel arrangements, or possible relocation; medical history concerning pregnancy or any questions relating to pregnancy; or whether there are children, how many, and their ages. One should use either first or last names for all candidates and persons involved in the recruitment.

Applicants with disabilities should also be asked questions relevant to the job. Whether the individual needs any reasonable accommodations or assistance during the hiring or interviewing process and the individual's ability to perform essential job functions with or without reasonable accommodations may be discussed. One should avoid discussions of past or present serious illnesses or physical or mental conditions; the nature or severity of an apparent disability; problems an individual may have had because of a disability; or how the person became disabled.

Because people are presumed innocent until proven guilty, records of arrest without convictions are meaningless. One may inquire about an applicant's conviction record for jobs where that is relevant.

When discussing the location, one should mention the special features: lakes, parks, and urban areas; sports, cultural, and other recreational features; and renting and buying options.

One should avoid references to the applicant's personal happiness and not suggest that one is interested in hiring a woman, minority person, or person with a disability as a statistic to improve the affirmative action/equal opportunity profile. Applicants are being considered for a position based on qualifications.

Interviews do have limitations. Reliability and validity are questionable. The same interviewer has higher interrater reliability than different interviewers. Interrater reliability is lower in unstructured interviews than in structured interviews. Even if the interview has reliability, it may not be a valid predictor of job performance. Validity tends to increase with a team approach. Interviewers seem to be more influenced by unfavorable than by favorable information. Attitudes and biases of interviewers affect how applicants are rated. Fortunately, there are interventions to reduce subjectivity. Multiple interviews using a team approach with a structured interview format for each job classification reduce biases. Training people how to do interviews is helpful. Scenarios can be used to check problem-solving ability of applicants (Arthur, 1998; Champy, 1995; Marquis and Huston, 2000; Sullivan and Decker, 2001).

Testing

Personality and interest testing is sometimes done but does require a trained psychologist. Ability tests are rarely used when hiring nurses. However, in-basket exercises, problem analysis, mock selection interviews, oral presentations, and debates have been used to select management personnel. Testing is useful for selecting clerical help. Tests can measure knowledge and skills possessed

R SEARCH Perspective 12-1

Data from Krugman M, Smith K, Goode CJ: A clinical advancement program: Evaluating 10 years of progressive change. *JONA* 30(5):215-225, 2000.

Purpose: The purpose of this study was to report the evolution of a clinical advancement program, UEXCEL, at a western teaching hospital and the outcomes associated with evaluation over time.

Methods: Structure and progression of program development and change were outlined. Evaluation data were collected using a 23-item clinical ladder satisfaction scale developed by Strzelecki. Data were collected in 1993, 1994, 1996, and 1998 using standard survey methods. The University of Colorado data were trended across units and time periods and were compared with other institutional evaluation data sets.

Results/conclusions: Improvement in nurse satisfaction with the UEXCEL program was steady and incremental. Satisfaction improved after each program revision. A significant demographic variable over time is the correlation between higher registered nurse education and program satisfaction. The authors concluded that successful clinical advancement programs need to balance professional dimensions and requirements for a clinical ladder with significant human resource rewards to create a model that motivates nurses to advance in their professional development, contribute to improved patient care outcomes, and commit to advancing the profession.

and estimate the rate at which the applicant can acquire the knowledge and skills required for the position. They measure clerical and mechanical aptitudes, general intelligence, and mental, perceptual, and psychomotor abilities.

EQUAL OPPORTUNITY AND AFFIRMATIVE ACTION

The employer is subject to a number of legal requirements that have been enacted to provide equal opportunity and affirmative action in the workplace. Requirements for providing equal opportunity are contained in Title VI and Title VII of the Civil Rights Act of 1964, Title IX of the Education Amendments of 1972, the Equal Pay Act of 1963, and the Age Discrimination in Employment Act of 1967. Affirmative action requirements are contained in Executive Order 11246, Section 503 of the Rehabilitation Act of 1973, and in Section 402 of the Vietnam Era Veterans Readjustment Assistance Act of 1974.

The Equal Pay Act of 1963 and as amended by the Education Amendments of 1972 makes it illegal to pay lower wages to employees of one gender when the jobs are of equal responsibility and accountability and are performed under similar working conditions when they require equal effort in mental and physical exertion and equal skill, experience, training, education, and ability (Yoder-Wise, 2003).

Title VI and Title VII of the Civil Rights Act of 1964, as amended by the Equal Employment Act of 1972, prohibit discrimination because of race, color, religion, gender, or national origin in any term, condition, or privilege of employment. Title IX of the Education Amendments of 1972 prohibits discrimination on the basis of gender in any educational program or activity receiving federal financial assistance. Prohibition of sexual discrimination applies to both males and females. A male successfully sued a skilled nursing facility for refusing to hire him in *Little Forest Medical Center of Akron v. Ohio Civil Rights Commission*

(1993). Discrimination is not an issue when bona fide occupational qualifications (BFOQs) are considered. For example, if an employee must be able to lift 150 pounds, any man or woman who could lift 150 pounds would be a viable applicant (O'Keefe, 2001).

The Age Discrimination in Employment Act of 1967 makes discrimination against older men and women employees by employers of 20 or more persons, employment agencies, or unions illegal. A 1986 amendment prohibits discrimination against persons older than 40 years. A 1978 amendment prohibited mandatory retirement under the age of 70 years and a 1987 amendment removed even that restriction except in certain job categories. Some possible exceptions include poor performance evaluations and limited occupational qualifications, such as lack of physical endurance. *Goodhouse v. Magnolia Hospital* (1996) involved a 53-year-old nurse who was terminated after 23 years of employment when there was a reduction in force. She applied for another position that was available in the facility but was not hired. She sued for age discrimination, she was awarded $100,000, and the hospital was ordered to reinstate her. Age discrimination settlements have averaged more dollars than cases involving disability, race, or gender discrimination. Age-based harassment, such as age-based comments, is also a violation of employee rights. In *Madel v. PCI Marketing, Inc.* (1997), the employer was held liable for using the word "old" with lewd language and for referring to the sleeping quarters as the "geriatric wing" (Grohar-Murray and DiCroce, 2003; O'Keefe, 2001; Sullivan and Decker, 2001; Yoder-Wise, 2003).

Executive Order (EO) 11246 (as amended by EO 11375) prohibits all government contracting agencies from discriminating against any employee or applicant for employment and requires that contractors take affirmative action to ensure that applicants are employed and that employees are treated during employment without regard to their race, color, religion, gender, or national origin.

Sections 503 and 504 of the Rehabilitation Act of 1973 prohibit discrimination because of handicap in employment and in programs and activities receiving federal funds. Section 503, in addition, requires contractors to take affirmative action to employ and advance in employment qualified handicapped individuals.

The Pregnancy Discrimination Act of 1978 prohibits sexual discrimination against women who are or could become pregnant. An employer may not refuse to hire a woman because of pregnancy if she is able to perform the major aspects of a job, and she must be allowed to work as long as she is able to do her job. However, the act does not mandate that pregnant women receive preferential treatment. A pregnant nurse was fired because of refusing to care for a patient with acquired immunodeficiency syndrome (AIDS) in *Alabama v. Flowers Hospital, Inc.* (1994). The Supreme Court ruled that policies that are written for fetal protection violate Title VII in the *UAW v. Johnson Controls, Inc.* (1991) case. Consequently employers can inform a job applicant or employee of risks, but the woman must be allowed to decide whether or not she accepts a job assignment. Disability benefits and sick leave for women unable to work because of pregnancy-related reasons are to be granted on the same basis as for employees unable to work for other medical reasons (Grohar-Murray and DiCroce, 2003; O'Keefe, 2001).

Section 402 of the Vietnam Era Veterans Readjustment Assistance Act of 1974 requires contractors to take affirmative action to employ and advance in employment qualified disabled veterans and veterans of the Vietnam era.

Affirmative action in Executive Order 11246 requires the employer to make extra efforts to recruit, employ, and promote qualified members of formerly excluded groups. It is based on the premise that unless action is taken to overcome systematic exclusion and discrimination based on national origin, race, color, gender, or religion, employment practices will perpetuate the status quo indefinitely. In addition to the elimination of all existing discriminatory practices, affirmative action requires actions beyond neutral nondiscrimination.

In 1980, the Equal Employment Opportunity Commission (EEOC) established guidelines indicating that sexual harassment in the workplace violates Title VII and making employers liable for an act of sexual harassment committed by an employee even if the employer had no prior knowledge of the reported sexual harassment. The guidelines define sexual harassment as including conditions for which (1) submission to sexual advances is explicitly or implicitly a condition of an individual's employment, (2) submission to or rejection of sexual advances is used as a basis for employment decisions, and (3) the sexual advances interfere with work performance or create an intimidating, hostile, or offensive work environment. The victim does not have to be of the opposite gender or the one harassed but can be anyone affected by the offensive behavior. Examples of a hostile working environment can include questions or comments about one's sexual life; e-mails of a sexual nature; computer screen savers that are sexually explicit and in view of others; offensive comments of a sexual nature; gossip, jokes, or stories with sexual content; cartoons, drawings, graphics, photographs, or posters of a sexual nature; obscene gestures; whistles; or touching the body (Grohar-Murray and DiCroce, 2003; O'Keefe, 2001; Sullivan and Decker, 2001).

The Immigration Reform and Control Act of 1986 mandates that employers verify the identity of employees and sanctions employers that knowingly hire an unauthorized alien (Grohar-Murray and DiCroce, 2003).

The Family and Medical Leave Act (FMLA) of 1993 provides job security for unpaid leave while a male or female employee is caring for a new infant of the employee or foster care placement or adoption; or is caring for a spouse, child, or parent who has a serious health problem; or is personally seriously ill. The act helps balance the demands of work and home for single parents or two-parent households where the single parent or both parents are employed full-time, putting job security and parenting at odds. Aging parents are also putting increasing demands on working children. To be eligible for the family and medical leave, the employee must have worked at least 12 months and at least 1250 hours during the previous 12 months. The employee is eligible for 12 weeks of unpaid leave in a 12-month period. The employer may require the employee to use all or part of any paid vacation, personal leave, or sick leave as part of the 12-week family leave. The employee's job and benefits are protected during the leave, and on return, the employee is to receive the original or equivalent job with equivalent pay (O'Keefe, 2001; Yoder-Wise, 2003).

Equal employment opportunity (EEO) policy concerns implementing employment practices that do not discriminate against or impair employment opportunities of protected groups. Affirmative action (AA) differs from EEO in that it enhances employment of protected groups. A major portion of an affirmative action program must recognize and remove barriers and establish affirmative measures to remedy past discriminatory practices. Such measures include additional aid to prepare disadvantaged people for jobs. It is noteworthy that Supreme Court rulings state that such measures are not restricted to workers who have individually been victims of discrimination.

Development of an affirmative action program includes the addition of affirmative action intent to the agency's philosophy; development of affirmative action policies and procedures; appointment of a manager responsible for the program; inclusion of affirmative action responsibilities in appropriate job descriptions; and publication of the affirmative action commitment internally to all employees and externally to sources for recruitment, to minority and women's organizations, to organizations of handicapped individuals, to appropriate veterans' service organizations, to community agencies, and to the community in general.

The affirmative action policy is disseminated internally by including it in the policy manual, annual reports, and other media, such as the agency newsletter. It can also be posted on bulletin boards. Nondiscrimination clauses are included in union agreements. Articles about the affirmative action program, its progress, and the activities of disadvantaged workers are published in agency publications. When employees are pictured in handbooks or advertising brochures, minority and nonminority men and women should be included.

Top administration should discuss the intent of the policy and individuals' responsibilities for its implementation with management personnel. Special meetings should be scheduled with all employees, and the policy should be discussed in orientation and management training classes.

A workforce analysis of job classifications by departments is the first step toward identifying where minorities, women, and men are currently employed and discovering areas of concentration and underuse. The availability of minorities, women, and handicapped persons having requisite skills is considered when determining whether there is underuse: How many minorities, women, and handicapped persons are in the geographical area from which the institution recruits? What percentage of the total workforce in the area are minorities, women, and handicapped persons? How many are unemployed? How many can be recruited from the local community or the nation? Are there training programs available to prepare minorities, women, and handicapped people with skills the agency can use? Can the agency prepare minorities, women, and handicapped personnel? An agency may be able to prepare nurses' aides or assistants but would need to rely on other institutions to prepare licensed practical, or vocational, nurses (LPNs or LVNs) and registered nurses (RNs). Are there disadvantaged people already employed by the agency who are transferable or promotable? Programs to correct underuse must be developed when there are fewer minorities, women, and handicapped persons in a job classification than would be expected by their availability.

Once management has completed its use and availability analysis, it establishes goals and timetables to improve use. To correct identifiable deficiencies, management needs goals that are measurable and attainable. Goals for minorities and women are presented separately. Those goals and the timetables for completion, along with supportive data and analysis, are major parts of the written affirmative action program.

Programs to achieve these goals must be developed and implemented next. This phase begins with a review of the employment process to identify barriers. Recruitment procedures and the selection process—including job requirements, job descriptions, application forms, testing, and interviewing—are examined. The upward mobility system, including training, assignments, job progressions, seniority, transfers, promotions, and disciplinary action policies, is reviewed. Wage and salary structure, benefits, conditions of employment, and union contracts are also studied. Appropriate changes are made, and an internal audit and reporting system to monitor and evaluate the affirmative action program is implemented. Records of referrals, placements, transfers, promotions, and terminations should be maintained for 3 years. Formal reports regarding attainment of goals and timetables are prepared on a regular basis. The manager of the affirmative action program reviews the reports with other managers, advises top administration of the program's effectiveness, and submits recommendations for improvement of unsatisfactory performance.

Compliance status is not judged solely by whether goals have been met by the time set for achieving them. A review of the program's content and the efforts made toward realization of the goals are factors that are considered in determining its effectiveness.

It is important to keep in mind that goals are not inflexible quotas that must be met but are targets that are reasonably attainable through good faith efforts. Goals therefore should be realistic, measurable, and achievable by the time established (Doverspike, Taylor, Arthur, 2000).

LEGAL INTERVIEWING QUESTIONS

When interviewing applicants for positions, one should remember that some employment inquiries are acceptable, whereas others are not (Table 12-2). The purpose of the question determines its propriety. Appropriate inquiries have a

TABLE **12-2** Legal Interviewing Guidelines

SUBJECT	MAY ASK:	MAY NOT ASK:
Age	Nothing	Any question to determine age
Arrest record	Nothing	Any questions to determine arrests
Availability for Saturday, Sunday, or holiday work	Whether the applicant can meet the work schedule	Any question about religious observance
Availability for weekend or evening work or travel	Whether the applicant can meet the work requirements	Any question unrelated to work requirements
Citizenship	Whether the applicant is legally able to work	Questions to identify country of origin
Convictions	Whether the applicant has pled guilty to, pled "no contest" to, or been convicted of anything other than a misdemeanor or summary offense	Whether the applicant has pled guilty to, pled "no contest" to, or been convicted of a crime
Disability	Whether the applicant, with or without reasonable accommodation, is able to perform the functions of the job	Whether the applicant has ever been disabled, suffered from a work-related injury, received workers' compensation, had a major illness, missed work because of illness, has any physical defects that interfere with some work or the position for which the person is applying
Education	About the vocational, academic, or professional education and schools attended	Any question designed to determine protected status
Family status	Whether the applicant can attend orientation and meet the requirements of the job	Whether the applicant is married, single, or divorced; ages of children or parents; plans to have children; spouse's job; family responsibilities
Languages	What foreign languages are read, spoken, or written and degree of acquired fluency	How or where the skill was acquired
National origin	Nothing	Any questions about lineage, ancestry, national origin, descent, or place of birth
Organizations	About memberships in professional organizations related to the job	Any questions about membership that would indicate race, creed, gender, national origin, religion, or an affiliation with a labor organization
Pregnancy	About the applicant's anticipated duration of time on the job or ability to meet orientation or attendance requirements	Any questions designed to learn about current, past, or future pregnancies
Relatives	About the names of applicant's relatives employed with the agency or competitor	The names and addresses of relatives other than those employed by the agency or competitor
Religion	Nothing	Any questions about religious denomination, church, pastor, or religious holidays observed
Gender	Nothing	Any questions

direct relationship to the applicant's capacity to do the job. Inappropriate questions may receive answers that will limit the person's opportunities because of ancestry, race, color, age, religion, gender, marital or parental status, or handicap. Some information needed for payroll or personnel purposes—such as age, proof of citizenship, and number of dependents—can be obtained after the person has been hired. Questions about the applicant's religious preferences, gender, marital status, credit rating, number and ages of dependents, or marital and family plans are not appropriate. Questions that would identify the person as being over 40 years of age or general questions about disabilities are not acceptable. Applicants may be asked to prove they are over 18 years of age and able to perform job-related functions. One can ask for an address and length of residence in a city or state but not for rental or home ownership information. Questions about ability to read, write, or speak a language are acceptable, but questions about one's primary language or the way one acquired the ability to use a language are unacceptable. One's legal right to remain in the United States can be questioned, but questions about naturalization of parents or spouse are unacceptable. The applicant may be asked to list membership in clubs, organizations, societies, and associations, excluding those that would indicate the national origin, race, color, or religion of the membership. Requests for all memberships are not appropriate. General questions about military service are inappropriate.

When interviewing minority candidates, one should not pretend interest in, or knowledge of, an ethnic culture or use ethnic vernacular or a foreign language one does not speak well. It is inappropriate to talk about one's minority friends or to expect the candidate to know all other minority members. Lack of eye contact should not be judged negatively, because some cultures interpret direct eye contact as disrespectful. The interviewer should be aware that body language and voice tone give messages that provoke confidence or mistrust and suggest support or indifference.

The manager should be aware that some minority applicants may not have well-defined aspirations and career goals because their opportunities may have been limited and they may feel they have little control over their careers. Minority applicants often have frequently changed jobs in search of better pay. Therefore steady work and work progression histories may be of little use in evaluating minority applicants who have had limited opportunities (Cahn, 2002; Cox, 2001).

MULTICULTURAL WORKFORCE

Multiculturalism is about working together toward a cohesive society while understanding, respecting, and protecting cultural differences. Diversity comes in many forms: race, ethnicity, culture, age, gender, sexual preference, education, income, physical attributes, skills, learning styles, mental abilities, and parental status.

Prejudice is an unreasonable bias that is formed before facts are known. It is an opinion or judgment that is often unfavorable. It may be suspicion, intolerance, or even hatred of others who are different from the opinion holder. It may result in judgments or actions that are harmful to another. To stop and overcome prejudice and to be open minded, do the following: Try to get to know people who are different from you. Eat at foreign restaurants. See some foreign films. Check the library for books, films, and videotapes about other countries and cultures. Attend diversity training. Attend a college course on diversity. Learn a new language. Participate in community work with organizations serving people who are culturally different. Travel to other countries. Write to a pen pal, and tell each other about your lives. Invite someone to your home. See the person not the label. Even if you have had a bad experience with a group, give everyone a chance. Do not judge everyone in a classification the same. Recognize feelings of prejudice, and deal with them (Cox, 2001).

Discrimination is the act of treating someone unfairly because of differences. That may be based on stereotypes. Stereotypes are fixed patterns so we may see everyone in a classification as alike instead of as individuals.

Ethnocentrism is a tendency to view other groups or cultures in terms of one's own. It is a belief of inherent superiority of one's own group or culture that is often accompanied by a feeling of contempt for other groups and cultures.

To create and maintain a diversity-friendly workplace there should be recruitment of diverse individuals, implementation of policies and procedures that support diversity, and no tolerance of "isms" (Cox, 2001; Tayeb, 1996).

CULTURAL DIVERSITY

People bring with them assumptions, attitudes, and behaviors related to their cultural heritage. The recognition of and respect for cultural differences help foster positive relationships. Leaders and managers need to have an awareness of how their own cultural background affects their performance.

Individuals within a cultural group vary widely, but the majority of individuals within a cultural group generally agree on common norms and traits. Communication is an important aspect of one's culture. It includes spoken and nonverbal expressions. Misunderstandings can result from silence, words used, tone of voice, pitch, and body movements. What a person says and does can be interpreted in a variety of ways. Unless the person's cultural heritage is understood, an interpretation could be wrong. Someone speaking loudly with animation might be misinterpreted as being aggressive, pushy, or rude. Someone speaking in a soft, low voice may be viewed as passive, afraid, or shy.

Context of speech refers to use of emotion in communications. Mexican Americans, Irish, and Italian Americans often use emotions, whereas African Americans, German Americans, and Jewish people rarely do. Kinesics is the use of gestures, stances, and eye movements when communicating. Alaskan Eskimos blink to indicate agreement. Irish and Italian Americans use

gestures, stances, and eye movements to emphasize points. Persons in certain socioeconomic groups in India are to avoid eye contact with persons in lower or higher socioeconomic groups and persons of the opposite gender.

Dialect and language styles often differ among cultural groups. Some cultures convey feelings and emotions through touch. Others find touch intrusive or consider it to have sexual connotations.

There are four zones of interpersonal space: (1) intimate, (2) personal, (3) social consultative, and (4) public. Each zone has distinctive distance and intimacy techniques for verbal and nonverbal communication. The intimate zone is 0 to 18 inches, is reserved for close personal relationships, and is considered taboo in some cultures.

The personal space, 18 inches to 4 feet, is where touching family and friends and some counseling interactions are permitted. The social consultative zone, 4 to 12 feet, is for casual social interactions. The public zone, beyond 12 feet, is beyond the sphere of personal involvement, and verbal communication is usually formal. The preferred space between people in the United States is 2 to 3 feet. In general, Asians do not mind closer spaces, whereas African Americans do not want their personal space invaded.

People tend to be past, present, or future oriented. People who value the past maintain tradition and are not likely to set goals for the future. People who focus on the present tend to be unappreciative of the past and do not plan for the future. People with future orientations plan and organize for the future.

People in the United States tend to be individualistic and desire to control their own lives. Chinese, Mexican, Vietnamese, and Puerto Rican Americans tend to consider the family as the most important social organization. Some cultural groups, such as Italians and Appalachian people, extend their family beyond blood lines.

Environmental control relates to the ability to control nature and direct the environment. Some groups believe they can control nature; others feel controlled by it. Still others, such as many Native American nations, believe humanity should attempt to live in harmony with nature.

There are also biological variations among cultures. Features, skin color, body size, and enzyme differences are related to cultural heritage. Understanding cultural variables can help leaders and managers recruit, retain, direct, and evaluate personnel. Understanding cultural variables can help one understand oneself better, as well (Giger and Davidhizar, 1990).

SEXUAL PREFERENCE AND GENDER

Sexuality characteristics concerning sexual orientation is about gender identification of the individual not about human sexuality. *Transgender* is an umbrella term used to include transsexuals, intersexuals, cross dressers, transgenderists, and others. Transsexuals' gender identity does not match their biological gender. Males may identify with females and females with males. They are often motivated to change their anatomy to more closely match their gender identity. Transgenderists are similar to transsexuals but choose to not have genital surgery. Cross dressers' gender expression is sometimes different from their biological gender. Intersexuals are not typically male or female. Gay men are biological males who identify as men and are attracted to other men. Gay men who dress in women's clothing are called drag queens. There are also female to male transsexuals, but it is more common for women to wear men's clothing than for men to wear women's clothing. Lesbians are biological females who identify as females and are attracted to other women.

Individuals go through three phases of coming out. First is comparison when people compare what they hear, see, and feel and start to reassess their own sexuality. Second is support and changes from tolerance to acceptance to support. Third are incorporation or integration and a sense of pride. Gays typically have more in common with straights than differences.

Organizations also have three phases of coming out. The first phase is acknowledgement that gay people exist in workplaces. Second are accommodations by such actions as offering partner benefits to same-gender and unmarried opposite gender couples and substituting the word *partner* for *spouse* in policies. Third is incorporation when sexual orientation is a fact of life. It includes nondiscrimination policies, education programs, brown bag meetings, change agent methodologies, mentoring, coming-out coaches, referral services, community outreach initiatives, dealing with spirituality and religion issues, a hot line to report harassment and discrimination, awards for promoting a safer work environment, and encouraging gay employees to bring their partners to events. Organization leaders should be clear and articulate about the mission, vision, values, and philosophy of the organization (Winfeld and Spielman, 2001).

GENERATIONAL DIFFERENCES

People born around 1925 to 1945 are known as traditionalists, matures, veterans, seniors, and the silent generation (Table 12-3). Their career goal was to build a legacy, and they were rewarded by the satisfaction of a job well done. They considered no news as good news and learned the hard way. They see retirement as a reward. They valued honesty, integrity, family, and work and were loyal hard workers. They lived unbalanced lives because they were consumed by work. They often lacked formal education. They lived through the depression, World War II, the Korean War, the New Deal, radio, and the silver screen, and they saw the rise of labor unions. Heroes included Lindbergh, Amelia Earhart, Joe Louis, and Babe Ruth. In their early years they listened to big band, swing, Bing Crosby, Tommy Dorsey, Duke Ellington, Ella Fitzgerald, Benny Goodman, Frank Sinatra, and Kate Smith. Cultural memorobilia included radio shows, Saturday-afternoon matinees, cowboy and Indian movies, serial movies, and the swimming hole. They were motivated by the message, "Do it!"

TABLE **12-3** Generational Differences

YEARS	1925-1945	1946-1964	1965-1980	1981-1984
Title	Traditionalists, matures, veterans, seniors, silent generation	Baby boomers	Generation X, baby busters, postboomers	Generation Y, nexters, millennial generation, Internet generation
Career goals	Build a legacy	Build a stellar career	Build a portable career	Build parallel careers
Rewards	Satisfaction of a job well done	Money, title, recognition, corner office	Freedom	Meaningful work
Feedback	No news is good news	Once per year with lots of documentation	Frequent feedback	Feedback when desired
Training	Learn the hard way	Train them too much and they will leave	The more they learn, the more they stay	Continuous learning is the way of life
Balance	Support for shifting the balance	Balance others, find meaning for self	Balance now, not at age 65 years	Give flexibility to balance own activities
Retirement	Reward	Retool	Renew	Recycle
Core values	Honesty, integrity, work, family	Optimism, team orientation, personal gratification, health and wellness, personal growth	Diversity, thinking globally, balance, techno literacy, self-reliance, informality	Optimism, civic duty, confidence, achievement, sociability, morality, diversity
Assets	Loyalty, hard worker	Service oriented, driven, good team players	Adaptable, techno literate, independent, creative	Collective action, multitasker, techno savvy, tenacity
Liabilities	Unbalanced life, consumed by work, lack of formal education	Not budget minded, uncomfortable with conflict, reluctant to go against peers, sensitive to feedback, self-centered	Impatient, poor people skills, inexperienced, cynical	Need for supervision and structure, inexperience
Defining events	Depression World War II, Korean War, New Deal, radio, silver screen, rise of labor unions	Assassinations, Vietnam, civil rights, cold war, women's liberation, space race, Woodstock, love-in, laugh-in	Watergate, Challenger disaster, fall of Berlin Wall, Persian Gulf, computers, birth control pills, latchkey kids, single-parent homes	Schoolyard violence, Oklahoma City bombing, terrorism, multiculturalism, crack cocaine, AIDS epidemic, computers, TV talk shows
Heroes	Lindbergh, Amelia Earhart, Joe Louis, Babe Ruth	Gandhi, Martin Luther King, John Kennedy, John Glenn	None	Princess Diana, Mother Teresa, Bill Gates, Tiger Woods, Christopher Reeve

TABLE **12-3** Generational Differences—cont'd

YEARS	1925-1945	1946-1964	1965-1980	1981-1994
Cultural memorabilia	Radio shows, Saturday afternoon matinees, cowboy and Indian movies, serial movies, swimming hole, work	*The Ed Sullivan Show,* fallout shelters, Slinkies, TV dinners, poodle skirts, pop beads, hula hoops, peace sign	Platform shoes, pet rocks, Cabbage Patch dolls, ET, *The Brady Bunch, Dynasty, The Simpsons*	American Girl dolls, Barney, Beanie Babies, Teenage Mutant Ninja Turtles, virtual pets, Oprah, Rosie, the Spice Girls, the X Games
Messages that motivate	The switch; I want you to...; Do it	We need you; you are important, I approve of you, you are valued	We don't have many rules; do it your way; we have the latest technology	You can be a hero here; you can help turn this company around; you will work with creative people
Spending style	Cautious, conservative, necessities	Buy now, pay later, pay with plastic	Cautious, conservative	Spend parents' money as fast as you can

Modified from Lancaster LC, Stillman D: *When generations collide,* New York, 2002, HarperCollins Books; Zemke R, Raines C, Filipczak B: *Generations at work: Managing the clash of veterans, boomers, Xers, and nexters in your workplace,* New York, 2000, American Management Association.

accompanied by a switch. This group tended to welcome retirement after long years of hard labor. They saw retirement as a time for leisure and a chance to do things they had not had the time or money to do before. Social Security helped make that possible. Unfortunately, some early retirees have reported that their standard of living has declined since retirement, and some are not confident that they will have enough money to remain comfortable for the rest of their lives. Their spending style is cautious and conservative, and they buy mainly the necessities (Bennis and Thomas, 2002; Goldberg, 2000; Lancaster and Stillman, 2002; Zemke, Raines, and Filipczak, 2000).

People born about 1946 to 1964 are known as the baby boomers. They want to build a stellar career and are rewarded by things such as money, title, recognition, and a corner office. Feedback once per year with lots of documentation suits them. Supervisors are afraid that if you train them too much, they will leave the organization. Baby boomers want to find meaning for themselves in their work and view retirement as a time to retool. They tend to value optimism, team orientation, personal gratification, health

and wellness, and personal growth. Their service orientation, drive, and being good team players are assets while the lack of budget mindedness, discomfort with conflict, conformity, sensitivity to feedback, and self-centeredness are considered liabilities. They have lived through assassinations, the Vietnam War, Chappaquiddick, Kent State, civil rights, the cold war, women's liberation, the space race, sit-ins, love-ins, and laugh-ins. In their early years they listened to rock 'n' roll, acid rock, the Beach Boys, the Beatles, the Grateful Dead, Bob Dylan, Elvis, Jimi Hendrix, Janis Joplin, the Supremes, and the Temptations. Many moved to suburbs and worked 60-hour weeks; about one half ended up divorced. Their heroes include Gandhi, Martin Luther King, John Kennedy, and John Glenn. Cultural memorabilia of this generation include *The Ed Sullivan Show,* fallout shelters, Slinkies, TV dinners, poodle skirts, pop beads, hula hoops, and the peace sign.

They are motivated by messages such as "We need you." "You are important." "I approve you." "You are valued." They have a spending style of buy now and pay later with plastic. As they near retirement, they need more opportunities that will challenge them since many are likely to work until about age 70 years. Many retirees would prefer to work at least part-time. Although they have worked excessive hours during the past few decades, many would like a slower pace now. They are willing students if treated respectfully. Adult education programs are up significantly. Older workers apparently are as productive as younger ones and have fewer on-the-job accidents. With the shortage of nurses and the cost of recruiting, hiring, and developing new employees, it is appropriate to encourage the most experienced nurses even with the highest pay to continue to work. A phased-out retirement by gradually reducing the number of days worked or perhaps the number of hours per day has possibilities. Besides the full-time permanent work, we can consider options such as part-time permanent work, full-time or part-time temporary work, contract work, consultation, telecommuting from home, and on-call work. Intelligence is believed to remain constant until at least age 70 years (Goldberg, 2000; Karp, Fuller, and Sirias, 2002; Lancaster and Stillman, 2002; Raines and Hunt, 2000; Zemke, Raines, and Filipczak, 2000).

Generation X, baby busters, or postboomers were born around 1965 to 1980. They want to build a portable career, are rewarded by freedom, and like frequent feedback. The more they learn, the more likely they are to stay. They want balance in their lives now. They see retirement as a period of renewal. Their core values include diversity, global thinking, balance, techno literacy, self-reliance, and informality. Their assets are adaptability, techno literacy, independence, and creativity, whereas impatience, poor people skills, inexperience, and a cynical nature are viewed as liabilities. They have lived through Watergate, the Challenger disaster, the fall of the Berlin Wall, the Persian Gulf War, computers, birth control pills, latchkey kids, and single-parent homes. In their early years they listened to disco, rap, Guns 'N' Roses, Michael Jackson, Elton John, Bon Jovi, Prince, Reggae, Bruce Springsteen, Tina Turner, and U2. They apparently have no heroes.

Some admire their mothers, especially after getting older and understanding the demands of parenting better. Cultural memorobilia include platform shoes, pet rocks, Cabbage Patch dolls, ET, *The Brady Bunch*, *Dynasty*, and *The Simpsons*.

They are motivated by statements such as "We don't have many rules." "Do it your way." "We have the latest technology." The Gen Xers are self-reliant, are seeking a sense of family, and want balance between work and family. They like informality, approach authority casually, and have a nontraditional orientation to time and space. They may do well with management by objectives rather than needing to be in a specific place at a specific time. They want a fun, relaxed workplace. They want ideas to be evaluated on merit not by years of experience. They appreciate hands-off supervision. They do not read as much as the matures but use computers more and like their freedom. Thus one should make a variety of learning materials, such as books, computer programs, CD-ROMs, sound, video, and face-to-face instruction, available but not mandatory. Be available to answer their questions when they come to you. Encourage them to think about what they have learned on a regular basis. It is good to give them mentors and lots of positive constructive feedback. Development is important to Gen Xers so let them know that is part of the job. An employee assistance program, particularly for low-wage workers, including transportation, child care, language skills, financial literacy, transition to home ownership skills, and filling out paperwork for food stamps and immigration matters can help retention. Employees may appreciate not only child care but also convenient postage, banking, dry cleaning, shoe repair, and the possibility to pick up carry-out dinner on the way home from work. Their spending habits tend to be cautious and conservative. Many are struggling to make ends meet. They are the first generation that probably will not be able to improve on their parents' lifestyle. They will lose money in Social Security. They are willing to work hard but want fair pay for the hours worked and want a life beyond work (Karp, Fuller, and Sirias, 2002; Lancaster and Stillman, 2002; Raines and Hunt, 2000; Tulgan, 2000; Zemke, Raines, and Filipczak, 2000).

People born around 1981 to 1994 may be called generation Y, the nexters, the millennial generation, or the Internet generation. They are interested in building parallel careers. They are rewarded by meaningful work and like feedback when they ask for it. They view continuous learning as a way of life and want to be given flexibility so they can balance their own activities. They see retirement as a time to recycle. Their core values include optimism, civic duty, confidence, achievement, sociability, morality, and diversity. Their assets include collective action, multitasking, technological savvy, and their tenacity, whereas their need for supervision and structure and their inexperience are seen as liabilities. They have lived through schoolyard violence, the Oklahoma City bombing, crack cocaine, the AIDS epidemic, multiculturalism, computers, and TV talk shows. They listened to alternative rap, the Backstreet Boys, Toni Braxton, Garth Brooks, Puff Daddy, Savage Garden, Spice Girls, Hanson, Jewel, Alanis Morrisette, and Will Smith. Their heroes include Princess Diana, Mother Teresa, Bill Gates, Tiger Woods, and Christopher Reeve. Cultural memorobilia of this generation include American Girl dolls, Barney, Beanie Babies, Teenage Mutant Ninja Turtles, virtual pets, Oprah, Rosie, the Spice Girls, and X Games.

They are motivated by the following messages: "You can be a hero here." "You can help turn this company around." "You will work with creative people here." The majority of the nexters were planned, and many appreciate being wanted. Like their grandparents, they have a stricter moral code and consequently rates of teenage pregnancy, teen abortions, drug use, drunk driving, and high school dropouts are down. Unlike their parents, they expect to work more than 40 hours per week to achieve their goals. They have an optimistic, can-do spirit. They will need plenty of orientation to the job. Make clear the long-term goals of the organization. Learn the goals of the personnel, and try to integrate those with the organizational goals. This generation does "gender bending" as men do more of the household tasks and women do more traditional male tasks. Generation Y has a new confidence, is the most education-minded generation in history, is leading a wave of volunteerism, and is paving the way to a more open, tolerant society. Gen Yers are comfortably self-reliant, want technology and other things right now, and want opportunities. There is a greater generation gap than between other generations. Their spending style is to spend their parents' money as fast as they can (Bennis, Spreitzer, and Cummings, 2001; Blanchard, Lacinak, Tompkins, et al, 2002; Lancaster and Stillman, 2002; Raines and Hunt, 2000; Zemke, Raines, and Filipczak, 2000).

Tulgan and Martin (2001, p. 63) have identified the 14 expectations of generation Y as follows:

1. Provide challenging work that really matters.

2. Balance clearly delegated assignments with freedom and flexibility.

3. Offer increasing responsibility as a reward for accomplishments.

4. Spend time getting to know staff members and their capabilities.

5. Provide ongoing training and learning opportunities.

6. Establish mentoring relationships.

7. Create a comfortable, low-stress environment.

8. Allow some flexibility in scheduling.

9. Focus on work, but be personable and have a sense of humor.

10. Balance the roles of "boss" and "team player."

11. Treat Yers as colleagues, not as interns or "teenagers."

12. Be respectful, and call forth respect in return.

13. Consistently provide constructive feedback.

14. Reward Yers when they've done a good job.

AMERICANS WITH DISABILITIES ACT

Three categories of individuals with disabilities are protected by the Americans With Disabilities Act (ADA): (1) individuals who have a physical or mental impairment that substantially limits one or more major life activities; (2) individuals who have a record or history of a physical or mental impairment that substantially limits one or more major life activities; and (3) individuals who are regarded as having such an impairment whether they have the impairment or not. Disability in a major life activity includes caring for oneself, walking, breathing, hearing, seeing, speaking, and learning.

Physical impairments include but are not limited to orthopedic, visual, speech, and hearing impairments; cerebral palsy, epilepsy, muscular dystrophy, multiple sclerosis, cancer, diabetes, tuberculosis, and HIV-positive status; drug addiction; and alcoholism.

Mental impairments include but are not limited to mental retardation, organic brain syndrome, emotional or mental illness, and specific learning disabilities.

Other conditions covered by the ADA include homosexuality or bisexuality; transvestism, transsexualism, pedophilia, exhibitionism, voyeurism, gender identity disorders, compulsive gambling, kleptomania, and psychoactive substance use disorders. ADA excludes current drug users from coverage when an adverse action is taken against an individual based on such use.

Temporary conditions may be considered a disability depending on the duration and the extent to which one or more major life activities are limited. Qualified individuals with a disability must meet the essential eligibility requirements of the agency, with or without (1) reasonable modification to the agency's rules, policies, or practices; (2) removal of architectural, communication, or transportation barriers; or (3) provisions of auxiliary aids or services.

People who pose a direct threat to the health or safety of others are not qualified for protection under the ADA. Determination may not be based on generalizations or stereotypes but must be based on an individualized assessment that relies on current medical evidence or the best available objective evidence to assess (1) the nature, duration, and severity of the risk; (2) the probability that the potential injury will actually occur; and (3) whether reasonable modification of policies, practices, or procedures will mitigate or eliminate the risk. Modifications that fundamentally alter the nature of the program, service, or activities are not required.

An agency should have procedures by which people who identify potential difficulties with meeting essential performance standards can receive appropriate assistance and guidance. When a person believes that she cannot meet one or more of the standards without accommodations or modifications, the agency must determine on an individual basis whether or not the necessary accommodations or modifications can be made. Reasonable accommodations are defined by the ADA to include (1) making existing facilities readily accessible to and usable by individuals with disabilities and (2) job restructuring; part-time or modified work schedules; acquisition or modification of equipment or devices; appropriate adjustment or modification of examinations, training materials, or policies; the provision of qualified readers or interpreters; and other similar accommodations for individuals with disabilities. Each agency should rely on its legal resources to make informed decisions.

The ADA does mandate that people with disabilities not be disqualified just because of an easily accommodated disability, but it does not mandate that people with disabilities be hired before fully qualified people without disabilities. In the case of *Zamudio v. Patia* (1997), the court required the employer to inform Ms. Zamudio when a position became available for which the reasonable accommodations she required could be done but did not require the employer to hire her before better qualified people or people with more seniority. Nor does the court require job restructuring when the person needing accommodation qualifies for other jobs that do not need accommodation, such as in the *Mauro v. Borgess Medical Center* (1995) case. The Michigan court denied an operating surgical technician accommodations to continue working in the operating room. Mauro was human immunodeficiency virus (HIV) positive and consequently moved to an equivalent position that did not require patient contact.

The ADA also provides for essential job functions that a person must be able to do to be qualified for a position. The court found that ability to restrain patients is an essential job function for a psychiatric nurse in the case of *Jones v. Kerrville State Hospital* (1998). Ability to work rotating shifts was considered an essential job function in the case of *Laurin v. Providence Hospital and Massachusetts Nurses Association* (1998).

There have been numerous lawsuits filed under the Americans With Disabilities Act. Some other relevant cases are as follows: *Howard v. North Mississippi Medical Center* (1992) found that migraine headaches and latex allergies are not disabilities; *Jessie v. Carter Health Care Center, Inc.* (1996) found that pregnancy is not a disability; *Webb v. Mercy Hospital* (1996) found that erratic behavior does not give notice to the employer that the individual has mental impairment; *Thompson v. Holy Family Hospital* (1997) found that a nurse with a lifting disability is not qualified for protection under the ADA; *Wilking v. County of Ramsey* (1997) found that a nurse taking medications for depression is not disabled; and *Cody v. Cigna Healthcare of St. Louis, Inc.* (1998) found that depression and anxiety are not disabling conditions (Grohar-Murray and DiCroce, 2003; O'Keefe, 2001; Sullivan and Decker, 2001; Yoder-Wise, 2003).

JOB REDESIGN

JOB ANALYSIS

Job analysis affects employee recruitment, hiring, orientation and training programs, performance appraisal, placement, transfers, and promotions; it consequently influences nursing care. It can determine equitable rates of pay and grade nursing positions within the total agency personnel system. By reviewing national, state, regional, and local wage surveys and using wage scales and performance appraisal, nursing personnel can be compensated satisfactorily for performance. It is the nurse administrator's responsibility to inform the analyst of the scope of authority in nursing positions so that they might be upgraded. This is especially pressing in the nursing profession, because nursing positions have long been rated lower than those of other professionals with comparable education, experience, and responsibility.

Job analysis is the study of a position to determine what knowledge, skill, aptitude, and personal characteristics are needed to perform certain responsibilities successfully. Analysis does not include any attempt to change the task. Rather, one starts by locating or developing a job description and position requirements. Questionnaires, interviews, observation, and logs furnish information about the job title and summary, duties performed, type of supervision given and received, equipment used, working conditions, and relationship to other positions. Job analysis determines minimum requirements (type and level of knowledge, skill, aptitude, and personal characteristics) and consequently sets standards for factors such as education, experience, intelligence, personality, and physical strength (Swansburg and Swansburg, 2002).

JOB EVALUATION

Job evaluation is a process of measuring the remunerative worth of a job in relation to other positions, both internal and external to the organization. On the assumption that workers will be more satisfied if they perceive pay rates as consistent, the objective of evaluation is to compare jobs and establish a consistent pay base, providing employees in responsible positions with more pay than those with less demanding jobs. A point system, ranking of jobs, job grading, and job-to-job comparison are used. Consideration is given to education, mental and manual skills, responsibility for resources (personnel, materials, finances), mental and physical effort, and working conditions, such as exposure to dangerous or disagreeable elements.

With the point system the nurse manager assigns numerical values to specific qualifications. An example appears in Box 12-3.

Once point values have been assigned to various job factors, they can be added to determine a grade. The grades for various jobs can be ranked, and job-to-job comparisons can provide a basis for determining pay.

Job evaluation is a systematic rather than a scientific process, and its high reliability does not ensure validity. The management values used to choose and weigh factors may not be consistent with the values of other personnel, or the selected values may differ among work groups. Although relative pay rates can be determined by job evaluation, the absolute levels are often negotiated by the individual or unions.

The number of grievances related to pay rates commonly increases after the introduction of job evaluation because personnel now have an objective basis for a grievance. Before job evaluation, employees had little concrete justification on which to file grievances. They complained that they were not getting paid enough; management insisted that they were. With job evaluation, employees have criteria on which to base grievances.

The transition period is especially troublesome. Problems related to adjusting the worker's present pay to the new pay structure may interfere with traditional lines of promotion. Adjusting a worker's pay upward to the new rate is acceptable to employees, but some may then file grievances for back pay. Back pay, however, could undermine the agency's budget. Therefore management may decide that back pay is retroactive only to a specified date. The case of an employee who has previously been overcompensated creates a more difficult situation. To prevent dissatisfaction, personnel can be assured that no one's pay will be reduced as a result of the new pay schedule. However, it is possible to deny any pay increase to the individual who was overcompensated until others' salaries have been raised and all have been realigned to the new pay schedule. That, of course, can be demoralizing to the overpaid individual, but the previous situation is demoralizing to other employees. More acceptable options may be to promote the individual to a job commensurate with the pay or give the overpaid employee additional responsibilities in the present position to make the current job commensurate with the salary. After the individual vacates the position, the salary for the job can be realigned at a lower salary level according to the pay schedule.

JOB DESIGN

Job design specifies the job content (what the job requires), job methods (how to do it), and the relationship among the organizational, social, and personal needs of the worker. It involves observation, recording, and analysis of current jobs to make work more efficient and to provide incentives for the workers, thereby reducing costs and improving job satisfaction.

JOB SIMPLIFICATION

Another technique, job simplification, removes the more difficult parts of the job so that the worker can do more of what remains. For example, a nurse can be hired to start all intravenous (IV) lines. The treatment nurse, team leader, and primary nurse, then, do not have to start any IV lines but can give other medications and treatments to more patients. Work simplification, however, tends to lead to further boredom.

Personnel may also be assigned more tasks. For instance, staff nurses can teach aides to do additional treatments. This may relieve some monotony, but many workers are already very busy, and the new tasks may prove to be no more meaningful than the others.

JOB ROTATION

Job rotation is another horizontal job-enlargement technique. Nurses may rotate shifts and assignments among different units and different

BOX **12-3** Job Evaluation

QUALIFICATIONS	POINTS

EDUCATION

Less than a high school diploma	10
High school diploma	20
High school diploma plus a special training course	30
Associate degree or 3 years in work study program and passage of accrediting examinations	40
Baccalaureate degree and passage of accrediting examinations	50
Master's degree in area of specialty needed for the position	60
Doctorate in area of specialty appropriate for the position	70

MENTAL SKILLS

Work is simple and repetitive and is performed according to instructions	10
Work involves a variety of duties that are performed according to procedures but require alertness to identify needed changes	20
Work involves a variety of complicated duties and some independent actions in adapting procedures to specific situations	30
Work involves planning, organization, implementing, and evaluating actions related to patient care	40
Work involves development of policies and procedures, organization of functions, development of staffing patterns, and budget preparations	50

MANUAL SKILLS

Work involves the normal manual skills, such as lifting, pushing, folding, writing, filing	10
Work involves about-normal manual skills, such as accurate measurements, administration of medications and treatments, manipulation of instruments, typing, bookkeeping	40
Work involves considerable manual skill, such as administering complex treatments and manipulation of complex equipment	50

RESPONSIBILITY FOR RESOURCES
Personnel

Supervises no one	10
Supervises fewer than 10 people	20
Directs up to 25 people	30
Directs up to 50 people	40
Directs up to 100 people	50
Directs more than 100 people	60

Finances

No responsibility for budget	10
Responsible for budget up to $10,000	20
Responsible for budget up to $25,000	30
Responsible for budget up to $100,000	40
Responsible for budget over $100,000	50

EFFORT
Mental

Requires little thinking or judgment	10
Requires some alertness while performing repetitive tasks according to directions	20
Requires mental effort for problem solving	30
Requires considerable mental effort for decision making and problem solving	40
Requires continuous mental effort for dealing with the most difficult situations	50

BOX **12-3** Job Evaluation—cont'd

QUALIFICATIONS	POINTS
Physical	
Light work requiring little physical effort, usually seated	10
Light physical effort, use of light materials, frequently seated	20
Sustained physical effort, seldom seated, continuous activity	30
Considerable physical effort, continuous activity, lifting	40
Working conditions	
Good working conditions—light, ventilation, freedom from disagreeable elements such as dirt, heat, wetness, odors, noise	10
Average working conditions with occasional exposure to disagreeable elements and danger	20
Fair working conditions with frequent exposure to disagreeable elements and danger	30
Poor working conditions with continuous exposure to disagreeable elements and danger	40

---

patients on the units, but this practice complicates continuity of care and often leads to additional frustration. Community health nurses may be rotated through clinic assignments. For instance, a nurse may work well-baby clinics one month; family planning the next; and immunization, tuberculosis, or venereal disease clinics at other times. Again, this can disrupt continuity of care.

JOB ENRICHMENT

Job enrichment is a vertical approach to job design that uses a fuller range of abilities and skills of the personnel. When planning job enrichment, one should consider skill variety—the number of different talents and skills needed to do a job; task identity—the degree to which one can do a job from beginning to end with a visible outcome; task significance—the degree to which the job has an impact on others; autonomy—the degree of independence and discretion one has to plan and implement the job; and feedback—the degree to which one receives clear feedback about the effectiveness of one's performance. These core job dimensions contribute to the psychological states that affect the work outcomes. Skill variety, task identity, and task significance contribute to the experience of

meaningfulness of work. One may experience responsibility for outcomes through autonomy and knowledge of the results through feedback. That should contribute to motivation, high-quality work performance, and satisfaction, which in turn contribute to lower absenteeism and turnover.

For example, community health nurses may have "their own" assortment of clinics in addition to their family caseload. Continuity is preserved because nurses are always at that clinic. They need to develop their expertise, knowledge, and skill in all the clinical areas. Previously hospital units have switched from functional or team nursing to primary nursing so nurses could give total patient care and so nurses could assume additional responsibility and accountability.

Job enrichment is intended to increase motivation and productivity while reducing absenteeism and turnover. It can, however, increase anxiety, conflict, and feelings of exploitation. Skill levels of personnel limit the amount of job enrichment possible, because some workers lack managerial skills and may not be able or willing to plan and control their jobs. Supervisors may not be willing to trust workers, and personnel may feel they are being exploited.

JOB DESCRIPTIONS

Job descriptions are derived from job analysis and are affected by job evaluation and design. They generally contain specifications that are the requirements for the job, major duties and responsibilities, and the organizational relationships of a given position. The title of the job indicates the major responsibilities and sets that job apart from others. The job description is a summary of primary duties in a complete but not detailed fashion. Job relationships and professional affiliations may be cited. Education, experience, and worker traits, such as aptitude, interests, and temperament, may be included. The physical demands and working conditions of the job may be mentioned. Job descriptions should be up to date, accurate, and realistic in terms of the resources available. Standard forms for all jobs within a category facilitate comparison.

Job descriptions should arrange duties in a logical order, state them separately and concisely, and use verbs to describe the action. They should be specific rather than vague and should avoid generalizations by using quantitative words whenever possible. To indicate frequency, one can note daily, periodically, or occasionally when the percentage of total time spent on a specific activity cannot be determined.

Job descriptions are useful for recruitment, placement, and transfer decisions. They can also be used to guide and evaluate personnel. Job descriptions help prevent conflict, frustration, and overlapping of duties. Box 12-4 provides a sample job description.

CAREER LADDERS AND PERFORMANCE MANAGEMENT PLANS

Marie Zimmer (1972) designed a clinical ladder to create a work environment that would nurture and challenge professional growth and recognize clinical excellence to meet the professional's needs for growth and recognition and the institution's requirement for a stable, experienced nursing staff. It was a ladder for clinical advancement with rungs for vertical advancement that provided recognition for nurses who chose to stay at the bedside. Clinical ladders evolved into career ladders and proliferated during the 1970s and early 1980s. Career programs varied from simple two-level clinical ladders to multitrack and multileveled systems that include provisions for evaluation.

Advantages of career ladders include potential to increase positive self-image, increase motivation, improve personal and professional satisfaction, provide opportunity for professional growth, provide a system of rewards for accomplishments, encourage development of peer review, improve recruitment and retention, and improve cost-effectiveness through lower attrition rate and retention of experienced nurses.

Potential problems with career ladders include the difficulty of designing them and their potential negative psychological effect. A newly hired experienced nurse may enter the career ladder at the same level as an inexperienced, newly graduated nurse; there may be fewer monetary rewards between clinical levels than administrative levels. Competency is difficult to define, and nurses on tracks may be evaluated by administrators instead of peers (McKay, 1986; Zimmer, 1972).

During the 1990s career management plans based on management by objectives emerged. They could involve identifying the vision, mission, strategies, and core competencies needed to accomplish the strategies that are consistent with the values of the organization. Forms can be developed to help identify the desired outcomes or objectives, desired behaviors, tracking sources such as reports, self-assessment and others' feedback, actual behavior, and degrees of achievement when the actual behavior is compared with the desired behavior. Then a developmental plan can be prepared by identifying the behavior to be enhanced, developmental activities, and what is to be done by whom by when. An interim review and coaching log can be maintained. There can be an end-of-cycle review noting employee's and manager's comments with the dated signature of each.

BOX **12-4** Sample Job Description

NURSING SERVICE DIRECTOR
Description of Work

General statement of duties: Performs administrative work in planning, coordinating, and directing the nursing service.
Supervision received: Works under general direction of the hospital administrator.
Supervision exercised: Supervises assigned personnel as a significant part of the duties.

Examples of Duties

(Any one position may not include all of the duties listed, nor do the listed examples include all tasks that may be found in positions of this class.)

Directs and administers the nursing service, including inpatient and ambulatory care; develops and implements policies and patient care standards for all nursing service areas.

Participates in the planning and development of hospital policies and practices; works closely with administrative and medical personnel in coordinating nursing service functions with those of all other hospital departments and services.

Develops and implements staffing and ratio patterns to meet patient care and medical service needs; directs the broad planning of in-service training and orientation programs for nursing staff; directs research activities for continuing education and coordinates the clinical experience of nursing students.

Develops nursing service philosophies and goals in accordance with hospital policies; encourages and provides channels for staff participation in achieving these goals; interprets nursing service objectives to administrative and medical staff.

Serves on various hospital and community committees for the coordination of nursing services with other patient care and educational services; participates in professional organizational activities and represents the hospital in working with various service agencies and volunteer groups.

Directs the preparation of budget for nursing service staffing, equipment, and supplies; develops systems and standards for patient care records and reports.

Directs the recruitment, selection, transfer, and promotion of nursing personnel and the maintenance of personnel records.

Performs related work as required.

Qualifications for Appointment

Knowledge, skills, and abilities: Extensive knowledge of professional nursing theory and practice. Extensive knowledge of modern principles and practices of hospital operation and nursing administration. Ability to plan, organize, and direct large-scale and comprehensive nursing activities. Ability to supervise, train, and motivate employees. Ability to communicate effectively orally and in writing. Ability to establish and maintain effective working relationships with administrative and medical personnel, employees, the public, and other agencies.
Education: Graduation from a 4-year college with attainment of a master's degree in nursing and major course work in nursing administration or education.
Experience: Five years' professional nursing experience including 3 years in an administrative capacity.
Necessary special requirement: Possession of a license to practice as a registered nurse as issued by the state board of nursing.

CLINICAL SPECIALIST I
Description of Work

General statement of duties: Performs advanced professional nursing work in a recognized medical specialty field.
Supervision received: Works under the general supervision of an administrative superior.
Supervision exercised: Supervises personnel as assigned, or full supervision incidental to the other duties.

Examples of Duties

(Any one position may not include all of the duties listed, nor do the listed examples include all tasks that may be found in positions of this class.)

Continued

BOX 12-4 Sample Job Description—cont'd

Performs advanced professional nursing work in specialized medical fields such as mental health, respiratory care, and other recognized medical specialties in accordance with standard nursing procedures and medical direction.

Interviews patient to obtain general background information and problem identification; evaluates patient's behavior and assesses immediate and long-range needs; schedules and conducts individual and group psychotherapy sessions.

Participates as a member of a professional medical, psychiatric, or social public health team in evaluating, developing, and implementing health care plans.

Makes rounds with physician to review condition of patients; develops nursing care plans; participates in the care of the critically ill.

Participates in the orientation and in-service training of professional nursing personnel in teaching new, advanced, or complicated methods and procedures; interprets nursing services to patients and hospital personnel.

Performs related work as required.

Qualifications for Appointment

Knowledge, skills, and abilities: Thorough knowledge of professional nursing theory and practice. Thorough knowledge of modern nursing care principles and practices in a recognized medical specialty. Ability to motivate and train employees. Ability to communicate effectively orally and in writing. Ability to establish and maintain effective working relationships with patients, employees, the public, and other agencies.

Education: Attainment of a master's degree in nursing.

Experience: Two years' experience in an appropriate nursing clinical specialty.

Necessary special requirement: Possession of a license or permit as a registered nurse by the state board of nursing.

Modified from Job Descriptions, Denver General Hospital.

RESEARCH Perspective 12-2

Data from Laborde SA, Lee JA: Skills needed for promotion in the nursing profession. *JONA* 30(9):432-439, 2000.

Purpose: The purpose of this research was to identify interpersonal versus technical skill importance to promotion within the nursing profession and the difference between perceived and actual importance of the skills.

Methods: A stratified random sample of 219 nurse administrators from a large southeastern United States hospital rated hypothetical candidates for managerial positions from mailed scenarios. The assignment of respondents into upper, middle, and lower management was based on considering top management responsible for the operations of multiple services; middle management for coordinating nursing units, and first-line managers as responsible for the production of nursing services. The

regression equation's beta weights were used to test the hypotheses. The chi-square test conducted for interpersonal skills did not find a statistically significant relationship between position and number of skills used.

Results/conclusions: At the lowest level management position studied, a greater number of technical skills significantly influenced promotion decision than at middle management. Interpersonal skills seem important at all levels of management. Significant differences were found between decision makers' perception of skill importance and the skill's actual importance to promotion decisions.

ORIENTATION

Induction is the first 2 or 3 days of orientation. It can be done by personnel department employees for all new employees. It includes a history of the organization, the vision, purpose, structure, working hours, holiday time, vacation, sick time, paydays, performance standards and evaluation, labor contracts, grievance procedures, parking facilities, eating facilities, health services, and education opportunities. That is more information than new employees can remember. It is advisable to have the information in a handbook and to reference the handbook during the induction. Both the new employees and experienced nurses in new positions need orientation. The manager introduces the nurse to the new job, agency policies, facilities, and coworkers. Orientation is important, and the manager who does not take the time to assist a new employee is making a serious mistake. Communicating regulations and exactly what is expected of the nurse diminishes uncertainty, relieves anxiety, and prevents unnecessary misunderstandings. One's security usually increases when someone is considerate enough to help one adjust to a new situation. The manner in which nurses are treated during their first day at a new job may be critical to their future job satisfaction and performance.

Because of information overload, induction and further orientation should be conducted over time. A checklist for orientation that indicates the content, time frame, and who is responsible to teach it can be helpful (Box 12-5). It is appropriate to use an orientation schedule (Box 12-6).

BOX **12-5** Sample Orientation Checklist

ACTIVITY	TIME FRAME	WHO IS RESPONSIBLE
History of organization	Day 1	Personnel department
Vision, purpose of organization	Day 1	Personnel department
Structure of organization	Day 1	Personnel department
Payroll information	Day 1	Personnel department
Tour of facilities	Day 1	Staff development department
Introduction to unit heads and purpose of departments	Day 1	Staff development department
Employee and organizational responsibilities, rules of conduct	Day 1	Personnel department
Fire and safety video	Day 1	Staff development department
Personnel policies	Day 2	Personnel department
Tour of unit	Day 2	Preceptor
Introductions to unit personnel	Day 2	Preceptor
Work schedules, staffing, scheduling policies	Day 2	Preceptor
CPR recertification	Day 2	Staff development department
Universal precautions update	Day 2	Staff development department
Workload assignments	Day 3	Preceptor
Introductions to charting	Day 3	Preceptor
Reporting of accidents	Day 3	Preceptor
Use of services such as nutrition, OT, PT, pharmacy, x-ray, clinical lab	Day 3	Preceptor
Job description	Day 3	Preceptor
Standards of performance	Day 3	Preceptor
Staff development	Day 3	Preceptor
Employee appraisal system	Day 3	Preceptor
Promotion and transfer policies	Day 3	Preceptor
Work with preceptor while assuming more responsibility	Week 2	Preceptor

CPR, Cardiopulmonary resuscitation; *OT,* occupational therapy; *PT,* physical therapy.

BOX **12-6** Sample Orientation Schedule

DAY 1

8:00-10:00 AM	Welcome by personnel department
	Employee handbook distributed; overview of organizational history, vision, purpose, structure, payroll information
10:00-10:15 AM	Bread, coffee, and fruit provided
10:15-11:30 AM	Tour of facilities by staff development department
11:30 AM–12:00 PM	Introduction of unit heads and purpose of units by staff development department
12:00-1:00 PM	Lunch with unit heads
1:00-2:15 PM	Employee and organizational responsibilities, rules of conduct by personnel department
2:15-2:30 PM	Break, refreshments provided
2:30-4:00 PM	Fire and safety video by staff development department

DAY 2

8:00-10:00 AM	Personnel policies by personnel department
10:00-10:30 AM	Report to unit, have break with preceptor
10:30 AM–12:00 PM	Tour unit with preceptor
	Introduction to unit personnel
	Work schedules, staffing, scheduling policies
12:00-1:00 PM	Lunch with unit personnel
1:00-3:30 PM	CPR recertification by staff development department
3:30-4:00 PM	Universal precautions update by staff development department

DAY 3

Work all day with preceptor on unit and shift
Workload assignment
Introduction to charting
Reporting of accidents
Use of services such as nutrition, physical therapy, occupational therapy, pharmacy, x-ray, clinical laboratory services

DAY 4

Work all day with preceptor on unit and shift
Job description
Standards of performance

DAY 5

Work all day with preceptor on unit and shift
Staff development
Employee appraisal system
Promotion and transfer policies

WEEK 2

Work with preceptor on unit and shift, gradually assuming more responsibilities to full workload day 5 of week 2

CPR, Cardiopulmonary resuscitation.

Orientation to the institution typically includes a tour of the facilities; a description of the organizational structure; a discussion of different departmental functions; a presentation of the philosophy, goals, and standards; an interpretation of administrative policies and procedures; and possibly an explanation of hospital relationships with the community. Next, the nurse will need an orientation to the nursing service, including interdepartmental relationships, departmental organization, administrative controls, philosophy, goals, policies, procedures, and job descriptions.

After the general orientation, new nurses may be assigned to an experienced nurse for orientation to their specific job. New nurses will need a tour of the unit so that they know the location of supplies, equipment, and policy and procedure books. Information about how the unit is run, specific methods of practice, and communication systems is important. Introductions to other personnel can help the new person feel welcome.

Frequent visits to see that the nurse is comfortable and that the orientation is progressing satisfactorily are helpful. Documentation of the orientation process is useful. The documentation may be a simple checklist that itemizes information such as the organizational structure, specific policies, fire and disaster plans, tour of the facilities, and procedures, with space for a signature. It can be retained in the personnel file.

Nurse internship programs are common to assist newly graduated nurses in making the adjustment from the student role to a staff nurse position. The instructor and head nurse usually work together to identify teaching-learning needs, plan rotation schedules, and evaluate the intern's performance. Classes are held on a regular basis for orientation, role adjustment, problem solving, and information about pathophysiology. There is a concentration on the mastery of technical skills. Some programs also present leadership instruction. Nurse internship programs help new graduates build self-confidence, lower frustration levels, increase nursing care planning, improve patient care, improve job satisfaction, and reduce turnover.

In-service education helps keep employees' skills and knowledge up to date. It usually involves how to use new equipment, new patient care procedures, and new services. The Joint Commission on Accreditation of Healthcare Organizations (JCAHO) requires that nursing in-service sessions be offered on a continuing basis and that employee attendance be documented.

Near the end of the probationary period, it is advisable to have a systematic evaluation. The nurse should know what characteristics will be evaluated. Two independent judgments, such as those of the manager and a head nurse, may be secured and used to check reliability of the evaluation. The results of the evaluation are indicative of the success of the selection process.

Orientation alone does not socialize people to the organization. Socialization is the sharing of attitudes and values through role modeling, myths, and legends. It is less structured than orientation. All employees need socialization. Instilling clarity of the value system throughout the organization is the socialization process for team spirit found in excellent organizations. It is correlated with reduced dissatisfaction, absenteeism, and attrition (Marquis and Huston, 1998, 2000; Sullivan and Decker, 2001).

STAFF DEVELOPMENT

"To encourage others is to strengthen the team."
—Anonymous

Staff development goes beyond orientation. It is a continuing liberal education of the whole person to develop her potential fully. It deals with aesthetic senses, as well as technical and professional education, and may include orientation, preceptorships, mentorships, skill checklists, internships, in-service education, courses, conferences, seminars, journal or book clubs, programmed learning, and independent study and refresher courses.

Nurse managers play an important role in the support of staff development and have a responsibility to review the goals for the staff development program and to provide a budget for those activities. They can do coaching by sharing ideas and telling stories about what it takes to succeed. They invest in relationships and plan stretch goals collaboratively with staff. They participate in needs identification and analyze how education effects change in nursing services. They then develop doable projects and actions to deal with the identified needs, delegate to people according to their interest and talents, and give feedback (Hargrove, 2000).

In addition, they must be careful to differentiate staff development needs from administrative needs. If staff nurses know how to do a procedure properly but do not do it because the necessary supplies and equipment are not available to them, the need is administrative rather than educational. Nursing managers are legally liable for the quality of nursing services. Their ability to document staff development provides strong supportive evidence for them. Conversely, the reception of staff development will be largely related to the reward system developed. Positive reinforcement through recognition, such as oral praise on the unit or acknowledgment of accomplishments in a newsletter, is useful. Staff development can also be related to retention, pay raises, advancement to other positions, or termination. The novice to expert theory can be used to guide staff development (Haag-Heitman, 1999; Hargrove, 2000).

PRECEPTORSHIP

Preceptorships may be used to help recruit, retain, orient, and develop staff. They may be used before students graduate to orient them to the agency and to recruit them for hire. If students have worked at an agency before graduation and are familiar with it, they can make sounder decisions about where to work, are not as likely to be unprepared for the work situation, and, consequently, are likely to be retained longer. The preceptorship also gives agency personnel an opportunity to evaluate students and determine if they are suitable candidates for employment.

During the preceptorship faculty members facilitate, monitor, and evaluate student learning. Faculty members direct students to resources, offer suggestions regarding patient care problems, and lead discussions at conferences. Faculty members are responsible for student learning and encouraging students to apply class content.

The preceptor is responsible for the quality of patient care and facilitates the student's learning. Preceptors are liaisons between students and the agency. They help students learn skills and learn how to organize their work. They provide real-life experiences for students before graduation to help reduce the difficulties of transition from school to work.

The professional nurturance of a preceptorship can be likened to the "good old boy" network or godfathers who look after godsons. It allows students to use and increase their knowledge and skills so they can assume increasing responsibilities. They gain experience with a variety of patients and different levels of staff. They have opportunities to discuss and adjust to professional-bureaucratic conflicts. Preceptorships are a potential recruitment tool for the agency and can increase the job satisfaction of nurses. Preceptors may even learn from the students and are likely to find the preceptor role challenging and stimulating.

There are also disadvantages to preceptorships. They add to staff nurses' responsibilities and require time. Sometimes busy nurses have little time to spend with students. It becomes difficult for faculty members to evaluate students because they have little direct observation of the students' work. The use of preceptors requires considerable planning and coordination. Role descriptions should clarify who chooses learning experiences for the student, who supervises the student, and who evaluates the student. Practical evaluation tools of the student, preceptor, and faculty should be developed and used. Educational and service administrative support is needed.

The faculty member serves as a preceptor of preceptors. A workshop to prepare preceptors is desirable. It is appropriate to discuss and clarify role descriptions, skill inventory lists for students, and guidelines for preceptor evaluation of students. Information about teaching methods, counseling, and evaluation is useful. Finding a time and place for the workshop and getting release time for the preceptors may create problems. Awarding continuing education credits for the workshop and preceptor experience may be considered as a way to reward preceptors.

The preceptor model can also be used by the staff development department and nurses after a graduate has been hired. The staff development faculty may present formal content in orientation and development programs that are reinforced by preceptors on the units.

MENTORSHIP

"I hear and I forget. I see and I remember. I do and I understand." —Confucius

Preceptors are role models who may become mentors. Mentors give their time, energy, and material support to teach, guide, assist, counsel, and inspire younger nurses. It is a nurturing relationship that cannot be forced. Close, trusted counselors, usually in their 40s or 50s, acquaint younger nurses, usually in their 20s or 30s, with the values, customs, and resources of the profession. The mentor is a confidant who personalizes role modeling and serves as a sounding board for decisions. The mentor is a resource person who supports the development of the younger person through influence and promotion.

There are phases to the mentoring process (Box 12-7). At first, during the invitational stage, mentors must be willing to use their time and energy to nurture someone who is goal directed, willing to learn, and respectfully trusting of the mentor. The younger professionals have a career goal, a vision of what they want to become; the mentors are people who have reached that goal and are willing to share the secrets of their success. Then there is a period of questioning, when the younger person has self-doubt and fears of being unable to meet the goals.

BOX **12-7** Phases of the Mentoring Process

Invitational:	Mentor uses time and energy to nurture a younger professional who is goal directed, willing to learn, and respectfully trusting of the mentor.
Questioning:	Mentee experiences self-doubt and questioning of goals. Mentor helps clarify goals and provides guidance.
Transitional:	Mentor helps student personalize learning and become aware of own strengths and uniqueness. Mentee is now prepared to be a mentor.

The mentor helps clarify those goals through self-discrimination. Next, mentors share information about power and politics, tell how they became successful, and serve as a sounding board. The transitional phase is the final phase, when mentors help students personalize learning and become aware of their own strengths and uniqueness. Younger nurses are then prepared to be mentors and to tell others how they became what they are.

Mentorship should provide an opportunity to share information, review work, provide feedback, explore issues, plan strategies, and solve problems. It helps socialize novices into professional norms, values, and standards. Career advancement and success are promoted, thus increasing self-confidence, self-esteem, and greater personal satisfaction.

CAREER PLANNING

CHOOSING A FIELD OF NURSING

There are many opportunities in nursing. From the 1930s until the 1990s about 70% of nursing was done in hospitals. Hospital nurses can do medical, surgical, obstetrical, pediatric, and psychiatric nursing or nursing in subspecialties, such as intensive cardiac care. Community health nursing, home care, hospice care, industrial nursing, school nursing, working in a physician's office or clinic, rehabilitation nursing, long-term care, and health promotion are other opportunities. The federal government offers additional options, such as a career in the U.S. Army, Navy, or Air Force and working for the nursing service of the Veterans' Administration or the Indian Health Services. Teaching, consulting, conducting research, serving as a staff member of a professional organization, and being an independent nurse practitioner are possibilities.

To set short-term and long-range goals, one considers the importance of salary, fringe benefits, retirement plans, work hours, and opportunities for advancement. Desirable climate and geographical location are also considerations. Short-term goals help position one for long-range goals. It is advisable to get some clinical experience before applying for teaching or consultation positions. Trends should be taken into consideration for long-term goals. The population is growing older and acquiring chronic diseases; health care reform is focusing on access to high-quality, economical care; care is moving from the hospital to the community; ambulatory care and home care are increasing; and health promotion is being encouraged.

LOCATING JOB OPENINGS

After deciding what type of nursing one wants to do and the geographical area where one wants to practice, one needs to locate job openings. Professional journals advertise positions, and college placement services and employment agencies maintain job listings. Recruiters are often at professional meetings. One can ask friends, acquaintances, and relatives if they know of openings. Employers can be contacted directly.

RESUME

A resume is a summary of information about one's education, employment, and professional and personal history. It is typically a prerequisite for an interview, because the employer uses the resume to determine who will be interviewed.

Consequently, the resume should be carefully developed and updated periodically.

Resumes should be printed on high-quality 8½ by–11 inch typing paper with a laser printer; they should never be handwritten. The contents should be well arranged, with major and minor headings to facilitate reading. The content should be concise yet complete, but not crowded. Resumes should contain the following information.

Identification

Full name, address, and telephone number should appear at the beginning of the resume.

Job Objective

Including or excluding a job objective is controversial. Some say it limits one's scope of employment, whereas others argue that the personnel manager should know what position the nurse is seeking. Separate resumes for each job, customizing the job objective, and accenting the characteristics that qualify the nurse for a particular job are appropriate.

Education

In reverse chronological order, one should list the names and locations of schools attended, dates of attendance, and diploma or degrees conferred. Continuing education, such as workshops, in-service education, and home study courses, indicates an interest in self-improvement and is appropriate to list. If the grade point average is high, it is appropriate to cite it.

Work Experience

Previous employment should be listed in reverse chronological order by identifying the name and location of each agency, dates of employment, position title, and responsibilities. New graduates can list their student clinical experiences. It is appropriate to give a reason for leaving the position.

Military Service

If the applicant has served in the armed forces, a summary of the military record should be included. Branch of service, years in the service, rank achieved, awards and distinctions, special assignments, skills, and knowledge acquired are some of the items appropriate to include.

Affiliations

Memberships, offices, committee activities in professional organizations, learned societies, and civic and social groups may be listed. Religious and political affiliations should be used with discretion.

Honors and Awards

Scholarships, honors, and awards may be cited by stating the honor, the organization that conferred it, the location, and the date.

References

If references are available, it should be stated that they will be provided on request. One should always check the willingness of people who might serve as references. One may also compile a letters of reference file by asking teachers, supervisors, or peers to write letters of reference "to whom it may concern" at the time of termination. This is an opportune moment to make such a request because the nurse's performance is vivid in the reviewer's mind. It may prevent the reviewer from having to write more than one letter when copies are acceptable, and the applicant does not have to be concerned about locating the person later. Compiling one's own letter file allows one to send the most informative and appropriate letters of reference. One keeps the original letters and sends the appropriate photocopies with the resume. Multiple copies with the original signature can be made to save time.

Cover Letter

The resume should be accompanied by a cover letter stating the applicant's interest in working for the specific agency, the special qualifications and interests the applicant brings, the applicant's availability, and how the applicant can be reached.

INTERVIEW

An interview allows the employer to determine if the applicant meets the requirements for the position being sought, and it allows the applicant to obtain information about the agency. First impressions are important. The interviewer will quickly assess the applicant's manners and appearance. The applicant may be questioned about dependability, responsibility, and ability to work with others. The compatibility of the applicant's goals with available opportunities may be explored.

JOB PROCUREMENT

A nurse is likely to apply for more than one job at a time. Once a position has been accepted, the other agencies should be informed of the decision in a friendly and professional way because the nurse may apply to those agencies again in the future.

CAREER MAPPING

"There are two educations, one should teach us how to make a living and the other how to live."
—John Adams

Career mapping is a strategic plan for one's career. It provides direction for formal education, experience, continuing education, professional associations, and networking. Nurses need to assess their own values and define success for themselves. Job security, sense of accomplishment, and opportunities for professional advancement are often considered important. Other issues to consider are work hours, salary, fringe benefits, retirement plans, organizational and geographical climate, and location.

Nurses also need to assess their skills. What do they do well, do poorly, want to do, not want to do, or have the potential to develop?

Once one has (1) assessed interests and skills, one should (2) determine goals, (3) develop a map, and (4) pursue strategies to maintain the map.

It is appropriate to make a list of interests and skills and to set 1-, 5-, and 10-year plans. The time frame can be illustrated in a career map with a 10-year time frame across the top of the paper. Then one can write in years of specific experience under "Dates" and types of education under "Experiences." One might focus on continuing education classes for a time or work on an advanced degree during certain periods.

Ongoing maintenance of the map will reflect advancement efforts: writing, personal presentations, networking, and professional development. The curriculum vitae (CV) and the resume are used interchangeably to present oneself in writing. The CV is a listing of educational, professional, and scholarly accomplishments most commonly used in academic settings. The resume is a concise history of education and experiences in a few pages. The vitae should have an attractive format and contain such information as professional goal, education, work experience, professional memberships, continuing education, research, publications, and presentations. If there have been no accomplishments in a category to date it is best to omit that category from the vitae. Resumes are updated periodically, especially when one is applying for a job. It is helpful to keep information files listing continuing education, organizational memberships, offices, committees, research, publications, and presentations so that accurate information is available for updating the resume. A cover letter should accompany a resume to introduce the sender and explain the purpose for sending the resume: interest in a position.

One must present oneself in person for an interview. One-on-one interviews are common. The applicant is typically asked the following questions: What are your goals? What are your strengths and weaknesses? Why do you want to work here? What do you have to offer this agency? In serial interviews the applicant sees one person after another. Looking attractive, having a positive attitude, remaining consistent, and treating each interviewer as if that person alone will make the decision are appropriate.

Serial interviews are increasingly common as one applies for jobs higher in the hierarchy. The interviewers are interested in the interrelationship with their specific area of responsibility. One's communication skills are tested during group interviews, when several people interview the applicant at once. Stress interviews are sometimes used to test an applicant's reactions to stress. They may leave a very negative feeling about the job; the applicant should try to remember such a test is not a personal attack. After the initial screening the most serious candidates may be asked back for an interview.

It is helpful to network with colleagues inside and outside the organization. Identify individuals who have influence over your career, who can serve as mentors, who can give you career guidance, and who can serve as references. Join professional organizations where you can meet colleagues with similar interests. Volunteer for committee work. Attend conventions and meetings. Have business cards made and swap them with colleagues. Keep in touch with your colleagues, ask for what you need, give feedback, and follow up with contacts.

Careers typically progress through stages of exploration, early career trial and establishment, middle career growth and maintenance, and later career plateau and decline. The exploration stage involves identifying the right career and getting the appropriate education. Early career involves getting the first job, adjusting to a daily work routine, choosing a specialty, transfers and promotions, and broadening one's perspective of the organization and profession. During the middle career people establish their professional identity, choose among alternative career paths, and take on more responsibility. In the later career people develop others, shape the future of the organization, plan for retirement, deal with a reduced workload and less power, and may help develop their replacement.

Exploration typically occurs during ages 15 to 22 years, early career during ages 22 to 38 years, middle career from 38 to 55 years, and later career from 55 to 70 years. However, some women raise a family before they start the exploration stage, and many interrupt their career to raise a family. It is more common for women than men to have discontinuous careers because of family responsibilities. People may change careers during their lifetime too (Steers and Black, 1994).

One progresses in professional development by systematically reviewing professional journals, collecting and filing articles and materials topically, developing a professional library, achieving professional certification, chairing a committee to develop leadership skills, presenting an in-service session, and fostering a support group.

GROUP PROCESS

Group process is critical for group development. How the group functions, communicates, and sets and achieves objectives is all related to group dynamics. Both task-oriented behavior and maintenance-oriented behavior are necessary for adequate group development.

People who assume group task roles coordinate and facilitate the group's efforts to identify the problem, explore alternative options, identify the ramifications of the options, choose the most viable option, and implement and evaluate the plan. There are numerous group task roles, and any member of the group may fulfill a number of these roles in successive participation (Box 12-8).

Initiator-contributors propose new ideas or different ways of approaching a problem. Their task is to identify the problem, clarify the objectives, offer solutions, suggest agenda items, and set time limits. The *information seeker* searches for factual information about the problem, whereas the *opinion seeker* clarifies values pertinent to the problem and its solutions. Unlike the information seeker, the *information giver* identifies facts, shares experiences, and makes generalizations. *Opinion givers* state their beliefs and what they think the group should value. Their focus is on values rather than on facts. The *elaborator* develops suggestions, illustrates points, and predicts outcomes. The coordinator clarifies relationships. The *orienter* summarizes the discussion, activities, and points of departure to provide perspective on the group's progress toward its goal. The *critic* may measure the group's achievement against a set of standards and evaluate the problem, content, and process. The *energizer* stimulates the group to increase the quantity and quality of their work. The *procedural technician* facilitates group action by arranging the room for the meeting, distributing the materials, working the audiovisual equipment, and generally functioning as the "go-for"—the person who goes for what is needed. The *recorder* keeps an account of the discussion, suggestions, and decisions.

BOX **12-8** Group Process Roles

GROUP TASK ROLES	GROUP MAINTENANCE ROLES	DYSFUNCTIONAL ROLES
Initiator-contributor	Gatekeeper	Aggressor
Information seeker	Encourager	Dominator
Opinion seeker	Harmonizer	Recognition seeker
Information giver	Compromiser	Special-interest pleader
Opinion giver	Follower	Blocker
Elaborator	Group observer	Self-confessor
Coordinator	Standard setter	Help seeker
Orienter		Playboy
Critic		
Energizer		
Procedural technician		
Recorder		

The roles of group building and group maintenance focus on how people treat each other while accomplishing a task. The *gatekeeper* regulates communication and takes actions to ensure everyone an opportunity to be heard. *Encouragers* radiate warmth and approval. They offer commendation and praise and indicate acceptance and understanding of others' ideas and values. *Harmonizers* create and maintain group cohesion, relieving tension through their sense of humor and helping others reconcile their disagreements. *Compromisers* promote group process by yielding status, admitting mistakes, modifying their ideas for the sake of group cohesiveness, maintaining self-control for group harmony, or generally making compromises to keep the group action oriented. The *follower,* acting as a passive audience, goes along with the group. The *group observer* keeps records of the group process and gives interpretations for evaluation of the proceedings. The quality of the group process is compared with standards by the *standard setters.*

Some members of the group may try to satisfy their individual needs irrespective of the group tasks or maintenance roles. For example, *aggressors* meet their needs at the expense of others by disapproving of others and deflating their status. The *dominator* asserts authority or superiority through flattery, interrupting others, and giving directions authoritatively. *Recognition seekers* call attention to themselves by boasting and acting in unusual ways. The *special-interest pleader* speaks for an interest group and addresses issues that best meet that need. The *blocker* is negative, resistant, and disagreeable without apparent reason and brings issues back to the floor after the group has rejected them. The *self-confessor* uses the group to express personal feelings, whereas the *help seeker* expresses depreciation, insecurity, and personal confusion that elicit sympathetic responses. The *playboy* has a lack of involvement in the group process and appears nonchalant. A high incidence of individual roles in a group requires self-diagnosis to suggest

what group-training efforts are needed. Having a trained observer record who is fulfilling what roles during a meeting can be revealing. An observer records each time a participant plays a certain role. A form with a list of roles down the left side and columns with the names of participants across the top can be helpful.

TEAM DEVELOPMENT

Groups go through stages of development (Box 12-9). They typically form, organize, solve problems, implement solutions, and disband. During the forming stage, individuals are likely to feel anxious, fearful, doubtful, and self-protective. The leader concentrates on putting the members at ease, explaining the purpose, developing a workable climate, and exerting leadership. Tension tends to be high; suspiciousness, hostility, and resistance are common; and disagreement emerges with the power struggles that occur during the organizing, or storming, phase. The leader needs to clarify goals, policies and procedures, code of conduct, and communication patterns to help the members' progress. Loyalty, trust, confidence, dignity, pride, and group cohesiveness develop during problem solving. The leader seeks to approve recommendations by consensus through a systematic and logical approach. The group has structure and purpose, roles are clarified, and interpersonal relationships are stabilized during the performing stage. The leader should help the group

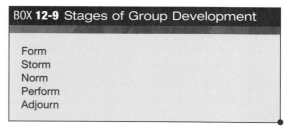

BOX **12-9** Stages of Group Development

Form
Storm
Norm
Perform
Adjourn

Data from Drinka TJK, Clark PG: *Health care teamwork: Interdisciplinary practice and teaching,* Westport, Conn, 2000, Auburn House; Parker GM: *Team players and teamwork: The new competitive business strategy,* San Francisco, 1996, Jossey-Bass.

BOX **12-10** Differences Between Groups And Teams

GROUP	TEAM
Sharing of information	Collective performance goals
Members not necessarily accepting common objectives	Objectives understood and accepted by members
Tending to have majority and minority opinion	Decisions by consensus with members heard and valued
Destructive criticism	Dialogue with resolution
Hidden personal feelings	Free expression accompanied by listening
Little discussion about how the group is functioning	Self-examination about team functioning
Individuals protecting their role and niche	Understood roles
Individual accountability	Individual and mutual accountability
Varied and random skills	Complementary skills
Neutral and sometimes negative energy	Synergy
Leadership that is appointed or elected	Shared leadership

Modified from Mears P, Voehl F: *Team building: A structured learning approach*, Delray Beach, Fla, 1994, St Lucie Press; Robbins SP: *Organization behavior: Concepts, controversies, applications*, ed 9, Upper Saddle River, NJ, 2000, Prentice Hall.

focus on issues, behaviors, or problems, not on a person. The leader should encourage group members to help build self-confidence and self-esteem of others, maintain constructive relationships, and take initiative to make things better. The leader should lead by example. Members may have positive or negative feelings about disbanding. The leader should express appreciation and give positive reinforcement.

According to James Lundy (1992) TEAMS means Together Each Achieves More Success. Dilenschneider has said, "In our age, independence and the ability to get things done are often mutually exclusive" (Lucas, 1998). David Coleman and Raman Khanna (1995) have compared individualism with sprinters who are uncoordinated individuals working toward a goal. The coordination level of group work is like a relay where there is coordinated but independent effort. Group dynamics level resembles a rowing crew that puts a concerted effort toward a goal. Just as there are differences between individuals and groups, there are differences between groups and teams (Box 12-10).

The team is empowered to do what is required. The team members need to know the purpose of the team, the goals, and the targets for accomplishment. Goal setting and planning

strategies to meet the goals are important. There should be plans to measure accomplishments (Box 12-11).

The leader should recruit and hire talented people. The inventory of talent on the team should be known. Team members should know each other's strengths and weaknesses. Team members need to continually develop their knowledge and skills. Although the organizations should use selection procedures and provide training and education opportunities, individual team members have responsibility for updating their own knowledge and skills too. Team members

BOX **12-11** Key Components of Effective Teams

Clear sense of direction
Talented members
Clear and enticing responsibilities
Efficient operating procedures
Constructive interpersonal relationships
Active reinforcement system
Constructive external relationships

Data from Huszczo GE: *Tools for team excellence: Getting your team into high gear and keeping it there*, Palo Alto, Calif, 1996, Davies-Black.

should know their roles and develop themselves to fulfill those roles. Listening, problem solving, conflict management, communication skills, assertiveness, and basic teamwork are important skills to learn.

Teams need policies and procedures for a disciplined but not overly rigid way to get things done. Ground rules help facilitate process and may include the following: One person speaks at a time. Wait for a person to finish speaking. Do not interrupt others. Keep comments to the point. Avoid lengthy stories and examples. Express views openly and honestly. Speak for yourself and use "I" statements. Maintain confidentiality of opinions expressed in the meeting. Focus on issues not on individuals. Stay on the topic. Encourage everyone to participate. Respect differences of opinion (Payne, 2001).

It is also helpful for team members to be familiar with their own and each other's personalities. Knowledge of the Myers-Briggs Type Indicator can help team members plan strategies for resolving conflicts among themselves. Validating different values and motives, building respect for diverse points of view, and integrating a range of perspectives into decision making by ensuring that all team members participate are important. Symbols such as shirts, jackets, or hats can be used to emphasize team identity.

Team members should respect and appreciate each other. It is also important for the organization to have an evaluation and reward system for reinforcing desirable behaviors. Team members need to understand that they will not badmouth each other. They also need to develop diplomatic ties with key players outside their own team (Carr, 1996; Harrington-Mackin, 1996; Huszczo, 1996; Parker, 1996; Porter-O'Grady, 1998; Robbins, 2000).

Organizational cultures that are people oriented, goal directed, and quality driven are conducive to team development (Box 12-12). The role of the manager in the development of self-managing teams is as follows:
- Show a willingness to help establish teams.
- Set goals and expectations.
- Monitor performance.

BOX 12-12 Characteristics of Cultures That Support Teams

Value employees' interpersonal requirements
Promote cooperative rather than competitive relationships
Encourage individual accountability and responsibility
Recognize individual contributions
Have positive visions of the future
Have short- and long-term goals
Have quality standards
Believe in their products and services
Are people oriented
Support the community

From Hicks RF, Bone D: *Self-managing teams*, Menlo Park, Calif, 1990, Crisp Publications.

- Give the team feedback to help it self-correct as it proceeds.
- Build relationships.
- Train and educate team members.
- Acquire needed resources, such as education, consultation, supplies, and equipment.
- Allow processing time.
- Protect the team from the political obstacles and roadblocks that may occur when people in the hierarchy feel threatened because they believe they are losing decision-making power.

Box 12-13 lists the benefits of self-managed teams.

The manager can help ensure the team's success through its infancy by selecting members who work well together, are mature problem solvers, have positive attitudes, are future oriented, are willing to take risks, and are interested in working on a self-managing team. The leader should meet privately with an ineffective team player and confront the person about the undesirable behavior. The leader should listen to understand the other person's point of view, reestablish team norms, and negotiate an agreement on a new behavior. Positive reinforcement should be given for desirable changes. If the person's behavior remains ineffective, reassignment for a better fit and dismissal are options.

Building a successful experience is also important. Documenting and communicating success make it easier to take the next steps. Verbal feedback to the organization about the successes of the team is very powerful. The manager should make sure that the commitment, time, and resources are available for success. She should encourage the team to go slowly enough to do it right and consequently move faster in the long run. Employees should then start feeling autonomy, responsibility, accomplishment, and belongingness that contribute to job satisfaction and synergy. The leader can educate team members so they know what to do; enable them so they know how to do it, and empower them by authorizing them to do it (Harrington-Mackin, 1996; McCoy, 1996; Parker, 1996).

It is appropriate to do a needs assessment to plan for staff development. First, identify the desired knowledge and skills. Then identify the present level of knowledge and skill and determine the discrepancy. Next, identify the resources available to meet the needs, plan and implement appropriate learning strategies, and evaluate the results. How did the learners react to the learning process? Was there behavior change indicating learning occurred? Was there an impact on the organization? Was the staff development cost-effective? Benefits of staff development could be improved job performance, less cost for rework and fixing errors, lowered supervision costs, enhanced service reputation, increased job security, increased job enrichment, enhanced cross training, higher morale, lower attrition, less expense for recruitment, more use of technology, faster implementation of strategic directions, and a more competitive strategic advantage. Benjamin Franklin said, "An investment in knowledge pays the best interest" (Bowsher, 1998; Davenport and Prusak, 1998, p. ix; Marquis and Huston, 2000).

Diversity should be considered when planning learning activities. Learners have diverse learning styles, so it is advisable to use a variety of teaching methods. Cultural variables should also be considered. People raised in a traditional hierarchical system may regard the teacher as an unquestionable authority and may be reticent to speak in class. Nonnative speakers of English may feel insecure to speak in group discussions or activities. Requesting their views may help them speak out. Leaders and managers should not underestimate the power of talk. A story is a good way to convey meaningful knowledge. Organizations should probably shift their focus from documents to discussions. We structure our reality with language. Consequently, Sue Hammond (1998) recommends appreciative inquiry, which appreciates and values the best of what is; envisions what might be; dialogues about what should be; and then innovates what will be. What we focus on becomes our reality. The use of successful history, tradition, and facts distinguishes appreciative inquiry from other visions based on dreams and wishes. People feel more comfortable taking what they know into the future. Dialogue is a powerful tool. It differs from debate, which uses power and knowing answers to prove and win a point. Dialogue uses questions to find out through respectful sharing and listening. Dialoging together can help build bonds and personal relationships (Davenport and Prusak, 1998; Marquis and Huston, 2000; McMaster, 1996; Odenwald, 1996; Zohar, 1997).

Pedagogy (teaching children) differs from andragogy (teaching adults). To teach children, it is appropriate to create an authoritative climate where the teacher makes the decisions, sets the goals, lectures, evaluates, and encourages competition. A more relaxed and informal climate is used for adults, where the teacher and the students make decisions, set goals, process activities, evaluate together, and encourage collaboration (Marquis and Huston, 1998, 2000).

There are several principles of learning and transfer of knowledge. People need to be able to attach what they are learning to what they already know. They need underlying knowledge and skills. They also need confidence to believe they can learn and to be willing to try new skills. They are more motivated to learn if they believe the learning will lead to desirable outcomes. Immediate and specific feedback improves performance. Self-monitoring and feedback become important as people increase their competency. Content can be taught in a concentrated or distributed way. Complex material that is learned over time is usually retained longer than material taught in a concentrated way. Storage of knowledge and skills in long-term memory is necessary to transfer it. Identical elements or training in a context similar to the real work environment facilitates transfer, as does stimulus variability, which incorporates a variety of situations one would encounter on the job into the training. General principles also enhance transfer of knowledge by having learners apply principles to a variety of situations they might encounter in the workplace. Relapse prevention then facilitates long-term maintenance of learned behaviors. People can identify high-risk situations and plan coping strategies to deal with them and can use "what if" scenarios to practice new knowledge and skills.

Numerous teaching methods and tools are available, including but not limited to lecture, discussion, role playing, case studies, simulations, games, small group activities, movies, audiotapes, videotapes, overheads, models, graphic materials, still pictures, drawings, graphs, posters, cartoons, and handouts. Technology has made Web pages, Internet, e-mail, listservs, chat rooms, telephone calls, telephone bridges, conference calls, voice mail, fax, audio conferencing, video conferencing, virtual instrumentation, interactive video, and multimedia possible. Videotelephone (a form of videoconferencing or desktop conferencing), videoconferencing, video/image mailboxes, image/fax transmission, and desk-to-desk conferencing, or integrated voice/data communications, are increasing (Billings and Halstead, 1998).

Chapter Summary

Chapter 12 covered the following:
Selection of Personnel
   Dealing with the Nursing Shortage
   Recruitment and Retention
   Screening of Potential Staff
      Application forms and resumes
      Letters of reference
      Interview
      Testing
Equal Opportunity and Affirmative Action
   Legal Interviewing Questions
Multicultural Workforce
Cultural Diversity
Sexual Preference and Gender
Generational Differences
Americans With Disabilities Act
Job Redesign
   Job Analysis
   Job Evaluation
   Job Design
   Job Simplification
   Job Rotation
   Job Enrichment
   Job Descriptions
   Career Ladders and Performance
      Management Plans
Orientation
Staff Development
   Preceptorship

On-line Resources

evolve   Additional critical thinking activities, worksheets, and case studies are available on-line at http://evolve.elsevier.com/Marriner/guide/

References

Alabama v Flowers Hospital, Inc, 33 F 3d 1308 A-1, 1994.

Arthur D: *Recruiting, interviewing, selecting & orienting new employees,* ed 3, New York, 1998, AMACOM.

Bennis W, Spreitzer GM, Cummings TG, editors: *The future of leadership: Today's top leadership thinkers speak to tomorrow's leaders*, San Francisco, 2001, Jossey-Bass.

Bennis WG, Thomas RJ: *Geeks & geezers: How era, values, and defining moments shape leaders,* Boston, 2002, Harvard Business School Press.

Billings DM, Halstead JA: *Teaching in nursing: A guide for faculty,* Philadelphia, 1998, WB Saunders.

Blanchard K, Lacinak T, Tompkins C, et al: *Whale done!! The power of positive relationships*, New York, 2002, The Free Press.

Bowsher JE: *Revolutionizing workforce performance: A systems approach to mastery,* San Francisco, 1998, Jossey-Bass Pfeiffer.

Cahn SM: *Affirmative action debate,* ed 2, New York, 2002, Routledge.

Carr C: *Choice, change & organizational change: Practical insights from evolution for business leaders & thinkers,* New York, 1996, American Management Association.

Champy J: *Reengineering management: The mandate for new leadership,* New York, 1995, Harper Business.

Cody v Cigna Healthcare of St. Louis, Inc, 139 F 3d 595 (8th Cir), 1998.

Coleman D, Khanna R: *Groupware: Technologies and applications,* Upper Saddle River, NJ, 1995, Prentice Hall.

Cox T: *Creating the multicultural organization: A strategy for capturing the power of diversity,* San Francisco, 2001, Jossey-Bass.

Davenport TH, Prusak L: *Working knowledge: How organizations manage to know,* Boston, 1998, Harvard Business School Press.

Doverspike D, Taylor MA, Arthur W: *Affirmative action: A psychological perspective,* Huntington, NY 2000, Nova Science Publishers, Inc.

Drinka TJK, Clark PG: *Health care teamwork: Interdisciplinary practice and teaching,* Westport, Conn, 2000, Auburn House.

Giger JN, Davidhizar R: Transcultural nursing assessment: *A method for advancing nursing practice, Int Nurs Rev* 37:199-202, 1990.

Goldberg B: *Age works: What corporate America must do to survive the graying of the workforce,* New York, 2000, The Free Press.

Goodhouse V: Magnolia Hospital 92F, ed 3: 248, 1996.

Grohar-Murray ME, DiCroce HR: *Leadership and management in nursing,* Stamford, Conn, 2003, Appleton & Lange.

Haag-Heitman B: *Clinical practice development using novice to expert theory,* Gaithersburg, Md, 1999, Aspen Publication.

Hammond SA: *The thin book of appreciative inquiry*, ed 2, Plano, Tex, 1998, Thin Book.

Hargrove R: *Masterful coaching fieldbook: Grow your business, multiply your profits, win the talent war!* San Francisco, 2000, Jossey-Bass Pfeiffer.

Harrington-Mackin D: *Keeping the team going: A tool kit to renew & refuel your workplace teams,* New York, 1996, American Management Association.

Harrington-Mackin D: *The team building tool kit,* New York, 1994, American Management Association.

Howard N: *North Mississippi Medical Center,* 939 F. Suppl 505, 1996.

Huszczo GE: *Tools for team excellence: Getting your team into high gear and keeping it there,* Palo Alto, Calif, 1996, Davies-Black.

Job descriptions, Denver General Hospital.

Joint Commission on Accreditation of Healthcare Organizations: *Health care at the crossroads: Strategies for addressing the evolving nursing crisis* (http://www.jcaho.org), accessed 7/23/03.

Jessie v Carter Health Care Center, Inc, 926 F Supp 613 (ED Ky), 1996.

Jones v Kerrville State Hospital, 142, Fed 3d 263 (5th Cir), 1998.

Karp H, Fuller C, Sirias D: *Bridging the boomer Xer gap:creating authentic teams for high performance at work,* Palo Alto, Calif, 2002, Davies-Black Publishing.

Lancaster LC, Stillman D: *When generations collide: Who they are, why they clash, how to solve the generational puzzle at work,* New York, 2002, Harper Collins Publisher.

Laurin v Providence Hospital and Massachusetts Nurses Association, 150 F3d 52 (1st Cir), 1998.

Little Forest Medical Center of Akron v Ohio Civil Rights Commission, 631 NE 2d 1068, 1993.

Lucas JR: *Balance of power,* New York, 1998, American Management Association.

Lundy JL: *Teams: Together each achieves more success: How to develop peak performance teams for world-class results,* Chicago, 1992, Dartnell.

Madel v PCI Marketing, Inc, 116 F 3d 1247 (8th Cir), 1997.

Marquis BL, Huston CJ: *Leadership roles and management functions in nursing: Theory and application,* Philadelphia, 2000, Lippincott.

Marquis BL, Huston CJ: *Management decision making for nurses:* 124 case studies, Philadelphia, 1998, Lippincott.

Mauro v Borgess Medical Center, 4:94 CV 05 (Michigan), 1995.

McCoy TJ: *Creating an open book organization... where employees think & act like business partners,* New York, 1996, American Management Association.

McKay DI: Career ladders in nursing: An overview, *Am J Nurs* 12:272-278, Sept-Oct 1986.

McMaster MD: *The intelligence advantage: Organizing for complexity,* Boston, 1996, Butterworth-Heinemann.

Odenwald SB: *Global solutions for teams: Moving from collision to collaboration,* Chicago, 1996, Irwin.

O'Keefe ME: *Nursing practice and the law: Avoiding malpractice and other risks,* Philadelphia, 2001, FA Davis.

Parker GM: *Team players and teamwork: The new competitive business strategy,* San Francisco, 1996, Jossey-Bass.

Payne V: *The team-building workshop: A trainer's guide,* New York, 2001, American Management Association.

Porter-O'Grady T: *The health care teambook,* St Louis, 1998, Mosby.

Raines C, Hunt J: *The Xers & the boomers: From adversaries to allies—A diplomat's guide,* Menlo Park, Calif, 2,000, Crisp Publications.

Robbins SP: *Organization behavior: Concepts, controversies, applications,* ed 9, Upper Saddle River, NJ, 2000, Prentice Hall.

Steers RM, Black JS: *Organization behavior,* ed 5, New York, 1994, Harper Collins College.

Sullivan EJ, Decker PJ: *Effective leadership and management in nursing,* ed 5, Upper Saddle River, NJ, 2001, Prentice Hall.

Swansburg RC, Swansburg RJ: *Introductory management and leadership for nurses:* An interactive text, Boston, 2002, Jones & Bartlett.

Tayeb MH: *The management of a multicultural workforce,* Chichester, NY, 1996, John Wiley & Sons.

Thompson v Holy Family Hospital, 122 F 3d 537 (9th Cir), 1997.

Tulgan B: *Managing generation X: How to bring out the best in young talent.* New York, 2000, WW Norton & Co.

Tulgan B, Martin CA: *Managing generation Y: Global citizens born in the late seventies and early eighties,* Amherst, Mass, 2001, HRD Press.

UAW v Johnson Controls, Inc, 55 Sup Ct 356, 1991.

Webb v Mercy Hospital, 102 E 3d (8th Cir), 1996.

Wilking v County of Ramsey, 983 F Supp 848 (D Kan), 1997.

Winfeld L, Spielman S: *Straight talk about gays in the workplace,* ed 2, New York, 2001, Harrington Press, Inc.

Yoder-Wise PS: *Leading and managing in nursing,* ed 2, St Louis, 2002, Mosby.

Zamudio v Patia, 956 F Supp 803 (ND Ill), 1997.

Zemke R, Raines C, Filipczak B: *Generations at work: Managing the clash of veterans, boomers, Xers, and nexters in your workplace,* New York, 2000, American Management Association.

Zimmer M: Rationale for a ladder for clinical advancement in nursing practice, *JONA* 2(6):18-24, 1972.

Zohar D: *Dewiring the corporate brain: Using the new science to rethink how we structure and lead organizations,* San Francisco, 1997, Berrett-Koehler.

13

Staffing and Scheduling

*"No person was ever honored for what he received.
Honor has been the reward for what he gave."*
—Calvin Coolidge

Chapter Overview

Chapter 13 presents assignment systems for staffing including case
management and managed care, staffing schedules, variable staffing,
variables affecting staffing, and staffing to meet fluctuating needs.

Chapter Objectives

- Identify at least five patient care delivery modes or assignment systems.
- Compare and contrast at least three patient care delivery modes or
  assignment systems.
- Discuss the relationship between case management and managed care if any.
- List at least six policy issues related to staffing schedules.
- Describe the pros and cons of centralized and decentralized scheduling.
- Identify at least three different staffing patterns and discuss the pros and
  cons of each.
- Describe how to calculate the number of full-time staff needed for vacation,
  holiday, and absentee coverage per year.

Major Concepts and Definitions

Case method assigning each patient to a nurse for total patient care
Functional nursing hierarchical division of labor
Team nursing RNs supervising auxiliary nursing staff
Modular nursing district nursing
Primary nursing RNs giving total patient care to a few patients
Managed care comprehensive health care system services through established networks of hospitals, physicians, and other health care providers to give population-wide access to economical, high-quality care
Case management management and coordination of the care a patient receives in all settings throughout an episode of illness
Collaborative practice cooperative interdisciplinary practice
Differential practice distinction between professional and technical nursing
Partners in practice interdisciplinary team
Staffing schedules work schedules for personnel
Centralized scheduling scheduling done in one location
Decentralized scheduling scheduling done in local areas
Self-scheduling staff coordinating their own work schedules
Rotating work shifts alternating work hours among days, evenings, and nights
Permanent shifts personnel working the same hours repeatedly
Block scheduling using the same schedule repeatedly
Variable staffing determining the number and mix of staff based on patient needs
Patient classification systems calculating staffing needs based on patient acuity
Staffing formulas calculations used to determine staffing needs

ASSIGNMENT SYSTEMS FOR STAFFING

Changes in assignment systems are a response to changing needs. In the 1920s the case method and private duty nursing were popular. By 1950 functional nursing was predominant in response to the shortage of nurses. During that decade team nursing was introduced to maximize use of the knowledge and skills of professional nurses and to supervise auxiliary workers. The late 1960s and 1970s witnessed a shift back to care of the patient by a professional nurse through primary nursing. Case management became popular during the 1980s, and managed competition emerged as an economic strategy guiding health care reform during the 1990s. It stimulated partners in practice, which is an interdisciplinary team. Each system involves leaders and managers

(Table 13-1) and has advantages and disadvantages (Table 13-2) (Grohar-Murray and DiCroce, 2003).

CASE METHOD

In the case method each patient is assigned to a nurse for total patient care while that nurse is on duty. The patient has a different nurse each shift and no guarantee of having the same nurses the next day. The patient care coordinator, with no obligation to assign nurses to the same patient, supervises and evaluates all care given on the unit. Popular during the 1920s along with private duty nursing, the case method emphasized following physicians' orders (Grohar-Murray and DiCroce, 2003).

FUNCTIONAL NURSING

In the 1950s, when few registered and only some practical nurses were available, nurses' aides

TABLE **13-1** Staffing Leadership and Management

LEADER	MANAGER
Is knowledgeable about staffing and scheduling	Develops fair scheduling policies and disseminates them
Is accountable for safe staffing	Assumes accountability for fiscal control and quality of staffing
Considers the impact of extraneous factors on staffing	Provides staffing to meet patient needs
Examines unit standard of productivity periodically to determine if changes are needed	Schedules staff in a fiscally responsible way
Encourages a team approach to staffing	Keeps policies in compliance with laws

Modified from Marquis BL, Huston CJ: *Leadership roles and management functions in nursing: Theory & application,* Philadelphia, 2000, Lippincott.

TABLE **13-2** Pros and Cons of Various Assignment Systems

ASSIGNMENT SYSTEM	PROS	CONS
Case method	Total patient care	Different nurse, different shifts, different days
Functional nursing	Efficiency	Nurses do managerial work
		Nurses' aides do patient care
Team nursing	Team effort	Time needed to coordinate delegated work
	Frees patient care coordinator to manage the unit	
	Nursing care conferences help problem solve and develop staff	
	Nursing care plan	
Modular nursing	Useful where there are few RNs	Paraprofessionals do technical aspects of care
	RNs plan care	
Primary nursing	RNs give total patient care	Confines nurse's talents to a limited number of patients
	Primary nurse has 24-hour responsibility	Associate nurse may change care plan without discussing with primary nurse
	Associate nurse works with patient while the primary nurse is off duty	
	Accountability in place	
	Continuity of care is facilitated	
	Reduces number of errors from relay of orders	
	Fewer patient complaints	
	Shorter hospitalization	
Managed care	Incorporates case management	Questionable continuity of care
	Can be used with any nursing care deliver system	
	Standard critical paths	
	Increases efficiency	
	Reduces costs	
Case management	Focuses on entire episode of illness	Effort to coordinate
	Emphasizes achievement of outcomes	
	Care is coordinated by a case manager	
	Second-generation primary nursing	
	Critical paths	
	Variation analysis	
	Intershift reports	
	Health care team meetings	
	Interdisciplinary approach	

gave much patient care. In functional nursing hierarchical structure predominates. The medication nurse, treatment nurse, and bedside nurse are all products of this system. The functional method implements classic scientific management, which emphasizes efficiency, division of labor, and rigid controls. It is an efficient system that is the least costly and requires few registered nurses (RNs). Procedural descriptions are used to describe the standard of care, and psychological needs typically are slighted. Care tends to be fragmented and depersonalized. RNs keep busy with managerial and nonnursing duties, and nurses' aides deliver the majority of patient care.

Although efficient, the functional assignment method does not encourage patient and staff satisfaction. Regimentation of tasks may bore nurses because they no longer have the satisfaction of seeing the effects of their total patient care. On the other hand, the functional system may work satisfactorily during critical staffing shortages. Routinized patient care for patients with similar needs may meet those needs more consistently than other systems, and some staff members may be satisfied by doing repetitious jobs well (Marquis and Huston, 2000; Swansburg and Swansburg, 2002; Yoder-Wise, 2003).

TEAM NURSING

After World War II RNs were still scarce, although the number of auxiliary personnel had increased. Team nursing was introduced during the 1950s to improve nursing services in hospitals and nursing homes by using the knowledge and skills of professional nurses and to supervise the increasing numbers of auxiliary nursing staff. The result was an improvement in patient and staff satisfaction. Team nursing is based on a philosophy that supports the achievement of goals through group action. Each team member is encouraged to make suggestions and share ideas. When team members see their suggestions implemented, their job satisfaction increases, and they are motivated to give even better care.

The team is led by a professional or technical nurse who plans, interprets, coordinates, supervises, and evaluates the nursing care. Team leaders assign team members to patients by matching patient needs with staff's knowledge and skills. They also do the work other members of the team are not qualified to perform. They set goals and priorities for patient care; centralize information through the use of a Kardex; direct the planning of care by directing care conferences and developing care plans; fix responsibility for the work; provide for coverage during absences, such as breaks, meals, and conferences; and coordinate and evaluate team activities. The team members report to the team leader, who reports to the patient care coordinator. This is a form of decentralization that frees the patient care coordinator to manage the unit.

One of the main features of team nursing is the nursing care conference. Its primary purpose is the development and revision of nursing care plans by providing an opportunity to identify and solve problems. Precision in the identification of problems is increased through information sharing. The belief that the total group has more information about a topic than any one person enhances the staff's appreciation of group work. A resulting consensus increases the commitment to the decisions made. Identification of the problem and determination of goals early in the conference necessarily precede planning intervention. During the conference, one care plan can be developed or the care plans for a caseload can be updated.

Team conferences also provide the opportunity to identify and work through staff educational needs. Nurses can review standards of care by comparing the actual patient's condition with the textbook example. They can review procedures and learn specialized nursing care and the operation of infrequently used equipment. By studying critical incidents, they may prevent problems from recurring and identify the contributing components of excellent care. Team conferences also provide an opportunity to discuss and resolve interpersonal problems and the chance to prevent future ones. Consequently, team spirit is fostered.

The team leader is responsible for planning and conducting the team conference, which should be limited in time and scope. Meeting for 15 to 30 minutes at the same time each day helps the conference become a part of the daily routine. A time that least interferes with other activities and a place away from the hub of activity are preferable. The team leader must arrange for coverage of the unit during the conference, because relief from patient care responsibilities is essential to prevent interruptions. Staff should be informed of the time, place, and purpose of the conference, so that they can plan their other work around the conference and be well prepared on arrival. Interest can be stimulated by allowing the staff to decide which patient they wish to discuss at the next conference and by having one of the team members record patient problems and solutions during the conference.

Preparation of the meeting area is also a responsibility of the team leader. Temperature, ventilation, lighting, and chair arrangements should be controlled. Refreshments may be appropriate. The team leader introduces the topic and starts the meeting on time to motivate latecomers to be more prompt. A brief review of the patient's condition is appropriate. The team leader monitors the group process, records problems and solutions on the nursing care plan or delegates that task, does appropriate teaching, and summarizes the major points. The nursing care plan is then available to the staff. The team leader serves as a role model by referring to the care plan while receiving and giving reports, making out assignments, and administering nursing care.

The nursing care plan is another main feature of team nursing. A care plan identifying present and potential problems and long- and short-term objectives should be developed for each patient. The care plan should be realistic to prevent morale problems that result from setting unattainable objectives. Care plans should be individualized, reflecting the interrelatedness of psychosocial and physiological needs and involving patient and family participation. Problems, mutually acceptable goals, objectives, actions, and responses are identified. The care is evaluated according to how well the objectives are met.

Team nursing contributes to the satisfaction of patient and staff needs. Each patient is treated as a unique individual. Staff can identify their contributions and the correlation between their work and patient outcomes. The closer interaction of staff contributes to *esprit de corps.*

Because each staff member does many tasks for a limited number of patients instead of a single task for a large number of patients, there is an increased likelihood of errors and a need to spend more time monitoring for them. It also takes time to coordinate delegated work. Although team leaders probably have the least contact with the patients, they are responsible for assessment, planning, and communicating with the physician. Continuity of care is not a given, because patients are not assigned to the same staff all the time and large assignments make individualized patient care difficult. Changing team membership makes it difficult for the team leader to know team members well enough to match their talents with patient needs. Team nursing is similar to functional nursing when the team leader administers medications and treatments other team members are not qualified to give. Team conferences are often omitted because they are difficult to fit into busy days, and care plans (if done) usually note functional duties relative to the physician's orders. Care plans rarely depict the patient as a total person and consequently are not comprehensive. Medication precautions, fluid intake requirements, dietary and environmental adaptations, protective measures, psychological support, teaching, rehabilitation, and referrals are seldom mentioned. In reality the key features of team nursing—nursing care conferences and nursing care plans—often receive inadequate attention, resulting in routinized care (Grohar-Murray and DiCroce, 2003; Marquis and Huston, 2000; Swansburg and Swansburg, 2002; Yoder-Wise, 2003).

RESEARCH Perspective 13-1

Data from Aiken LH, Clarks SP, Sloane DM: Hospital staffing, organization, and quality of care: Cross-national findings. *Nursing Outlook* 50:187-194, Sept/Oct 2002.

Purpose: The purpose of this study was to examine the effects of nurse staffing and organizational support for nursing care on nurses' dissatisfaction with their jobs, nurse burnout, and nurse reports of quality of patient care in an international sample of hospitals.

Methods: This was a multisite cross-sectional survey of 10,319 nurses working on medical and surgical units in 303 hospitals across the five jurisdictions to obtain data on hospital organizational attributes, managerial policies, staffing and resource availability, job satisfaction and burnout, and nurse-assessed patient outcomes. Logistic regression models were used to analyze the data.

Results/conclusions: Dissatisfaction, burnout, and concerns about quality of care were common among hospital nurses in all five sites. Adequate nurse staffing and organizational/managerial support for nursing are key to improving the quality of patient care, to diminishing nurse job dissatisfaction and burnout, and to improving the nurse retention problem in hospital settings.

MODULAR, OR DISTRICT, NURSING

Modular, or district, nursing is a modification of team and primary nursing. It uses smaller teams for patients who are grouped geographically. It is sometimes used when there are not enough RNs to practice primary nursing. Each RN, assisted by paraprofessionals, delivers as much care as possible to a group of patients. The RN plans the care, delivers as much of it as possible, and directs the paraprofessionals for the more technical aspects of care. The RN's role is closer to that of a coordinator and information processor than that of a charge nurse.

Modular nursing decreases the sense of isolation and unrealistic expectations often associated with primary nursing. When nurses are consistently assigned to the same module, continuity and quality of care can increase. More time may be spent in direct care. Closer monitoring is possible. Morale can improve when staff know they are making a difference. It is less costly than primary nursing but more costly and less efficient than team nursing.

Some physical changes may be necessary to implement modular, or district, nursing. For example, a medication cart may be placed in the hall instead of using a medication room. Kardexes may be kept on the medication cart. Charts may be moved to the patient's room. Patient Kardexes and staff identification badges may be color coded (Marquis and Huston, 2000).

PRIMARY NURSING

During the late 1960s and early 1970s, primary nursing was instituted in some hospitals by professional nurses who were unhappy with fragmented care and lack of direct patient contact. Based on the philosophy that patients, instead of tasks, should be the focus of professional nurses, primary nursing features an RN who gives total patient care to four to six patients. The RN remains responsible for the care of those patients 24 hours per day throughout the patient's hospitalization. The associate nurse cares for the patient by using the care plan developed by the primary nurse while the primary nurse is off duty. The associate nurse is expected to contact the primary nurse regarding changes in the care plan. The number of patients assigned to one nurse varies according to length of hospitalization, complexity of care, number of medical and paramedical personnel involved with the patient's care, availability of support systems, and the shift worked. Day-shift nurses are assigned the greatest number of patients; evening nurses have some; and night nurses are primarily auxiliary nurses because of their reduced contact with patients and families.

The primary nurse does the admission interview and develops the nursing care plan, including teaching and discharge planning, which is shared with the associate nurse. Primary nurses have autonomy and authority for the care of their patients. Consequently, accountability is placed and continuity of care is facilitated. Primary nursing decreases the number of people in the chain of command and reduces the number of errors that can result from a relay of orders. Other advantages include mobile use of auxiliary workers and increased satisfaction by both nurse and patient. Nurses can identify patient outcomes as a result of their work. Patients have the security of knowing the nurse is available and has to cope with fewer people than in other assignment systems. Research suggests that patients have fewer complications and a shorter hospitalization when cared for by a primary nurse.

Unfortunately, primary nursing confines a nurse's talents to a limited number of patients. Other patients cannot benefit, and if a patient has a nurse who is not capable, the patient may be worse off than if cared for by numerous people, some of whom might meet the patient's needs. Another problem occurs when the associate nurse changes the care plan without discussing the reasons with the primary nurse. Thus it is critical that the primary nurse communicate verbal and written plans to the associate nurse. The success of primary nursing seems to depend on the quality of the nursing staff and administrative support (Grohar-Murray and DiCroce, 2003; Marquis and Huston, 2000; Sullivan and Decker, 2001; Swansburg and Swansburg, 2002; Yoder-Wise, 2003).

CASE MANAGEMENT

Case management has its roots in psychiatry and social work that focused on chronic long-term

outpatient care in the 1920s. It was used by community health nursing in the 1930s, and it was adapted to acute-care settings and outpatient services during the mid-1980s. It focuses on an entire episode of illness, including all settings in which the client receives care. A case manager coordinates services for the patient and family. Options for alternative health care, living arrangements, and community and social services are considered. Arrangements with nonpreferred providers may be negotiated to reduce claim costs. Case management can cross departmental and disciplinary boundaries.

There are a variety of models for case management. The nurse may give care and coordinate it or just coordinate it. The nurse may work across agencies such as an ambulatory clinic, acute-care facilities, and long-term care facilities or may make site visits to the home or health care agencies. Case management emphasizes achievement of outcomes in designated time frames with limited resources. Case management is sometimes called second-generation primary nursing.

Case management involves critical paths, variation analysis, intershift reports, case consultation, health care team meetings, and quality assurance. Critical paths visualize outcomes within a time frame and have been developed for various diagnoses. Variation analysis notes positive or negative changes from the critical path, the cause, and the corrective action taken. This information is reported in intershift reports. Case consultation may be indicated when the client's condition differs from the critical path as noted in the intershift report. Case consultation is conducted about once each week for a few minutes immediately after intershift report to deal with variations. It can also be conducted informally whenever a staff member identifies a variation and consults others. The problem solvers focus on the variation and the desired outcomes, brainstorm ideas to achieve desired outcomes, and use open communication to evaluate a plan. A summary can be used to close the session.

Health care team meetings provide an interdisciplinary approach to problem solving.

The case manager needs to identify no more than three priority goals and decide what team members should be present after considering the patient, family, physician, social service, various therapists, and others involved. The case manager should set the time and place for the meeting, make the arrangements, and post the date, time, place, and people to attend in the Kardex. The case manager calls the meeting to order, states the goals, initiates discussion, documents the plans, and sets time limits for follow-through. The variance between what is expected and what happens is assessed for quality assurance. Collaboration is important (Cesta, 2002; Conger, 1999; Dykes and Wheeler, 1997; Grohar-Murray and DiCroce, 2003; Marquis and Huston, 2000; Poirrier and Oberleitner, 1999, Siefker, Garrett, and Genderen, 1997; Swansburg and Swansburg, 2002; Yoder-Wise, 2003).

COLLABORATIVE PRACTICE

Collaborative practice can include interdisciplinary teams, nurse-physician interaction in joint practice, or nurse-physician collaboration in caregiving. Collaboration is cooperative and assertive. The interaction between nurses and physicians or other health care team members in collaborative practice should enable the knowledge and skills of the professions to influence the quality of patient care provided synergistically. It is important to the managed care models that proliferated during the 1990s (Del Togno-Armanasco, 1993; Etheredge, 1993).

The American Nurses Association (ANA) and the American Medical Association (AMA) established the National Joint Practice Committee (NJPC) in 1972 with funding from the W.K. Kellogg Foundation. The committee's report supported collaborative practice and suggested that increased collaboration results in improved quality of care and patient and nurse satisfaction and a decreased need for physician supervision of nurses. Primary nursing, nurse decision making, integrated patient records, a joint practice committee, and a joint record review were found to enhance nurse-physician collaboration.

During the 1990s there was a rapid move of health care from the hospital to the community. With the rapidly aging population, accompanying increase in chronic diseases, interdisciplinary teams, and advancing technology, a computer- and network-based community infrastructure became increasingly important. A prototype of an information system in community nursing was developed in Delphi programming environment, and an international classification of nursing practice was published and is copyrighted by the International Council of Nurses.

A common classification system became increasingly important for communication. The first nurse-initiated classification system began in 1973 and is known as NANDA (North American Nursing Diagnosis Association). Nurses have worked at refining that over the decades, and a research team at the University of Iowa formed the Nursing Diagnosis and Extension Classification to refine, extend, validate, and classify nursing diagnoses in collaboration with NANDA to produce a comprehensive and validated taxonomy of nursing. Researchers have been leading the classification work through the Center for Nursing Classification at the University of Iowa College of Nursing. NIC (Nursing Interventions Classification) interventions have been linked with NANDA nursing diagnoses and the Omaha system problems and are being linked with NOC (Nursing Outcomes Classification). NOC has been recognized by the ANA Congress of Nursing Practice Steering Committee on Databases to Support Clinical Nursing Practice as useful for clinical nursing practice and has been included in the National Library of Medicine for inclusion in the Unified Medical Language System (UMLS) (Johnson, Bulechek, Dochterman, et al, 2001; Johnson, Mass, and Moorhead, 2000; McCloskey and Bulechek, 2000).

Staff and supervisors of the Visiting Nurses Association of Omaha developed the Omaha classification system. The three parts—(1) problem classification, (2) intervention scheme, and (3) problem rating scale for outcomes—were developed for community health nursing (Pesut and Herman, 1999). The 1999 ANA House of Delegates passed a recommendation to "advocate the timely implementation of ANA-recognized standardized nursing languages (SNLs) including the Nursing Management Minimum Data Set (NMMDS) to establish comparability nursing data across clinical settings, populations, geography and time" (ANA House of Delegates materials, 1999).

During the 1990s primary care became a focus of health care. Nurse practitioner programs had a marked increase in enrollment as advanced practice nurses played a key role in primary care. Medical education made some shift from specialties to general medicine. Health maintenance organizations (HMOs), preferred provider organizations (PPOs), and integrated health care systems increased.

MANAGED CARE

During the 1980s managed care referred to unit-based acute care, but over time it was transformed (Table 13-3). During the 1990s the focus shifted from acute care to promotion of health

and disease management of chronic and terminal care. Managed care involves financing care and risk management of acute, chronic, and terminal diseases as health maintenance organizations (HMOs), preferred provider organizations (PPOs), and integrated care systems proliferate. Managed care is shaped by fluid market forces and changes quickly and frequently. No single definition of managed care has endured for long, and continuous change is probable. There are several differences between traditional insurance programs and managed care. Traditional insurance allowed patients to see any health care professional with unlimited access to specialty providers and coverage for acute illness or injury only. Managed care uses a network of credentialed care professionals, covers primary and preventive care, and restricts access to specialty providers. Traditional insurance assumed all financial risk and used multiple providers to deliver care without knowledge of the total patient plan of care. Retrospective audits were done on claims data only. Managed care transfers risk to the providers, has the patient care

TABLE **13-3** Leader for Managed Care and Manager for Case Management

LEADERS FOR MANAGED CARE	MANAGERS FOR CASE MANAGEMENT
Facilitate the development of a managed care strategic vision and mission	Give and/or coordinate care
Facilitate the development of a managed care strategic plan	Emphasize outcomes in time frames
Communicate with and educate stakeholders in the integrated network	Serve as impartial patient advocate
Develop a continuum of care	Educate patient and family
Develop contracts with providers of care, and develop financial risk–sharing contracts	Work across agencies
Facilitate continuous quality improvement	Maintain relationship with referral source
Facilitate use of critical paths and care maps with management development of staff	Serve as liaison with insurance claims
Support case management and use of alternative care delivery as a way to control costs	Do variance analysis and evaluate outcomes
Facilitate development of integrated information management capabilities	Use case consultation as necessary
Lead a flexible organization that can make changes rapidly to meet quickly changing needs	Conduct team meetings as necessary

Modified from Cesta TG: *Survival strategies for nurses in managed care*, St Louis, 2002, Mosby; Conger MM: *Managed care: Practice strategies for nursing*, Thousand Oaks, Calif, 1999, Sage; Finkelman AW: *Managed care: A nursing perspective*, Upper Saddle River, NJ, 2001, Prentice Hall; Kongstvedt PR: *Essentials of managed health care*, Gaithersburg, Md, 2001, Aspen; Turner SO: *The nurse's guide to managed care*, Gaithersburg, Md, 1999, Aspen.

provider manage and coordinate the patient's care, and does prospective review of the costs, use, and quality of treatment (Knight, 2002; Kongstvedt, 2001).

DIFFERENTIATED PRACTICE

Differentiated practice generally refers to the difference between professional and technical nursing. Complexity of decision making, timeline of care, and structure of the setting are its main distinctive features. The Midwest Alliance in Nursing organization facilitated clarification of differentiated practice. Professional nurses have received a baccalaureate or graduate degree. They give direct care to patients with complex interactions of nursing diagnoses and relate to their families from preadmission time to postdischarge time in a variety of more or less structured settings. Until the 1990s the technical nurse received a diploma or an associate degree and gave nursing care to patients with common conditions and to their families in structured settings. With the movement of health care into the community and an attempt to lower health care costs, technical nurses, licensed practical nurses (LPNs), and unlicensed personnel are used in the community and less structured situations too.

The original Integrated Competencies of Nurses (ICON) model addressed entry into practice roles by developing a differentiated practice model. The baccalaureate degree–prepared nurses assessed, planned, and evaluated. The associate degree–prepared nurses implemented care. One professional and two or three associate nurses cared for 10 to 15 patients during the day. ICON II responded to the shortage of nurses by "grandfathering" all RNs into the professional role. LPNs then filled the technical role.

Mathey's Primary Practice Partners model responds to the nursing shortage by recommending former military corpsmen, emergency medical technicians (EMTs), and registered certified technicians (RCTs) with special technical training to be nurse extenders. These and other job categories may expand differentiated practice models.

The partners in practice models of the 1990s cross trained cleaning personnel, who had less downtime than previous nurses' aides, to be nursing assistants. Use of unlicensed personnel increased during the 1990s (Grohar-Murray and DiCroce, 2003, Marquis and Huston, 2000; Yoder-Wise, 2003).

LEVEL OF STAFF

The level of staff available greatly influences the assignment system used. When there are a few RNs and a few practical nurses, many aides are quickly oriented and used. This is an expensive and relatively dangerous mix, because aides do not have the educational background to do most of what is required or to recognize what should be reported. After the aides have done all they can, there is still much work to be done. Consequently, there is considerable downtime. This staffing mix lends itself best to functional nursing.

Team nursing is appropriate when there are some RNs, even more practical nurses, and fewer aides. The RNs plan and direct the care, pass medications, and do the more complicated treatments. Although this provides better physical care, the staff is still not adequately educated to understand the pathophysiological basis of symptoms, to plan nursing intervention, and to detect changes in the status of the patient at an early stage so staff members may promptly report pertinent information to the physician. There is also a dearth of patient education and response to psychosocial needs.

Modular nursing is appropriate when more RNs are available, and primary nursing works best with a staff of only RNs. Research regarding exclusively RN staffs indicates an increase in staff, patient, and physician satisfaction. There is an increase in professional orientation, personal liking of colleagues, and cooperation with others. Collegial relationships are more common, and there is more mobility on units because nurses can cover for each other. There is greater competence in skills, creative interventions, personalized care, and continuity of care.

All-RN staffing is economical. It has been found to save money through decreased turnover, sick leave, unpaid absences, float hours, and overtime. RNs can give better care in fewer hours. Patients have fewer complications, shorter hospitalizations, and lower readmission rates. Hospitals also generate more revenue when patients have shorter stays with a concentration of treatments. Unfortunately, frequent shortages of nurses make all-RN staffs unlikely.

Pure applications of case method, functional method, team nursing, modular nursing, and primary nursing are possible, but they seldom exist in pristine form. Rather, it is common to find elements from more than one assignment system combined and used at the same time. Case management is used across settings. During the 1980s managed care was considered unit based. During the 1990s disease management and case management became a part of managed care through community-focused, collaborative arrangements and structures such as HMOs.

STAFFING SCHEDULES

Staffing policies largely influence staffing schedules. To determine staffing policies, one must consider the following questions (Marquis and Huston, 1998, 2000; Swansburg and Swansburg, 2002):

- What is the best organization for staffing—centralized or decentralized to clinical areas or nursing units?
- Who is responsible for the original scheduling or daily adjustments?
- Where are nursing hours posted and an accurate copy kept?
- For what period will schedules be prepared—1, 2, 4, or 6 weeks?
- How far in advance will personnel know their work schedule?
- Will there be an adjustment in staffing based on the identification of patient needs?
- Will there be shift rotation?
- If there is shift rotation, how often—daily, weekly, monthly?
- How much time should elapse between rotated shifts?
- What day starts a calendar week—Sunday or Monday?
- Will there be 2 days off each week or an average of 2 days each week?
- How often are weekends off guaranteed?
- What days does a weekend comprise—Friday, Saturday, Sunday?
- Will days off be split or consecutive?
- What are the maximum and minimum work spans?
- How many holidays and vacation days are allowed?
- How far in advance of scheduling should employees request time off?
- How will holiday time off be determined?
- Will part-time help be used?
- If so, what is the most economical ratio between full- and part-time personnel?
- Will part-time help be allowed to specify when they can and cannot work?
- Will part-time help be required to work weekends? If so, how often?
- Will "float" personnel be used?
- What are the low-census procedures?
- Is there a policy for trading days off?
- What is the emergency request policy?

CENTRALIZED SCHEDULING

Two major advantages of centralized scheduling are fairness to employees through consistent, objective, and impartial application of policies and opportunities for cost containment through better use of resources (Table 13-4). Centralized scheduling also relieves nurse managers from time-consuming duties, freeing them for other activities. Centralized scheduling is not without its critics, however. Lack of individualized treatment of employees is a chief complaint, and centralized scheduling has brought to the surface previously unrecognized organizational and managerial problems.

Organizational and managerial problems can be reduced when (1) the philosophy and goals of the agency are identified; (2) the goals,

TABLE **13-4** Pros and Cons of Centralized and Decentralized Scheduling

SCHEDULING METHOD	PROS	CONS
Centralized	Fairness	Lack of individualized treatment
	Cost containment	Unfair treatment
Decentralized	Managers have authority	Schedule used to punish and reward
	Staff get personalized attention	Time consuming for managers
	Staffing is easier	Less efficient use of resources
	Staffing is less complicated	Cost containment is more difficult

objectives, and organizational structure are defined; (3) scheduling policies are stated; (4) standards of nursing care practices are set; (5) acuity of care as it relates to staffing needs is determined; (6) patient needs, personnel policies such as vacation and personal leave, and staff development are taken into account in personnel schedules; and (7) quality of care is measured.

Resistance to centralized scheduling may be reduced when head nurses prepare and control their own budgets, understand and approve the scheduling policies, and have open communication with the scheduler. Line and staff accountability should be carefully defined to prevent confusion over responsibility and authority when staff personnel make decisions where line managers are accountable. Line authority is accountable for decisions, and staff provides support to help line make decisions.

The staff functions of the scheduler include scheduling employees according to staffing policies, implementing procedures for position control and reallocation of staff, maintaining records for line managers, gathering information and preparing reports to help line authority prepare personnel budgets, and maintaining communications with other appropriate departments, such as personnel and payroll.

Line responsibilities of managers include developing a master staffing pattern; establishing procedures for adjustment of staff; clarifying requirements for each job description and staff position; hiring, developing, promoting, disciplining, and firing employees when appropriate; and defining and controlling the personnel budget.

Computers can be used for centralized scheduling. Before implementing a computer system, an analysis of policies and procedures is done and baseline data are collected. Agency policies regarding the nature of the schedule—straight, alternating, or rotating shifts; frequency of alternating or rotating shifts; work stretch; weekends-off sequence; and use of part-time help—are constants in the information processing system. Variables such as census, acute conditions of patients, special requests, special assignments, vacations, and holidays can be fed into the computer.

Advantages of centralized computer scheduling include cost-effectiveness through the reduction of clerical staff and better use of professional nurses by decreasing the time spent in non–patient-care activities; unbiased, consistent scheduling; equitable application of agency policies; an easy-to-read work schedule developed in advance so employees know what their schedules are and can plan their personal lives accordingly; and availability of data for monitoring the effect of staff size and composition, quality of care, and cost. However, staff may not trust the machine and nurse managers may feel a loss of control and may resist the use of technology (Englebardt and Nelson, 2002; Saba and McCormick, 2000; Sullivan and Decker, 2001; Yoder-Wise, 2003).

DECENTRALIZED SCHEDULING

When managers are given authority and assume responsibility, they can staff their own units through decentralized scheduling. Personnel feel that they get more personalized attention with decentralized scheduling. Staffing is easier and less complicated when done for a small area instead of for the whole agency. Each manager learns the responsibility and challenges of scheduling staff. With a philosophy of sharing and mutual trust, managers can work together to solve chronic staffing problems. Because of their knowledge and experience, managers can form a support system and offer each other informed advice. Nurse managers and charge nurses are freed from staffing responsibilities and have more time for other tasks.

Unfortunately, some staff members may receive individualized treatment at the expense of others, and work schedules can be used as a punishment-reward system. Scheduling staff, which is very time consuming, takes managers away from other duties or forces them to do the scheduling while off duty. Decentralized scheduling may use resources less efficiently and consequently make cost containment more difficult.

SELF-SCHEDULING

Self-scheduling is a system that is coordinated by staff nurses (Table 13-5). It is a process by which nurses and other staff collectively develop and implement work schedules, taking policies and variables affecting staffing into consideration. A process might allow about 2 weeks for staff to indicate the days, shifts, weekends, holidays, and vacation days that they want. Then about 2 weeks are needed for negotiations to finalize a schedule that accommodates both the staff's and the unit's needs. Staff may negotiate before and after work and during break and lunchtime. They may also write notes to each other and wait for responses.

Self-scheduling can help create a climate where professional nursing can be practiced. It saves the manager considerable scheduling time and changes the role of the manager from supervisor to coach. It increases the amount of time the staff spends on scheduling and helps develop a more accountable and professional staff. It also increases staff members' ability to negotiate with each other.

Self-scheduling has been associated with increased perception of autonomy, increased

job satisfaction, increased cooperative atmosphere, improved team spirit, improved morale, decreased absenteeism, reduced turnover, and shortened scheduling time. It has also been effective in recruitment and retention. Staff do need negotiation and conflict negotiation skills (Marquis and Huston, 2000; Sullivan and Decker, 2001; Swansburg and Swansburg, 2002; Yoder-Wise, 2003).

ALTERNATING OR ROTATING WORK SHIFTS

Although straight shifts are used by some institutions or for some personnel within institutions, rotating work shifts are common for staff nurses. The frequency of alternating between days and evenings, or days and nights, or rotating through all three shifts varies among institutions. Some nurses may work all three shifts within 7 days.

Alternating and rotating work shifts create stress for staff nurses. Environmental cues, such as sunrise and sunset, fluctuate in a predictable cycle. Instruments that designate hours, minutes, and seconds correspond to the natural daily cycle and allow knowledge of one's location in that cycle. Social and work routines synchronize with the internal circadian rhythms as the body rhythms are timed to coincide with the usual activities. Thus when environmental conditions are changed by altering work hours, sleep time, hour for rising, mealtimes, and social and recreational activities, the body must make accommodations for the environmental changes. Body rhythms need time to adjust to the discrepancy between the person's activity cycle and the new demands of the environment. The ability of the body functions to adjust varies considerably among individuals. It may take 2 to 3 days to 2 weeks for a person to adjust to a different sleep-wake cycle.

Alternating and rotating work shifts affect the health of nurses and the quality of their work. The rapid shift of work schedules causes stress. Nurses complain of restlessness and nervousness while trying to sleep, wakefulness or sleepiness at inappropriate times, anorexia, digestive disturbance, disruption in bowel habits, fatigue, slower

TABLE **13-5** Advantages and Disadvantages of Various Scheduling Methods

SCHEDULING METHOD	PROS	CONS
Self-scheduling	Coordinated by staff nurses Saves manager scheduling time Helps develop accountability Increased perception of autonomy Increased job satisfaction Improved team spirit Improved morale Decreased absenteeism Reduced turnover Effective for recruitment and retention	Increases amount of time staff spends on scheduling
Rotating work shifts	Can rotate teams	Rotate among shifts Increase stress Affect health Affect quality of work Disrupt development of work groups High turnover

Permanent shifts	Can participate in social activities
	Job satisfaction
	Commitment to the organization
	Few health problems
	Less tardiness
	Less absenteeism
	Less turnover
		Most people want day shift
		New graduates predominantly staff
		  evenings and nights
		Difficulty evaluating evening and
		  night staff
		Nurses may not appreciate the
		  workload or problems of other shifts

Block, or cyclical, scheduling	Same schedule repeatedly Nurses not so exhausted Sick time reduced Personnel know schedule in advance Personnel can schedule social events Decreased time spend on scheduling Staff treated fairly Helps establish stable work groups Decreases floating Promotes team spirit Promotes continuity of care	Rigidity
Variable staffing	Use census to determine number and mix of staff Little need to call in unscheduled staff	

reaction time, lower job performance, and error proneness. There are changes in the patterning of temperature, blood pressure, and urine excretory cycles and a possible lowered resistance to disease. Resultant increases in medication errors, equipment failures, and errors in problem solving are probable.

To guarantee that nurses work their share of weekends, holidays, and unpopular evening and night hours, alternating and rotating assignments currently focus on the time patterns of an individual nurse rather than on well-integrated work groups. The rotation of personnel on an individual basis is disruptive to the development of work groups.

The Federal Aviation Agency's (FAA's) rotation of teams of airport personnel may be used as a model by nursing services. The FAA rotates entire teams consisting of four or five controllers plus trainees and a leader, chosen because of their qualifications, amount of experience, and anticipated compatibility. Their schedules are planned 1 year in advance so that team members can plan their personal lives with confidence. Emergencies and vacations are handled within the team. Absenteeism affects the workload of the peers with whom one must continue to work; therefore team identification reduces absenteeism because of team pressure. Controllers have a low turnover rate.

In hospitals, rotation of teams instead of individuals could contribute to team development. If a group of personnel work together consistently, they can help each other through the dependence of the orientation phase of group development and the conflict experienced during the organizational phase, when the role negotiations of who will be responsible for what occur. The staff has a chance to become an interdependent, cohesive group with good communication and effective problem-solving abilities. Unfortunately, there is usually a high turnover of nursing personnel, which complicates team development. Perhaps more attention to team development would reduce turnover.

PERMANENT SHIFTS

Permanent shifts relieve nurses from stress and health-related problems associated with alternating and rotating shifts. They also provide social, educational, and psychological advantages. When nurses are able to choose the shift that best suits their personal life, they can participate in social activities (such as hobbies, sports, and community, professional, or church organizations) even when they require regular attendance. They may be able to continue their education by planning courses around their work schedule. Child care arrangements can be stable. Nurses may develop a sense of belonging to a shift and feel and work better because the shift suits them. In studies conducted with Montreal nurses, those working permanent shifts had higher averages on psychological scales such as mental health, job satisfaction, social involvement, and commitment to the organization. They had fewer health problems and less tardiness, absenteeism, and turnover.

Although the day shift is not always the preferred shift, it is likely to be. Consequently, assignment to preferred shift may have to be done on a seniority-priority basis. This usually results in a predominance of new graduates staffing the evening and night shifts. Managers may have difficulty evaluating the evening and night shift personnel unless they make some observations during those shifts; therefore it may be easier for evening and night supervisors to evaluate permanent staff on those shifts. One disadvantage of permanent shifts is that nurses may not develop an appreciation for the workload or problems of other shifts.

BLOCK, OR CYCLICAL, SCHEDULING

Block, or cyclical, scheduling uses the same schedule repeatedly. With a 6-day forward rotation, personnel are scheduled to work 6 successive days followed by at least 2 days off. The schedule repeats itself every 6 weeks.

Personnel can be scheduled with every other weekend off and 1 day during the week so that there are no more than 4 consecutive days of work. Several blocks are possible. Because nurses are not exhausted by working too many consecutive days, sick leave can be reduced. By having one team member at a time on vacation and by rotating holidays among the workers, vacations and holidays can be scheduled to avoid changes in the block. However, some nurses fear that 1 day off at a time is not adequate to feel rested. But nurses who currently do not work more than 4 consecutive days report that 1 day is adequate to refresh themselves.

There are several advantages to established rotations. Personnel know their schedules in advance and consequently can plan their personal lives. Absences because of social events decrease because staff can plan their social activities around their work schedules. There is a decrease in preoccupation with staffing, time for scheduling, time for maintenance of schedule, and conflict over preferred days off. Staff are treated more fairly by equitable distribution of popular and unpopular days on duty. The scheduling of appropriate number and category mix of personnel is simplified. Once the appropriate mix is determined, it is repeated. This helps establish stable work groups and decreases floating, thus promoting team spirit and continuity of care. The initial schedule is time consuming, and a decrease in flexibility of staffing may be perceived as a disadvantage, especially by people who need flexibility (Sullivan and Decker, 2001; Swansburg and Swansburg, 2002).

"I have not failed. I've just found 10,000 ways that won't work." —Thomas Edison

VARIABLE STAFFING

Variable staffing is a method that uses patient needs to determine the number and mix of staff. Time measures are done for direct and indirect patient care. A patient classification system is developed, and tables are designed to determine the number of nursing hours required, depending on the number of patients in each category. This provides the information to determine staff needs by skill levels. Nursing pools, floats, and part-time help can be used to supplement the regular staff to accomplish the variable staffing. With a study of previous staffing needs, redistribution of peak routine work, and slight overstaffing in some areas to create float personnel for last-moment needs, there may be little need to call in unscheduled staff (Table 13-6).

EIGHT-HOUR SHIFT, FIVE-DAY WORKWEEK

The 5-day, 40-hour workweek became popular during the late 1940s. It was a radical change from the 10-hour day, 5-day workweek that contained split shifts and few holidays. It has been a predominant pattern since then. The shifts are usually 7 AM to 3:30 PM, 3 PM to 11:30 PM, and

TABLE **13-6** Pros and Cons of Variable Staffing

	PROS	CONS
8 hours	Traditional	
10 hours	Time to complete work	Longer workday
	Long weekends	Fatigue
	Extra days off	Overlap
	Decreased overtime	Difficult to find substitute
	Cover peak workloads	
	Decreases costs	
12 hours	Lower staffing requirements	Overtime
	Lower cost per patient day	Exhaustion increases at end of workweek
	Increased knowledge of patients	Tension increases at end of workweek
	Get new admissions settled	Increases in minor accidents
	Not so rushed	Increases medication errors
	Better continuity of care	Home and social life suffers the week
	Team development is possible	worked
	Less daily reporting	
	Less time to do staffing	
	Reduced travel time	
	Less personal expenses for gas, meals, babysitting	
Baylor plan/weekend option	Few people need to work weekends	Illness increased
	Weekends off more frequently	Absences increased
	Work fewer hours for greater pay	
	Staffing improved	
	Morale improved	

11 PM to 7:30 AM, allowing for a half-hour lunch break and a half-hour overlap time between shifts to provide for continuity of care (Grohar-Murray and DiCroce, 2003).

TEN-HOUR DAY, FOUR-DAY WORKWEEK

The Intensive Coronary Care Unit at Saint Elizabeth Community Health Center in Lincoln, Nebraska, implemented the 10-hour day, 4-day workweek with an every-other-weekend-off staffing pattern. The shifts were 7 AM to 5:30 PM, 1 PM to 11:30 PM, and 9 PM to 7:30 AM. A cyclical schedule allowed at least 14 hours off between shifts and a 4-day weekend every 6 weeks for those who rotated. The workweek began on Sunday, and the weekend was Saturday and Sunday for all shifts. The main problem was fatigue, but it was not found to be as serious a problem as anticipated. The long weekends and extra days off were attractions (Bauer, 1971). In addition, there is time to finish work, peak workloads can be covered, and there is decreased overtime and decreased costs. Ten-hour days, however, are considered long workdays to some, and there is overlap (Grohar-Murray and DiCroce, 2003; Swansburg and Swansburg, 2002).

TWELVE-HOUR SHIFT, THREE DAYS ON AND FOUR DAYS OFF

The 12-hour shift, starting at 7 or 7:30 AM and ending at 7 or 7:30 PM, was adopted by some institutions. The better use of nursing personnel lowers staffing requirements; this consequently lowers the cost per patient day. Nurses find they get to know their patients better because they have more time to study charts and can visit patients more frequently. They have more time to get new admissions settled before the change of shift and feel that they can give better patient care because they are not so rushed. They find that there are fewer communication gaps and better continuity of care. Consequently, there are improved nurse-patient relations, job satisfaction, and morale.

Working relations are improved. Personnel work with the same group of people, so team development is possible. There is less friction and no 3 to 11 PM shift to blame for problems. Less daily reporting results in less confusion about physicians' orders and changes in procedures and routines. Less time is required for staffing, thus freeing supervisors and head nurses for other duties.

Total time off is increased, with an increased usefulness of time. Travel time is reduced. There is less personal expense for babysitting, gas, and meals. Nurses find they have more time to relax and enjoy their days off and are able to return to work refreshed. Flexibility for personal schedules improves staff morale.

Overtime pay has been of some concern. The 1966 Amendments to the Fair Labor Standards Act permit agencies to calculate overtime pay on a 14-consecutive-day work period. Consequently, overtime pay is required only for more than 80 hours in a 2-week period.

Some nurses complain that the extra time they have for learning and research becomes boring. Nurses also complain that their home and social lives suffer the days they work.

The wide variety of staffing practices suggests there is no right or wrong staffing schedule. Rather, there is much variability to consider when designing the best staffing schedule for a given situation (Grohar-Murray and DiCroce, 2003; Swansburg and Swansburg, 2002).

BAYLOR PLAN—WEEKEND ALTERNATIVE

Baylor University Medical Center in Dallas, Texas, started a 2-day alternative plan. Nurses have the option to work two 12-hour days on the weekends and be paid for 36 hours for day shifts, or 40 hours for night shifts, or to work five 8-hour shifts Monday through Friday. This plan required a larger nursing staff, filled weekend positions, and reduced turnover. Some hospitals have implemented the Baylor plan, indicating that the extra pay on weekends compensated for vacations, holidays, and sick time.

Some hospitals have nurses work 12-hour shifts when they work weekends. This way fewer people have to work weekends and, consequently, staff can have weekends off more frequently. Although illness and absences increased, recruitment and staffing improved (Grohar-Murray and DiCroce, 2003; Swansburg and Swansburg, 2002).

VARIABLES AFFECTING STAFFING

Although institutional and nursing service philosophy and objectives guide staffing, various patient, staff, and environmental factors also affect staffing patterns. The types of patients, their expectations, fluctuations in admissions, length of stay, and complexity of care complicate staffing (Box 13-1). Personnel policies, educational and experiential levels of staff, job descriptions, the mix of work titles or leveling, hour and rotation policies, absenteeism, and the competitive market also affect staffing. Environmental factors, such as the floor plan of the unit and hospital, number of patient beds, availability of supplies and equipment, the organizational structure, and support services from other departments and agencies, are also considered when planning staffing patterns.

Budget submission is done periodically by submitting a summarization of the revenue and expense sections of the budget for review. A narrative justification is used to negotiate changes in the budget.

Managers are responsible for implementation of the budget to meet the staffing needs of the unit, including weekends, holidays, vacations, and sick leave coverage through busy and slow periods (Yoder-Wise, 2003).

STAFFING STUDIES

Three major types of staffing studies are used to predict the number, level, and mix of personnel required for staffing. Nursing care needed may be predicted from patient classification systems by assigning patients to categories according to diagnosis, acuity of care, or amount of self-sufficiency. Number, level, and mix of staff needed can be determined by noting the

---

BOX 13-1 Variables That Affect Staffing

Workload budgets indicate the amount of work produced by a unit in terms of units of service, which are used to calculate expense budgets.

Activity reports measure statistics about current activity centering on the number of units of service given compared with the capacity.

Average daily census is the average number of patients cared for per day for a period of time.

Average length of stay is the average number of days that patients stay in the agency.

Adjusted units of service allow budgeting based on expected workload units of service adjusted for the expected mix of patients.

Care hours calculation determines the average required care hours per patient per 24 hours for each classification level and the sum or the total hours of care needed for all patients.

Personnel expense budget is the budget for all personnel assigned to a unit.

Fixed staff are employees who do not vary with the patient volume.

Variable staff are responsive to the projected number of care hours needed.

Establishing positions should involve the manager's discretion for use of full-time and part-time personnel to total the number of full-time equivalents needed to meet the care needs.

Labor costs are determined by calculating the dollar basis of the straight-time salary, differentials, overtime, raises, and fringe benefits for each employee used by the unit.

Expense budget (other than personnel) is a combination of the direct unit expenses plus the indirect overhead expenses.

Revenue budget is the unit's income.

Modified from Finkler SA, Kovner CT: *Financial management for nurse managers and executives*, Philadelphia, 1993, WB Saunders, pp. 315-347.

---

number of patients in each category. Then a cost-effective nursing personnel budget based on the needs of patients and the qualifications of nursing personnel can be determined. Patient classification systems can be combined with nursing care plans, and costs to individual patients can be determined. Systems that charge patients for the care they receive can be designed.

Time standards can be determined for nursing procedures by listing and analyzing the procedures required by each patient. The time required for each patient and the sum for all patients on a unit can then be calculated. Formulas deduced from statistical analysis of work sampling data can be used to predict the number of nursing care hours needed. However, staffing is a function of fiscal factors, market availability, creativity, and innovation.

"It is better to light a candle than to curse the darkness." —*Eleanor Roosevelt*

Principles of Nurse Staffing

The American Nurses Association (1999) identified the following principles for nurse staffing related to unit patient care: Staffing levels should reflect individual and aggregate patient needs. The concept of nursing hours per patient day should be questioned. Functions to support quality patient care should be used when determining staffing levels. Principles related to staff include the following: Patient needs should determine the required clinical competencies. Nurses need both nursing management support and representation at both the operational and executive levels. Clinical support should be readily available from experienced RNs for less proficient RNs. Principles related to the organization include the following: Organizational policy should reflect valuing employees. All organizations should have documented competencies for staff. Organizational policies should recognize the needs of both patients and staff.

PATIENT CLASSIFICATION SYSTEMS

Patient classification systems were introduced when managers realized that nurse staffing needs were more dependent on the patient's dependency on care than on the medical diagnosis. The three basic styles of patient classification systems are (1) descriptive, (2) checklist, and (3) time of relative value unit standard. In the descriptive style, the nurse classifies the patient in the category that most closely describes the care received. The tool used is a narrative on a concise acuity table. Category 1 may be self-care and category 4 complete care, including feeding, frequent skin care, complete bath, complete bed rest, and frequent positioning. The patient does not have to receive all the care in a category to be classified in that category. The nurse chooses the category that best describes the patient. The major problem with this style is interrater reliability, caused by the subjectivity of the interpretation of the patient's degree of care. The descriptive style is a quick-check guide, but the poor interrater reliability leads to a wide range of requested nurse/patient ratios. Many administrators have moved away from this subjective style of patient classification.

The checklist-style acuity table divides descriptions of care routines into activity categories, such as eating and bathing. Activity levels are described in each category. Levels in the eating category might be self-care, help setting up, feed, and frequent feedings. Each activity is assigned an activity level point score, such as 1 for routine care or self-care and 4 for comprehensive care. The nurse checks the activity level for each patient in each category and totals the points for each patient to determine the level of care. This is usually done at each shift or daily. It, too, is a subjective system.

Time standard, or relative value unit (RVU), systems assign a value unit (usually a measure of time) to various activities of patient care. Those activities are usually clustered according to categories, such as diet, bathing, and mobility. There is considerable variation in the complexity of these systems.

Medicus was one of the first patient classification systems developed and was introduced in the late 1960s. It is still used in the 2000s. It clusters patients into five categories with 5 being the greatest intensity of care. Indicators and the average hours of nursing care required determine the level. It reflects both direct and indirect care.

GRASP (Grace Reynolds Application and Study of PETRO) was introduced in 1970. It identifies about 50 direct care plus indirect patient activities. Time studies are done to validate that the time estimates are tailored to the organization. Interrater reliability is checked. Calculations are to be done every 12 hours and may be done by computerized form or manually with paper and pencil. Although GRASP is time consuming, it has common use even in the 2000s. It is a multidimensional nursing-management information system that includes staffing/scheduling, cost identification, budgeting, and quality evaluations.

The Sisters of Mercy Health Corporation developed ARIC (Allocation, Resource, Identification, and Costing) in the 1970s. This system recognizes the dependent and independent activities of nurses and classification information. It generates staffing reports based on the information entered including actual versus needed staffing, staff exceeding workload, and level of productivity. The credibility is questioned because of rapidly changing circumstances in health care.

TISS (Therapeutic Intervention Scoring System) puts numerous conditions and treatments into categories for 1, 2, 3, or 4 points and sums the points into four classifications: class I—less than 10 points; class II—10 to 19 points; class III—20 to 39 points; and class IV—more than 40 points. It works well for acute medical-surgical areas. Other classification systems have been developed for specialty areas such as hospice care and long-term care.

The matrix has become increasingly popular by the early 2000s. Census may be recorded as number of patients down the left-hand column. Then there may be columns for number of licensed (RN, LPN) and unlicensed (aides, techs) staff needed, including the unit secretary for days and nights for 12-hour shifts.

With increasingly sophisticated technology, computers can incorporate time and motion data plus expert nurse judgments, be used to predict the cost-effectiveness of patient outcomes, match patient needs with caregiver profiles, and track and monitor patient-caregiver interactions (Englebardt and Nelson, 2002; Sullivan and Decker, 2001; Swansburg and Swansburg, 2002; Yoder-Wise, 2003).

TIME STANDARDS

When figuring time standards for nursing care, one should consider both direct and indirect

RESEARCH Perspective 13-2

Data from Seago JA: A comparison of two patient classification instruments in an acute care hospital. *JONA* 32(5):243-249, 2002.

Purpose: The purpose of this study was to compare the predictive validity of two types of patient classification instruments commonly used in acute-care hospitals in California.

Methods: Two general types of systems commonly used are the summative task type of patient classification system and the critical incident or criterion type of patient classification system. Data were collected using medical record review only. Both types, criterion and summative, of patient classification systems' data collection instruments were completed for all patients at both collection points. Each patient had a before and after score for each type of instrument. Three hundred forty-nine medical records for inpatients meeting the inclusion criteria were examined.

Results/conclusions: The most significant finding of this study was that there were virtually no differences in the predictive ability of summative versus criterion patient classification instruments. Using the same patients, both types of instruments predicted the actual score more than 78% of the time.

care. Direct care involves the patient and includes feeding, bathing, treating, and giving medications. Indirect care involves all activities that are not direct care, such as preparation of and cleaning up after medications and treatments, clinical work, reporting, communications, and coffee and lunch breaks.

Once the number and kind of care activities required by each patient are identified and the length of time it takes to do the activities is calculated, one can add up the time required by all patients on a unit and divide by the number of productive work hours on a shift to determine the number of personnel needed. The mix of nursing personnel can be predicted by categorizing the care needed by the qualifications needed to give it, adding the time in each category, dividing by productive hours on a shift, and obtaining the number of specific types of personnel required to meet the patients' needs. Once this is accomplished, patients can be charged by the level of care required.

Public health nurses deal with health needs of aggregate groups in the community, whereas visiting nurses provide care to clients in their own homes. There are also health care clinics and nurse practitioner clinics in the community. For visiting nurse services and home health agencies, staffing is determined by the number of clients who need to be seen in a day. A standard amount of time is often allocated per visit. A standard of 45 minutes per visit for four to six clients depending on the amount of driving has been used, but the acuity of clients treated at home has increased. Thus an acuity system is merited.

STAFFING FORMULAS

When determining the number of staff to hire, one must consider hours for which coverage is required, vacations, holidays, absenteeism, and staff development time. If nurses work 5 days per week and coverage is needed for 7 days, it takes 1.4 nurses to have one nurse on duty 7 days and 2.8 nurses to have two nurses on duty for 7 days. This is calculated by multiplying the number needed on duty by days of the week for which coverage is required and dividing by the number of days each employee works per week to determine the number of personnel needed for coverage. Table 13-7 provides some examples. This figure does not allow for vacations, holidays, absenteeism, or staff development time.

To calculate vacation coverage, multiply the number of vacation days per year by the number of people at that skill level. Dividing the total number of vacation days per skill level by the total days worked per year per person determines the number of people needed for vacation coverage. For example:

$$\begin{array}{c}\text{Number of}\\\text{vacation days}\\\text{per year}\end{array} \times \begin{array}{c}\text{Number of}\\\text{full-time people}\\\text{at that skill level}\end{array} = \begin{array}{c}\text{Total vacation}\\\text{days by}\\\text{skill level}\end{array}$$

$$\begin{array}{c}\text{Total}\\\text{vacation}\\\text{days by}\\\text{skill level}\end{array} \div \begin{array}{c}\text{Total days}\\\text{worked per}\\\text{person per year}\end{array} = \begin{array}{c}\text{Number of}\\\text{full-time people}\\\text{needed for}\\\text{vacation}\\\text{relief coverage}\end{array}$$

To determine holiday coverage, multiply total number of personnel required (7-day coverage per skill level) by the number of holidays to determine the number of holiday days to be

TABLE **13-7** Staffing Formulas

NUMBER NEEDED		DAYS OF WEEK		NUMBER OF DAYS EACH WORKWEEK		NUMBER OF PEOPLE REQUIRED
1	×	7	÷	5	=	1.4
2	×	7	÷	5	=	2.8
3	×	7	÷	5	=	4.2
4	×	7	÷	5	=	5.6
5	×	7	÷	5	=	7.0

staffed. Then divide the total holiday relief days by the total days worked per year per person to obtain the number of personnel required per skill level for holiday coverage per year:

$$\text{Number of personnel} \times \text{Number of holidays} = \text{Number of holidays needing coverage}$$

$$\text{Number of holiday relief days} \div \text{Number of days worked per year per person} = \text{Number of personnel required for holiday coverage per year}$$

The percentage of absenteeism is used to calculate absentee relief coverage:

$$\text{Weeks/year} \times \text{Days worked/week} \times \% \text{ of absenteeism} = \text{Absentee days/person/year}$$

$$\text{Personnel requirements (7 days/week)} \times \text{Absenteeism days/person/year} = \text{Absentee coverage for staffing}$$

$$\text{Absentee coverage required} \div \text{Total days worked/person/year} = \text{Full-time personnel required for absentee coverage per year}$$

Personnel required for staff development relief per year can also be calculated:

$$\text{Number of hours required or recommended for staff development} \times \text{Number of staff} = \text{Number of hours per year for staff development needing relief coverage}$$

$$\text{Number of staff development hours needing coverage} \div \text{Hours worked/day} \div \text{Total days worked/person} = \text{Full-time personnel required for staff development coverage}$$

A staffing slide rule can be developed to save time when computing the number of budgeted positions needed to meet staffing standards by preparing a table that identifies the number of persons needed on duty, number of persons needed to cover days off, and number of persons needed to cover additional days off for vacation, holiday, sick, and personal leaves. Table 13-8 provides examples.

One full-time equivalent (FTE) is equivalent to 40 hours worked per week for 52 weeks. That equals 2080 hours per year. One person or a combination of personnel can fill an FTE. Fixed FTEs are scheduled to work no matter what the volume of work is. Variable FTEs are for employees who are scheduled according to workload needs (Sullivan and Decker, 2001; Yoder-Wise, 2003).

Computers are being used with increasing frequency for determining nurse staffing depending on such factors as system availability, reliability, capital resources, revenue resources available, resource consumption, system benefits, training, and implementation (Fralic, 2000).

STAFFING TO MEET FLUCTUATING NEEDS
Full-Time Staff

Full-time staff may be hired to meet the average staffing needs of an institution. The most common adjustment for an increased workload is to

TABLE **13-8** Staffing Formulas

NUMBER NEEDED ON DUTY	NUMBER NEEDED TO COVER DAYS OFF	15.6 EXTRA DAYS + 6%	18.2 EXTRA DAYS + 7%	20.8 EXTRA DAYS + 8%	23.4 EXTRA DAYS + 9%
1	1.4	1.46	1.47	1.48	1.49
2	2.8	2.92	2.94	2.96	2.98
3	4.2	4.38	4.41	4.44	4.47
4	5.6	5.84	5.88	5.92	5.96
5	7.0	7.30	7.35	7.40	7.45

transfer staff from a less busy area to the over-loaded area. This is economical for the agency but disrupts the unity of work groups, causes the transferred nurse to feel insecure, and contributes to job dissatisfaction and turnover. Some units require specialized knowledge and skill that not every nurse has. Cross training is helpful.

In the companion floor system, two units relieve each other. Staff nurses are oriented to the second unit and know that if they are transferred, it will be to the companion unit. Thus staff aggravation is minimized, flexibility is possible, and quality of care is maintained.

At best, a complementary, or float, staff is com-posed of full-time staff nurses who are oriented to many areas and like the challenge of different types of patients and settings. Unfortunately, most nurses prefer stability. Consequently, the float staff is likely to be part-time staff or new personnel waiting for a permanent assignment.

Having full-time staff work double shifts and overtime is another option. The nurse is already oriented to the area, and continuity of care is facilitated. There are also disadvantages, how-ever. Institutional costs increase. The nurses may become tired, errors are likely to increase with fatigue, and overtime may interfere with the nurses' personal lives (Sullivan and Decker, 2001; Swansburg and Swansburg, 2002).

Part-Time Staff

Flexible working hours can be an incentive for inactive nurses to start part-time employment and can thus reduce staffing shortages. Most nurses are women who have to combine their nursing role with many other roles, such as wife, mother, and homemaker. A part-time job can broaden the woman's horizons beyond her home, increase her income, give her ego satis-faction, and help her maintain her nursing skills. It is not uncommon for nurses to want to work part-time while continuing their educa-tion. Part-time nurses tend to work more than their share of unpopular hours, and some prefer evening and night duty exclusively. When part-time nurses' other responsibilities decrease, they

are likely candidates for full-time work. It is sometimes possible for two people to share a job.

There are, of course, disadvantages to the use of part-time nurses. Educational and adminis-trative expenses are higher proportionately for part-time than for full-time help. For example, it is likely to cost as much to orient a part-time nurse as a full-time nurse, thus costing more per hours worked. Maintaining continuity of care is complicated, because two or more part-time people may fill budgeted full-time positions. There are also disadvantages for the employee. The part-time nurse may not receive benefits, such as paid sick or vacation days, and is not likely to be considered for promotion. Sometimes benefits are prorated for part-time workers.

Temporary help is another option. Some institutions hire temporary help for the summer to give relief for vacations. Temporary bed and bath teams or a premium day has been used to reduce weekend staffing shortages. Staff nurses get an extra day off (a premium day) if they work one additional weekend within a 4-week schedule. Some nurses may be willing to work on an on-call basis year-round.

External temporary help agencies are avail-able in some areas. The use of such agencies can greatly reduce the amount of time middle management must spend on staffing. The super-visor merely calls the external agency and requests so many nurses, and the agency makes the necessary contacts. The agency has a registry of available nurses who are allowed to have highly flexible, self-determined schedules. This allows some nurses to work who could not otherwise and consequently helps those nurses maintain their skills. It is then more likely for those nurses to return to nursing practice on a full-time basis than if they had remained inac-tive. Their availability may boost morale, and they may introduce new ideas and stimulate creativity among the regular staff.

Unfortunately, there are also disadvantages to temporary help agencies. The matching of the nurses' credentials and qualifications with assign-ments and orientation to assignments are severe problems. Although some temporary help agencies do keep orientation information and procedure manuals for their client institutions on file, their use may still be optional. It is likely to take considerable time for the regular staff to orient the temporary help, errors are likely to increase, and continuity of care is jeopardized. The temporary nurses get preferred schedules, leaving the regular staff with more of the less-attractive hours. Consequently, morale may be lowered.

A central placement service run by the state board of nursing or the state nurses' association could be useful for matching nurses' qualifications and interests with actual or anticipated vacancies throughout the state.

There are many variables to consider when planning staffing schedules. The more accurately those variables are assessed, the better one is able to contain costs while providing high-quality care (Grohar-Murray and DiCroce, 2003).

Managers have several relatively undesirable options for handling a called-in absence or otherwise uncovered shift. They can consider the following:

Using a float, per diem, or agency nurse
Asking a nurse to work for the sick person and canceling a shift for that person later in the week
Asking a part-time person to work an extra shift
Substituting one type of classification for another, such as an LPN for an RN
Asking one staff member to work a few hours of overtime and another to come in a few hours early
Doing without a substitute
Covering the shift themselves

Mandatory Overtime

Mandatory overtime is requiring staff to stay on duty after their scheduled shift ends. Some managers may believe that a tired nurse is better than no nurse at all. The American Nurses Association and other professional organizations oppose mandatory overtime. There is fear that tired, overworked nurses may have compromised decision-making abilities and be more prone to making mistakes. Nurses fear litigation and risk of losing their nursing license. Mandatory overtime is a political issue and is often a negotiating point for unionized nurses. Some states have adopted legislation prohibiting mandatory overtime. Organizations often have policies about their right to mandate overtime. Some specify that refusing to work required overtime constitutes patient abandonment and is punishable. Some states have clarified that refusing mandatory overtime is not patient abandonment (American Nurses Association, 1999; Yoder-Wise, 2003).

REDUCTIONS IN FORCE

Declining inpatient activity and changing patient care patterns have caused some institutions to right size or downsize. Proactive right-sizing measures may eliminate or minimize the need for downsizing. Right sizing is a comprehensive and systematic process that studies ineffective, costly programs and generates ideas for replacing them with revenue-generating programs. Units that should be investigated include those where the occupancy rate is below 60%, where caregiver worked hours per patient have increased by several percentage points in a year, where fixed staffing levels have increased by a small percentage of the full-time equivalents, where productivity goals are not met, where costs exceed revenues, and where the units have been out of service (Bruce and Patterson, 1985).

Finding new work for present departments can delay the need for downsizing. Examples are contracting out continuing education and laundry services and attracting work through expanded or new services, such as geriatrics. Slow times can be used for in-service education for personnel to increase competence, for cross training personnel to work in more than one area, for carrying out special projects, and for updating policies and procedures. Reducing overtime; encouraging use of holidays, vacation time, and leaves of absence without pay; reducing temporary help; and deferring hiring can decrease the budgetary deficit (Borg and Jensen, 1985).

Use of attrition, temporary early retirement, and conversion of full-time to part-time positions may be considered before termination. When it becomes necessary to implement layoffs, there are many issues to consider: Will they be based on seniority, job skills, job classification, or a combination of those factors? It is beneficial to involve managers from the patient care coordinator position up in deciding the criteria for layoffs. If seniority is used, is there a bumping policy? Bumping through transfers, demotions, and layoffs makes layoffs much more complicated and time consuming and involves about five times more people than originally targeted. People who know their positions are in jeopardy may experience more stress than those who have actually been bumped. Nurses may be angry and frustrated that they are transferred outside their specialty area. They may not be suited to their new position and may file grievances that are time consuming and costly to both staff and management. Many nurses would rather be laid off and be eligible for unemployment compensation than work where they do not feel qualified. Orientation and training for the new positions also cost time and money. Nurses may be too angry to orient people who will replace them. Those who are staying may worry about being responsible for inexperienced nurses placed on their units. Those who retrain may leave the institution as soon as they find another position in their area of interest. Many qualified people may leave voluntarily but will discuss their unhappy experiences in the community.

There are also communication issues. Many people prefer to be informed about the layoff by personal communication rather than in writing. It is common to have a public meeting with immediate written follow-up. Many want information about why cuts are needed, the extent of the cuts, and the potential effects. They may want to be informed as soon as possible so they can make necessary arrangements.

Attention must be given to morale building through increased communication and input into decision making. A central communication office may be helpful by allowing personnel to call or stop in for clarification or information. A meeting may be scheduled to explain rules, present facts, and answer questions in an attempt to reduce anxiety. Discussion of the organization's bumping policy and procedures is particularly appropriate. Recall policy should also be discussed so that retained and laid-off personnel know their rights and responsibilities concerning future vacancies. Support groups can be formed to allow for venting anger and sharing feelings. Stress management workshops are appropriate.

A placement committee may be formed to match affected personnel to openings, or a review process may be implemented to respond to objections. Job skill evaluation and job counseling may be offered to affected personnel. Clear-cut procedures for matching personnel skills and openings are essential. Training opportunities to prepare people for new jobs should be provided, and prospective employees should be informed of the organization's layoff policies before they are hired (Meehan and Price, 1988). Public relations efforts for community image will require attention.

Productivity

Productivity is the product or work produced through a specific amount of resources, measured as outputs divided by inputs. For example, productivity can be measured as required staff hours divided by provided staff hours multiplied by 100. Improvements in productivity involve more work or product produced for less overall cost. Productivity can be increased by decreasing the staff hours provided while holding the required staff hours constant or increasing them. It is often measured through the patient classification system: average daily census, number of patient days per month, number of patients treated, and number of procedures performed are productivity measures.

Many actions can be taken to increase outputs while maintaining or reducing inputs. Recognizing the need to do better, involving staff, seeking staff ideas and recommendations, creating challenges, management interest in staff achievements and concerns, and praise and reward for good performance can help. Evaluating the problems, resources, and realities in the organization; using work flow analysis and work simplification procedures; and improving use of time by helping personnel keep and analyze time diaries and decreasing waiting time can make a difference. There are many ways to improve productivity: set a climate for productivity by asking personnel what would help them be more productive and implementing their ideas. Set targets for increasing outputs. Have personnel set personal objectives and measure performance against them. Seek new approaches to old problems and improve products and services. Staff development, attention to process, ethics, and aesthetics enhance productivity through attention to doing the right things the right way (Swansburg and Swansburg, 2002).

Chapter Summary

Chapter 13 covered the following:
Assignment Systems for Staffing
    Case Method
    Functional Nursing
    Team Nursing
    Modular, or District, Nursing
    Primary Nursing
    Case Management
    Collaborative Practice
    Managed Care
    Differentiated Practice
Level of Staff
Staffing Schedules
    Centralized Scheduling
    Decentralized Scheduling
    Self-Scheduling
    Alternating or Rotating Work Shifts
    Permanent Shifts
    Block, or Cyclical, Scheduling
    Variable Staffing
    Eight-Hour Shift, Five-Day Workweek
    Ten-Hour Day, Four-Day Workweek

    Twelve-Hour Shift, Three Days on and
        Four Days Off
    Baylor Plan—Weekend Alternative
Variables Affecting Staffing
    Staffing Studies
        Principles of nurse staffing
    Patient Classification Systems
    Time Standards
    Staffing Formulas
    Staffing to Meet Fluctuating Needs
        Full-time staff
        Part-time staff
        Mandatory overtime
    Reductions in Force
        Productivity

On-line Resources

evolve Additional critical thinking activities, worksheets, and case studies are available on-line at http://evolve.elsevier.com/Marriner/guide/

References

American Nurses Association House of Delegates materials, 1999.
American Nurses Association: *Principles for nurse staffing with annotated bibliography*, Washington, DC, 1999, American Nurses Publishing.
Bauer J: Clinical staffing with a 10-hour day, 4-day workweek, *JONA* 1:12-14, Nov-Dec 1971.
Borg JH, Jensen DL: Managing layoffs: A comprehensive approach, *Nurs Manage* 16:31-37, Aug 1985.
Bruce A, Patterson D: Resizing hospital nursing organizations, an alternative to downsizing, *Nurs Manage* 18:33-35, Aug 1985.
Cesta TC: *Survival strategies for nurses in managed care,* St Louis, 2002, Mosby.
Conger MM: *Managed care: Practice strategies for nursing*, Thousand Oaks, Calif, 1999, Sage.
Del Togno-Armanasco V, Hopkin LA, Harter S: *Collaborative nursing case management: A handbook for development and implementation*, New York, 1993, Springer.
Dykes PC, Wheeler K, editors: *Planning, implementing and evaluating critical pathways: A guide for health care survival into the 21st century*, New York, 1997, Springer.
Englebardt, Nelson: *Health care informatics: An interdisciplinary approach*, St Louis, 2002, Mosby.

Etheredge MLS, editor: *Collaborative care: Nursing case management,* New York, 1993, Springer.

Finkelman AW: *Managed care: A nursing perspective,* Upper Saddle River, NJ, 2001, Prentice Hall.

Finkler SA, Kovner CT: *Financial management for nurse managers and executives,* Philadelphia, 1993, WB Saunders, pp. 315-347.

Fralic M (Ed).: *Staffing management and methods: Tools and techniques for nursing leaders,* San Francisco, 2000, Jossey-Bass.

Grohar-Murray ME, DiCroce HR: *Leadership and management in nursing,* Stamford, Conn, 2003, Appleton & Lange.

Johnson M, Bulechek G, Dochterman, et al: *Nursing diagnoses, outcomes, and interventions: NANDA, NOC and NIC linkages,* St Louis, 2001, Mosby.

Johnson M, Mass M, Moorhead S: *Nursing outcomes classification (NOC),* St Louis, 2000, Mosby.

Knight W: *Managed care: What it is and how it works,* Gaithersburg, Md, 2002, Aspen.

Kongstvedt PR: *Essentials of managed health care,* ed 4, Gaithersburg, Md, 2001, Aspen.

Marquis BL, Huston CJ: *Leadership roles and management functions in nursing: Theory and application,* ed 3, Philadelphia, 2000, Lippincott.

Marquis BL, Huston CJ: *Management decision making for nurses: 124 case studies,* Philadelphia, 1998, Lippincott.

McCloskey JC, Bulechek GM, editors: *Nursing interventions classification (NIC),* St Louis, 2000, Mosby.

Meehan M, Price C: Managing layoffs with minimum loss of productivity, *Nurs Adm Q* 13:26-32, Fall 1988.

Poirrier GP, Oberleitner MG: *Clinical pathways in nursing: A guide to managing care from hospital to home,* Springhouse, Pa, 1999, Springhouse Corp.

Saba VK, McCormick KA: *Essentials of computers for nurses,* ed 3, New York, 2000, McGraw-Hill/Appleton & Lange.

Seifker JM, Garrett MB, Genderen AV: *Fundamentals of case management: Guidelines for practicing case managers,* St Louis, 1997, Mosby.

Sullivan EJ, Decker PJ: *Effective leadership and management in nursing,* Upper Saddle River, NJ, 2001, Prentice Hall.

Swansburg RC, Swansburg RJ: *Introductory management and leadership for nurse managers,* Boston, 2002, Jones and Bartlett.

Yoder-Wise PS: *Leading and managing in nursing,* ed 3, St Louis, 2003, Mosby.

14

Evaluation and Discipline of Personnel

Chapter Overview

Chapter 14 differentiates methods of performance management, appraisal interviews and reports, legal implications, principles of disciplinary action, penalties, components of a disciplinary action program, modification of employee behavior, problem employees, employee counseling, and outplacement counseling.

Chapter Objectives

- Recall at least five purposes of personnel evaluation.
- Explain at least six common errors in performance evaluation.
- Describe five methods of personnel evaluation.
- Discuss 360-degree evaluation.
- Explain various ways to arrange a room for performance evaluations.
- Defend at least five principles of disciplinary action.
- Relate at least three components of a disciplinary action program.
- Compare discipline without punishment with progressive discipline.
- Explain behavior modification.
- Judge at least three types of problem employees.
- Identify at least three types of employee counseling.
- Explain outplacement counseling.

Major Concepts and Definitions

Evaluation valuation, appraisal, determination of worth
Peer review group evaluation of a group member
Appraisal interview verbal evaluation
Appraisal report written evaluation
Discipline to train, control, punish
Penalties punishment; negative consequences
Behavior modification changes in behavior
Reinforcement actions that strengthen a behavior or increase its probability
Shaping reinforcing successive attempts at achieving the desired behavior
Extinction annihilation, destruction
Substance abuse misuse of drugs
Angry furious, raging, tumultuous
Withdrawn retreated, isolated
Productivity results
Absenteeism absence from work
Due process procedural requirements to ensure fairness
Termination end of something
Directive counseling counselor telling one what to do
Nondirective counseling client deciding what to do
Outplacement counseling helping dismissed personnel find another job

Leaders encourage peer review, promote motivation and growth through it, reduce the anxiety related to it, and develop trust by being honest and fair. Leaders facilitate two-way communication, facilitate growth through coaching, and support employees attempting to correct performance deficiencies. Managers use a formalized system, document standards, gather fair and objective data, determine educational and training needs, follow up on performance deficiencies, maintain documentation of the appraisal process, and give frequent informal feedback (Table 14-1).

PURPOSES

Performance appraisal is a periodic formal evaluation of how well personnel have performed their duties during a specific period. Purposes of the evaluation are as follows: (1) to determine job competence, (2) to enhance staff development and motivate personnel toward higher achievement, (3) to discover the employee's aspirations and to recognize accomplishments, (4) to improve communications between managers and staff associates and to reach an understanding about the objectives of the job and agency, (5) to improve performance by examining and encouraging better relationships among nurses, (6) to aid the manager's coaching and counseling, (7) to determine training and developmental needs of nurses, (8) to make inventories of talent within the organization and reassess assignments, (9) to select qualified nurses for advancement and salary increases, and (10) to identify unsatisfactory employees.

COMMON ERRORS IN EVALUATION

Criteria involving judgments are used for performance evaluation. Because human judgment

TABLE **14-1** Leadership and Management for Performance Management

LEADER	MANAGER
Encourages peer review process	Uses a formalized system for performance appraisal
Promotes motivation and growth through the appraisal process	Uses documented standards as bases for performance appraisal
Reduces anxiety inherent in the appraisal process	Gathers fair and objective data for performance appraisals
Develops trust by being honest and fair	Determines education and training needs from appraisal process
Facilitates two-way communications through appraisal interviews	Follows up on performance deficiencies
Encourages growth through coaching	Maintains documentation of the appraisal process
Supports employees attempting to correct performance deficiencies	Provides frequent informal feedback

Modified from Marquis BL, Huston CJ: *Leadership roles and management functions in nursing: Theory and application*, ed 2, Philadelphia, 2000, Lippincott.

is subject to the influences of prejudice, bias, and other subjective and extraneous factors, the attempt to get objective, accurate evaluations is extremely difficult. A number of errors may affect performance ratings. The manager should be aware of the most common ones and try to minimize them.

The halo error is the result of allowing one trait to influence the evaluation of other traits or of rating all traits on the basis of a general impression. A logical error is rating a nurse high on one characteristic because the nurse possesses another characteristic that is logically related. Sometimes employees are given a good rating in the recent past because they did good work in the distant past, or outstanding performance on a recent job may offset a mediocre performance during the rest of the evaluation period. A manager is likely to rate personnel who are compatible with the manager higher than they deserve and may not see certain types of defects that are like the manager's. The person who does not complain is likely to have higher ratings than the person who does.

The horns error is the opposite of the halo effect. The evaluator is hypercritical. Managers who are perfectionists may rate personnel lower than they should. Managers may compare how they used to do the job with how it is done now and are more likely to rate people doing jobs with which they are familiar lower than those with whose jobs they are not familiar. Good workers on weak teams are more likely to get lower ratings than if they were working on a better team. Persons who are not well known may be judged by the company they keep. A recent mistake may offset a year's good work. If the worker is contrary, managers may vent their irritation by lowering the rating. The nonconformist or person with a personality trait that is not appreciated is likely to be rated lower than that person's work merits.

The contrast error is produced by the tendency of managers to rate the nurse opposite from the way they perceive themselves. A small range of scores may be a result of the central tendency error. When the rating on a preceding characteristic influences the rating on the following trait, a proximity error exists. Because raters tend to have their own built-in set of standards or frame of reference on which to make evaluations, it becomes a major problem comparing different raters' scores. Some managers may be easy and lenient, whereas others may be severe in their judgments.

The manager can take precautions to minimize judgment errors. For instance, a forced-distribution technique may be used to overcome the leniency and central tendency errors. A critical incident checklist can reduce the halo effect and logical rating errors. Ranking systems, paired comparisons, and forced-choice techniques may be used (Marquis and Huston, 2000; Sullivan and Decker, 2001).

METHODS OF PERFORMANCE MANAGEMENT

ANECDOTAL NOTES

Anecdotal records are objective descriptions of behavior recorded on plain paper or a form. The notations should include who was observed, by whom, when, and where. The notation comprises a description of the setting or background and the incident, and interpretation and recommendations may be included. Value-laden words such as good and bad should be avoided.

Characteristic behavior cannot be determined without several incidents depicting similar behavior. The director or patient care coordinator may use time sampling to accumulate observations. The time that is set aside specifically for observations may be divided by the number of staff to be observed. The manager then concentrates on the scheduled staff member for a short period. It is advisable to make several brief observations over a time span to allow for temporary variables and to identify patterns of behavior.

An advantage of anecdotal recordings is that the description is not coerced into a rigid structure. However, this latitude becomes a problem when the interpreter tries to develop relationships between notations that may have little or no relationship to each other. Although anecdotal records provide a systematic means for recording observations, they do not guarantee that observations will be made systematically or that specific, relevant behaviors will be observed. It also takes considerable time to record the observations.

CHECKLISTS

With a checklist the manager can categorically assess the presence or absence of desired characteristics or behaviors. Checklists are most useful for tangible variables, such as inventory of supplies, but they can be used for evaluation of nursing skills as well. It is advisable to list only the behaviors essential to successful performance, and it is advantageous to determine the behavior to be observed in advance. The same criteria can then be used in each situation. Unfortunately, this does not guarantee that the observed behavior is a persistent one or that a representative situation is being observed, nor is the checklist practical for evaluating interpersonal relations (Marquis and Huston, 2000).

RATING SCALES

The rating scale does more than just note the absence or presence of desirable behavior. It locates the behavior at a point on a continuum and notes quantitative and qualitative abilities. The numerical rating scale usually includes numbers against which a list of behaviors is evaluated:

Observation of working hours   1 2 3 4 5
Ability to get along with others   1 2 3 4 5

This is not a very reliable tool because of the inconsistent value attributed to the number. That fault can be partially overcome by adding a few quantitative terms, as shown in Box 14-1.

The tool can be made even more reliable by developing a standard scale using comparative examples to establish a set of standards. The difficulty is finding appropriate comparative standards. A nurse-to-nurse comparison scale might be developed (Figure 14-1).

BOX 14-1 Rating Scale

Rate the staff member on the items below. Responses have the following values:
1 = Never
2 = Sometimes
3 = About half the time
4 = Usually
5 = Always
A. Observation of working hours   1 2 3 4 5
B. Ability to get along with others   1 2 3 4 5

Nurse	Observation of working hours				
	Lowest (1)	Below average (2)	Average (3)	Above average (4)	Highest (5)
Betty Green	X				
Sara Smith		X			
Pam Peterson			X		
Sue Jones				X	
Anita Anderson					X

Figure 14-1 Nurse-to-nurse comparison scale.

As long as the managers can agree on the qualifications of a few nurses known to all of them, a comparison scale that gives a common reference for rating the rest of the staff nurses can be developed.

The graphic rating scale differs from the numerical rating scale in that words rather than numbers are used (Figure 14-2).

Graphic rating scales usually list extremely broad and general personal characteristics that are to be rated from poor to excellent or from low to high. Raters are given little if any guidance about what work behavior qualifies a person for a particular rating and must consequently use their own judgment about how to classify the behaviors.

The descriptive graphic rating scale is similar to the graphic rating scale except that it presents a more elaborate description of the behavior being rated (Figure 14-3).

BARS is an acronym for behaviorally anchored rating scales, sometimes known as BES, or behavioral expectation scales. They are similar to graphic rating scales in that a person is rated on a series of dimensions or qualities. However, BARS differ from graphic rating scales in the ways that the criteria are identified and the alternative responses along the rating scale are anchored or described. BARS evaluate behavior relevant to specific demands of the job and provide examples of specific job behaviors corresponding to good, average, and poor performances. This reduces the amount of personal judgment needed by the rater.

The major disadvantage of BARS is the time and expense required to involve large numbers of employees in determining the dimensions of effective performance and behavioral examples of various levels of performance of each variable. Separate BARS are needed for each job. It is primarily applicable to physically observable behaviors rather than to conceptual skills. However, it should reduce rating errors and provide more reliable, valid, meaningful, and complete data. Employees give more acceptance and commitment to this appraisal system because of their

Unsatisfactory | Below average | Average | Above average | Outstanding

Observation of working hours

Figure 14-2 Graphic rating scale.

Usually late | Sometimes late | Usually on time

Observation of working hours

Figure 14-3 Descriptive graphic rating scale.

involvement in designing it. They have full knowledge of the requirements of the job, and they evidence less defensiveness and conflict because people are evaluated on the basis of specific behaviors rather than personalities. This system thereby identifies performance deficiencies and needs for development.

BOS is an acronym for behavioral observation scales (Box 14-2). This system capitalizes on some of the strengths of BARS while avoiding some of the disadvantages. BOS also use critical incidents of worker behavior. The evaluator lists a number of critical incidents for each performance dimension and rates the extent to which the behavior has been observed on a five-point scale ranging from almost never to almost always. It too is relatively reliable, is well accepted and understood, and provides useful feedback, but it is relatively time consuming and expensive to develop.

Instead of a descriptive choice, a percentage rating scale provides a quantitative choice. The manager may rank the employee's behavior on any given criterion as among the bottom 10% of staff, next 20%, middle 40%, next 20%, or top 10% of staff (Figure 14-4).

To maintain perspective, the manager may list staff names down the side of a paper and the behavior to be rated across the top. Rating one behavior at a time, the manager checks for variation in evaluations because one expects variation in performance. Forced distribution should be used cautiously. It is based on a normal bell-shaped curve with a few people ranked high, a few ranked low, and the majority ranked in the middle. However, this assumes that the group is representative of the total population, and this is not true for a group of nurses (Marquis and Huston, 2000; Swansburg and Swansburg, 2002).

RANKING

"He who spares the guilty threatens the innocent."
—*Legal maxim*

Ranking forces managers to rank staff in descending order from highest to lowest even if they do not think there is a difference. Ranking implicitly requires the manager to compare each nurse with others, but that comparison is not systematically built into the method. Paired comparison forces the supervisor to compare each nurse with each other nurse. As shown in Table 14-2, if managers are ranking four nurses, they must deal with six possible pairs; this number can be calculated as follows:

$$N(N-1)/2 = 4(3)/2 = 12/2 = 6$$

Then each pair is presented to the manager, who must determine which of the two she thinks is better. Choices should be marked (Figure 14-5).

Tally marks can be placed in a matrix to help visualize the ranking (Figure 14-6).

The major disadvantages of paired comparisons are that they do not lend themselves to large numbers of staff and they demand considerable time of the manager (Marquis and Huston, 2000).

MANAGEMENT BY OBJECTIVES

"Success comes in cans; failure in can'ts."
—*Anonymous*

Management by objectives (MBO) is a tool for effective planning and appraisal. It emphasizes the achievement of objectives instead of personality characteristics. It focuses attention on individual achievement, motivates individuals to

---

BOX 14-2 Behavioral Observation Scale

Circle the number that most closely approximates your assessment of the staff member on the following qualities:

Punctual	Almost never	1 2 3 4 5	Almost always
Gets along well with coworkers	Almost never	1 2 3 4 5	Almost always

Figure 14-4 Percentage rating scale.

accomplishment, and measures performance in terms of results. MBO is a managerial method whereby the manager and staff nurse identify major areas in which the nurse will work, set standards for performance, and measure results against those standards. It determines the results that the nurse is to achieve in a given time frame.

To develop MBO, nurses should first review the mission and group objectives. They can determine the mission and objectives by analyzing what they do or what they think they should do. They describe their job and clarify its purpose. This helps identify major job responsibilities.

Next, they list their major job responsibilities. Results expected, rather than activities, should be listed. This can be accomplished by asking themselves why the activity is being done or why it is important. For example:

What is the task?   To help team members organize their work for the day
Why?   To improve use of their time
Why?   To be as productive as possible
Why?   To give good, cost-effective nursing care by completing the work identified on nursing care plans efficiently

Major job responsibilities of a nurse manager are related to productivity, quality of care, morale, turnover, staff development, self-development, and affirmative action.

Once the major job responsibilities are identified, expected levels of accomplishment are determined. Criteria for expected levels of accomplishment should be results oriented, established before the fact, time bound, realistic and attainable, measurable and verifiable, written, and agreed on by both the manager and the staff associate. Common errors to avoid when developing objectives are writing too many objectives or too complex objectives; having too high or too low standards; using too long or too short a time period; and having imbalanced emphasis, objectives that are not measurable, or objectives for which the cost of measurement is too high.

After staff associates have reviewed the mission and group objectives and determined their major job responsibilities and the expected levels of accomplishment, they should meet with the manager to establish priorities and to develop plans for the accomplishment of the objectives. The manager will determine whether the objectives are compatible with the overall goals of the organization. The manager and staff associate should hold periodic reviews to check the progress and make adjustments. An annual review should be held to compare the actual results with the expected levels of accomplishment and to set the objectives for the next period.

The underlying philosophy is a belief that people perform best and develop most in an

TABLE **14-2** Example of Ranking Using Paired Comparison

NURSES	POSSIBLE PAIRS	
Anita Anderson	AA with SJ	SJ with PP
Sue Jones	AA with PP	SJ with SS
Pam Peterson	AA with SS	PP with SS
Sara Smith		

Figure 14-5 Paired comparisons.

Figure 14-6 Visualizing rankings.

environment of participative management, high performance standards that build on individual strengths, prompt feedback that accentuates the positive, and appropriate rewards. Staff are encouraged to "do their thing" while maintaining individual accountability. The manager is a listener and clarifier who readjusts responsibilities on the basis of individual differences.

Higher frequencies of appraisal are associated with a more favorable attitude toward MBO, higher goal success, improvement of manager–staff associate relationships, clarity of goals, an opinion that the manager was helpful and supportive, the attitude that staff associates had influence in matters affecting them, and esteem for and satisfaction with the manager. More praise and less criticism of the objectives by the manager are associated with higher goal success. It is advisable to use an incentive system that rewards effective planning, as well as goal achievement, when using MBO.

Advantages of MBO for the staff nurse are that the standard of evaluation is based on the characteristics of a specific person and job; nurses have input and some control over their future; nurses know the standard by which they will be judged; nurses have knowledge of the manager's goals, priorities, and deadlines; staff nurses have a greater understanding of where they stand with the manager in relation to relative progress; there is a better basis for evaluation than personality traits; MBO emphasizes the future, which can be changed, instead of the past; and it stimulates higher individual performance and morale.

Advantages for the manager include a reservoir of personnel data and performance information for updating personnel files, an indication of personnel development needs within the agency, a basis for promotion and compensation, a relationship with the staff that makes the manager a coach rather than a judge, and better managerial planning and use of the employee.

MBO directs work activities toward organizational goals, facilitates planning, provides standards for control, provides objective appraisal criteria, reduces role conflict and ambiguity, and uses and motivates human resources.

MBO is limited because it is not an easy system to implement and requires hard work for maintenance; the process must be taught and reinforced for managers to become and remain proficient in applying the principles of the system; the MBO system assumes that staff nurses and managers will define suitable standards that will serve the agency; it presumes that managers understand their limitations; managers are responsible for assessing actual results rather than activities that seem to indicate results; some managers are unable to manage by objectives; some staff nurses may not want to be involved in setting goals; managers and staffs may give lip service to MBO, although managers really set the goals; staff nurses may set their goals according to what they know their managers expect; MBO stresses results but does not supply the methods for achieving them; nurses can become frustrated if they believe that increasingly higher goals will be expected of them; overlapping objectives are difficult to evaluate; MBO lends itself to quantitative assessment but may neglect qualitative factors; and MBO does not provide comparative data for promotions and salary increases (Marquis and Huston, 1998, 2000; Odiorne, 1965, 1969).

R SEARCH Perspective 14-1

Data from Meretoja R, Leino-Kilpi H: Instruments for evaluation nurse competence. *JONA* 31(7/8):346-352, 2001.

Purpose: The purpose of this study was to review the literature to help nurse administrators locate and evaluate existing instruments to ensure safe and qualified nursing care.

Methods: Data collection procedures included literature searches from MEDLINE and CINHAL.

Results/conclusions: Of the studies reviewed, seven were conducted to develop or to test a new instrument; six were conducted to differentiate job performance by education, experience, and career commitment; four reported development of new instruments; and two dealt with item identification for performance standards and assessment models and were regarded as early stages of instrument development. All the instruments were designed to assess practicing nurses. The method of nurse competence assessment was nurses' self-evaluation in 11 studies; was supervisor, preceptor, or manager evaluation in seven studies; and was the single method used in two studies. Patient evaluation was used in one study.

SELF-APPRAISAL

Self-appraisal promotes dignity and self-respect. It is a less structured approach used in participative organizations that promotes employee acceptance of plans for improvement and uses the manager as a coach instead of a judge. Personnel are the best source of information about their work. Self-appraisal ensures that the person is prepared for the discussion, and it increases the perception of fairness. Personnel may be fearful of punishment; rate themselves low to avoid disagreement with the boss; or evaluate themselves high to influence the supervisor. Sometimes employees undervalue their achievements or feel uncomfortable giving themselves high ratings. If used alone, self-appraisal could provide an inaccurate picture. If the self-appraisal is not consistent with other available data, the manager should confront the differences (Grote, 1996; Marquis and Huston, 2000; Rocchiccioli and Tilbury, 1998; Swansburg and Swansburg, 2002).

PEER REVIEW

Peer review is a process whereby a group of practicing registered nurses (RNs) evaluates the quality of another RN's professional performance. It provides a feedback mechanism for sharing ideas, comparing the consistency of the nurse's performance with standards, recognizing outstanding performance, and identifying areas in which further development is required. This process can increase personal and professional growth and job satisfaction because of the recognition from peers.

Once it has been decided that an institution will use peer review, appraisal tools must be developed. A review of the evaluation tools currently used and the literature on evaluation tools is in order. Various standards may also be reviewed. The tool developed may address technical competence and human relationship, communication, organizational, leadership, and other skills. The process must also be determined, and then staff must be oriented to the system.

The staff should be oriented to the components of the peer review before it is implemented and thereafter during orientation. It is appropriate to give them copies of the peer review process and forms used for peer review. Opportunities to learn how to fill out the forms, how the peer review committee uses the materials, and what questions are to be expected during the peer review interview should be provided.

The peer evaluation process typically includes a review of an employee's self-evaluation form (including short- and long-term goals), reference letters, committee work, special projects, additional education, and contributions to nursing; a performance evaluation by the nurse's immediate manager; a review of past performance; care plans and charting done by the nurse; assessment; observation of the nurse; interviews with clients; a summary of the findings; a presentation of the findings; and recommendations to the nurse. It is appropriate to allow the candidate some agency time to prepare a review folder. A leader is assigned to the nurse to help clarify policy and procedures and to check the documents for completeness.

Who will evaluate whom must be determined. A committee may be appointed, elected, or randomly selected, but it should represent a number of job titles and a wide variety of specialty areas. The members should be familiar with committee responsibilities. The committee's recommendations should be made by consensus, with dissenting opinions recorded.

Once the candidate has been evaluated, there should be a peer review interview for feedback. All feedback must be well documented in the review materials. Hearsay reports are not permitted. The review committee chairperson or designee is responsible for arranging the interview and helping the candidate feel welcome and comfortable. The interview may provide recognition of outstanding performance, identification of areas in which further development is required, recommendations regarding learning needs, and possibly a recommendation for classification.

Peer review can be threatening and time consuming. There is a risk of rating candidates too high or too low. Friends may inflate evaluations. Peers may omit suggestions for improvement for people with whom they work. Managers may feel threatened. However, nurses will be held accountable and responsible for their nursing performance when they are measured against realistic and attainable standards (Marquis and Huston, 1998, 2000; Rocchiccioli and Tilbury, 1998; Swansburg and Swansburg, 2002).

RESEARCH Perspective 14-2

Data from Hyrkas K, Paunonen-Ilmonen M: The effects of clinical supervision on the quality of care: Examining the results of team supervision. *The Journal of Advanced Nursing* 33(4):492-502, 2001.

Purpose: The purpose of this study was to ascertain the conceptions of five ward teams having clinical supervision of its effects on the quality of care.

Methods: Data were collected using group interviews and analyzed using phenomenography.

Results/conclusions: The following categories describing the conceptions related to clinical supervision and to the quality of care emerged: knowledge, change, and "I and we as providers of quality." Conceptions of the effects varied among and within the teams and sometimes contradicted each other. The importance of knowledge was underlined on three of the five wards. The patient's point of view emerged only on one ward. It can be concluded that clinical supervision has effects on the quality of care, and it can be considered a quality-improving intervention in nursing practice.

CUSTOMER OR SUBORDINATE EVALUATION

Student evaluation of teachers is common in education. Patients can evaluate their care. Staff can evaluate their managers and leaders (Rocchiccioli and Tilbury, 1998).

360-DEGREE FEEDBACK

Three hundred sixty-degree feedback is a multisource system of assessment including self-appraisal and subordinate, peer, and administrative feedback. It creates credible feedback, reduces supervisor bias, supports a team environment, supports career development, moves from a seniority to a performance system, and allows rewarding high performers. Unfortunately, friendships or competition may bias the process; some people may collude; some respondents are more critical than others; and some teams are harder than others. Computers with safeguards for confidentiality can be used for on-line assessment (Edwards and Ewen, 1996; Grote, 1996).

APPRAISAL INTERVIEW

There are several kinds of appraisal interviews. They include tell and sell, tell and listen, problem solving, and goal setting. When using the tell-and-sell technique, the manager does most of the talking while the staff associate listens. The manager reports the results of the evaluation to the employee and tries to persuade the staff associate to improve. This assumes that managers are qualified to evaluate staff associates and that staff associates will want to correct their weaknesses. In this role of judge, the interviewer risks losing the loyalty of the employee and inhibiting independent judgment. Face-saving problems are created. Employees usually suppress defensive behavior and attempt to cover their hostility to protect themselves. The tell-and-sell method uses positive and negative extrinsic motivation and is most likely to be successful when the employee respects the interviewer. It tends to perpetuate existing values and practices. The tell-and-sell method works best with young or new employees or individuals who are new

to an assignment. These employees may want advice and assurance from an authority figure. Under these conditions managers are most likely to be respected because of their position, knowledge, and experience. Unfortunately, the tell-and-sell method fosters either dependent and docile or rebellious behavior. After a tell-and-sell style evaluation, the employee often feels like looking for another job.

When using the tell-and-listen method, the manager speaks for about half the time and lets the staff associate speak for the remainder. The interviewer outlines the strong and weak points of the staff associate's job performance and then listens to the interviewee's response. Although still in the role of judge, the interviewer listens to disagreement and allows defensive behavior without attempting to refute any responses. This tends to remove defensive behavior. The employee expresses defensiveness and feels accepted while the interviewer listens, reflects, and summarizes. Thus resistance to change is reduced, and the staff associate develops a more favorable attitude toward the manager. Although this method fosters upward communication and allows the interviewer to learn and change views, the need for change may not be developed in the employee. Tell and listen works best when there is a good relationship between the interviewer and interviewee. Interviewers can learn about staff associates' needs and aspirations, but the latter may not know where they stand. There are no plans for personnel development.

With the problem-solving method, the interviewer assumes the role of helper to stimulate growth and development in the interviewee. It assumes that change can occur without correcting faults and that discussing problems can lead to improvements because the discussion develops new ideas and mutual interests. The staff associate does most of the talking while the interviewer listens, reflects ideas and feelings, asks exploratory questions, and summarizes. Intrinsic motivation is stimulated through increased freedom, increased responsibility, and problem-solving behavior; thus change is facilitated. Both the manager and staff associate learn from each other. Staff associates may view their job in relation to others more accurately, and managers gain insights into staff associates' working conditions. Unfortunately, the employee may lack ideas, and change may be other than what the interviewer had planned. Although this method is excellent for problem solving and personnel development, it does not warn staff associates or let them know where they stand, evaluate them for lateral transfers or promotional purposes, provide a rating or furnish an evaluation record, or supply top administration with an inventory of talent.

Goal setting is future oriented. It focuses attention on the employee's achievement and consequently stimulates accomplishment. The philosophy behind MBO is teamwork. Top administration sets the organization's objectives, and employees set individual objectives. This method integrates institutional and personal achievement goals. It clarifies objectives and, because it focuses on results and not methods, encourages the person closest to a job to decide how to do it. MBO involves participative management. An autocratic leader is likely to dictate goals to a staff associate. Although that is not consistent with a participative management philosophy, it is better for staff associates to know what is expected of them than not to know.

Which appraisal interview style is used largely depends on the purpose of the evaluation, the manager's philosophy of management, and the institutional guidelines. The manager can create an atmosphere during the interview that is consistent with the appraisal interview style. To create an authoritative image for the tell-and-sell method, managers should have the interview in their office and sit behind a desk, preferably looking down on the staff associate (Figure 14-7).

To create an atmosphere of equality for the tell-and-listen, problem-solving, or goal-setting style, the interviewer and employee may sit at a corner table looking at each other (Figure 14-8).

Figure 14-7 Tell-and-sell arrangement.

Sitting at a table helps create a working situation for problem solving and goal setting. Sitting either side by side or at the corner of the table helps create a sense of equality and a working relationship (Figure 14-9).

Nonverbal communication is important and should be consistent with verbal communication. Active listening can be expressed through eye contact, a responsive posture, and facial expressions and lets the interviewee know that the interviewer is trying to understand the employee's attitudes and feelings. Pauses give the employee time to think and respond. The interviewer may restate what the employee said. Although this helps the interviewee know the

Figure 14-8 Problem-solving arrangement.

Figure 14-9 Goal-setting arrangement.

interviewer is listening, it does not guarantee that the meaning of the message was understood. Paraphrasing states the message in fewer and simpler words. If the interviewee says, "I don't understand! One minute she tells me to do it this way, and the next minute she tells me to do it that way," the interviewer may paraphrase, "She confuses you." One should ask for clarification if the intent is not clear or say, for example, "Do you mean…?" Reflection of feelings, such as "You sound proud of that," helps show understanding. Summarizing what has been said at the end of the interview is particularly important.

The manager's assessment of the staff nurse's performance should be continuous rather than annual. This maximizes feedback for learning. The manager and staff nurse should have an appointment to do the appraisal interview when both are unhurried and should meet where they have privacy. Adequate time should be allowed and interruptions prevented. The purpose of the interview should be clear; both should enter it ready to compare notes, knowing that the counseling notes will not become part of the personnel file. Emphasis should be on the growth of the nurse and on accomplishments related to specific targets. Actual, observed behavior rather than broad personality traits should be discussed during the exchange of ideas between the manager and the staff nurse. The staff nurse should be encouraged to take the initiative in setting goals for improving performance, with the manager supporting, guiding, and validating the nurse's plans.

If managers find it necessary to make unfavorable comments, they should insert them between favorable comments. It is important that the managers not create an atmosphere in which they appear to be sitting in judgment. When the manager enumerates needed improvements, the staff nurse's self-esteem is threatened, and the nurse may become defensive. The greater the threat to the self-image, the poorer the attitude toward evaluations will be, and less improvement in job performance results. If the staff nurse becomes defensive or aggressive, the manager should accept comments without a fight. Keeping quiet and not exposing alibis can help the staff nurse save face.

Before the interview is terminated, ways in which the manager can help the staff nurse accomplish goals should be explored. Staff nurses will probably approach their work with more enthusiasm and confidence if they believe they have the respect and support of the manager (Maier, 1976).

APPRAISAL REPORTS

The appraisal report is to be written jointly by the manager and staff nurse. It should be reliable, valid, and accurate, showing progress made by the nurse and giving illustrations to substantiate value judgments. If both have kept notes that they have periodically assessed, and if the staff nurse believes the manager's intent is to help rather than to blame, the nurse will feel more free to be honest in an evaluation of strengths and weaknesses. If staff nurses have not been functioning satisfactorily, they will already be aware of it. If their performance has not improved adequately since previous interviews, they should be informed that the weakness will be included in the report. Any improvements are to be noted, and staff nurses should know exactly where they stand. It may be necessary to tell them they have to make certain improvements within a definite time period or they will be fired.

Permanent, cumulative evaluation records can be used to assess how the nurse can best be used in the agency. They can be used as a basis for pay increases and promotions or terminations.

LEGAL IMPLICATIONS FOR PERFORMANCE APPRAISALS

The Equal Pay Act of 1963, which prohibits paying personnel of one gender at a different rate from personnel of the other gender for the same work; the Civil Rights Act of 1964, which prohibits discrimination on the basis of race, color, religion, gender, or national origin; and the Age Discrimination in Employment Act of 1967, which prohibits discrimination against persons 40 to 70 years of age, all require that employers document the quality of employee performance before making decisions about selection, training, transfer, retention, and promotion.

The most legally defensible content of performance appraisals should be based on job analysis, should be objective and verifiable, and should be specific and job related rather than global. Individual traits such as attitudes should not be evaluated. Legally defensible procedures should be a formal, standardized system and uniform for all personnel in a job category. Performance standards, performance results, appeal process, and antidiscrimination laws should all be communicated to personnel. Raters should have written instructions for how to do an unbiased appraisal. Using more than one rater is desirable, and raters should observe the worker firsthand. Documentation requirements should be consistent for all personnel within a job category, documentation of critical incidents for extreme ratings should be required, and a thorough written record of evidence should be collected about evaluations, counseling about performance deficits, and help to take corrective actions before termination decisions are made (Sullivan and Decker, 2001).

DISCIPLINE OF PERSONNEL

NEED FOR DISCIPLINE

Lack of knowledge about policies and procedures is a major cause of the need for disciplinary action. Management should provide orientation from the first day of employment. Nurses cannot be expected to follow rules that are unknown to them, vague, or loosely enforced. Consequently, each new employee should be given an employee's handbook. The handbook itemizes the rules and procedures of the agency and specifies the type of discipline that will be imposed for infractions. New employees should be encouraged to read the handbook and ask questions about it.

During orientation the manager should explain in detail the most frequently violated rules and discuss their significance and rationale. It is recommended that the manager conduct regularly scheduled meetings with staff to discuss changes or to review policies. Rules and regulations also may be posted in a consistent and conspicuous manner.

Most employees are not disciplinary problems, but a minority requires more than positive stimuli. These few cases are potentially explosive. About one half of the grievance cases appealed to an arbitrator by labor unions involve disciplinary action. In about one half of those cases, management either reversed or modified its decision when the individual's appeal was upheld. Consequently, it is of utmost importance that disciplinary action be undertaken in a judicious manner. The disciplinary action program and grievance procedure must be uniform for all personnel of a specific grade or classification. A standard disciplinary action program with procedures outlined and forms provided should be available to managers.

PRINCIPLES OF DISCIPLINARY ACTION
Have a Positive Attitude

The manager's attitude is very important in preventing or correcting undesirable behavior. If personnel are treated as suspect, they are more likely to provide the trouble that the manager anticipates. People tend to do what is expected of them; therefore it is the manager's duty to maintain a positive attitude by expecting the best from the staff.

Investigate Carefully

The ramifications of disciplinary action are so serious that managers must proceed with caution. They should collect the facts, check allegations, talk to witnesses, and ask accused employees for their side of the story. Managers should accept the employee's account until and unless the allegations are proven. The manager may wish to consult other managers or the director. If the situation is serious enough to require action before a full investigation can be conducted, it is better to suspend the employee subject to reinstatement after investigation than to take more drastic action.

Be Prompt

Managers should not be so expeditious that they neglect to be thorough in ascertaining the facts. If a staff nurse is disciplined unfairly or unnecessarily, the effects on the entire staff may be severe. However, if the discipline is delayed, the relationship between the punishment and the offense may become less clear. Because of the distastefulness of disciplinary action, the manager may tend to postpone the punishment as long as possible. The longer the delay, the more the staff forget their actions, the more likely they are to feel that the discipline is not deserved, and the fewer are the positive educational effects for the future.

Protect Privacy

Disciplinary action affects the ego of the staff nurse. Thus it is better to discuss the situation in private. By helping the nurse save face, there is less possibility of future resentment and a greater chance for future cooperation. However, a public reprimand may be necessary for the nurse who does not take private criticism seriously.

Focus on the Act

When disciplining a staff nurse, the manager should emphasize that it was the act that was unacceptable, not the employee. If the employee is not acceptable, the person should be fired.

Enforce Rules Consistently

Offending employees should be treated equally or consistently for similar transgressions. Equal treatment is based on rules with specific penalties for various acts and the number of offenses. Consistency reduces the possibility of favoritism, promotes predictability, and fosters acceptance of penalties.

Be Flexible

Consistent implementation is complicated by the fact that individuals and circumstances are never the same. A penalty should be determined only after the entire record of the employee is reviewed. The manager should consider length of service, past accomplishments or problems, level of skill, and expendability to the organization. The intent of the staff nurse, the extenuating circumstances, and whether this situation constitutes a test case and will set precedent for the future should also be taken into consideration. If managers enforce identical penalties for seemingly similar offenses, they may be excessively severe with one person and lenient with the other.

Advise the Employee

The employees must be informed that their conduct is not acceptable. Personnel files containing anecdotal notes can be a useful management tool, but they are of little value in upholding disciplinary action if the staff nurse is not informed of the contents promptly.

Take Corrective, Constructive Action

The manager should be sure that the staff nurse understands that the behavior was contrary to the organization's requirements and should explain why such regulations are necessary. The staff nurse should be counseled as to what behavior is required and how to prevent future disciplinary action.

Follow Up

The manager should quietly investigate to determine whether the staff nurse's behavior has changed. If the staff nurse continues to invite disciplinary action, the manager should reevaluate the situation to try to determine the reason for the nurse's attitude. The manager must try to come to terms with the offender and the reasons for the transgression.

PENALTIES

Oral Reprimand

For minor violations that have occurred for the first time, managers may opt to give an oral warning in private. They might tactfully correct the deviation by telling the staff nurse the proper way to deal with the situation or by rebuking the nurse. An oral reprimand is of limited value beyond alerting the nurse in a relatively friendly way to a need for correction. Because nothing is in writing and the reprimand is given in private, it is difficult to prove that a warning was given. Over time the manager may become unsure and inexact about what was said to whom and under what conditions. When an oral warning is given, the manager is advised to make an anecdotal note of the time, place, occasion, and the gist of the reprimand. Oral comments may be easily forgotten, but too formal handling of initial minor offenses can be counterproductive.

Written Reprimand

If the offense is more serious or repeated, the reprimand may be written. It is suggested that the manager and staff associate develop a written plan for improvement that defines what the staff associate will do to make the performance acceptable and what the manager will do to change the environmental situation if appropriate. A time limit should be set. Additional penalties may be defined in case the employee's behavior does not adequately improve during the allowed time period. The written notice should include the name of the worker, the name of the manager, the nature of the problem, the plan for correction, and the consequences of future repetition. It is recommended that the worker sign the report to indicate that she has read it, received a copy of it, or both. A copy should be given to the employee and one retained for the personnel file. If the employee believes that signing such a document would be considered an admission of guilt and hence refuses to sign, the manager may ask another managerial person to sign as witness to the fact that the document was discussed with the worker and that a copy was given to the worker. It is appropriate for higher management and the personnel department to review this report. At the end of the designated time, the manager and worker should have another conference to determine if the terms of the agreement have been met. It is hoped that the nurse can be complimented for having made progress and that no further action is deemed necessary. However, if no change or inadequate change has occurred, the continuing nature of the problem should be identified and documented. Additional penalties will probably be necessary.

Other Penalties

Fines may be charged for offenses such as tardiness. Loss of privileges might include transfer to a less desirable shift and loss of preference of assignment.

Layoff, demotion, and discharge are the most serious penalties and require approval beyond the manager. Layoff may be appropriate in situations where it is best to remove the nurse while an investigation is conducted. The staff nurse may be reinstated with no loss of pay if cleared through the investigation or may be suspended if found guilty of a serious offense. Demotion is a questionable solution. It creates hard feelings, which may be contagious, and more than likely places offenders in a position for which they are overqualified. Termination becomes necessary as a last resort (Marquis and Huston, 2000).

COMPONENTS OF A DISCIPLINARY ACTION PROGRAM

Codes of Conduct

Employees must be informed of the nature and meaning of codes of conduct. Agency handbooks, policy manuals, and orientation programs may be used. The staff nurse must understand that the rules are reasonable and directly related to efficient, effective operation of the agency.

Authorized Penalties

During disciplinary action the personnel record should indicate that a fair investigation was made of charges before the assessment of guilt and determination of penalties. The agency's disciplinary action program should indicate that the current action is being administered without bias and is directly related to the offense.

Records of Offenses and Corrective Measures

Records are of utmost importance when disciplinary action is appealed. The personnel record should clearly indicate the offense, management's efforts to correct the problem, and resulting penalties.

Right of Appeal

Formal provision for the right of employee appeal is a part of each disciplinary action program. Appeal beyond the manager ensures equitable treatment and encourages more employee acceptance of the disciplinary process. At the same time, fair managers need not fear a review of their actions by others.

DISCIPLINE WITHOUT PUNISHMENT

"Justice is better when it prevents rather than punishes with severity." —*Legal maxim*

Progressive discipline starts with an oral reprimand, then a written reprimand, then suspension without pay, and if no corrective action is taken, the last step is termination. Discipline without punishment gives disciplinary suspension with pay to demonstrate that management is sincere in the desire to see the worker change and stay. It starts with complete documentation to recognize and reinforce desirable performance, to confront the few who do not meet the standards, and to support workers to correct problems while maintaining self-esteem. The system is designed to influence the worker to accept responsibility, to change behavior, and to return to an acceptable standard of performance. Without punishment there is an oral reminder, a written reminder, and a leave during which the employee makes a decision about taking responsibility for her behavior. This allows solving problems and enhancing relationships. It focuses on personal responsibility and decision making. Initially the manager lets the employee know what is expected and the employee's responsibility to do what is expected. A memo is used to document the interaction. By making the correction, the employee can "wipe the slate clean" and have information about the incident removed from the record. Otherwise, the employee gets 1 day with pay to take responsibility for her behavior and do what is best for her and the organization. That helps reduce the anger associated with the final step. If necessary, people are discharged from the organization fairly, humanely, and permanently. The decisions to perform well or poorly and to follow the rules or not are the employee's. Requiring employees to take responsibility for their own behavior is more effective than punishing. Punishment can produce compliance but not commitment. Seeking agreement about why a problem must be solved and the logical consequences to the employee if it is not helps get commitment (Grote, 1995).

MODIFICATION OF EMPLOYEE BEHAVIOR

Can an employee's behavior be changed by changing the manager's behavior? Is behavior that recurs in the presence of the manager being reinforced by the manager? Is it possible that doing nothing is doing something? In all three instances the answer is yes. Behavior leads to consequences, and the consequences that follow the behavior affect the probability of recurrence of that behavior. Because behavior is a function of the consequence, it is important for nurse managers to identify the contingency relationship.

Consequences may be favorable, punitive, absent, or insufficient. Positive consequences increase the probability of recurrence of the behavior that preceded them. Absence of consequences decreases the probability, and insufficient consequences have little effect. Punishing consequences have varied and unpredictable effects. Punishment is not the opposite of a favorable consequence. Having no consequence is the opposite of a favorable one.

REINFORCEMENT

Positive reinforcement increases the probability of a recurrence of desired behavior. It is more effective the sooner it follows the desired behavior, and it should be clearly connected to the behavior that the manager wishes to increase. Positive reinforcement may be as subtle as a smile or a nod of the head when someone speaks. Whatever is being said when the manager smiles or nods is reinforced and will recur with increasing frequency. Recognition is a powerful reinforcer. "Mr. Jones must feel so much better now since you have completed his morning care" and "You collected a lot of valuable information during your interview with Mrs. Smith" are examples. "I'm glad to see you here today" reinforces attendance, whereas "I see you were absent again yesterday" gives attention to the absence.

The nurse manager can even stimulate new behavior by verbal acknowledgment of the desired response. Words are used to describe the behavior the nurse manager wants to encourage. A comment such as "I really appreciate nurses' attending in-services" is likely to increase attendance at in-services. A number of stimuli—such as feedback, attention, praise, avoidance of punishment, merit pay increases, special assignments, assistance with tuition, or tickets to a ball game

or play—can be used to reinforce behavior. However, nurse managers must consider that any stimulus can be reinforcing or aversive depending on the person and the situation, so they should carefully select stimuli that are reinforcers for the individual in a given situation. For example, tickets to a ball game may be reinforcing to some and aversive to others. Recognition is one of the easiest, cheapest, and most universally effective reinforcers.

SHAPING

Shaping is a behavior-modification technique used when the response does not meet the criteria. By systematically reinforcing successive approximations, the nurse manager can shape the responses into the desired behavior and get the nurse to do something new. The manager provides favorable consequences after any attempt at the desired behavior and then withholds consequences until improvement is made. When working with the staff nurse who is chronically absent or late, the manager may acknowledge that the nurse is at work: "I see you were only 30 minutes late today." Later, "I see you were only 15 minutes late today." Still later, "I noticed you were only 5 minutes late today." The manager may initially praise a new employee for attempting a new task and then note improvements in skill as they occur. Once the level of desired performance has been reached, it can be maintained by providing favorable consequences intermittently. Too many positive consequences cause satiation, and they lose their effect on the behavior. Performance that has been intermittently reinforced is most resistant to extinction.

EXTINCTION

Withholding reinforcers will decrease the probability of the occurrence of the behavior and contribute to its extinction. Therefore if the manager does not mention or otherwise reward undesirable behavior, the lack of action should contribute to extinction. Conversely, any reinforcer that is presented frequently but not paired with another reinforcer will lose its effectiveness.

Promises of "raises" or "hiring more help and getting some relief" become meaningless if not paired with a pay increase or recruitment and selection of personnel. Managers who praise everyone for everything all the time will find that their words lose their effectiveness as reinforcers. When the consequences are not worth the effort, the behavior will decrease also.

PUNISHMENT

The manager can decrease the probability of a response by pairing the behavior with an aversive stimulus. People who are late to work will not be paid for the time they are absent. There will be no overtime pay for people who did not complete their work on time. Employees who do not meet work standards will be fired. Firing a few workers who were not meeting standards can have an immediate impact on the remaining personnel, who initially work harder to avoid being fired. However, if management does nothing to reinforce the more productive work behavior, avoidance behavior is likely to occur. Employees may cover up for each other, steal from the agency what they rationalize is theirs, or resign. By using aversive stimuli to control behavior, management pairs itself with those stimuli and becomes viewed as aversive.

Once managers have started an aversive stimulus, they should not stop it until the behavior has been corrected or the cessation may act as a positive reinforcer. Absences, tardiness, excuse making, rationalizing, placing blame elsewhere, and other avoidance behaviors will increase if they successfully reduce the aversive stimuli. If the manager gruffly asks a nurse why some work has not been done (aversive stimulus), and the manager backs off when the staff nurse replies that she thought someone else was doing it, blaming others is reinforced. Although punishment causes behavior to occur less frequently, it does not teach new behaviors and is likely to increase avoidance behaviors. Most motivation problems are caused by punishment, absence of consequences, or insufficient consequences.

BEHAVIOR MODIFICATION FOR THE EMPLOYEE WITH A PERFORMANCE PROBLEM

Besides being aware of the subtle ways that one's behavior may reinforce, shape, or reduce behavior of others, the nurse manager may apply behavior modification to personnel with performance problems. First, one must identify the performance problem and analyze the antecedent, behavior, and consequence. What happened before the behavior occurred? Each time nurse A was late to work, she had worked the evening shift the night before. Each time nurse B yelled at her staff, an emergency treatment was being performed. Head nurse C was condescending to her staff after a physician had scolded her. What happened after the behavior occurred? Someone had already done part of nurse A's work by the time she got to the ward. Staff nurses responded quickly when nurse B yelled at them during an emergency procedure. Nurse C's staff avoided her.

Once the performance problem has been identified, the baseline frequency is determined. The baseline measure is the frequency before any attempts to change it. If nurses are interested in modifying their own behavior, they may collect the baseline data themselves. The behavior must be precisely defined, observable, and consequently countable. Written records should be kept, preferably on a portable recording system that is present when the behavior occurs, so the nurse can record it immediately. A tailor-made tally sheet is useful because one can see data in relation to time. If the behavior occurs daily, it should be recorded for 1 week. If there are large variations in the behavior from one day to the next, observations should be recorded for 2 weeks. A time-sampling technique can be used by busy managers by randomly selecting short periods to observe and tally behaviors. This is effective only for high-frequency behavior. The manager must consider if the period of data collection was representative of the normal situation and use a stable baseline rate as a cue to start the intervention (Figure 14-10).

If one transfers the information from the tally sheet to a graph that depicts frequency over

	M	T	W	Th	F	Sat	Sun
7:00	I I I	I I	I I	I I I	I I		
8:00			I				
9:00	I I			I	I		
10:00		I		I			
11:00			I		I		
12:00				I	I		
1:00		I	I		I		
2:00	I I	I	I I	I I	I		
3:00	I I I	I I	I I I	I I	I I I		

Figure 14-10 Tally sheet.

time, it is easy to visualize the effect of the intervention strategy. One can put a wavy vertical line on the graph to depict the point where intervention was started (Figure 14-11).

After identifying the relevant variables, the supervisor and nurse select appropriate reinforcement, extinction, punishment, or any combination of intervention strategies to decrease the frequency of the undesirable behavior. If the desired performance is punished, the punishment should be removed. Instead of making fast workers finish everyone else's work, they can be allowed time to do what they choose, such as read in the library or meditate in the chapel, receive a bonus day at a specified frequency, or be given a merit pay increase specifically for

doing more than their share of the work. If undesirable behavior is rewarded, the reward should be removed. Instead of having slow employees' work completed by others, the manager should inform the workers that they are responsible for so much work by themselves, must have that work completed before going home, and will receive no overtime pay for completion of the normal workload.

If desired behavior has not been rewarded, the manager should arrange a consequence. This may be as simple as orally acknowledging a nurse's accomplishment occasionally. Nurses' accomplishments can be acknowledged in the agency's newsletter. Awards can be created to recognize desirable behavior.

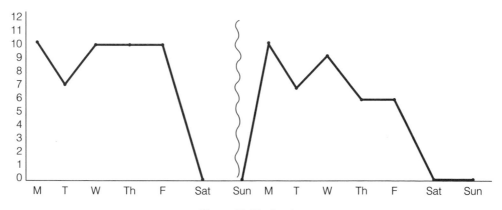

Figure 14-11 Graph.

If obstacles are identified, they should be removed. Nurses can be referred to professional counseling to help them work through situational crises that are interfering with their work performance. The manager can try to get the resources nurses need to do their job. Nurses should also have the necessary education to do what is expected of them. They may need formal education, on-the-job training, practice sessions, or simply feedback. The staff associate is the best source of information for what can serve as a positive reinforcer because what may be desirable for the manager may be aversive to the staff associate.

Once the intervention strategy has been planned, it should be implemented and the response frequency recorded. The strategy should be evaluated for effectiveness. If it is not working, it should be analyzed and revised. Once the desired behavior is obtained, it should be maintained through intermittent reinforcement (Marquis and Huston, 2000).

PROBLEM EMPLOYEES

Substance abusers, angry or withdrawn workers, personnel with excessive absenteeism, and the terminating employee provide challenges to nurse managers. In each case the manager must be alert to symptoms of problems, help the employee solve the problem, and evaluate the results.

SUBSTANCE ABUSERS

Substance abuse is not uncommon among nurses. It affects all socioeconomic classes, cultures, and races. Only 5% or less of all persons with alcoholism are skid-row bums. Among alcoholic nurses studied, most had been in the top one third of their class, held advanced degrees, held responsible and demanding jobs, and had an excellent work history.

Nurses with alcohol or other drug addictions often exhibit psychosocial problems (Box 14-3). Personality changes may be noted as the nurse becomes more irritable, withdrawn, and moody. Because of a decreased interest in outside activities, isolation increases. Related social changes include eating alone and avoiding social gatherings.

Changes in personal appearance become apparent. Changes in dress, an unkempt appearance, flushed complexion, red eyes, swollen face, and hand tremors are common. Mental status changes include forgetfulness, confusion, and decreased alertness.

General behavior changes too. Inappropriate responses and irritability occur more frequently. Excuses for behavior become more elaborate. Intolerance and suspicion of others and nervousness increase. Avoidance of others is noted. Work efficiency drops, there is a decline in the quality and quantity of work, and the work pace becomes uneven. Some assigned tasks are forgotten. Arriving late and leaving early and extended lunch hours and break times become patterns of behavior. Accidents increase. It is important for staff to know the importance of their reporting chemical abuse, because it is often

---

BOX 14-3 Signs and Symptoms of Possible Substance Abuse

SIGNS

Psychosocial problems
  Irritability
  Moodiness
  Tendency to isolate self
Social changes
  Eating alone
  Avoiding social
    gatherings
Changes in personal
  appearance
  Changes in dress
  Unkempt appearance
  Flushed complexion
  Red eyes
  Swollen face
  Hand tremors
Mental status changes
  Forgetfulness

Confusion
Decreased alertness
General behavior
  changes
Inappropriate
  responses
Elaborate excuses
  for behavior
Intolerance of others
Suspiciousness
Nervousness

SYMPTOMS

Odor of alcohol
Slurred speech
Unsteady gait
Errors in judgment

not the manager who identifies the problem, especially if the manager covers more than one unit (Hutchinson, 1987a).

When a nurse reports to work in a state of acute intoxication, the manager notes the signs objectively and asks a second person to validate the observations. The odor of alcohol, slurred speech, unsteady gait, and errors in judgment are symptoms of intoxication. The intoxicated nurse is removed from the situation, confronted briefly and firmly about the behavior, and sent home to rest and recuperate. Then the incident is recorded. The manager describes the observation, states the action taken, indicates future plans, and has the employee sign and date the memo after returning to work. Refusal to sign and date the memo should be noted by the manager and a witness.

Sally Hutchinson (1986) has described three stages in the self-annihilation trajectory that nurses experience as they become addicted: the experience, the commitment, and the compulsion. The experience is the nurse's introduction to alcohol or drugs and involves the three phases of initiating, connecting, and experimenting. Initiating is the first experience with drugs and is often experienced as a patient. The use of alcohol or drugs is associated with the relief of pain in the connecting phase. During the experimenting phase the person uses a variety of drugs to find the one of choice.

The commitment stage has three phases too: dialogue with self, disengaging, and routinizing. Commitment is the decision to use alcohol or drugs in one's lifestyle. It requires finding a source. After finding the chemical of choice, the person dialogues with self to justify the use of the chemical to alleviate psychological or physical pain. Denying, bargaining, and justifying are common dialogues. After the self-diagnosis, a disengaging process occurs. People disengage from their conscience and their usual behavior. They disengage from their family, friends, and colleagues and from the values of nursing and society. They transform themselves into alcohol or drug users. They start using chemicals

routinely to relieve their distress. Alcoholism is easier than drug addiction. The alcoholic nurse is more likely to miss work because of hangovers, whereas the drug-addicted nurse is likely to work overtime to have additional access to drugs. Many conning strategies are used to obtain chemicals.

The third stage, compulsion, has two phases—craving and surrendering. It is when the physical addiction becomes dominant. Some people stay in the experience stage for up to 1 year, but once they become committed, the compulsion stage follows.

Chronic performance problems are more common than acute intoxication. Each time performance problems are observed, they should be documented, including date, time, who was observed by whom, and a description of the incident and circumstances. At a prearranged conference, the nurse is confronted with the observations and how they affect job performance and patient care. The nurse is allowed to give an explanation. Alternatives are explored, and a course of action is planned. When substance abuse is identified as the problem, the offender is encouraged to take voluntary action. The manager refers the nurse to a local treatment facility and meets with the nurse periodically to monitor progress. The manager is not to serve the role of therapist.

Hutchinson (1987b) has identified four phases of recovery: premotivation, breakthrough, early recovery, and extended recovery. During the premotivation phase the person may decide to stop using drugs to please someone. The person may hope to use chemicals only occasionally and employ a strong denial system. Denial decreases, and the person admits to an addiction problem during the breakthrough phase. The person begins to cope with loss of the chemical, rediscovers values, and gains an image of self as a drug-free person during early recovery. The extended recovery begins after about 6 months in early recovery. People acknowledge their feelings about themselves and their relationships. They gain respect for themselves and their skills. They acquire control of their lives. This is the stage when the nurse can return to work and be productive.

Instead of disciplining and firing personnel whose job performance is impaired, more and more health care organizations are trying to help them regain their health and productivity through employee assistance programs (EAPs). At first EAPs focused on alcohol and drug abuse, but the services have broadened to include financial, legal, and marital problems; gambling; work addiction; and eating disorders. EAPs have increased productivity, reduced absenteeism, and lowered insurance costs. Assessment, diagnosis, and early intervention benefit the employee and the organization.

Many state nurses associations have started peer assistance programs. Ideally the association intervenes early in the addiction process before legal action is necessary. Often reports of impairment are made through a confidential telephone call or as a referral to the chairperson of the peer assistance program. The chairperson verifies that an impairment exists and may coach the nurse manager about documentation, verification, and intervention. A regional representative or local intervener contacts the person in question and makes an appointment.

The local intervener typically outlines the purpose of the visit with the impaired person, presents information about chemical abuse, and identifies behavior and circumstances in which the impairment has been evident. The fact that the disease is progressive is stressed. Various treatment options are presented. Issues such as hospitalization, insurance coverage, use of sick time and accrued vacation time, and family responsibilities are discussed. If the person denies impairment or refuses treatment, the impaired nurse may be reported to the state board of nursing by the employer.

When an impaired nurse participates in a peer assistance program, an advocate is assigned. The advocate maintains contact with the impaired nurse during treatment and until a solid recovery is established. A contract made by the peer review program advocate and the impaired nurse typically identifies employment restrictions, random urine screens, attendance at Alcoholics Anonymous or Narcotics Anonymous meetings, attendance at nurses' support groups, and contacts with the advocate.

When alcoholic or drug-abusing nurses refuse counseling or fail to follow the plan of care, they are told treatment is mandatory for continued employment. If they still refuse mandatory participation in the treatment, they are terminated in accordance with the hospital's policies.

ANGRY OR WITHDRAWN EMPLOYEES

Nurse managers often deal with angry or withdrawn employees. Anger and withdrawal are the fight and flight responses to anxiety. The angry nurse is more likely to be considered a troublemaker. The withdrawn person may be viewed as nice. However, both need help.

Anxiety occurs from the frustration of unmet expectations or loss of self-respect. The anxiety is transformed into feelings or actions, and relief is felt. Angry, hostile, and destructive behavior is a primary response to frustration. It is intended to gain mastery over the situation. The angry employee may become hostile and use critical, sarcastic, and obscene language with others. Consequently, interpersonal relationships suffer, and productive work may be impaired. Anger can also be displaced to patients and others.

Withdrawn persons do not invest emotional energy in others. Fear of self-disclosure or having others become attached to them is frightening. Withdrawal is a protective mechanism to avoid hurt. Withdrawn persons sit through meetings without becoming involved. They are not assertive and do not protect their rights. They may be delegated more than their fair share of the work because they are so cooperative and polite. This leads to more feelings of use, abuse, and helplessness.

Nurse managers need to recognize aggressive and passive behaviors among employees, teach and display assertive behavior, and encourage problem solving. They should help personnel understand themselves and their job responsibilities, develop trust, and promote group harmony. Employees should be encouraged to express themselves without fear of reprisals. Managers should be sincere, firm, and fair. Job expectations should be clear and personnel rewarded liberally and disciplined justly.

DECREASED PRODUCTIVITY

Decreased productivity is a side effect of personnel problems. Managers should make sure that desired performance is not being punished or undesirable behavior rewarded. Expectations are clarified. Employees are taught how to do what they are expected to do. If boredom is a problem, job rotation and special projects are considered.

ABSENTEEISM

Absenteeism is also a side effect of personnel problems. Ineffective management, poor working relationships, boredom, lack of control over decisions affecting one's life, and overwork are contributing factors. Some workers are immature and lack the self-discipline to get themselves to work. Others stay away to avoid an unpleasant or boring job. Some are poorly motivated, do as little as possible to prevent being fired, and do not see their job as a means toward an end. The hypochondriacal employee uses absenteeism to get attention and sympathy from others. Abusive absenteeism may be used to get even with a manager. Some personnel are exhausted from overwork, have lost their enthusiasm for the job, or are burned out.

Managers should make sure that there are attendance policies, that the policies do not reward nonattendance, and that they are enforced consistently. Attendance records should be maintained, and grievance procedures should be established.

Documented attendance policies greatly influence absence rates. Traditional sick leave policies have rewarded employees for absenteeism and have encouraged them to be dishonest to collect sick pay or be punished by losing it. Employees who receive sick pay are absent considerably more than those who do not. Some agencies have required a physician's excuse before an employee can receive sick pay to decrease the dishonest use of sick time. Because most people are sick only 1 or 2 days at a time, some hospitals do not compensate for the first 2 days of any sickness. The third and successive days are compensated. Other agencies have gone to paid time off. Each employee receives a certain amount of paid time off inclusive of holiday, vacation, and sick leave with few restrictions as to its use. It is typically collected at a rate calculated by length of continuous service. It simplifies record keeping but provides incentive to use the days whether sick or not.

Absenteeism data should be collected and analyzed to determine trends and patterns of individuals and personnel in general. Recording the date of absence, the reason and whether excused or unexcused, day of the week, preceding or following a day off, the employee's job classification, shift, tenure, age, gender, marital status, or any other information thought to be useful provides information to detect trends and pinpoint problems. Absenteeism often occurs more frequently in certain job classifications or departments, on specific days or shifts, or among a group working under a specific manager. Problems need to be identified so managers can develop control measures. Baseline data are also useful to determine the success of the control program.

A progressive discipline policy that imposes increasingly severe penalties is appropriate. Such a policy allows employees to know in advance the consequences of their behavior. Progressive discipline often starts with an oral reprimand that is documented and progresses through a written warning, pay deduction, suspension without pay, and dismissal.

TERMINATING EMPLOYEES

Working with a terminating employee (whether voluntary or involuntary) is also challenging for the nurse manager. The manager must help the employee deal with the related feelings. A sense of loss and grief is common. A period of shock or denial that is then followed by disorganization, anger, guilt, and loneliness is normal. This is followed by a deorientation period and a reestablishment phase. A termination checklist can help the manager through the termination process (Box 14-4).

The manager can help terminating employees by providing an opportunity to talk about their feelings. Airing feelings about leaving, self-image, not working anymore or filling another position, and other interests that may be pursued helps relieve the anxiety. Helping the employee plan for the future is also useful.

It is not uncommon for terminating employees to detach themselves from the job and do little for some time before the termination. The manager can assign tasks that are considered important that can either be finished or transferred to someone else at the time of the employee's termination.

Rituals such as best wishes cards and going away parties serve to acknowledge the termination and provide a rite of separation that facilitates the termination process.

EMPLOYEE COUNSELING

Counseling helps improve employees' mental health, thus enhancing understanding, self-control, self-confidence, and consequently their ability to work effectively. Counseling accomplishes several activities on a directive to nondirective scale. It provides an opportunity to give advice, offer reassurance, improve communication, release emotional tension, clarify thinking, and reorient.

When giving advice, a counselor tells the employee what the counselor thinks the employee should do. Unfortunately, it is almost impossible to understand another person's complicated problems, and consequently the advice may not be sound. Advice may foster feelings of inferiority and dependence on the counselor.

Reassurance provides courage to face a problem and confidence that one is handling the situation appropriately. False reassurance is dangerous. It may prevent the employee from getting the professional help needed. It offers little comfort when the counselee knows that the counselor cannot predict the outcome. Even if there is some comfort obtained, it tends to dissipate when the person faces the problem again.

Counseling improves both upward and downward communication. It allows employees to express their feelings to management. Although individual names must be kept confidential, feelings can be grouped into categories and

---

BOX 14-4 Termination Checklist

DATE COMPLETED	ACTION TAKEN
_____	Review termination plan for consistency with laws, policies, and procedures with Human Resources.
_____	Get supervisor's approval for termination.
_____	Have witness present for termination conference.
_____	Terminate access to information technology.
_____	Notify security.
_____	Collect department's property, such as keys, disks, manuals, and so on.
_____	Collect agency's property, such as employee badge, handbooks, parking pass, and so on.
_____	Complete necessary forms.
_____	Arrange for employee to remove personal property from the premises.
_____	Advise employee he or she will not be permitted back on the premises.
_____	Advise employee of employee assistance program.
_____	Advise employee that the final paycheck will be mailed. Confirm mailing address.
_____	Forward employee file to Human Resources.

interpreted to higher management. The counseling session allows the counselor to explain company policies and activities to the employee, thus achieving downward communication.

Catharsis, or the release of emotional tension, often occurs when people have the opportunity to talk about their frustrations. They become more relaxed, and their speech becomes more coherent and rational as they explain their problems to a sympathetic listener. Then, as emotional blocks to clear thinking are eliminated, thinking becomes more rational. People may realize that their emotions are not appropriate for the situation. This may help people recognize and accept their limitations and bring about a reorientation or change in values and goals. The manager should refer an employee to professional help when reorientation is needed.

Directive counseling occurs when the counselor listens to the employee's problems, decides how to solve the problems, and tells the employee what to do. The counselor predominantly gives advice. This type of counseling does give some emotional release, can be reassuring, and fosters communication. Thinking may be clarified in a limited way. Reorientation seldom occurs.

Nondirective counseling is client centered. The counselor listens and encourages employees to explain their problems, identify alternatives, explore the ramifications of each option, and determine the most appropriate solution. Emotional release occurs more frequently in nondirective than in directive counseling. Clear thinking and reorientation are fostered. Reassurance may be used, but advice should be limited. This approach can be very beneficial, but managers must be cautious not to neglect their normal directive leadership responsibilities.

Nondirective counseling is more time consuming and costly than directive counseling. To be effective, the employee must have the intelligence to identify problems and assess solutions and the emotional stability to deal with them. The nondirective counselor must be cautious not to allow emotionally dependent employees to avoid their work responsibilities.

Cooperative counseling is a compromise between directive and nondirective counseling. It is the cooperative effort by the counselor and employee through an exchange of ideas to help solve the problem. The cooperative counselor starts by listening, as would a nondirective counselor. As the interview progresses, however, the cooperative counselor offers information and insight and is likely to discuss the problems with a broad knowledge of the organization's point of view. This may help change the employee's perspective. Cooperative counseling combines the advantages of both directive and nondirective counseling and avoids most of the disadvantages.

Because of employees' rights to privacy, it is appropriate for the manager to refer an employee to professional help when personal problems are interfering with job performance or when a person needs reorientation (Swansburg and Swansburg, 2002).

OUTPLACEMENT COUNSELING

Although not many RNs are fired, during economic recessions the incidence of reduced workforces increases. Outplacement counseling can be used to minimize the emotional and professional scarring that results from being dismissed from one's position.

Poor job performance, tardiness, absenteeism, substance abuse, inappropriate behavior, and staff reduction are the most common reasons for discharging nurses. A termination of this nature is usually a progressive process. However, for some offenses nurses can be terminated immediately. These are likely to include abuse of patients and visitors, insubordination, intoxication, possession of drugs, theft, gambling, disorderly conduct, willful destruction of property, sleeping on duty, or falsification of records.

The termination procedures used must be consistent with agency policies. Termination usually involves several steps, beginning with an oral warning. If the employee does not change the offending behavior in response to the oral warning, written warnings with corrective interviews are used. There should be well-documented, sufficient grounds for termination. The nurse manager can use anecdotal notes to record both strong and weak attributes of the worker. These notes should contain factual information about who was observed by whom, where, and the background of the incident. There should be a sufficient number of observations to establish a pattern of behavior.

Written warnings used with corrective interviews should state the expected level of performance and the consequence if that standard is not met. Suspension is typically used before termination. The counseling note should be signed by both the nurse manager and the worker. If the worker refuses to sign, a witness can validate that the worker has read the counseling notes and refuses to sign them.

Poor job performance should be analyzed. Have employees been taught how to do what is expected of them? If not, they should be taught. Do they practice the skill often enough to keep their talents refined? If not, practice sessions could be made available. Specific, descriptive feedback should be given. Demonstrations and return demonstrations are appropriate. The feedback should be as close to the act as possible. Positive reinforcement for what was done well is as important as identifying weaknesses and making plans to overcome them. Follow-up by noting changes is also important.

A problem-solving approach can be used for tardiness and absenteeism. Why is the person late or absent so often? If a person has difficulty getting children to a babysitter and herself to work by 7 AM, could that person's hours be changed to 8 AM to 4:30 PM? This will allow the employee to fulfill her parental responsibilities, and it will also help provide a smooth transition at the change of shift. If the person is a night owl who has difficulty getting up in the morning, could that person be assigned the evening shift? Is the person working two jobs to make ends meet? Are financial assistance and counseling available? Are family problems

interfering with attendance? Is the person hung over when reporting to duty? The social services that are available for patients should also be used for staff, for example, self-help groups such as Alcoholics Anonymous, single parents, and shelters for women. Social services, the chaplain, or family counseling is also useful.

Repeated failure to meet performance standards, lack of compliance with company policies, and staff reductions are just causes for termination. Each should be a progressive process. The employee should know what level of performance is expected to prevent termination and the risk of termination.

Support services are needed by people who are terminated. The agency should have termination policies regarding severance pay, terminal vacation, accrued holidays and sick time, and insurance. The person may need information about unemployment. This is an opportune time for a counselor in personnel to help terminating employees reassess their location and vocation. Where do they want to live? What type of climate do they like? What type of work interests them and provides the most satisfaction? What do their educational background and skills prepare them to do? What can they do to prepare themselves better to reach their goals? How important are salary, fringe benefits, retirement plans, work hours, and opportunities for advancement?

Once terminating employees decide what they want to do and where, they may need assistance to locate job openings. Professional journals, employment agencies, and college placement services are sources of information. Recruiters are often present at professional meetings. Friends, relatives, and acquaintances may help locate positions, and employers can be contacted directly.

Terminating employees are likely to need help preparing resumes, writing marketing letters, and interviewing. They do not need to state the reason that they left the last job on this marketing letter, resume, or job application. However, they should be prepared to address the issue during an interview. They should be honest about the reason for termination, speak about the treatment they have had, if any, and focus on the knowledge and skills they have learned on the last job that they can transfer to the new one. They should not be critical of the last employer.

The sooner one accepts the fact that one has been fired, the sooner one can put the pieces back together and move on. The boss should be very clear about the reason. The termination should not come as a surprise. With the progressive process the employee should know the consequences of not meeting the performance standards. Any reduction in workforce should be done with fair warning and target dates. Employees should be informed of the grievance policy and procedure when reflecting if they have been fairly treated. The outplacement counseling can help the person know what questions to ask about pay and benefits, how to tell the family, how to solicit help from friends and acquaintances, and how to budget to protect securities until another job can be obtained. Career counseling and job placement counseling are useful.

Being fired initiates stress and can be quite devastating. Outplacement counseling can help reduce the related personal and professional scarring that inevitably results from being dismissed.

"Keep away from people who try to belittle your ambitions. Small people always do that, but the really great make you feel that you, too, can become great." —Mark Twain

Chapter Summary

Chapter 14 covered the following:
Purposes
Common Errors in Evaluation
Methods of Performance Management
  Anecdotal Notes
  Checklists
  Rating Scales
  Ranking
  Management by Objectives
  Self-Appraisal
  Peer Review

Customer or Subordinate Evaluation
360-Degree Feedback
Appraisal Interview
Appraisal Reports
Legal Implications for Performance
  Appraisals
Discipline of Personnel
  Need for Discipline
  Principles of Disciplinary Action
    Have a positive attitude
    Investigate carefully
    Be prompt
    Protect privacy
    Focus on the act
    Enforce rules consistently
    Be flexible
    Advise the employee
    Take corrective, constructive action
    Follow up
  Penalties
    Oral reprimand
    Written reprimand
    Other penalties
  Components of a Disciplinary Action
    Program
    Codes of conduct
    Authorized penalties
    Records of offenses and corrective
      measures
    Right of appeal
  Discipline Without Punishment
Modification of Employee Behavior
  Reinforcement
  Shaping
  Extinction
  Punishment
  Behavior Modification for the Employee With
    a Performance Problem
Problem Employees
  Substance Abusers
  Angry or Withdrawn Employees
  Decreased Productivity
  Absenteeism
  Terminating Employees
Employee Counseling
Outplacement Counseling

On-line Resources

evolve Additional critical thinking activities, worksheets, and case studies are available on-line at http://evolve.elsevier.com/Marriner/guide/

References

Edwards MR, Ewen AJ: *360 feedback: The powerful new model for employee assessment & performance improvement,* New York, 1996, American Management Association.

Grote D: *The complete guide to performance appraisal,* New York, 1996, American Management Association.

Grote D: *Discipline without punishment,* New York, 1995, American Management Association.

Hutchinson S: Chemically dependent nurses: Implications for nurse executives, *JONA* 17:23-29, Sept 1987a.

Hutchinson S: Chemically dependent nurses: The trajectory toward self-annihilation, *Nurs Res* 35: 196-200, July-Aug 1986.

Hutchinson S: Toward self integration: The recovery process of chemically dependent nurses, *Nurs Res* 36:339-343, Nov-Dec 1987b.

Maier NRF: *The appraisal interview: Three basic approaches,* La Jolla, Calif, 1976, University Associates.

Marquis BL, Huston CJ: *Leadership roles and management functions in nursing: Theory and application,* ed 3, Philadelphia, 2000, Lippincott.

Marquis BL, Huston CJ: *Management decision making for nurses: 124 case studies,* Philadelphia, 1998, Lippincott.

Odiorne GS: *Management decisions by objectives,* Englewood Cliffs, NJ, 1969, Prentice Hall.

Odiorne GS: *Management by objectives: A system of managerial leadership,* Belmont, Calif, 1965, Pitman Publishing.

Rocchiccioli JT, Tilbury MS: *Clinical leadership in nursing,* Philadelphia, 1998, WB Saunders.

Sullivan EJ, Decker PJ: *Effective leadership and management in nursing,* Upper Saddle River, NJ, 2001, Prentice Hall.

Swansburg RC: *Introductory management and leadership for clinical nurses: A text-workbook,* Boston, 1993, Jones and Bartlett.

Swansburg RC, Swansburg RJ: *Introductory management and leadership for nurse managers,* Boston, 2002, Jones and Bartlett.

15

Continuous Quality Improvement, Risk Management, and Program Evaluation

*"The greater the difficulty the more glory in
surmounting it. Skillful pilots gain their reputation
from storms and tempests."* —Epicurus

Chapter Overview

Chapter 15 identifies quality management heroes; outlines history, tools, and
processes for continuous quality improvement (CQI); and discusses program
evaluation, regulatory influences, risk management, and liability issues.

Chapter Objectives

- Compare and contrast the roles of leaders and managers regarding quality
  improvement.
- Discuss trends in the history of continuous quality improvement.
- Identify three quality management heroes and their contributions to the field.
- Identify and describe at least five tools that can be used to facilitate continuous
  quality improvement.
- Outline a process for continuous quality improvement.
- Itemize activities that could be on a calendar of events for program evaluation.
- Identify and discuss at least six internal and six external sources of invalidity.
- Identify and discuss at least six research designs. In the discussion identify which
  sources of invalidity the design controls for and which could still be a problem.
- List the five steps in the risk management process.
- Identify at least three sources for identifying potential risks.
- Describe the importance of customer satisfaction in relation to risk management.
- Describe the research process as applied to quality improvement.
- Discuss the relationship among torts, negligence, and malpractice.
- Discuss at least one liability issue.

Major Concepts and Definitions

Continuous quality improvement preventive problem solving that results in exemplary service

Risk management development and implementation of strategies to prevent patient injury, minimize financial loss, and preserve agency assets

Customer satisfaction risk management of public relations is striving for customer satisfaction

Evaluation valuation

Validity measurement of what is to be measured

Internal invalidity extraneous variables that confound the effects of the experimental variable

External invalidity factors that reduce the findings' generalizability

Statistics facts or data of a numerical kind that are assembled, classified, and tabulated so as to present significant information about a given subject

Torts legal wrongs

Negligence unintentional tort where harm results by not behaving in a reasonable and prudent manner

Malpractice negligent acts of people with professional education

Legally liable legally responsible

Plaintiff complaining party

Defendant answering party

Leaders envision high-quality care, encourage others to be involved in quality improvement, encourage setting high standards, are proactive, facilitate interdisciplinary quality, and consequently build a culture of quality. Managers organize quality-driven services; select standards, measures of those standards, and tools to measure them with others; facilitate collecting and analyzing data; determine discrepancies between care provided and standards; and facilitate ongoing quality improvement (Table 15-1).

HISTORY OF CONTINUOUS QUALITY IMPROVEMENT

In the late 1950s planning, organizing, and evaluating health care services became a public concern. In 1952 the Joint Commission on Accreditation of Hospitals—now the Joint Commission on Accreditation of Healthcare Organizations (JCAHO)—was formed. The American Nurses Association (ANA) and the National League for Nursing (NLN) both published manuals

---

TABLE **15-1** Quality Improvement Leadership and Management

LEADER	MANAGER
Envisions high-quality care	Organizes quality-driven services
Encourages others to be involved in quality improvement	Selects standards and measures of those standards with others
Encourages setting high standards	Selects tools with others
Is proactive versus reactive	Facilitates collecting and analyzing data
Facilitates interdisciplinary quality improvement	Determines discrepancies between care provided and standards
Builds a culture of quality	Facilitates ongoing quality improvement

Modified from Marquis BL, Huston CJ: *Leadership roles and management functions in nursing: Theory and application,* ed 3, Philadelphia, 2000, Lippincott.

in 1959 to help establish standards for health care.

During the 1960s the ANA started a division of nursing practice to develop standards for nursing practice, which became the basis for quality assurance programs. The ANA also developed a process to evaluate the quality of patient care.

In October 1972 the Ninety-second Congress passed Public Health Law 92-603, an amendment to the Social Security Act that mandated the establishment of professional standards review organizations (PSROs) to review the quality and cost of care received by clients of Medicare, Medicaid, and Maternal Child Health programs. Health care facilities were to develop quality control programs by 1976, or the government would do it for them. Consequently, quality assurance has received considerable attention. The ANA developed guidelines for standards of nursing practice under the PSRO system; the American Hospital Association and the JCAHO developed a retrospective review of care. Individuals and agencies developed criteria and processes for the measurement of quality of care.

JCAHO required audits of care, delivered in its initial quality assurance standards, and increased the number of multidisciplinary audits required in 1975. Nursing then became a major contributor for evaluation of documentation. During the 1990s, JCAHO had nursing examine a nursing care problem quarterly, document assessment of the problem, develop and implement the plan for correction, and evaluate the effectiveness of the implemented actions.

Instruments for measuring nursing care were developed during the 1970s, but limited data were generated or published in quality assurance studies. The quality assurance program recommended by JCAHO was a retrospective review of patient care through a closed-chart audit that focused on patient-care outcomes.

Cost containment became a major issue in the 1980s. The federal prospective payment system (PPS), which uses a series of diagnostic related groups (DRGs) to determine a hospital's reimbursement for care provided to Medicare patients, was introduced. Outpatient services that were often uncovered for reimbursement in the 1970s became the preferred alternatives to health care in the 1980s. Outpatient services, long-term care, and home care were less expensive ways to deliver some care. The power in health care shifted from the provider to the consumer, primarily the third-party payers and insurers (Koch and Fairly, 1993).

Total quality management as the right thing to do the first time, on time, all the time was introduced in health care during the 1980s for improvement and customer satisfaction. Factories in Europe during the Industrial Revolution used measurement and standardization. Industry in the United States adopted quality management and product inspection after the turn of the century. During World War II industry in the United States produced large quantities of military products with declining quality. The boom in industry continued after World War II. The Japanese started focusing on quality through total workforce training and participation in quality improvement efforts. They called upon quality experts from the United States to train Japanese personnel. W. Edwards Deming, Joseph Juran, Philip Crosby, Avedis Donabedian, and Donald Berwick were important in the quality improvement movement. Deming (1982), with his 14-point management philosophy, was primarily responsible for training engineers in the United States to improve quality of military goods during World War II and was a key figure in training the Japanese. Juran (1981, 1989) and his trilogy of interrelated processes of quality planning, quality control, and quality improvement were also used to train Japanese. Crosby (1992) has 14 steps that emphasize training all employees, using teams, setting goals, and recognizing employees for their involvement. He is known for his zero defects concept. Donabedian and Berwick applied quality management principles to health care. Donabedian (1986) is known for his structure, process, and outcome criteria for quality assessment. Berwick (1989) stressed the importance of improving process toward quality improvement.

Quality became the issue in the 1990s. The objective became to provide quality health care in the most appropriate health care setting at the most economical cost. Customers started wanting involvement in decision making and wanted information about quality and costs. This brought intense competition among health care providers, and quality improvement became the key to survival and success.

QUALITY MANAGEMENT HEROES

Deming is the genius who revitalized Japanese industry with his focus on total quality management and CQI. The Deming chain reaction is as follows: (1) improve quality, (2) decrease costs with fewer mistakes, less rework, fewer delays, and better use of time and materials, (3) improve productivity, (4) capture the market with better quality at lower prices, (5) stay in business, and (6) provide jobs. Box 15-1 outlines the 14 key points of the Deming management method (Aguayo, 1990; Mears, 1994; Walton, 1986, 1990).

Juran is an advocate for total quality management (TQM). His quality trilogy is composed of three activities: quality planning, control, and improvement (Juran, 1988, 1989, 1992; Juran, Goyna, and Bingham, 1988) (Box 15-2).

Crosby defines quality as conformance to requirements. He believes that the system for

---

BOX **15-1** Fourteen Points of the Deming Management Method

1. Create constancy of purpose for improvement of products and services. Deming suggests that the purpose is to stay in business and provide jobs through maintenance, research, innovation, and constant improvement.
2. Adopt the new philosophy. Mistakes and negativism should be unacceptable.
3. Cease dependence on mass inspection. Deming maintains that quality arises from improvement in the process rather than from inspection and that workers should participate in improvement in the process. When quality is addressed at the inspection phase, workers are paid to make the mistake and then paid to correct it, which is very expensive.
4. End the practice of awarding business on the price tag alone. Buyers should get the best quality in a long-term relationship with a single supplier for any specific item rather than purchasing the lowest-priced and often poor-quality items from the cheapest vendor.
5. Constantly improve the system of production and service. Management must always look for ways to reduce waste and improve quality.
6. Institute training. Workers cannot be expected to do their jobs well if no one tells them how to do so.
7. Institute leadership. Deming believes that people who do not do well are just misplaced. It is the leader's responsibility to identify workers who need individual attention, find an appropriate place for them in the organization, and help them do a better job.
8. Drive out fear. Many workers are afraid to ask questions or point out problems for fear of being blamed for the problem. They may continue to do something wrong or not at all. For the best quality and productivity, people need to feel secure.
9. Break down barriers between staff areas. Often departments compete with each other or have goals that conflict. It is better to have teamwork to solve problems.
10. Eliminate slogans, exhortations, and targets for the workforce. It is better for workers to develop their own slogans.
11. Eliminate numerical quotas because they deal with numbers, not quality. They often contribute to inefficiency and high cost because workers meet quotas at any cost to keep their jobs.
12. Remove barriers to pride of workmanship. People are eager to do a good job. Barriers such as faulty equipment, defective materials, and misguided managers should be removed.
13. Institute a vigorous program of education and retraining. Both managers and staff need to be educated about new methods and teamwork.
14. Take action to accomplish the transformation. Managers and staff need a plan of action to carry out the quality mission. A critical mass of people must understand the 14 points about continuous quality improvement.

Modified from Walton M: *The Deming management method*, New York, 1986, Putnam; Walton M: *Deming management at work*, New York, 1990, Putnam's Sons.

BOX 15-2 Juran's Quality Trilogy

QUALITY PLANNING

1. Determine who the customers are.
2. Determine the needs of the customers.
3. Develop product features that respond to the customers' needs.
4. Develop the processes that produce those product features.
5. Transfer the resulting plans to the operating forces.

QUALITY CONTROL

1. Evaluate actual quality performance.
2. Compare actual performance with quality goals.
3. Act on the difference.

QUALITY IMPROVEMENT

1. Establish the infrastructure needed to secure annual quality improvement.
2. Identify the specific needs for improvement, which become the improvement projects.
3. Establish a project team with responsibilities for bringing the project to successful closure.
4. Provide the resources and training needed by teams to diagnose the problems, develop a remedy, and establish controls to maintain the gains.

Modified from Juran JM: *Juran on leadership for quality: An executive handbook*, New York, 1989, Free Press.

BOX 15-3 Crosby's 14 Steps to Quality Improvement

1. Commitment from management
2. Use of quality improvement teams composed of people with process knowledge and commitment to actions
3. Quality measurement to identify areas that need improvement and change
4. Measuring the cost of quality and nonquality
5. Quality awareness by all personnel
6. Corrective actions through opportunities for improvement
7. Zero defects planning—do it right the first time
8. Employee education for quality improvement
9. Zero defect day as demonstration of commitment to quality
10. Goal setting toward zero defects
11. Error-causal removal by removing barriers
12. Recognition for meeting goals
13. Quality councils to assist people in quality improvement
14. Do it all over again

Modified from Crosby PB: *Let's talk quality*, New York, 1989, McGraw-Hill; Crosby PB: *Quality is free: The art of making quality certain*, New York, 1992, McGraw-Hill; Crosby PB: *Quality without tears: The art of hassle-free management*, New York, 1995, McGraw-Hill.

---

creating quality is prevention of errors instead of appraisal. He has identified 14 steps to quality improvement, some of which are parallel (Crosby, 1989, 1992, 1995) (Box 15-3).

Quality improvement differs from quality assurance (Table 15-2). The process of quality improvement includes the following steps:

- Identify the customers and their expectations and the outputs using brainstorming, focus groups, and interviews.
- Describe the current process using flow charts and focus groups.
- Measure and analyze the discrepancy between desired expectations and reality using check sheets, logs, time charts, trend charts, histograms, and surveys.
- Focus on an improvement opportunity using decision matrix, Pareto charts, and voting.
- Identify root causes of inefficiencies through brainstorming, affinity charts, cause-and-effect diagrams, tree diagrams, relationship diagrams, force-field analysis, and focus groups.
- Generate and select solutions to the problem by brainstorming and using decision matrices and tree diagrams.
- Map out a trial run through brainstorming, force-field analysis, action planning, tree diagrams, and flow charting.
- Implement the trial run using check sheets, logs, and histograms.
- Evaluate the results using check sheets, logs, surveys, focus groups, histograms, and trend charts.
- Draw conclusions using Pareto diagrams, focus groups, and force-field analysis.
- Standardize the change using force-field analysis, brainstorming, action planning, tree diagrams, and flow charting.

TABLE **15-2** Comparison of Quality Assurance and Quality Improvement

QUALITY ASSURANCE	QUALITY IMPROVEMENT
Detection oriented	Prevention oriented
Reactive	Proactive
Narrow focus	Cross-functional
Getting by	Raising standards
Tradition and safety	Experimentation and risk
Busyness	Productivity
Leadership not vested	Leadership leading
Leader as director	Leader as empowerer
Employee as expendable	Employee as customer
Responsibility of few	Responsibility of all
Problem solving by authority	Problem solving by all
We-they thinking	Organizational perspective
Cynicism	New optimism

- Monitor holding the gains through check sheets, trend charts, surveys, histograms, and control charts.

CONTINUOUS QUALITY IMPROVEMENT

Deming introduced the *plan-do-check-act cycle* (PDCA) (Walton, 1990). FOCUS-PDCA is an acronym for the following (Walton, 1990, p. 107):

Find a process to improve.

Organize a team that knows the process.

Clarify current knowledge of the process.

Understand causes of process variation.

Select the process improvement.

Plan the improvement and continue data collection.

Do the improvement, data collection, and analysis.

Check the results and lessons learned from the team effort.

Act to hold the gain and to continue to improve the process.

The basic assumptions for the PDCA cycle are that (1) decisions should be based on facts instead of on hunches and intuition, (2) people who perform the work know it best, (3) teams can have more success than individuals working alone, (4) teams need to be trained in problem-solving processes, and (5) it helps to display information graphically (Sandras, 1995; Walton, 1990).

PDCA cycle methods include the following (Cofer and Greeley, 1998; Ritter and Brassard, 1998):

Plan

Plan the change.
Identify opportunities.
Develop vision statement.
Collect data to define problems and opportunities.
Use CQI tools to organize data and thinking.
Decide on improvement initiatives.

Do

Implement the planned change.
Implement initiatives.
Test with a trial run.
Identify costs, people, and materials.
Educate staff and management about changes in process.

Check

Observe the effect of the change.
Monitor progress of initiatives.
Meet with staff to discuss changes.
Delegate staff to monitor results.
Compare new data with original data, using CQI tools.
Use CQI tools to monitor results.

Act

Adjust as necessary.
Incorporate changes into department policies.
Inform and educate all involved.
Distribute new policies to key individuals.
Look for new opportunities.

The planning phase involves identifying customers, their needs, areas not meeting those needs, and improvement proposals. Deming identified the following seven helpful charts: cause-and-effect chart, flow chart, Pareto chart, histogram, run (trend) chart, scatter diagram, and control chart. Other tools that can be used to display information graphically include checklists, pie charts, time charts, decision matrices, affinity charts, tree diagrams, relationship diagrams, force-field analysis, and bar graphs. Processes that can be used to envision and make decisions include benchmarking, observations, interviews, questionnaires, record audits, nominal group technique, brainstorming, quality circles, focus groups, action planning, and voting.

TOOLS AND PROCESSES FOR CONTINUOUS QUALITY IMPROVEMENT

A *bar graph* is a series of bars representing successive changes in the value of a variable or different data sets. A simple bar graph can measure one set of data that does not need to be subcategorized (Figure 15-1). The cluster bar graph can divide simple bar graph totals into subtotals (Figure 15-2). The histogram and Pareto chart are bar graphs (Cofer and Greeley, 1998).

Benchmarking is a process of identifying best practices and comparing them with the agency's practices to improve performance. It is learning and borrowing from others. The process is as follows: (1) identify the benchmark team, (2) identify what to benchmark, (3) gather information through search of the literature, (4) survey

Errors

Figure 15-2 Cluster bar graph.

benchmark partners through written or telephone surveys or site visits, (5) compare benchmark data with organization's current practices and outcomes, (6) borrow ideas from the best and adapt them to important processes within the organization, and (7) monitor the results (Gift and Mosel, 1994; Stowell, 1997; Swansburg and Swansburg, 2002).

Brainstorming is a process of creating a free flow of ideas without fear of criticism and then thinking about the good in the wild ideas generated (Cofer and Greeley, 1998; Ritter and Brassard, 1998). (See Chapter 3.)

A *cause-and-effect diagram,* or *fishbone diagram,* is used to identify the root causes of a problem or outcome. Identify a problem, and then use brainstorming to identify root causes. Start with the outcome and then identify causal categories, such as facilities or equipment, materials or supplies, methods, and people, and items within those categories that cause the problem. Ask "why" four or five times. Identify first-, second-, and third-level causes until the causes become narrow enough to address. This can be outlined to look like a fish skeleton or can be done as hierarchical outlining on the computer (Brassard and Ritter, 1994; Cofer and Greeley, 1998; McCloskey and Collett, 1993; Oddo, 1995; Rocchiccioli and Tilbury, 1998; Yoder-Wise, 2003) (Figure 15-3).

Check sheets are grids that can be used to collect and classify raw data. They are good tools for monitoring key performance indicators. That raw data can be used to generate histograms,

Figure 15-1 Simple bar graph.

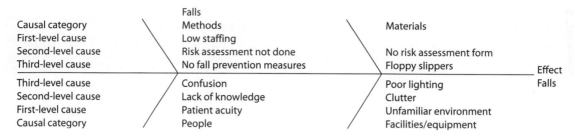

Figure 15-3 Cause-and-effect diagram, or fishbone diagram.

Pareto charts, run charts, and other tools that display information graphically (Band, 1994; Cofer and Greeley, 1998; McCloskey and Collett, 1993; Oddo, 1995; Sandras, 1995; Thomas, Gallace, and Martin, 1992; Wheatley, 1997) (Table 15-3).

A *decision matrix* is a grid that helps prioritize options. First, there is brainstorming to identify options. Those options are then evaluated, and unfeasible options are eliminated, leaving viable alternatives. The viable options are then listed down the left side of the grid. Criteria for evaluating each option are identified at the top of columns. How well the item meets the criterion can be rated as follows: 1 = poorly, 2 = adequately, and 3 = well. The criterion can be weighted as follows: 1 = unimportant, 2 = important, and 3 = very important. Then a weighted score can be calculated by multiplying the score by the criterion weight. The score can be recorded to the left of the diagonal dividing the score box, with the weighted score to the right of the diagonal (Band, 1994; Cofer and Greely, 1998; Sandras, 1995) (Table 15-4).

A *histogram* is a bar graph that can be used to compare patterns of occurrence over time. It displays the frequency with which comparable events occur and illustrates the variations in the occurrences. It can be used to identify trends and analyze variations. The measurement should occur at least 25 times during the period studied to get useful data. Raw data are gathered possibly using a checklist to plot the histogram. The range of the data is calculated by subtracting the smallest from the largest data point. The square root of the total number of data points collected will determine how many bars to use in the histogram. Divide the overall range by the number of bars to determine the interval for each bar. Use the check sheet to group the raw data by intervals. The number of data points per interval determines the height of the bar for that interval. A histogram that peaks in the middle with a narrow base indicates little performance variance. A histogram that peaks in the middle with a wide base indicates much performance variance. Histograms that peak to the right or left are skewed histograms and probably indicate that something unexpected happened during the process. Histograms with two peaks are bimodal and probably contain incompatible data sets that

TABLE **15-3** Check Sheet

STAFF/DAY	SUNDAY	MONDAY	TUESDAY	WEDNESDAY	THURSDAY	FRIDAY	SATURDAY	WEEKLY TOTAL/PERSON
Ann		///	//	/	/		/	8
Betty	/	//	//	//	//			9
Carol		//	///	///	////	///		15
Daily total	1	7	7	6	7	3	1	32

TABLE **15-4** Decision Matrix

	CRITERIA						
	EASE OF IMPLEMENTATION 2	COST 3	TIMELINESS 2	VALUE ADDED 3	QUALITY IMPACT 3	WEIGHTED SCORE	RANK
Surveys	3 / 6	3 / 9	3 / 6	2 / 6	3 / 9	36	1
Interviews	1 / 2	1 / 3	1 / 2	3 / 9	2 / 6	22	2
Observations	1 / 2	1 / 3	1 / 2	2 / 6	2 / 6	19	3

should be separated. Recalculate abnormal histograms before considering defective processes (Band, 1994; Cofer and Greely, 1998; McCloskey and Collett, 1993; Oddo, 1995) (Figure 15-4).

A *flow process chart* helps analyze how a task is being performed (Figure 15-5). Flow process chart symbols include O for operation, → for transportation, □ for inspection, **D** for delay, and Δ for storage. An operation is the actual performance of the work, such as giving an injection. Transportation represents physical movement—the relocation of a person or thing from one place to another, such as movement of the syringe from the medication room to the patient's bedside. Inspection is to determine whether the necessary work has been properly performed. Nurses make sure that they are giving the right medication to the right patient and using the right mode at the right time. A delay is an unplanned interruption

in the flow of the process. Storage is an anticipated interruption in the process or at the end of it. When making a flow process chart, one must decide whether to follow the flow of material or the activities of the worker, because they may not be the same.

As a result of methods improvement, one should eliminate activities or combine steps when possible and change the sequence of activities as necessary to improve the performance of various steps. The proposed method is then analyzed using flow charting. The potential impact on people is considered. Trial runs are conducted, and debugging is done (Band, 1994; Cofer and Greeley, 1998; McCloskey and Collett, 1993; Oddo, 1995; Rocchiccioli and Tilbury, 1998).

A *Gantt chart* is a grid with a time frame across the top that could be in minutes, hours, days, weeks, months, years, or decades depending on

Figure 15-4 Histogram.

	Present		Proposed		Savings	
	No	Hr	No	Hr	No	Hr
Operation	8					
Transportation	2					
Inspection	2					
Delay	0					
Storage	1					

Procedure: Injection   Distance traveled   Present ☐ Proposed ☐

Person ☐

Material ☐

Steps in procedure	○ → ☐ D △	Distance (ft)	Time (hr)	Remarks
Read medication order	○ → ☐ D △			
Collect vial and syringe	○ → ☐ D △			
Open vial	○ → ☐ D △			
Open disposable syringe	○ → ☐ D △			
Draw up solution	○ → ☐ D △			
Recheck medication order	○ → ☐ D △			
Put vial in medication drawer	○ → ☐ D △			
Take shot to patient	○ → ☐ D △			
Check patient identification	○ → ☐ D △			
Administer shot	○ → ☐ D △			
Return to medicine room	○ → ☐ D △			
Dispose of syringe	○ → ☐ D △			
Chart medication	○ → ☐ D △			
Store chart	○ → ☐ D △			

Key:
○ Operation
→ Transportation
☐ Inspection
D Delay
△ Storage

Figure 15-5 Flow process chart.

the time frame of the process. Tasks to be accomplished are listed down the left side of the grid. An X is put in the cell when a certain task is to be done. A line is drawn through cells when the task takes a period of time. This tool is used for managing production activities to complete a project (Swansburg and Swansburg, 2002). (See Chapter 3.)

Nominal group technique is a process for developing team goals and priorities. Individuals list ideas on a paper during silent generation of ideas. Each participant may give one idea at a time during a round-robin session. The ideas are written onto a chalkboard or paper. Ideas are expressed around and around the circle until all ideas have been expressed. Then there is a discussion for clarification before the preliminary vote. Participants may rank the first five to seven items, with the highest number being the highest weighting. Then the votes are weighted by multiplying the number of votes per priority for each item. If more than nine items surface as priorities, there can be further discussion and a second vote weighting the top items. Once items have been identified, brainstorming can be used to address the issues (Cofer and Greeley, 1998; Oddo, 1995). (See Chapter 3.)

A *Pareto chart* is a bar graph that displays categories of data in descending order of frequency or significance from the left to right. It is named after Pareto, an economist who noticed that 80% of the wealth in Italy in the nineteenth century was controlled by 20% of the population. The Pareto principle is that most effects come from a few causes (Figure 15-6). Once the major cause of a problem is identified, it can be problem solved, leading to considerable impact (Band, 1994; Brassard and Ritter, 1994; Cofer and Greeley, 1998; McCloskey and Collett, 1993; Oddo, 1995; Sandras, 1995; Yoder-Wise, 2003).

Pie charts compare relative size of different data sets in a circle instead of as bars on graphs. Data are collected and assigned percentages of the whole (Figure 15-7). A circle is drawn and divided into proportional pieces equal to the percentage of each indicator subtotal. Different segments can be shaded differently (Cofer and Greeley, 1998).

Program evaluation and review technique (PERT) is a system model for planning that identifies key activities in a project and sequencing of those activities in a flow diagram with duration of each phase of the program assigned (Swansburg and Swansburg, 2002). (See Chapter 3.)

Radar charts are circular displays of before-and-after data to demonstrate progress made or lost. Decide what indicators to measure. Draw a circle and divide it into equal segments numbering the number of indicators. Establish the rating scale. Rate each indicator using the rating scale, and post the finding on the segment line for that indicator. Draw a line connecting the posted ratings. Repeat the process later, use a different type line to connect the second posted ratings, and compare the old and new ratings (Cofer and Greeley, 1998; Oddo, 1995) (Figure 15-8).

Figure 15-6 Pareto chart.

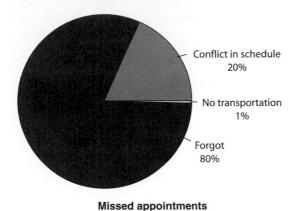

Missed appointments

Figure 15-7 Pie chart.

A *run chart* is a line graph that displays the variations in data over time. It allows a quick assessment of patterns and trends. It is good for monitoring time-related trends and shifts in processes (Cofer and Greeley, 1998; McCloskey and Collett, 1993; Oddo, 1995; Yoder-Wise, 2003) (Figure 15-9).

Scatter diagrams help determine relationships between two variables. They reflect correlations but do not explain causation. Identify two variables to compare. Collect the data, and note the highest and lowest values for each variable. Draw axes for each variable ranging from the lowest to the highest value for each variable.

Plot each data point where the two measurements intersect, and analyze the pattern. If the points are clustered together from the lower left to the upper right, there is a positive correlation. If the points are clustered together from the upper left to the lower right, there is a negative correlation. If the points are scattered randomly, there is no correlation between the variables (Band, 1994; Cofer and Greeley, 1998; McCloskey and Collett, 1993; Oddo, 1995; Sandras, 1995) (Figure 15-10).

Several authors of the 1990s have outlined processes for risk management and change for quality improvement. Otto Lerbinger (1997, pp. 343-350) outlines lessons learned from crises as follows:

Assess personal and organizational vulnerability. ...

Look for ways to reduce vulnerability. ...

Exercise constant vigilance and establish monitoring systems. ...

Communicate with and relate to a wide range of stakeholders. ...

Speed up and broaden the decision-making process. ...

Apply a variable time perspective. ...

Examine immediate, short-term, and long-term impacts. ...

Recognize the importance of the corporate culture and its supporting structures.

Figure 15-8 Radar chart.

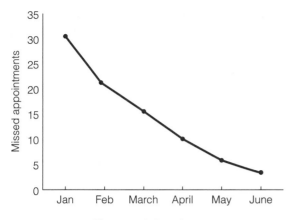

Figure 15-9 Run chart.

Michael Hammer (1996, p. 104) said, "Superior process performance is achieved by having a superior process design, the right people to perform it, and the right environment for them to work in." Jim Fuller (1997, pp. 8-13) outlined the five steps in the process of project definition as follows:

Step One: Identify the project. …

- Define why something must be done. …

- Define what would be done and the intended outcomes. …

- Create a preliminary cost-benefit analysis. …

- Analyze the risk. …

- Define the project's relationship to other performance improvement projects. …

- Evaluate future opportunities. …

- Assess organizational readiness. …

Step Two: Create a written definition document. …

Step Three: Create a project objective statement. …

Step Four: Validate the definition. …

Step Five: Create a project priority matrix. …

Jack Hagan (1994) says a quality plan requires a framework. The following basic model can be applied to any plan:

Phase One—A Philosophy for Quality. This phase includes the establishment of:

a. A vision.

b. A clear policy.

c. Primary quality objectives.

d. Guidelines for meeting those objectives.

Once these are established, a company quality philosophy exists.

Phase Two—Tactics. This phase provides the ways and means for putting the philosophy into operation through:

a. Specific programs and projects.

b. The creation of an ongoing review process to help the business to understand its progress and make necessary adjustments when appropriate.

This basic model can be specifically adapted to a quality plan using the following eight-step process (pp. 60-62):

1. Obtain management commitment through sponsorship. …

2. Form the team. …

3. Develop a vision. …

4. Develop a policy statement. …

Positive

Negative correlation

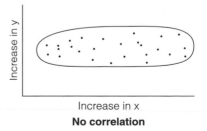

No correlation

Figure 15-10 Scatter diagrams.

5. Develop objectives and guidelines. …

6. Review current programs and projects. …

7. Develop and implement a formal review process. …

8. Implement the plan. …

Hagan (1994, p. 63) recommends the following guidelines:

Plan it right—keep it short and simple.

Make it fun—be innovative.

Implement it—involve everyone.

Monitor it—show results.

Make it last—stress continuous improvement.

Make it rewarding—recognize excellence.

Sustain its success—focus on customer enthusiasm.

Rolf Smith (1997, p. 3) has identified seven levels of change as follows:

Level One: Effectiveness—doing the right things

• Set priorities.

• Focus.

• Do what is important first.

• Become more effective.

Level Two: Efficiency—doing the right things right

• Follow procedures.

• Understand standards.

• Clean up your mess.

• Become more efficient.

Level Three: Improving—doing things better

• Think about what you are doing.

• Find ways to improve things.

• Listen to suggestions.

• Help, coach, and mentor others.

Level Four: Cutting—doing away with things

• Stop doing what does not count.

• Simplify.

• Ask "why?"

• Refocus continuously.

Level Five: Adapting—doing things other people are doing

• Notice and observe more.

• Read about best practices.

• Think before you act.

• Copy!

Level Six: Different—doing things no one else is doing

• Think about thinking.

• Ask "Why not?"

• Combine new technologies.

• Focus on different, not similar.

Level Seven: Impossible—doing things that cannot be done

• Question assumptions.

• Defocus: Get a little crazy.

• Break the rules!

• What is impossible today, but…?

• Wouldn't it be amazing if…?

• Where will it take real magic?

PROGRAM EVALUATION

Program evaluation is an essential part of effective administration. It is the evaluation of a set of activities designed to determine the value of the program or of the program elements. Evaluative research is the use of scientific research methods to make an evaluation. Program evaluation may be formative or summative. Formative evaluations provide information about the program during the developmental stages. Summative evaluations provide information for judging a developed program. Evaluation may be descriptive or comparative.

Programs are evaluated for any number of reasons. Federal, state, or local agencies may require program evaluation. Program evaluation can be used to improve programs systematically or to determine the state of the programs. It can be used to evaluate the effect of new technologies on programs and help determine if parts responsible for success in one program can be used in other parts of the system.

Once the program to be evaluated and the purpose for its evaluation have been decided, someone should be made accountable for the evaluation. Credibility is the major argument in favor of an external evaluator. A person who is part of the program may have difficulty in being objective about the program's strengths and weaknesses because of pride, loyalty, or job security. On the other hand, an internal evaluator may be as objective as an external one and has knowledge about the program, its history, and circumstances; such knowledge facilitates the evaluation.

CALENDAR OF EVENTS

One of the first things the evaluator should do is develop a calendar of events that depicts the tasks to be done, the schedule, and organization of the project. A calendar of events for program evaluation itemizes activities to be done down the left margin and projected dates across the top. The projected date for each activity is estimated. This is a valuable tool for planning and judging the progress of the program evaluation (Table 15-5).

COMMITTEE SELECTION AND FUNCTIONS

Each agency needs multidisciplinary committees to establish criteria and a process for continuous quality improvement and to evaluate care, make recommendations, and do follow-up work. A chairperson with enthusiasm and attention to detail helps ensure a successful program. Members also need to be interested in quality assurance and knowledgeable about channels of communication, hospital resources, patient population, and nursing needs. Representation of nurses, physicians, pharmacists, therapists, nutritionists, and housekeepers from various units helps produce a wide variety of ideas. Preset meeting times allow for staffing to accommodate attendance, and large committee membership supplies personnel to do the work.

CONCEPTUAL FRAMEWORK

Structure, process, and outcome or any combination of these is the common approach to evaluation. The structure approach focuses on the delivery system by which nursing care is implemented. Committee members evaluate policies, procedures, job descriptions, orientation

TABLE **15-5** Calendar of Events

	JAN.-FEB.	MARCH-APRIL	MAY-JUNE	JULY-AUG.	SEPT.-OCT.	NOV.-DEC.
Inform personnel of purpose of the evaluation and who is responsible	X					
Define goals	X					
Determine criteria	X					
Develop instrument		X				
Train data collectors		X				
Pilot test			X			
Collect data			X			
Analyze data				X		
Report findings				X		
Correct deficiencies					X	
Reassess (follow up)						X

schedules, in-service schedules, and charting. The process approach measures what the nurse does while delivering patient care. Both nurse and patient may be interviewed to collect evidence of professional judgment and functions. The outcome approach measures the results of the care administered to the patient and evaluates whether the goals were reached by considering clinical manifestations, patient knowledge, and the client's self-care. Outcomes became the focus of accreditation standards during the 1990s.

Audits may be concurrent or retrospective. Concurrent audits evaluate care as it is being administered and may include observation of staff; inspection of patient; open-chart auditing; staff and patient interviews; and group conferences including participation from the client, family, and staff. Retrospective audits judge care after it has been delivered through the study of patient charts or care plans after the patient has been discharged, postcare questionnaires, patient interviews, or all of these.

REVIEW OF THE LITERATURE

A review of the literature locates instruments, criteria, and standards that have been developed and allows committee members to benefit from others' accomplishments and mistakes.

PROGRAM EVALUATION MODEL

The formulation of program goals is essential for program evaluation. The goals should be clear, specific, and measurable. The evaluator will need to develop indicators to measure the extent to which the goals are achieved. These program-outcome indicators are the dependent variables of the study. The standards set by accrediting agencies such as the American Nurses Association (ANA), the National League for Nursing (NLN), and the Joint Commission on Accreditation of Healthcare Organizations (JCAHO) can be used to determine goals and criteria (American Nurses Association, 1996a and b).

Methods of data collection should be decided next. There are numerous sources for the collection of data, including questionnaires, interviews, observations, ratings, government statistics, instructional records, policy and procedure manuals, financial records, documents such as minutes of meetings or transcripts of trials, and tests.

INSTRUMENT DEVELOPMENT

An operational definition of quality of care gives direction to instrument development. Instruments may be general and appropriate for all patients or structures or applicable only to a specific process or to a homogeneous group in which differences in scores are due to variations in the concept being evaluated rather than to other factors. Medical diagnosis, symptoms, acuity, age, and health care settings often are used to determine homogeneity. A taxonomy of nursing diagnoses is evolving. Identification of homogeneous patient groups for the development and application of instruments necessitates the development of numerous tools.

Once the patient group or specific process has been identified, selection of goals, criteria, and items is the priority. The goal is a statement of the end that one strives to attain. Criteria are the standards or scales against which judgments are made. Criteria describe what is implied in the goal in concise, measurable statements of desired structure, process, or outcome. They are written for a specific condition and are understandable, clinically sound, and achievable.

Brainstorming is a common approach for identifying items. Actual problems (those that patients generally experience) and potential problems (those with a high risk of occurring) are identified, and the structure, process, or outcome to resolve or prevent them is determined. The generation of as many ideas as possible without immediate evaluation is recommended initially. Later, items can be eliminated, checked for comprehensiveness, put into a uniform format, precisely defined, and quantified. A pilot study to collect data with the instrument can clarify which items should be retained, discarded, or rewritten.

Scales and measurements must be developed. A checklist to determine whether a characteristic is present; ratings to give each item a measure of worth such as good, average, or poor; and ranking by comparison, such as more or less than the standard, are common measurements. Scales are nominal, ordinal, interval, or ratio. The simplest type is the nominal. Its categories are collectively exhaustive, and each is mutually exclusive, meaning that there is a category for all the observations and that each observation can fit only one category. Gender, marital status, and the presence or absence of a condition are examples. Ordinal scales classify observations into a specific order of more or less, such as good, average, or poor. Interval scales are ordered with equal measurement between each class, but the unit of measurement is determined arbitrarily. Examples are the thermometer and sphygmomanometer. Ratio scales contain the properties of the other scales plus an absolute-zero point. Multiplication and division are possible because each number has a relationship to any other number. Currency systems are examples.

SOURCES OF INTERNAL AND EXTERNAL INVALIDITY

Establishment of validity and reliability is important. Validity is the measurement of what is supposed to be measured and is difficult to establish. Face validity is an analysis of the instrument's appearance as valid. Someone simply looks at an instrument and decides if it has face validity. It is the easiest assessment of validity but is a questionable criterion because of its high degree of subjectivity. Content validity is a judgment that the content of the instrument is appropriate and closely related to what is to be measured. It is best determined by a jury of experts. Construct validity is particularly important when phenomena or concepts that are not directly observable, such as intellectual skills, human characteristics, and personal adjustment, are involved. The construct is a hypothetical definition that clearly defines observable phenomena. Construct validity is theory oriented. An instrument contains predictive validity to the extent that it predicts future behavior. It can be determined by checking the prediction after a

RESEARCH Perspective 15-1

Data from Burke TA, McKee JR, Wilson HC, et al: A comparison of time-and-motion and self-reporting methods of work measurement. *JONA* 30(3):118-125, 2000.

Purpose: The purpose of this study was to compare the results from a time-and-motion study with those using self-reporting.

Methods: A single observer observed eight nurses during five shifts or 40 hours per nurse. After completion of the time-and-motion study, participants were to self-report their work activities during their ensuing five shifts.

Results/conclusions: For analysis, 290 hours of time-and-motion study observations and 338 hours of self-reporting data were available. Comparable amounts of total time were reported within the various activity categories using time-and-motion and self-reporting methods. A significantly higher number of activities were reported using time-and-motion. Mean activity times were significantly longer using the self-reporting method compared with time-and-motion. The researchers concluded that nurse executives should consider continuous self-reporting as a low-cost means of quantifying allocation of time among nursing personnel. Self-reporting is not recommended for estimating the total number of activities or the mean time per activity because of perceptual differences between participants of what constitutes an activity.

period of time. Concurrent validity reveals the behavior that is being demonstrated presently and is particularly important for concurrent audits.

When designing research, the evaluator gives careful consideration to sources of internal and external invalidity. Extraneous variables can confound the effects of the experimental variable and are therefore sources of *internal invalidity*. Factors that reduce the generalizability are sources of *external invalidity*.

There are several sources of *internal invalidity*. *History* is a problem when an event extraneous to the purpose of the study occurs between the pretest and posttest and confounds the effect of the experimental variable. It is a hidden treatment or a change-producing event that occurred in addition to the treatment. The problem of history is a more plausible explanation of the change the longer the time lapse between pretests and posttests. It can be controlled with experimental isolation, which can almost never be used when human subjects are involved. For example, a group-training technique to reduce racial prejudice against African Americans has been developed. A group of prejudiced individuals is convened, pretested, trained, and posttested. If an African American political leader is assassinated during that time, one would suspect that history confounded the experimental effect. The reduced prejudice can probably be attributed to sympathy for the assassinated African American politician rather than to the therapy.

Maturation is another internal invalidity problem. It is a systematic change over time in a person's biological or psychological condition, including growing older or becoming tired or hungry. Prescribed plan activities to promote walking for 12- to 15-month-olds or bladder control for 2- to 3-year-olds would be questionable because children normally learn those skills during those times.

Testing is a practice effect or the effect on the scores of the posttest of taking the pretest. The practice effect is larger for the same test than for an alternative form of the test. The practice effect is a form of test wiseness that lasts about

3 months. People taking an achievement, intelligence, or personality test for a second time within a 3-month period will usually do better than people taking it for the first time, although it is unlikely that they have become brighter or better adjusted.

Instrumentation becomes a problem when there are changes in the measuring instrument over time. Changes in tests, judges, measuring devices, or calibrations cause instrumentation problems. Results from one test cannot usually be compared with results of a different test. Instrument decay or the fatiguing of spring scales causes invalidity problems. Observations produce instrumentation problems. There are intrahuman differences of the observer through fatiguing, the process of learning, the process of increased skill with practice, and learning to establish rapport. There are differences in observations by the same person at different times. One may be more lenient at one time than at another. One becomes more skillful with experience. There are also interhuman differences, such as knowledge and skill. Researchers observing disruptive behavior in psychiatric patients before and after a treatment may become more aware of disruptive behavior by the second observation and record more behaviors, or they may record fewer minor disruptions the second time because of the high level of disruptive behavior they had observed. In either case, the treatment effect is difficult to determine.

Statistical regression becomes a problem when groups have been selected because of their extreme scores. The phenomenon of regression toward the mean is the inevitable tendency of persons whose scores are extreme (far above or below the norm) on the first test to be less extreme on the second test. Patients chosen for a therapy group because of their high anxiety would show less anxiety on a second test regardless of the treatment.

Selection is a problem when the experimental group differs from the control group. For example, a selection problem may exist when one is trying to compare a control ward with an experimental ward because patients were assigned as a function of systematic characteristics, such as presenting symptoms or histories. Randomization is a control for selection. This problem often occurs when the subjects are already formed into groups for reasons other than the study.

Experimental mortality is a differential loss of subjects from comparison groups. It includes lost cases, cases on which only partial data are available, and cases who refuse to participate. The experimental group may appear stronger or more intelligent only because the weak and stupid members dropped out of it. People who smoke or drink heavily are likely to be the first to drop out of therapy groups to reduce smoking and drinking, leaving the clients who appear most successful with the therapy.

Researchers must also be aware of *external invalidity* problems that complicate the generalizability of the findings. Subjects who are available to the experimenter may not represent the population, and consequently the results of the research are not generalizable. Random *sampling* solves this problem. The independent variable needs to be operationally defined so that replication of the research is possible. Multiple-treatment interference, Hawthorne effect, novelty effect, and experimenter effect are considered. When two or more treatments are given consecutively to the same subjects, it is difficult, if not impossible, to know the cause of the results, and *multiple-treatment interference* occurs. The person who knows he or she is a subject may change behavior, not because of the treatment, but because the person knows he or she is being observed. This is the *Hawthorne effect*. The subject may react either positively or negatively because of the newness of the treatment, thus producing the *novelty effect*. The *experimenter effect* occurs when the subject is influenced by the experimenter. Such subtle behavior as smiling and nodding one's head during an interview may unintentionally influence the subject.

Pretest sensitization is the same as the testing internal validity problem except as it relates to generalizability of the results, which makes it an external validity problem. Identification of the dependent variables and selection of instruments to measure those variables are necessary for external validity. One must also consider if the effect will be lasting or if one is likely to get different results at different times. In the situation where the African American political leader was assassinated, thereby reducing prejudice against African Americans among those in group therapy, we had a history internal validity problem. Now we have an *interaction-of-treatment-with-time* external validity problem. The racial prejudice may have been temporarily reduced as a result of the assassination but will probably not be maintained for long. Treatments to reduce smoking may appear most successful right after a cancer scare but not as successful later. One must have internal validity to obtain external validity, which is the ability to generalize the research results. With program evaluation there may be little intent to generalize the results.

Reliability is repeatability and is easier to determine than validity. Scores obtained by different raters' observations of the same event at the same time or by the same rater at different times can be compared. The *test-retest method* involves administration of the same test again after a period of time with the hope that the results will be consistent. The fact that people may remember items from the first administration or that people change over time is a problem. This method is appropriate for stable characteristics but is problematic for unstable traits. The *split-half method* compares halves of the test to determine internal consistency. Reliability is suggested when the results of both halves are similar. To use the split-half method, both halves need to contain enough items to be reliable. *Statistical methods* to check reliability include the Kuder-Richardson test for internal consistency and the Spearman-Brown formula for a coefficient for the total test (Campbell and Stanley, 1963).

RESEARCH DESIGNS

Next, the evaluator should design the evaluation. Will the evaluation be one shot only or a continuous process? Will a program be assessed, or will programs be compared? Will an experimental or a quasiexperimental design be used? The pretest-posttest control group, posttest-only control group, Solomon four group design, and factorial design are experimental designs.

Experimental Designs

In the *pretest-posttest control group*, experimental subjects are randomly divided into two comparison groups as follows:

R O X O

R O   O

where:

R = Randomly assigned individuals

O = Observation

X = Experimental treatment

The control and experimental groups are randomly assigned. The two groups are considered equivalent during initial observation. During final observation, the difference between groups should be the result of a variable being applied to one group but not to the other. The pretest-posttest control group true experimental design controls for history, maturation, testing, instrumentation, regression, selection, and mortality. One should consider the Hawthorne and novelty effects because the interaction of the testing and the experiment is not controlled.

In the *posttest-only control group*, experimental subjects are randomly divided into two groups to be compared as follows:

R X O

R   O

The control and experimental groups are randomly assigned. A pretest is not administered. A treatment is applied to one group only. Because of the random selection, it is assumed that the groups are equivalent before the treatment is administered to one group and that the

difference noted on the posttest is due to the treatment. This design controls for history, maturation, testing, instrumentation, regression, selection, mortality, and the interaction of the testing and the experiment. It is superior to the pretest-posttest control design unless there is a question about the randomness. This design is appropriate when a pretest is awkward and is convenient for maintaining anonymity. The Solomon four group design is a better design but may not be worth more than double the effort.

The *Solomon four group design* uses four randomly selected groups. It combines the pretest-posttest control group and the posttest-only control group designs as follows:

R O X O

R O   O

R   X O

R   O

It is considered the most desirable of the experimental designs because it allows the investigator to examine the effects of the treatment in four independent comparisons. The Solomon four group design controls for history, maturation, testing, instrumentation, regression, selection, mortality, and the interaction of testing and the experiment. However, it may not be worth the effort.

Factorial design allows for observation of some subjects at all levels of all experimental variables and can be used when the situation is under the complete control of the experimenter, which is rarely the situation.

Quasiexperimental Designs

The evaluator usually cannot control the time and subjects to whom experimental variables are applied. However, the evaluator may be able to select the time and persons on whom observations will be made and can consequently gain some control through the use of quasiexperimental designs.

A *time series* involves a series of measurements over a period of time with an experimental variable introduced at some point in the sequence as follows:

O O O O X O O O O

Maturation is controlled because it is not likely to cause the difference among each of the observations. Testing, regression, and selection are controlled. History is the most probable problem, and the longer the time over which the observations are made, the more probable the problem. Instrumentation is also a potential problem. It is important not to change the instruments or their calibration. It is best if this design is repeated by several researchers in separate situations.

When the *equivalent-time-samples design* is used, the time available for making the observations is divided into equal time periods as follows:

XO XO XO XO XO

The times to make observations are randomly selected. This design controls for history, maturation, testing, instrumentation, regression, selection, and mortality. The multiple-treatment effect is a problem, and generalization of the findings is limited to similar populations.

In the *nonequivalent control group*, the broken line (- - - -) means the groups are not equivalent samples:

O X O

- - - - -

O   O

For this design a control and an experimental group are both given a pretest and posttest. However, the groups are not randomly selected and do not have sampling equivalence. It is better than a one-group pretest-posttest design because it controls for history, maturation, testing, and instrumentation. Regression, mortality, and interaction between selection and maturation need to be considered as potential problems.

The *counterbalanced designs* are sometimes called Latin square, switchover designs, crossover designs, and rotation experiments. The following is an example:

$$X_1O \ X_2O \ X_3O \ X_4O$$

$$X_2O \ X_4O \ X_1O \ X_3O$$

$$X_3O \ X_1O \ X_4O \ X_2O$$

$$X_4O \ X_3O \ X_2O \ X_1O$$

Four experimental treatments are applied in a random manner in turn to four individuals or groups. Counterbalanced designs control for history, maturation, testing, instrumentation, regression, selection, and mortality. Multiple-treatment interference is a problem. Strength can be obtained through replication.

For *separate-sample pretest-posttest design,* a pretest is given on one group and a posttest on another as follows:

R O (X)

R   X O

This simulated before-and-after design is weak, but it is better than a single-group pretest-posttest design because it controls for testing, regression, and selection. History, maturation, and mortality are not controlled, and the instrumentation needs to be questioned.

For the *separate-sample pretest-posttest control group,* two groups are pretested, one receives the experiment, and the two are posttested. This excellent design controls for history, maturation, testing, instrumentation, regression, selection, and mortality. Because it is an expensive design, it has probably never been used.

R O (X)

R   X O

R O

R O

For the *multiple time-series design,* a series of measurements is taken over a period of time on two separate groups with an experimental variable introduced at some point in the sequence of one of the groups as follows:

O O O X O O O

- - - - - - - - - - -

O O O   O O O

This excellent design can be used to compare one agency with a similar one. Controlling for history, maturation, testing, instrumentation, regression, selection, and mortality, it is the best of the more feasible designs. Power is increased through repeated measures.

The *recurrent institutional cycle design* is a patched-up design that starts with an inadequate design and adds features to control for sources of invalidity. It becomes an accumulation of precautionary checks that approaches experimentation.

X O

- - - - - - -

O X O

In *regression-discontinuity analysis design,* the broken line (--) means the groups are not equivalent. They differ by known amounts along a variable. The treatment is applied to individuals or groups that exceed a certain level of a variable rather than randomly. This design controls for history, maturation, testing, regression, and selection. Instrumentation and mortality would need to be questioned.

X O

———

X O

———

X O

———

O

———

O

———

O

(Campbell and Stanley, 1963).

METHODS OF DATA COLLECTION

Observation, interviews, questionnaires, and content analysis of charts and care plans are the most common methods for data collection. When *observation* is used, the quality assurance committee determines what to observe, develops observational procedures, and trains observers. Observations should be planned and recorded systematically and subjected to controls. Observation is suitable for concurrent audits. Behavior is observed and recorded as it occurs, and the process can be noted. Because observation does not demand participation of the observed, it is relatively independent of the subject's willingness to cooperate and therefore makes subjects readily available. Observation is a comparatively inexpensive method that lends itself to simple data-gathering instruments and recording equipment. Although it can be stopped at any time, it is limited to the length of the occurrence. The timing of an event may be difficult to predict, and consequently the observer may waste time waiting for something to happen. The presence of an observer also may influence the subject's behavior. Observations may be difficult to record, are subject to observer bias, and may vary among observers. Consequently, observers need training. Specifications of observer tasks; detailed instructions; sharp, measurable categories; immediate, detailed recording; observation averaging; and the use of recording equipment such as cameras and tape recorders help overcome observer bias and variability.

Interviews of both clients and staff may be used to evaluate care. Interviews may be (1) nondirective—subjects talk about whatever they desire; (2) focused—the subject speaks to a list of topics; (3) nonstandardized—the interviewer makes up the questions; (4) semistandardized—the interviewer asks a specific number of questions and probes; or (5) standardized—the interviewer conducts each interview in exactly the same manner using the same wording without probing. The interviewer can minimize misunderstanding by probing, clarifying, pursuing topics in depth, and observing nonverbal communication. Subjects do not need to be literate. Interviewing provides more flexibility and a greater response rate than questionnaires. However, it is an expensive method because it requires so much time. The subject may be nervous or may attempt to please the interviewer, and the recording of answers is problematic.

Questionnaires are less time consuming and consequently less expensive than interviews. They are particularly useful when subjects are dispersed over a large geographical area. Less skill is needed to administer a questionnaire than to conduct an interview. Questionnaires put less pressure on the subject for immediate response, standardize instructions and questions, and offer anonymity. The participants, however, must be literate. Unfortunately, often only a small percentage of questionnaires are returned, and the effect of nonrespondents is difficult to evaluate. Items may be omitted or misunderstood. A forced choice may not be an actual choice, and probing is not possible.

When preparing a questionnaire, the subjects' frame of reference and information level and the social acceptability of the item should be considered. Language should be gauged to the level of the subjects. Lengthy or leading questions and double negatives are to be avoided, and each question should contain only a single idea. Questions are arranged from general to specific. A pretest is helpful for identifying problems with the instrument. A high proportion of omissions, "other," "don't know," or all-or-none responses suggests poor questions. Added qualifications and comments and variation in answers when questions are reordered also suggest problems.

The percentage of returns of the questionnaires is influenced by a personal cover letter requesting cooperation, sponsorship by the health care agency, attractive format, short length, ease of filling out and returning, and inducements for replying. The best response is from people interested in the topic.

Content analysis of charts and care plans is a common method of data collection. It is a method of observation and measurement that is systematic, objective, and quantitative. Frequency of occurrences usually is noted on a check-off list. Descriptive statements can then be given about frequency of occurrences and changes in conditions. Unfortunately, it can take a long time to review records; classification systems may be too ambiguous for a phenomenon to fit a category; the chart chosen may not represent the phenomenon; and prejudices in the scoring method can bias the results.

SAMPLING

Sampling is a technique of selecting a sample from the whole population being studied. Evaluators want to be able to generalize their conclusions concerning the quality of care given the total population. Adequacy of sample size is important, especially with small samples, if the quality assurance committee members are to have confidence in their inferences. The more homogeneous the population, the smaller the sample size necessary to be representative. Budgetary and time restrictions greatly influence sample size.

The best sampling technique is *random sampling,* which allows each patient an equal chance to be included in the sample. A table of random numbers that can be located at the back of most statistics books is frequently used. To use this method, patient records are numbered. Evaluators close their eyes and point to a number on the table to start the selection. They then systematically progress by row or column until the appropriate number of records is selected. A roulette wheel can be used. The wheel is spun, and the charts of the patients whose numbers are chosen by the pointer are selected for review. The wheel is repeatedly spun until the desired sample size has been reached. A third possibility is to put pieces of paper with a chart number or patient name on each into a large container. The evaluator draws a piece of paper, rotates the papers, and draws another until the desired sample size is reached.

Systematic sampling consists of selecting every-*n*th patient. Selection can be according to admission, discharge, or an alphabetical listing. The evaluator makes a random start and then selects systematically. The size of the interval is determined by the percentage of the population desired in the sample size. For example, if one wants the sample to be 10% of the population, the evaluator chooses every tenth patient.

Stratified sampling divides the population into sections and then takes a random sample from each section to ensure that important variables are represented. For instance, patients may be classified according to body systems by the major diagnosis. If 30% of hospital admissions are classified as cardiovascular cases, 30% of the sample would be drawn from those cases.

Cluster sampling uses small samples from various sections of the population. A certain number of audits may be selected from each hospital unit. Instead of randomly selecting 100 patient charts, 10 charts may be randomly selected from each of 10 hospital units.

Multistage sampling randomly selects some percentage of the population and then randomly samples smaller subunits. For instance, in a large hospital system, the evaluator would randomly select which hospitals are to be audited. Next, the specialty area to audit within the selected hospitals is randomly selected. Finally, the specific units within those specialty areas and the specific patients on those units are randomly chosen.

Incidental or *convenience sampling* uses readily available subjects. The families of patients who happen to be in the coffee shop at a particular time or patients who happen to be in their rooms at a particular time may be interviewed.

The sample mean is not truly representative of the total population average. It is an attempt to approximate it. The difference between the mean or average of the sample and the total population is the sampling error.

ANALYSIS OF DATA

Simple scoring is preferred and can be subjected to descriptive measures. Frequency distribution indicates how many times observations were assigned to specific categories. Measures of central tendency can be calculated from the frequencies. The *mean* is the average. It is calculated by adding all the scores and dividing that sum by the total number of scores. The *mode* is the most frequently occurring score, and the *median* is the score in the middle with one half the number values above it and one half below it (Burns and Grove, 2001; Campbell and Stanley, 1963; Polit-Beck, and Hunger, 2001). Evidence-based practice is a combination of research and continuous quality improvement (Craig and Smyth , 2002; Hamer and Collinson, 1999).

EVIDENCE-BASED NURSING

Evidence-based nursing uses research methodology to identify best practices for quality assurance (Craig and Smyth, 2002; Hamer and Collinson, 1999; Kelly-Heidenthal 2003; Smith, James, Lorentzon, 2004).

HISTORY OF REGULATORY INFLUENCES

Health insurance can be traced to the seventeenth century in London where workers could pay to ensure that their family members would receive health care if needed. That worked well until the cholera epidemic in 1831, when there were insufficient funds to meet the needs of so many sick people.

Health care in the United States was simple before the depression of the 1930s. Most of the medical practices were simple remedies, since there were no medicines or advanced technologies. The fee for service was typically paid at the end of the visit and may have been a trade, such as a chicken, for the health care. Most people could afford the medical care. Hospitals were supported by charitable donations, but people who received charitable care often got less quality of care than those who paid did. However, during the depression most people in the United States could not afford medical care, and many hospitals closed because of the drop in charitable donations. There was no insurance or local, state, or federal funding to defray costs. There was some disability insurance where the employer continued to pay a portion of a sick employee's salary, but there was no assistance for medical costs.

Technological advances and the development of antibiotics during the 1940s advanced the ability to improve health, but unfortunately the cost was prohibitive for most people in the United States. A prepaid payment system that would relieve the burden on the sick person during an illness and ensure that the physician and hospital expenses were paid was envisioned. The first known insurance in the United States was in Oklahoma in 1927 when a physician had people in the community buy shares from the physician to build the hospital and then qualify to receive any needed medical care. A prepaid program for teachers was started at Baylor University Hospital in Dallas in 1929. A prepaid program for municipal employees underwritten by a Kaiser insurance company was also started that year in Los Angeles. Although physicians, hospitals, and legislators resisted prepaid health care programs, the American Hospital Association (AHA) developed national standards to govern those programs in 1933. Physicians, legislators, and hospitals collaborated to introduce the Blue Cross Plan in 1939.

There was a period of health care expansion from the 1940s through the 1960s, much of which was supported by the federal government. The Hill-Burton Act (The Hospital Survey and Construction Act of 1946) was the beginning of extensive federal subsidization for health care resources. That facilitated medical education and research and technological progress. Policies focused on an increase in access to quality health care. The Hill-Burton Act stimulated hospital

building. Medicare and Medicaid were introduced in 1965 to support the right to quality health care for individuals who were elderly, poor, or 65 years or older and entitled to Social Security or a railroad retirement. The Social Security survey of 1963 found that about one half of the retirees had no private health insurance, and it was common for a worker to lose employer-sponsored health insurance at retirement.

Whereas insurance companies were afraid to insure the elderly population, legislation was passed to extend Medicare coverage to permanently and totally disabled people in 1973. Part A is totally funded by federal funds and covers inpatient care. Part B is voluntary, is partially funded, and covers outpatient services. The large enrollment, inflation, and increasing technology increased the costs to the federal government. Medicaid, which aids states in providing health care to the poor, is a companion to Medicare. Although it provides federal funding to states, states are responsible for the administrative operation.

By the early 1970s the federal government understood that it could not afford unlimited coverage for unlimited numbers of enrollees in Medicare. Cost containment policies such as utilization review, rate control, and control of capital expenditures were addressed. In 1972 the Social Security Act was amended to create the professional standards review organization (PSRO). Physicians reviewed Medicare patients to control health care utilization and costs. The Economic Stabilization Program, which was a federal program to control rates with individual states responsible for rate control, was in effect from 1971 to 1974. The National Health Planning and Resources Development Act of 1974 authorized and established a national certificate-of-need (CON) program to control capital expansion in health care.

The federal government could not meet the health care costs by regulations alone, so it started combining market and regulatory strategies in the early 1980s. The Omnibus Budget Act of 1981 and the Tax Equity and Fiscal Responsibility Act

(TEFRA) of 1982 combined the strategies. These laws permitted health maintenance organizations (HMOs) to offer competitive medical plans and encouraged competition. The TEFRA Act of 1982 set operating cost per case and required development of a prospective pricing system. The Peer Review Improvement Act of 1982 repealed the PSRO program and started the peer review organization (PRO). The Social Security Amendment of 1983 encouraged prospective pricing based on diagnostic related groups (DRGs) to control utilization and costs. The National Health Planning and Resource Development Act was repealed in 1986, consequently repealing the CON requirement. Civilian Health and Medical Programs of the Uniformed Services (CHAMPUS) was given authority to reimburse institutional providers based on DRGs in 1984. The Consolidated Omnibus Budget Reconciliation Act of 1985 went into effect in January 1987 and required all Medicare-participating hospitals to accept patients from CHAMPUS. The PRO reviews Medicare and CHAMPUS using the same generic screening tools. Legislation was facilitating competition among health care services (Koch and Fairly, 1993).

For nearly a century various groups have recommended proposals for health care reform. In 1915 a group recommended a focus on prevention and sharing of health care costs by employers, employees, and the government. In 1932 a commission encouraged doctors to form group practices to share responsibility for cost-effective, high-quality health care. In 1933 President Franklin Roosevelt initiated the Social Security Act, which he intended to include national health insurance. In 1946 President Harry Truman introduced a plan for national health reform, declaring that health is a right, not just a privilege. In 1972 President Richard Nixon advocated that employers take responsibility and contribute to their workers' health care. In 1993 President Bill Clinton advocated a bold health care reform.

President Clinton outlined six principles basic to the Health Security Act: (1) security—guaranteeing comprehensive benefits to everyone in the United States; (2) simplicity—cutting red tape and consequently simplifying the system; (3) savings—controlling the costs of health care; (4) quality—making health care better; (5) choice—preserving and increasing the options available; and (6) responsibility—making everyone responsible for health care.

Security is accomplished by providing every person in the United States with a comprehensive health benefits package that cannot be taken away. Simplicity is achieved by reducing paperwork, which wastes time and costs billions of dollars. Savings can be achieved through group purchasing. Quality involves emphasizing keeping well and giving consumers information to judge quality themselves. Choice means the right to choose one's health care provider to protect the doctor-patient relationship. Responsibility means that every employee and every employer contribute to the cost of health care (White House Domestic Policy Council, 1993).

The Clinton health care reform plan was complex and coherent, with interlocking parts that fit together logically. There was an emphasis on universal health care coverage and broad, comprehensive coverage that includes preventive care, prescriptive medications, mental health services, home health benefits, and long-term care. It was designed to slow the current rate of increase in health care costs until they are comparable to the rate of inflation while providing access to economical, high-quality health care. The Clinton plan did not pass legislation, but it did facilitate the momentum toward managed care, including health maintenance organizations (HMOs), individual provider arrangements (IPAs), and preferred provider organizations (PPOs), which are characterized by prepayment, comprehensive coverage, and preventive care.

Quality standards are often set by professional bodies and promulgated through codes of ethics, standards of care, standards of performance, and practice guidelines, which can be monitored through accreditation, peer review, and certification processes. State boards of nursing help enforce standards under each state's nurse practice act. Multiple associations in nursing have developed standards using different criteria and formats that have lead to confusion. The American Organization of Nurse Executives, American Association of Colleges of Nursing, National League for Nursing, and the American Nurses Association (ANA) have joined efforts to coordinate and standardize formats and criteria for certification and practice standards (Rocchiccioli and Tilbury, 1998). The ANA has a set of ANA nursing standards, including Standards of Clinical Nursing Practice and standards for areas of nursing such as addictions, nurse administrators, advanced practice, cardiac rehabilitation, college health, community health, continuing education and staff development, correctional facilities, developmental disabilities or mental retardation, diabetes, forensics, genetics, gerontological nursing practice, home health, nursing informatics, oncology, otorhinolaryngology, parish nursing, pediatric clinical nursing, psychiatric-mental health, and respiratory nursing. They outline standards of care including the following: (1) assessment, (2) diagnosis, (3) identification of outcomes, (4) planning, (5) implementation, and (6) evaluations. Their standards of professional performance include the following: (1) quality of care, (2) performance appraisal, (3) education, (4) collegiality, (5) ethics, (6) collaboration, (7) research, and (8) resource utilization. ANA (1995, 1996a, 1996b, 1998) has also published *Nursing Quality Indicators, Nursing Care Report Care for Acute Care Standards of Clinical Practice* to help assess risk and improve quality of care.

The three voluntary accrediting agencies for community health nursing are the Community Health Accreditation Program (CHAP) of the National League for Nursing, the National Home Caring Council, and Joint Commission on Accreditation of Healthcare Organizations (JCAHO). Community Health Accreditation Program (CHAP) is one of two organizations nationwide authorized to provide home care accreditation, and in 1998 it became the first accrediting organization in the nation to be deemed an authority for Medicare hospices (National League for Nursing, 1998). JCAHO accreditation is also voluntary for long-term care. Nursing homes are required to meet state and federal licensing standards. Federal and state surveys and regulatory activities have increased since the Omnibus Budget Recognition Act (OBRA) was passed in 1987 and implemented in 1990.

RESEARCH Perspective 15-2

Data from French P: What is the evidence on evidence-based nursing? An epistemological concern. *Journal of Advanced Nursing* 37(3):250-257, 2002.

Purpose: The purpose of this study was to use symbolic interactionism to analyze the concept meaning of evidence-based nursing as a distinct construct or process.

Method: An epistemological analysis was conducted on a sample of concept clarification statements taken from popular literature, defining the nature of "evidence" and "evidence-based practice."

Results/conclusions: A frequency analysis of relevant key words in one publication database revealed the increasing use of "evidence-based medicine." The earliest use of the phrase "evidence-based" was in 1992. Most of the related papers have been published since 1995. "Evidence-based practice" was commonly used as a euphemism for information management, clinical judgment, professional practice development, or managed care. There was insufficient evidence to demonstrate that evidence-based nursing is a single construct or process. The term adds little more to the existing long-standing traditions of quality assurance and research-based practice.

JOINT COMMISSION ON ACCREDITATION OF HEALTHCARE ORGANIZATIONS

The Joint Commission on Accreditation (JCOA) was established in 1948. It became the Joint Commission on Accreditation of Hospitals (JCAH) in 1951 and was renamed the Joint Commission on Accreditation of Healthcare Organizations (JCAHO) in 1987. This voluntary, independent accrediting organization published the first hospital accreditation standards in 1953. In 1965 the Health Care Financing Administration (HCFA) gave the joint commission deemed status and gave their standards the benchmark of quality and meeting most of Medicare standards. In 1970 the JCAH changed its standards from review of minimum requirements to optimum level of care, and in 1975 it required every hospital to have a plan for quality assurance using explicit, measurable criteria that could be used in retrospective audits of care documented in medical records. In 1979 the standards were written that stressed a coordinated, organization-wide program for medical and nursing quality assurance. The structure and process standards stressed quality assurance activities that focused on problems whose solutions would have a big effect on patient care outcomes. It established a quality assessment standard in 1980 that has since been revised. In 1985 standards replaced the broad, problem-based approach with narrower systematic monitoring and evaluation of important aspects of patient care. The standards focused on specific departments, with each conducting its own systematic monitoring and evaluation that were conducted by concurrent audits of both patient care processes and medical records so that problems could be resolved while the patient was still hospitalized. In 1988 the quality assurance standards for nursing were revised to be evaluated objectively against preestablished standards and criteria. The results needed to be analyzed to determine problem areas and a plan developed to correct practice deficiencies. Reevaluation of the effectiveness of the corrective action was expected. In 1991 JCAHO published a 10-step process for the assessment, measurement, and improvement of quality of care: (1) assign responsibility, (2) delineate scope of care, (3) identify important aspects of care, (4) identify indicators, (5) establish thresholds for evaluation, (6) collect and organize data, (7) evaluate care, (8) take action to improve care, (9) assess actions and document improvement, and (10) communicate information.

By 2000 there were enormous changes in response to a rapidly changing environment and health care arena. There was a focus on continuous monitoring of performance; use of active, collaborative multidisciplinary teams; more randomized data selection for review; reporting of aggregate data; use of computers to manage and analyze data; linkages among patient, organization, and structure functions; sentinel events; root causes; performance improvement and sustained performance leading to continuous quality improvement; surveying physician practices that are part of a system; and random, unannounced surveys.

OUTCOME AND ASSESSMENT INFORMATION SET

Home health agencies, nursing facilities, and skilled nursing facility units certified to participate in Medicare and Medicaid Services (CMS) are required by federal regulations to collect, encode, and transmit the Minimum Data Set (MDS) Outcome Assessment Information Set (OASIS) to the State Repository at the Oklahoma State Department of Health. The Quality Improvement and Evaluation Services area is responsible for coordinating activities and database functions that fall under the umbrella of the national QualityNet system developed by the Centers for Medicare and Medicaid Services (CMS) that used to be called the Health Care Financing Administration (HCFA) (CMS website, accessed June 1, 2003).

RISK MANAGEMENT

Health care risk management is quite new. Losses were low before 1965, when the case of *Darling v. Charleston Community Memorial Hospital* set a precedent for holding hospitals directly liable for failure of administrators or staff to properly monitor and supervise health care delivery in the hospital. States also began to liberalize their workers' compensation laws into no-fault programs that facilitated an increase in claim settlements. Hospitals then started creating alternatives to commercial malpractice insurance including self-insurance. Medicare required self-insured hospitals to have risk management programs. The Joint Commission started requiring risk management programs in 1989. Several states require reporting of any event that resulted in harm to the safety or life of a patient or employee.

Risk management involves the development and implementation of strategies to prevent patient injury, minimize financial loss, and preserve agency assets. Risk management focuses on liability control. It assesses areas in which claims can be prevented. By reducing the frequency and severity of injuries to patients, the likelihood of litigation can be decreased and litigation costs lessened. The risk management process includes risk identification, analysis, treatment, evaluation, and follow-up.

The first step in risk management is identifying potential risks for accidents, injury, and financial loss. Energy should be put into preventive activities such as providing a safe physical environment, fostering customer satisfaction, and providing high-quality service. The present institution-wide monitoring system should be reviewed. The completeness of the monitoring system should be evaluated, including audits, committee minutes, incidence reports, patient questionnaires, and oral complaints. Whether additional systems need to be implemented to provide data for risk management control should be determined.

After data have been collected, they should be analyzed to determine the frequency and severity of problems in general categories. One should consider the severity or consequence of a failure, the occurrence or frequency of the problem, and the detection or the probability of detecting the problem before the impact of the effect is realized to set priorities. Then a plan to reduce the risks as much as possible should be developed and implemented. Safety procedures should be reviewed, and laws and codes related to patient care, consent, and safety should be monitored. Needs for personnel, patient, and family education should be identified and education implemented. The results of the risk management program should be evaluated and reported to appropriate groups. Risk management programs should include customer satisfaction, safety and security, continuous quality improvement, and liability control (Grohar-Murray and DiCroce, 2003; Martin and Tate, 1997; McDermott, Mikulak, and Beauregard, 1996; Rocchicciolo and Tilbury, 1998; Sullivan and Decker, 2000; Swansburg and Swansburg, 2002; Yoder-Wise, 2003).

Nurses should be able to recognize sentinel events. A sentinel event is an unexpected outcome involving a death or serious physical or psychological injury that needs immediate investigation and response. Accredited organizations are expected to identify and respond to all sentinel events occurring in the organization by doing a thorough and credible root-cause analysis, implementing improvement to reduce risk, and monitoring the effectiveness of the improvements. Asking "why" at least five times helps discover underlying problems that might otherwise be overlooked. Sentinel events could include but are not limited to death or major permanent loss associated with a medication error; inpatient suicide; elopement; any procedure performed on the wrong patient, wrong side, or wrong body part; perinatal death; assault or homicide; patient falls; or hemolytic transfusion reaction involving blood group incompatibilities. Other high-risk areas include infant abduction, restraints/seclusion, and falls (Ammerman, 1998; Joint Commission on Accreditation of Healthcare Organizations, BOJ's Guide to 1990 Standards and Scoring, p. 13; Joint Commission on Accreditation of Healthcare Organizations [AMH 1/98-2/94]).

Medical errors are believed to result in thousands of preventable events annually.

To improve the situation we need to create a culture of safety in the health care system instead of the culture of secrecy and the name, blame, and shame game that exists. When one is punished for reporting an error the probability of reporting the error is decreased. In fact, errors are often an accumulation of several systematic factors such that if one element in the chain had been changed, the harm to the patient might have been prevented. A safety culture assumes that to err is human, and good people often make errors in a flawed system. It distinguishes between blameworthy errors (those errors made out of vindication, carelessness, or recklessness) and those that are unintentional. Reporting of errors is rewarded instead of punished. Accountability involves acknowledging the error, apologizing, repairing the harm, uncovering the causes of the error, and correcting the process or system. About 2% of reported medical errors are medication related.

Pape (2001) reports the results of several research studies of medication administration errors. A medication error has been defined as "any preventable medication-related event occurring as a result of actions by a health care professional that may cause or lead to patient harm while the patient is in the care of the health care provider" (Pape, 2001, p. 154). Prescribing, transcribing, dispensing, and administering errors are common. Medication errors include omitting a medication, giving medication at the wrong time, to the wrong patient, in the wrong dose, by the wrong route, or to a patient with a known allergy, or giving repeated medication without an order, or discontinuing medication without an order. Illegible handwriting, improper abbreviations, not putting a zero before a decimal point or putting one after an unnecessary decimal point following a whole number contribute to errors. "D/C" could mean discontinue or discharge; "HS" could mean hour of sleep or half strength; "cc" for cubic centimeter has been mistaken for "u" for units; and "1.0" often looks like "10." Lack of knowledge or application of knowledge, use of wrong drug name, incorrect calculations or unit expressions,

distractions, interruptions, identifying patients by room numbers instead of identification bands, and fatigue can contribute to errors. System factors that can contribute to errors include but are not limited to the following: excessive workloads, inexperience, crowded spaces, noise, distractions, interruptions while preparing medications, and failure to follow policies, procedures, and protocols.

Barriers to reporting errors include fear of punishment, reduced self-esteem, and perceived decrease in level of professionalism. Sometimes doctors are relaxed about medication errors and write orders to erase the error. Teaching staff policies, procedures, and guidelines; labeling "medication error" as "drug variance"; and rewarding instead of punishing reporting may increase accuracy of reporting medication errors. Computerized systems for physician order entry system and drug compatibility check and including pharmacists in planning and prescribing patient care can be helpful. Asking nurses to identify all causes of medication errors, doing a root-cause analysis, and using an interdisciplinary team approach to identify problems from different perspectives and to recommend solutions may help reduce errors through continuous quality improvement (Pape, 2001).

CUSTOMER SATISFACTION

"Anger is only one letter short of danger."
—Anonymous

The dissatisfied customer is the one most likely to pursue litigation. Therefore it is important to identify incidents that might lead to claims, educate patients and their families about the care, and handle patient complaints. To handle complaints, listen and let the patients express themselves before speaking. Do not become defensive. Avoid reacting emotionally. Negotiate. Ask for the patient's expectations, and explain what you can or cannot do. Agree on actions to be taken and a time frame. Follow through. A caring attitude can be very effective. It is also important to teach personnel about customer relations and how to prevent and handle complaints.

SAFETY AND SECURITY

A safety and security program should provide safety for patients, their families and other visitors, and personnel. Risks from custodial negligence should be controlled. There should be plans for natural disasters, fire, electrical shock, power loss, and bioterrorism. There should be an equipment maintenance program.

Regarding terrorism, clinicians need necessary information to make diagnoses, manage care, prevent further problems, and report actions. They need to maintain their personal safety, manage scarce resources, isolate as necessary, treat acutely ill, and decide who needs treatment and who can wait. Public health officials have to interpret surveillance data, investigate outbreaks, use epidemiologic measures, and issue surveillance alerts.

The American Nurses Association encourages the development of policies that release registered nurses as part of organized medical rescue teams during disasters. The agency should keep a listing of all nurses who have been educated in disaster and emergency preparedness and who are members of emergency preparedness teams. The registered nurse should keep the employer informed of competency in disaster and emergency preparedness and give the employer copies of disaster/emergency preparedness education competence. The nurse should inform emergency teams if the employer denies or withdraws consent for emergency deployment (see ANA Position Statement on Work Release During a Disaster—Guidelines for Employers, www.nursingworld.org, accessed 5/21/03).

NATIONAL SAFETY COUNCIL

The safety movement began in ancient times with the Egyptians, Greeks, and Romans, and in the Middle Ages guidelines were established regarding working conditions. The safety movement became a major force in industry during the industrial revolution. In 1913 the National Council for Industrial Safety (later renamed the National Safety Council and still later renamed the Center for Medicare and Medicaid Services) was founded. It developed a forum to develop national standards. Other groups also formed and started keeping statistics on accident and injury rates in industry.

Occupational diseases and safety issues were identified, and methods to control hazardous and toxic materials and to protect the people who handle them were developed. On-the-job safety issues received serious attention. Since World War II, the safety movement not only has reduced injuries and deaths but also has shown administrators that money spent on safety measures returns a profit of up to several hundred percent.

The National Safety Council encouraged cooperation among labor, management, and government to develop legislation and upgrade safety standards. The National Safety Council sought to improve investigative methods and supported special research projects. Changes in the workforce, new technologies and their hazards, environmental hazards, blood-borne diseases, and drug and alcohol abuse are challenges.

OCCUPATIONAL SAFETY AND HEALTH ACT

The purposes of the Occupational Safety and Health Act of 1970 and the Mine Safety and Health Act of 1977 are to ensure safe and healthful working conditions and to preserve the nation's human resources. They established nationwide guidelines and standards for the first time. The Secretary of Labor and the Occupational Review Committee are responsible for administration and enforcement of the acts. Research and education activities are the responsibility of the Secretary of Health and Human Services and are implemented by the National Institute for Occupational Safety and Health (NIOSH). The Assistant Secretary of Labor for Occupational Safety and Health acts as the chief of the Occupational Safety and Health Administration (OSHA). OSHA monitors the following: (1) development of standards about occupational health and safety, (2) development of health and safety regulations, (3) inspections and investigations to check the status of compliance, and (4) citations and proposals for penalties for noncompliance with the standards.

OSHA's primary responsibilities are as follows: (1) to promulgate, modify, and revoke health and safety standards; (2) to approve or reject state plans for programs; (3) to require employers to keep records of safety and health data; (4) to conduct investigations and inspections and to issue citations and propose penalties; (5) to petition the courts to restrain imminent danger situations; and (6) to provide educational programs, consulting, funding for state plans, and statistical records of illnesses, injuries, and accidents.

The Occupational Safety and Health Review Commission (OSHRC) is a three-member quasi-judicial board that hears cases when OSHA actions are contested by employees and employers. The committee decisions can be reviewed by state and federal courts.

NIOSH is the federal agency responsible for research, education, and training. The representatives can inspect agencies and ensure compliance but are not authorized to enforce OSHA regulations. The main functions of NIOSH are as follows: (1) to develop educational programs, (2) to develop occupational health and safety standards, and (3) to conduct research. The responsibility to establish research methods and conduct statistics surveys belongs to the Bureau of Labor Statistics.

With few exceptions, OSHA applies to every employer in all 50 states and all U.S. possessions who has one or more employees and who engages in business affecting commerce. All local, state, and federal government employees and mine operators and their employees are exempt from coverage.

Under OSHA the employer is responsible for providing a safe, healthful work environment and for complying with the applicable standards. The employees must comply with applicable standards. The employer is liable for the state and federal sanctions for violating standards.

Employees are subject to their employer's sanctions.

All standards promulgated by OSHA are published in the *Federal Register*. OSHA requires employers to keep records of all occupational illnesses and accidents and to report either to OSHA or to the state plan within 48 hours. OSHA can grant two types of variances from the standards: temporary and permanent. Employers must show just cause for either variance and inform the employees of the application.

Workplace inspections are usually conducted without prior notice. Investigations of imminent dangers are top priority, followed by catastrophic and fatal accidents, followed by employee complaints regarding hazards and reinspections. General inspection procedures include an opening conference, a walk-through documenting alleged violations, interviews with workers, and a closing session. Citations and penalties vary according to the seriousness of the violation. Violation citations are to be posted near where the violation occurred. If an employer wants to contest a case, the area office that initiated the action should be contacted. OSHA encourages states to assume responsibility for administering and enforcing occupational safety and health laws. Areas needing regulations include but are not limited to blood-borne pathogens, lifting guidelines, confined-space regulations, ergonomic guidelines, respiratory guidelines, and egress.

Administrators need to identify the tasks to be performed, identify the tools necessary, evaluate the environment in which the tasks will be performed, assess the organization in which this takes place, and make necessary changes to provide a safe work environment for the employee (Kavianian and Wentz, 1997).

SOURCES OF LAW

There are four sources of law and parallel systems at the state and federal levels. The four sources of law are constitutions, statutes, administrative agencies, and court decisions that contribute principles for common law.

The constitution is the highest law in the United States. It defines the structure, power, and limits of government, and it guarantees citizens certain fundamental rights. It is interpreted by the U.S. Supreme Court and gives authority to the other sources of law. It has little direct involvement in malpractice.

Statutory law or legislative law is law passed by local, state, or federal legislators, such as the U.S. Congress, state legislatures, and city councils, that must be signed by the mayor, governor, or president. Statutory law can be expanded, amended, or repealed by action of the legislature. Nurse practice acts vary among states but must be consistent with provisions or statutes established at the federal level. Nurse practice acts define and limit the practice of nursing and determine what constitutes unauthorized practice. Before 1970, very few federal or state laws dealt with malpractice. Since then, many statutes affect malpractice.

Administrative agencies are given authority to act by legislative bodies. They create rules and regulations that enforce statutory laws. Administrative laws are valid only when they are within the scope of the authority granted to them by the legislative body. State boards of nursing are administrative agencies created to implement and enforce the state nurse practice act. The state board members write rules and regulations and conduct investigations and hearings to ensure that law's enforcement. The National Labor Relations Board and health and safety boards can affect nursing practice.

Court decisions are called tort laws. Initial trial courts usually have a single judge or magistrate make the decision. Intermediary appeal courts have three justices, and the highest courts of appeal have nine justices. They interpret legal issues that are in dispute and set precedents. There are two levels of court in the United States: trial court and appellate court. The courts interpret most malpractice law (Marquis and Huston, 2000; Pozgar, 1999; Sullivan and Decker, 2000).

CATEGORIES OF LAW

Laws are categorized into two basic types: public law and private or civil law. Public law is composed of constitutional law, administrative law, and criminal law. Private law is also classified into tort law, contract law, and protecting and reporting law (which is sometimes categorized as criminal law). The most common law affecting nursing practice is tort law.

Tort law is the branch of civil law that concerns legal wrongs committed by one person against the person or property of another. Tort law is categorized into two categories: unintentional and intentional. Negligence and malpractice, which is professional negligence, are considered *unintentional torts*.

Negligence is the failure of a person not to perform an act (omission) or to perform an act (commission) that a reasonable person would or would not do in a similar situation. Negligence is an unintentional tort that involves harm resulting from the failure of people conducting themselves in reasonable and prudent ways. Carelessness is not thinking before one acts or not paying attention. One can be careful and still be negligent for not acting as prudently as others would in the same circumstances (Grohar-Murray and DiCroce, 2003; O'Keefe, 2001; Marquis and Huston, 2000; Pozgar, 1999).

Malpractice is negligent acts of people with specialized education. Malpractice reflects negligence, but not all negligence is malpractice. When people are held legally responsible for their negligent acts, they are legally liable and may be required to pay for damages. Medical malpractice refers to the negligent acts of any health care professional when conducting patient care responsibilities. Nursing malpractice refers specifically to nurses conducting their patient care responsibilities. Common causes of malpractice claims against nurses are medication errors from misreading the medication order or not clarifying an incomplete or ambiguous order and technique in giving injections.

Negligent conduct depends on the act itself and the surrounding circumstances, including the following: (1) the nature of the nursing function, (2) the nurse's qualifications to perform the function, (3) the urgency of the situation, and (4) the foreseeable harm if the care is not implemented. The emergency room nurse is not held to the same standards of care expected under more normal circumstances. Being a minor does not exempt a nurse from liability for acts of malpractice, and the nurse's state of mind and physical condition are not considered relevant.

The rule of personal liability means that people are responsible for their own tortious conduct even when someone else may share that liability under some other law. Supervisors will not usually be held liable for the negligent acts of those they supervise because all professional persons are held liable for their own negligent behavior. However, a supervisor may be found guilty of negligence for making an assignment beyond a worker's capabilities without giving adequate supervision in carrying out the delegated functions. If a supervisor believes that certain staffing will jeopardize patient safety and potentially precipitate litigation, the position should be documented and the hospital administrator informed.

The doctrine of respondeat superior applies to the U.S. government because the government has agreed to be sued for negligent acts of its employees under the Federal Tort Claims Act (FTCA). By virtue of special statutory enactments, nurses employed by the Veterans Administration and the U.S. Public Health Service have complete immunity from personal liability for acts of negligence in the implementation of their government responsibilities. However, the aggrieved patients may sue the government for injuries they have sustained. Occupational health nurses are potentially exposed to a greater risk of being sued for negligent conduct than other nurses because of the joint effect of the doctrine of respondeat superior and workers' compensation laws. Workers' compensation laws usually prevent an employee from suing an employer, so the aggrieved employee can sue only the nurse.

A nurse is legally required to implement medical procedures ordered by a licensed physician or a physician assistant acting on behalf of the physician employer unless the nurse has reason to believe harm would result from doing so. Failure to carry out the physician's order will subject the nurse to liability for subsequent harm to the patient if there is not reason to question the order. Consequently, nurses must know how to implement the procedure and the effect of the procedure on the patient. When nurses question physician's orders, they should tactfully question the physician. If the physician is insistent, the nurse should take the matter to the supervisor or responsible hospital official. Patient safety is of utmost concern. The nurse has a legal responsibility not to follow the order when there are reasonable grounds to believe that the action would harm the patient.

Malpractice is professional negligence that involves any misconduct or lack of skill in carrying out professional responsibilities. Duty, breach of duty, causation, and injury must be present for malpractice to exist. If one of these factors cannot be proved beyond a reasonable doubt, the malpractice claim maybe dismissed (Grohar-Murray and DiCroce, 2003; O'Keefe, 2001; Yoder-Wise, 2003).

Intentional torts have an intent to harm and include the following: assault, battery, false imprisonment, invasion of privacy, libel, slander, and defamation of character. *Assault* involves mental disturbance of personal integrity, including fright and humiliation. It does not include actual contact (Killion and Dempski, 2000; O'Keefe, 2001; Pozgar, 1999; Swansburg and Swansburg, 2002).

Battery is an intentional tort involving unpermitted and intentional contacts with one's person or extension of the body to clothing, object in the hand, car, and so forth. A hostile intent of the defendant is not necessary. It is the absence of the plaintiff's consent to the defendant's contact that is the issue. Direct contact with the plaintiff is not necessary, and the personal integrity exists even when the plaintiff is under anesthesia or asleep. The defendant is liable for all harm, including unforseeable consequences from the conduct (Killion and Dempski, 2000; O'Keefe, 2001; Pozgar, 1999; Swansburg and Swansburg, 2002).

Grounds for civil actions regarding assault and battery include forcefully handling an unconscious patient, forcing a patient out of bed to walk, forcing a patient to submit to treatment even if a consent had been signed because resistance implies withdrawal of consent, lifting a protesting patient from bed to a stretcher or chair, threatening to strike or striking a child or adult unless in self-defense, and in some states performing alcohol, blood, urine, or other health tests for presumed drunken driving without consent. Some mental health patients and nursing home residents have brought suits for assault and battery against their health care providers. Assault, battery, and false imprisonment are considered intentional torts. Intentional torts such as assault and battery often are not covered in malpractice insurance (O'Keefe, 2001; Pozgar, 1999; Swansburg and Swansburg, 2002).

False imprisonment is willful detention without consent or authority of law. It is an intentional infringement of the right of a person to move freely and without hindrance. Actual physical force is not necessary. All that is necessary is for a person who is physically confined to a given space to experience fear that force, which may be implied by words, threats, or gestures, will be used to detain the person or to intimidate him or her without legal justification. Most false-imprisonment cases in health care involve locking mentally ill patients in their rooms. An agency can be held liable for the conduct of a nurse-employee who unlawfully confines or detains a patient against the patient's will because of the doctrine of respondeat superior. Some mental health patients and nursing home residents have brought suits for false imprisonment against their health care providers (Killion and Dempski, 2000; O'Keefe, 2001; Pozar, 1999; Swansburg and Swansburg, 2002).

Privacy and confidentiality are very important. Invasion of privacy is a tort violation of a person's right to make personal choices without interference and to not be subjected to uninvited publicity. The information disclosed by patients is confidential and only to be available to authorized personnel. Nurses should be discreet about the release of information over the telephone because of the difficulty of identifying the caller and may not use photographs, videotapes, or research data without the explicit permission of the involved patient. The nurse must even obtain permission to release information to family members and close friends. The patient can sue for invasion of privacy when confidential information is directly or indirectly communicated to unauthorized people.

The Health Insurance Portability and Accountability Act (HIPAA) was enacted by the federal government in 1996 to give people portability of their health care coverage and control over how their personal information is used and disclosed; it also made organizations that create or receive personal information accountable for protecting it. HIPAA is composed of three different sets of rules: (1) the Privacy Rule, effective 4/14/2003; (2) the Electronic Transactions/Code Sets Standards, effective 10/21/2005; and (3) the Security Rule, which goes into effect 4/21/05. Some believe that you cannot keep information private if it is not secure.

Health care providers covered under HIPAA must follow strict guidelines to protect health information including the following:

1. Provide all patients with a written notice on how their information may be used or disclosed.
2. Restrict use and disclosure of health information except as permitted by law.
3. Establish safeguards to limit incidental disclosures of health information.
4. Establish policies and procedures to protect and safeguard protected health information.
5. Train all workforce members on safeguarding health information.

The privacy rule creates rights for individuals to do the following:

1. Request restriction on the use or disclosure of health information
2. Inspect and obtain copies of protected health information
3. Request changes in health information
4. Request an accounting of disclosures of protected health information

Telehealth raises challenges to privacy and confidentiality. It uses telecommunications and information technologies to provide care at a distance and to transmit health care information. Teleconferencing cameras can be used to diagnose, treat, monitor, and educate patients from a distance. X-ray films and electrocardiograms (ECGs) can be transmitted and viewed. Electronic dermoscopes and stethoscopes can allow health care providers to look at eyes, ears, skin, and wounds and to listen to heart, lungs, and bowel sounds. This allows ready access to expert advice and patient information that is especially beneficial in rural areas. E-mail can be used to deliver health services, and the World Wide Web can be a valuable resource for health education (Saba and McCormick, 2000).

The Uniform Health Care Information Act of 1997 governs the flow of health care information. Under it, patients are to have access to health care information to make informed decisions, provide informed consent, and correct inaccurate or incomplete information in the record. The legal implications for telenursing, which uses communications technology to transmit health information from one location to another, includes the reasonableness standard for disclosure, nurses' potential for civil or criminal liability, and the elements necessary to obtain a valid disclosure authorization from the patient. The patient has a right to privacy via the telephone, cordless telephone, cellular telephone, and computer. Under the 1992 Amendment to the Federal Wiretap Statutes, cordless telephone communications are protected the same as land-based telephone communications. Unfortunately, unintended interceptions of cordless health care communication can happen through devices such as other cordless telephones, baby monitors, and FM radios. Cellular telephones are similar to cordless telephones in that they broadcast the communication to a receiving station that transmits the communication over a land-based telephone line. Unfortunately, cellular telephone communications are commonly intercepted inadvertently by other cellular telephones. Since 1986, cellular telephone communications have the same legal protection and right to privacy as the land-based telephone communications. Considering the ease with which cellular and cordless telephone communications can be intercepted, the provider must consider the risks of harm versus the benefits to the patient. When the risk of harm is greater than the benefit, the provider should inform the patient of the potential risks of disclosure of the health care information and get agreement in writing for the provider to use the telephone. The use of the Internet to communicate health care information also has an expectation of privacy. A fax sent by computer or telephone between two providers is an electronic digital communication sent over a land-based telephone line and is subject to the right of privacy and confidentiality.

Confidentiality is the right to privacy of records. Patients have the right to believe that the information they disclose to health professionals will be used strictly for diagnosis and treatment and will not be shared with others without permission of the person.

There are a few exceptions to confidentiality. All 50 states require disclosure in cases of child abuse when certain professionals suspect abuse. The identified professionals vary from state to state but usually include nurses, physicians, child-care providers, and school teachers. Elder abuse and abuse of the disabled may also require disclosure. Case law helps guide professional actions when clients are dangerous to themselves or others. In the case of *Tarasoff v. Regents of the University of California,* a 1976 decision created the Tarasoff duty, or the duty to warn. If a client revealed an intent to harm another person, the health care provider has a legal obligation to notify the intended victim. The *Gross v. Allen* (1994) decision informed mental health professionals that they must tell the patients' caregivers of any intent of suicide or intent to harm others. Although these cases involved psychologists, there is relevance to advanced practice nurses (American Bar Association, 2001; Grohar-Murray and DiCroce, 2003; Guido, 2003; Marquis and Huston, 2000; O'Keefe, 2001; Sullivan and Decker, 2001; Sullivan and Mattera, 1997; Swansburg and Swansburg, 2002; Yoder-Wise, 2003; Yount, 2001).

Defamation is verbal or written communication that injures someone's reputation. It usually involves hatred, contempt, or ridicule and may cause someone to be avoided or shunned. It often harms the reputation of another by lowering the estimation toward that person. Oral defamation is slander, and written defamation is libel. Defamation, slander, and libel as well as invasion of privacy are quasiintentional torts.

To be held accountable for the tort of *libel*, the plaintiff has to show that the defendant published a defamatory statement about him or her. However, the defendant may not have intended to communicate the defamatory statement to anyone or may not have intended the statement to be defamatory. The statement may not be defamatory until put together with facts unknown to the writer. The writer may have thought the information was factual or made a general statement that was taken personally by someone. In *Olson v. Molland* (1930) and *Weidman v. Ketcham* (1938), when the defendant did not intent to publish the statement, the law did not impose liability. However, when the truth of the statement is questioned, there are many rules that vary from state to state. Absolute privilege and qualified privilege may provide a defense to an action for defamation. The first, absolute privilege, attaches to statements made during judicial or legislative proceedings as well as confidential communications between spouses. The second, qualified privilege, attaches to statements that result from a legal or moral duty to speak in the interests of third parties when the statement is made in the absence of malice such as ill will, hatred, or monetary gain. The case of *Judge v. Rockford Memorial Hospital* (1958) demonstrates the defense of privilege. A director of nurses wrote a letter to a nurse's professional registry stating that the hospital did not want to have a specific nurse's services available to them because of losses of narcotics during times that nurse was on duty. The director of nurses' letter was considered a privileged communication because of the director of nurse's legal duty to write the communication in the interests of society.

There are fewer *slander* than libel lawsuits because it is more difficult to prove, the awards are small, and the legal fees are high. A person bringing a slander suit usually must prove special damages. However, a professional does not need to prove that the words caused damage because it is presumed that slander toward one's professional capacity is damaging. However, if the person making an injurious comment cannot prove the statement is true, the person can be held liable. Consequently, health professionals should avoid making slanderous remarks about other health professionals. However, reporting alleged professional misconduct is not grounds for defamation because of qualified privilege to report complaints to the professional's supervisor (Killion and Dempski, 2000; O'Keefe, 2001; Pozgar, 1999).

LIABILITY CONTROL

Policies and procedures for handling incidents and claims should be developed and implemented. Some incidents may relate to medication errors, falls, procedures (particularly invasive procedures), patient or family refusal of treatment, and patient or family dissatisfaction with care. Because of the negative connotation of the word *incident*, some agencies use the term *event, occurrence,* or *situation* instead. Filing an incident report is not admitting guilt. It is reporting something that is not a part of routine care.

It is preferable that incident report forms contain questions that can be answered yes or no or by multiple choice. Narrative should be limited. The observer should give a factual, nonjudgmental account of what was seen, heard, felt, or smelled. No impressions, interpretations, or opinions should be stated. All information needed should be in one place.

Documentation is critically important. When documenting, the nurse should use the appropriate form and black ink, putting the patient's name and identification number on each page. Each entry should be specific, record the date and time, and use only approved abbreviations. The nurse should document nursing actions taken in response to identified patient problems, patient's responses to medications and treatments, and safeguards to protect the patient. The nurse should write on every line without inserting notes between lines or leaving empty spaces. To correct an error, the nurse should draw a line through it and write "error" above it with the date, time, and nurse's initials. Never erase or obliterate an entry. The nurse should always follow the institution's policies and procedures and give care that is appropriate according to the standard of care as defined in the state nurse practice act. There should be no entry in the patient's record about the existence of an incident report, and the incident report should not be left in the chart. Incident reports that are inadvertently disclosed are no longer considered confidential and can consequently be subpoenaed in court (Marquis and Huston, 2000).

The quality of the documentation often determines the outcome of lawsuits. Medical records are legal documents that can be introduced in court. Nurses and other personnel must be well versed in accurate and comprehensive documentation. Nurses should also know how to testify in court and how to serve as expert witnesses, Bernzweig, 1996).

LIABILITY ISSUES

NURSE LICENSURE

The usual organizational pattern for nurse licensing authority in each state is the establishment of a separate board that is organized and operated within the guidelines of specific legislation to license all professional and practical nurses; to determine eligibility for initial licensure and relicensure; to enforce licensing statutes, including suspension, revocation, and restoration of licenses; and to approve and supervise educational institutions (Pozgar, 1999). Members of the state board of nursing are typically appointed by the governor.

NURSE PRACTICE ACTS

Nurse practice acts are the policing power of the state. The laws typically have rules and regulations that are implemented by state boards of nursing. The nurse practice acts define nursing, set standards for licensure, mandate licensure examinations, set standards for curricula of schools of nursing, regulate schools of nursing, regulate advanced practice nurses, and allow state boards of nursing to investigate reports of violations, and discipline violators. Discipline may include probation, revocation of license, and referral to criminal courts (Swansburg and Swansburg, 2002).

The nurse practice act typically defines nursing, delineates the scope of practice, and outlines the activities nurses licensed in that state can legally perform. The mutual recognition model allows jurisdictions to retain the rights to govern practice within the jurisdiction even with mutual recognition agreements with other compact states. The nurse practice acts outline requirements for initial licensure and renewal. Licenses are generally valid for 2 to 3 years. In 1976, California was the first state to institute mandatory continuing education for renewal of the nursing license. Several states now require continuing education, typically with a requirement of 20 to 40 hours of continuing education over 2 to 3 years. Some states require specific continuing education content such as specific health problems, and others allow the nurses wide latitude in meeting the requirements (Cherry and Jacob, 2002).

NURSING STANDARDS

The standard of care is generally defined as the degree of care, expertise, and judgment used by a reasonable and prudent nurse under similar circumstances. It is established by expert testimony in nursing malpractice cases. Experts use a variety of sources. Not all the sources have the same information, and there is no single standard of care. Nurse practice acts, American Nurses Association (ANA) standards, Joint Commission on Accreditation of Healthcare Organizations (JCAHO) standards, institutional policies and procedures, nursing literature, and physicians' orders may be used to establish standards for court cases. Common causes of nurse liability include failure to assess, failure to plan and implement a plan of care based on the patient's condition, and failure to follow the organization's policies and procedures (O'Keefe, 2001; Sherman, 1999; Tucker, Canobbio, Paquette, et al, 2000).

PATIENT CARE ISSUES

PATIENT'S BILL OF RIGHTS

Patients retain their basic fundamental rights as identified in the Constitution and courts of law when they are admitted to a health care system. They are often given the Patient's Bill of Rights as they enter the health care system. The American Hospital Association published that document in 1992. Revisions to it were being discussed in 2003.

INFORMED CONSENT

Informed consent is given by patients who fully understand what is being consented to. It involves legal individual capacity to consent, voluntary freedom of choice, and access to understandable information. If the patient is not a competent adult, the following may give consent: a legal guardian; emancipated, married minor; mature minor; parent or legal guardian of a child; minor for diagnosis and treatment of specific disease states or conditions, and court order. Consent may be given orally or in writing. Both are legally effective, but it is advisable to get the consent in writing. The patient or legal consenter must be told the suspected diagnosis, nature of the proposed treatment, expected outcomes, benefits and risks, and alternative treatments possible. A statement that the patient

can withdraw consent at any time should be provided, and the patient should be given an opportunity to ask questions (Guido, 2003; Marquis and Huston, 2000; O'Keefe, 2001; Pozgar, 1999; Sullivan and Decker, 2000; Swansburg and Swansburg, 2002; Yoder-Wise, 2003).

Consent is not legally required when immediate care is necessary to save the life and consent cannot be obtained either from the patient or an authorized legal representative. Constructive consent or consent implied by law is effective. Minors are not legally capable of giving valid consent to medical treatment, but minors who live apart from their parents and are married are considered emancipated and are capable of giving consent. The law presumes every adult is mentally competent until adjudicated otherwise. After people have been declared mentally incompetent in a judicial proceeding, they cannot give valid consents. When patients have been deemed clinically incompetent but not legally incompetent, nurses should seek the participation of the patient's next of kin in making decisions. When family members cannot agree, treatment should be postponed until a legal guardian is appointed with the authority to make the necessary medical decisions.

RIGHT TO REFUSE TREATMENT

Competent adults have the right to refuse treatment. That is guaranteed by the Constitution and has been tested in court cases. More recently, most states have passed statutory laws to protect the right to refuse treatment and to protect the health care provider who agrees to not treat even when treatment could be considered indicated. Those laws are related to advanced directives, living wills, and durable power of attorney (Sullivan and Decker, 2000).

Advanced directives are documents that allow the competent person to make choices such as being put on life support, stopping treatment, or refusing treatment before the need for medical treatment. Advanced directives do not need to be signed by an attorney. However, they are to be signed by two witnesses preferably who are not heirs, relatives, or physicians. They are only effective when the patient is not able to make decisions and can be changed or cancelled at any time. A *living will* is a document signed by a competent adult indicating what health care the person wants in the future. Those decisions are to be upheld even if the adult's decision-making capacity is lost. The *durable power of attorney* permits a competent adult to appoint a proxy to make decisions for that person if that person becomes incompetent. It has broader applications than a living will because it can be applied to any injury or illness that leaves a person incapacitated. Health care providers are to follow the wishes stated in these documents. In the absence of these documents, family members are asked to make those decisions. However, the family members do not have the legal authority to make those decisions unless they are legally appointed as guardians or are the parents. The Patient Self Determination Act of 1990 is a federal law that requires all health care facilities that receive Medicare or Medicaid funds to provide written information to adult patients concerning their right to make health care decisions (Sullivan and Decker, 2001). The American Nurses Association (ANA) supports the patient's right to self-determination and indicates the role of the nurse includes public education, education of the profession, in-service education of other health care providers, research, and patient care. The ANA recommends that questions about advanced directives be part of the nursing admission assessment (see www. nursingworld.org).

Do-not-resuscitate (DNR) orders state the patient will not receive cardiopulmonary resuscitation (CPR) or other aggressive treatments if the heart stops beating. It should be given to family members, the physician, and designated proxy and taken to the health care facility during admission. The order should be placed where it can be easily found during an emergency. Families often call 911 during a medical emergency. However, emergency medical staff may not be required to follow the order in some states (American Bar Association, 2001).

FREEDOM FROM CHEMICAL OR PHYSICAL RESTRAINTS

The Omnibus Budget Reconciliation Act (OBRA) of 1987 also provides patients a right to be free from chemical or physical restraints for the purpose of convenience or discipline not required to treat medical symptoms. Restraining patients without consent and sufficient justification can be interpreted as false imprisonment. This law applies to health care organizations that receive Medicare or Medicaid funds. Health care providers are to consider alternatives to restraints. Physicians' orders are to specify duration and circumstances required when using restraints on a patient. No per rate needed (PRN) restraints are allowed. Patients are to be monitored and reassessed frequently to evaluate the continued need for the restraints. Physical restraints have been associated with injuries and deaths. Psychotropic drugs, often used as chemical restraints, are no longer legal for the purpose of controlling behavior. They may only be used for diagnosis-related conditions. Psychotropic drugs have caused patients to become deeply sedated, agitated, and combative (Sullivan and Decker, 2000).

ORGAN DONATION

Congress enacted the National Organ Transplant Act (NOTA) in 1984. Consequently organ procurement organizations (OPOs) were created. They keep a list of possible recipients and train hospital staff about getting family consent. There are no costs to the organ donor for donating organs. However, the funeral and burial expenses are still the responsibilities of the donor's family. The United Network for Organ Sharing maintains a national computer list of patients waiting for transplants. Organs are offered to local patients first and then to the regional and national levels. Efforts are made to select patients regardless of their race, gender, religion, or other personal information.

Anatomical gift is the legal term for organ donations (kidneys, hearts, livers, lungs, pancreases) and tissues including corneas, eyes, bones, bone marrow, skin, and heart valves. Bone marrow and kidneys can be donated while the donor is still alive. If the person did not indicate whether organs were to be donated, the family makes the decision after the patient dies. The National Organ Transplant Act makes it illegal to buy or sell organs for profit. A child or incompetent person cannot consent to be an organ donor so that people needing organs will not be able to prey on vulnerable people.

A person must be at least 18 years old and of sound mind to be an organ donor. Removal of anatomical parts involves a surgical procedure that rarely interferes with funeral or burial arrangements. Even if a person has signed an organ donor card or indicated organ donation in an advanced directive, the next of kin will probably be asked for permission to take parts. If the next of kin refuses, the authorities will probably not remove parts even if the patient has volunteered parts. A desire to donate organs should be discussed with the family and written into advanced directives, as well as put in a will. It is usually too late to donate organs by the time the will is located (American Bar Association, 2001).

ASSISTED SUICIDE

The American Nurses Association (ANA) believes that nurses should not participate in assisted suicide or active euthanasia because such acts violate the Code for Nurses, ethical traditions, goals of the profession, and its covenant with society. Nurses have an obligation to provide compassionate and comprehensive end-of-life care that includes promotion of comfort, relief of pain, and sometimes forgoing life-sustaining treatments (see www.nursingworld.org). Hospice organizations do not endorse taking medications in doses that cause the patient's death. However, letting death come naturally does not mean the patient will not be given medication to ease the pain. Pain management is not the same as committing suicide by taking large doses of pain medications (American Bar Association, 2001).

Euthanasia is classified as active or passive. Active euthanasia is intentional and thought of as suicide. If someone helps a person take his or her own life, the person assisting could be subject to criminal sanctions for aiding and abetting suicide. Passive euthanasia occurs when life-saving measures are withdrawn or withheld, allowing the person to die a natural death. Those acts are generally accepted pursuant to legislative acts and judicial decisions (Pozgar, 1999).

PERSONNEL ISSUES

"Hatred and anger are powerless when met with kindness." —Anonymous

EMPLOYMENT-AT-WILL

Employment-at-will means that an employee is free to accept or not accept a job at will, and the employer is free to hire or discharge an employee at will for any reason. However, case law has provided exceptions to the employment-at-will doctrine for defamation, public policy issues, retaliatory discharge, contractual relationships, and fairness to the extreme that employment-at-will has little applicability today. Public policy exception is the first exception and involves cases in which an employer discharges an employee in direct conflict with public policy, such as for serving on a jury, whistle blowing by reporting the employer's illegal actions, or filing a workers' compensation claim.

There have been several court cases related to retaliation for the employer for whistle blowing, such as for speaking out against unsafe practices, reporting a violation of federal laws, or filing lawsuits against employers. In *Roulston v. Tendercare (Michigan) Inc.* (2000), a social services director was fired for confronting the director of nursing about patient abuse. The court supported the social services director's lawsuit against the nursing home for retaliation. In *UTMB v. Hohman* (1999), a nurse felt wrongfully discharged for reporting a physician's alleged abuses. In *Fleming v. Correctional Healthcare Solutions, Inc.* (2000), a nurse was discharged for reporting financial mismanagement. Both courts upheld the right for the nurses to sue for retaliation.

In *Taylor v. Memorial Health Systems, Inc.* (2000), the conditions that must be present to file a valid employer retaliation lawsuit were enumerated as "(1) The whistleblower must disclose or threaten to disclose an allegation in writing and under oath to the state department of professional regulation. (2) The allegation must have been about the activity, policy, or practice of the employer that is or was a violation of a state or federal law, rule, or regulation. (3) The employee must have given the employer written notification and reasonable time to correct the problem. (4) The employee must have suffered retaliation in the form of some actual harm (*Taylor v. Memorial Health Systems, Inc.*, 2000, p. 755)" (Guido, 2003, pp. 64-65). These may vary from state to state.

Courts may uphold implied contracts. In *Watkins v. Unemployment Compensation Board of Review* (1997) the court treated employee handbooks, company policies, and oral statements made at the time of employment as setting the employment relationship. In *Trombley v. Southwestern Vermont Medical Center* (1999) the court found the procedure for progressive discipline in the employee handbook must be followed before terminating a nurse for giving incompetent care.

Employee handbooks and departmental policy and procedure manuals are implied contracts if they are without disclaimers. Handbooks that do not contain disclaimers may alter an employer's or employee's at-will status. A disclaimer is the denial of a right that is alleged to belong to someone. In *Simonson v. Meader Distribution Co.* (1987) the court found the employer's disclaimers clear. The disclaimers included the following: "Management reserves the right to make any changes at any time by adding to, deleting, or changing any existing

policy. The rules set out below are as complete as we can reasonably make them. However, they are not necessarily all-inclusive, because circumstances that we have not anticipated may arise. Some currently unanticipated circumstances may warrant the application of discipline, including discharge. Management may vary from the above policies if, in its opinion, the circumstances require" (Pozgar, 1999, p. 472).

The purpose of the good faith and fair dealing exception is to prevent unfair or malicious termination. In *Fortune v. National Cash Register Company* (1977) an employee was discharged just before a final contract was signed for which the employee was to receive a large commission. The court found that the discharge was in bad faith to prevent payment of the commission.

The nurse manager needs to know related state and federal laws. Managers should review employee handbooks, departmental policy and procedure manuals, and recruitment materials for unwanted statements and to consider adding disclaimer clauses. Managers should take corrective action to whistleblowers' complaints and monitor the treatment of the employee after the complaint is filed, making sure that employee performance evaluations are performed according to the policies and that appropriate paperwork is in appropriate files (Guido, 2003; Pozgar, 1999).

COBRA

The Consolidated Omnibus Budget Reconciliation Act of 1985 (COBRA) is a federal law that amends the Employee Retirement Income Security Act of 1974 (ERISA), which is a federal law that controls how the employee benefit plan is administered. COBRA is a complex law that allows an employee and dependents to continue the group insurance coverage at about the same cost for a specific period of time after the employment status changed. The employer that employees 20 or more people on a typical business day and sponsors group health plans for the employees must inform the employee within 14 days of the qualifying event that the employee has the right to continue coverage under COBRA. COBRA must be elected for coverage within 60 days of the qualifying event and is retroactive to the qualifying event. Coverage by a spouse's health care plan does not disqualify a person if that person was covered before the qualifying event. If the new health care plan does not cover a preexisting condition, a person may still be able to continue on the former health plan under COBRA. Qualified beneficiaries qualify for COBRA when the employee died, was fired except for gross misconduct, had hours reduced, became divorced or legally separated, became eligible for Medicare, or the child is no longer considered a dependent under the health plan. If the person lost a job or had hours reduced, continued coverage lasts for 18 months or until the person gets other insurance. In the event of death, the spouse and dependents may pay for coverage for another 36 months. In the cases of divorce or a child no longer being a dependent, continued coverage lasts for 36 months or until the spouse or child finds other insurance (American Bar Association, 2001).

DIVERSE WORKFORCE

There are legal considerations to managing a diverse workforce. People are protected from overt and subtle discrimination by Title VII of the Civil Rights Act of 1964. People have a responsibility to be fair and just. Diversity in language, word meanings, accents, and dialects leads to misunderstanding. People from unassertive cultures may be reluctant to ask questions. Cultural differences can lead to conflict and unfulfilled expectations. Managers can learn about cultural diversity and increase their own sensitivity, role model cultural sensitivity, and develop a comprehensive cultural diversity program for staff (Marquis and Huston, 1998).

TESTIFYING

Testifying under oath can be a terrifying experience, but understanding procedures and a few rules can make the experience less stressful. Appearance is important. One should dress neatly and conventionally. A business suit is usually appropriate. If one is testifying just before, after, or during a shift, a uniform is appropriate.

A pleasant demeanor is also important. One should project a polite, sincere, and cooperative image. One should know the facts before testifying. It is appropriate to review the record, particularly the part one is responsible for. The health care agency record should never be falsified. It may be helpful to make a sketch or diagram if placement of persons and objects is important.

The court recorder records everything said, so one should enunciate clearly. Questions must be answered orally because nodding the head and other nonverbal responses are difficult to record and subject to interpretation. One is likely to be asked for personal and professional information, such as residence, age, marital status, educational background, grades received, and employment history. One should be sure the question is understood before answering it. Making an inaccurate response because the question was not understood can adversely affect the outcomes. Pausing before answering the question is appropriate to formulate an answer and to allow time for an attorney to raise objections. If the attorney objects to a question, one should refrain from responding until the issue is resolved. The lawyer will direct the witness if an answer is required. One should keep answers brief, tell the truth, and answer only the question asked. One should try to give favorable facts and avoid questionable words such as think, guess, and maybe. Sometimes matters of amount, distance, and time are crucial. One should not be forced into guessing. If unable to make a reliable judgment, "I don't know" is an appropriate response. When asked to identify an exhibit such as a medical record, one should scrutinize it carefully and indicate whether it is recognized or not. Whoever calls one as a witness has the first opportunity to ask questions. Afterward, the opposing party's attorney has the opportunity to ask questions (Kilmon, 1985; O'Keefe, 2001; Pozgar, 1999).

EXPERT WITNESSES

Because malpractice litigation has increased and physicians are serving as expert witnesses for nursing less than they did before the 1970s, nurses are increasingly acting as expert witnesses. Some state nurses associations are developing resource banks of nurse expert witnesses. Nurses may need to submit a letter of intent describing their qualifications as a nurse expert, resume, and letters of reference. Some state nurses associations provide continuing education regarding legal issues and being an expert witness to ensure a pool of adequately prepared expert witnesses.

Attorneys often want to meet experts before selecting them. They also need resumes and letters of reference. Attorneys often contact experts by telephone and provide brief case summaries. Then the nurse must decide which cases to accept. The case must match the expert's area of expertise. Experts should review only records that are within their specialty. The expert compares the facts of the case with standards of care and offers a professional opinion. The expert should understand clearly whether the attorney wants the expert to defend the nurse or dispute the nurse's credibility. The cases selected should not involve matters concerning places where the expert has worked or people with whom the expert has worked because the issue of bias could be raised. Fees negotiated should include time required to review the records, write a report, and provide testimony (Pozgar, 1999; Salmond, 1986).

Chapter Summary

Chapter 15 covered the following:

History of Continuous Quality Improvement
Quality Management Heroes
Continuous Quality Improvement
    Tools and Processes for Continuous Quality
        Improvement
Program Evaluation

Calendar of Events
Committee Selection and Functions
Conceptual Framework
Review of the Literature
Program Evaluation Model
Instrument Development
Sources of Internal and External
    Invalidity
Research Designs
    Experimental designs
    Quasiexperimental designs
Methods of Data Collection
Sampling
Analysis of Data
Evidence-Based Nursing
History of Regulatory Influences
Joint Commission on Accreditation of
    Healthcare Organizations
Outcome and Assessment Information Set
Risk Management
Customer Satisfaction
Safety and Security
    National Safety Council
    Occupational Safety and Health Act
Sources of law
Categories of Law
Liability Control
Liability Issues
    Nurse Licensure
    Nurse Practice Acts
    Nursing Standards
Patient Care Issues
    Patient's Bill of Rights
    Informed Consent
    Right to Refuse Treatment
    Freedom From Chemical or Physical
        Restraints
    Organ Donation
    Assisted Suicide
Personnel Issues
    Employment-at-Will
    COBRA
    Diverse Workforce
Testifying
Expert Witnesses

On-line Resources

evolve Additional critical thinking activities, worksheets, and case studies are available on-line at http://evolve.elsevier.com/Marriner/guide/

References

Aguayo R: *Dr. Deming: The American who taught the Japanese about quality,* New York, 1990, Carol Publishing.

American Bar Association: *Complete and easy guide to health care law,* New York, 2001, Three Rivers Press.

American Nurses Association: *Nursing care report card for acute care,* Washington, DC, 1995, The Association.

American Nurses Association: *Nursing quality indicators: Definitions and implications,* Washington, DC, 1996a, The Association.

American Nurses Association: *Nursing quality indicators: Guide for implementation,* Washington, DC, 1996b, The Association.

American Nurses Association: *Standards of clinical nursing practice,* ed 2, Washington, DC, 1998, The Association.

Ammerman M: *The root cause analysis handbook,* Portland, Ore, 1998, Productivity.

Band WA: *Touchstones: Ten new ideas revolutionizing business,* New York, 1994, John Wiley & Sons.

Bernzweig EP: *The nurse's liability for malpractice: A programmed course,* ed 6, St Louis, 1996, Mosby.

Berwick DM: Sounding board: Continuous quality improvement as the ideal in health care, *N Engl J Med* 320(1):53-56, 1989.

Brassard M, Ritter D: *The memory jogger II,* Methuen, Mass, 1994, GOAL/PAC.

Burns N, Grove SK: *The practice of nursing research: Conduct, critique, & utilization,* ed 4, Philadelphia, 2001, WB Saunders.

Campbell DT, Stanley JC: *Experimental and quasi-experimental designs for research,* Chicago, 1963, Rand McNally.

Cherry B, Jacob SR: *Contemporary nursing; Issues, trends, & management,* St Louis, 2002, Mosby.

CMS Website, accessed June 1, 2003.

Cofer JI, Greeley HP: *Continuous quality improvement for health information management,* Marblehead, Mass, 1998, Opus Communications.

Craig JV, Smyth RL: *The evidence-based practice manual for nurses,* St Louis, 2002, Churchill Livingstone.

Crosby PB: *Completeness: Quality for the 21st century,* New York, 1992, Dutton.

Crosby PB: *Let's talk quality,* New York, 1989, McGraw-Hill.

Crosby PB: *Quality is free: The art of making quality certain,* New York, 1992, Mentor Books.

Crosby PB: *Quality without tears: The art of hassle-free management,* New York, 1995, McGraw-Hill.

Deming WE: *Quality, productivity, and competitive position,* Cambridge, Mass, 1982, Massachusetts Institute of Technology Press.

Donabedian A: Criteria and standards for quality assessment and monitoring, *Qual Rev Bull* 3:99-108, 1986.

Fleming v Correctional Healthcare Solutions, Inc, 751 A2d 1035 (NJ), 2000.

Fortune v National Cash Register Company, 272 Mass 96, 264 NE2d 1251, 1977.

Fuller J: *Managing performance improvement projects: Preparing, planning, and implementing,* San Francisco, 1997, Pfeiffer.

Gift RG, Mosel D: *Benchmarking in health care: A collaborative approach,* Chicago, 1994, American Hospital Publishing.

Grohar-Murray ME, DiCroce HR: *Leadership and management in nursing,* Stamford, Conn, 2003, Appleton & Lange.

Gross v Allen, 22 Cal App 4th 354, 1994.

Guido GW: Legal and ethical issues. In Yoder-Wise P: *Leading and managing in nursing,* St Louis, 2003, Mosby.

Hagan J: *Management of quality: Strategies to improve quality and the bottom line,* New York, 1994, Business One Irwin.

Hamer S, Collinson G: *Achieving evidence-based practice: A handbook for practitioners,* St Louis, 1999, Bailliere Tindall.

Hammer M: *Beyond reengineering: How the process-centered organization is changing our work and our lives,* New York, 1996, Harper Business.

Health Care Financing Administration: *OASIS overview* (http://www.hcfa.gov/medicare/hsqb/oasis/hhoview.htm), accessed Feb 18, 1999.

Joint Commission on Accreditation of Healthcare Organizations: *BOJ's guide to 1999 standards and scoring.*

Joint Commission on Accreditation of Healthcare Organizations: *CAMH: Comprehensive accreditation manual for hospitals—The official handbook, CAMH Updates,* Oakbrook Terrace, Ill, Jan 1998–Feb 1999, The Commission.

Judge v Rockford Memorial Hospital, 150 NE 2d 202 (Ill App Ct), 1958.

Juran JM: *Juran on leadership for quality: An executive handbook,* New York, 1989, Free Press.

Juran JM: *Juran on planning for quality,* New York, 1988, Free Press.

Juran JM: *Juran on quality by design: The new steps for planning quality into goods and services,* New York, 1992, Free Press.

Juran JM: Product quality: A prescription for the West. I. Training and improvement programs, *Man Rev* 70: 8-14, 1981.

Juran JM, Goyna FM Jr, Bingham RS Jr, editors: *Quality control handbook,* New York, 1988, McGraw-Hill.

Kavianian JR, Wentz CA: *Occupational and environmental safety engineering and management,* New York, 1997, John Wiley & Sons.

Kelly-Heidenthal P: Nursing leadership and management. Clifton Park, New York, 2003, Delmar.

Killion SW, Dempski KM: *Legal and ethical issues,* Thorofare, NJ, 2000, Slack.

Kilmon EL: Do you swear to tell the truth? *Nurs Econ* 3:98-102, March-April 1985.

Koch MW, Fairly TM: *Integrated quality management: The key to improving nursing care quality,* St Louis, 1993, Mosby.

Lerbinger O: *The crisis manager: Facing risk and responsibility,* Mahwah, NJ, 1997, Lawrence Erlbaum Associates.

Marquis BL, Huston CJ: *Leadership roles and management functions in nursing: Theory and application,* ed 2, Philadelphia, 2000, Lippincott.

Marquis BL, Huston CJ: *Management decision making for nurses: 124 case studies,* Philadelphia, 1998, Lippincott.

Martin P, Tate K: *Project management memory jogger,* Methuen, Mass, 1997, GOAL/PAC.

McCloskey LA, Collett DN: *A primer guide to total quality management,* Salem, NH, 1993, GOAL/QPC.

McDermott RE, Mikulak RJ, Beauregard MR: *The basics of FMEA,* Portland, Ore, 1996, Productivity.

Mears P: *Healthcare teams: Building continuous quality improvements,* Delray Beach, Fla, 1994, St Lucie Press.

National League for Nursing: *National League for Nursing 1998 annual report,* New York, 1998, The League.

Oddo F, editor: *Coach's guide to the memory jogger II,* Methuen, Mass, 1995, GOAL/QPC.

O'Keefe ME: *Nursing practice and the law: Avoiding malpractice and other legal risks,* Philadelphia, 2001, FA Davis Co.

Olson v Molland, 232 NW 625 (Minn), 1930.

Pape TM: Searching for the final answer: Factors contributing to medication administration errors, *J Contin Educ Nurs* 32(4):152-160, 2001.

Phillips JJ: *Handbook of training evaluation and measurement methods,* ed 3, Houston, 1997, Gulf.

Polit DF, Beck CT, Hunger BP: *Essentials of nursing research: Methods, appraisals, and utilization,* Philadelphia, 2001, Lippincott.

Pozgar GD: *Legal aspects of health care administration,* ed 7, Gaithersburg, Md, 1999, Aspen.

Ritter D, Brassard M: *The creativity tools memory jogger: A pocket guide for creative thinking,* Lawrence, Mass, 1998, GOAL/PAC.

Rocchiccioli JT, Tilbury MS: *Clinical leadership in nursing,* Philadelphia, 1998, WB Saunders.

Roulston v Tendercare (Michigan), Inc, 608 NW 2d 525 (Mich App), 2000.

Saba VK, McCormick KA: *Essentials of computers for nurses: Information for the new millennium,* ed 3, New York, 2000, McGraw-Hill/Appleton & Lange.

Salmond SW: Serving as an expert witness, *Nurs Econ* 4:236-239, Sept-Oct 1986.

Sandras WA: *Just-in-time: Making it happen,* New York, 1995, John Wiley & Sons.

Sherman VC: *Raising standards in American health care: Best people, best practices, best results,* San Francisco, 1999, Jossey-Bass.

Smith P, James T, Lorentzon M, et al: *Shaping the facts. Evidence-based nursing and health care.* St. Louis, 2004, Churchill Livingstone.

Smith R: *The 7 levels of change: Create, innovate and motivate with the secrets of the world's largest corporations,* Arlington, Tex, 1997, Summit.

Stowell DM: *Sales, marketing, and continuous improvement: Six best practices to achieve revenue growth and increase customer loyalty,* San Francisco, 1997, Jossey-Bass.

Sullivan EJ, Decker PJ: *Effective leadership and management in nursing,* ed 5, Upper Saddle River, NJ, 2001, Prentice Hall.

Sullivan GH, Mattera MD, editors: *RN's legally speaking,* Montvale, NJ, 1997, Medical Economics.

Swansburg RC, Swansburg RJ: *Introductory management and leadership for nurses: An interactive text,* ed 3, Boston, 2002, Jones and Bartlett.

Tarasoff v Regents of the University of California, 17 Cal 3d 425, 444, 1976.

Taylor v Memorial Health Systems, Inc, 770 So2d 752 (Fla App), 2000.

Thomas PR, Gallace LJ, Martin KR: *Quality alone is not enough,* New York, 1992, American Management Association.

Trombley v Southwestern Vermont Medical Center, 738 A2d 103 (Vt), 1999.

Tucker SM, Canobbio MM, Paquette EV, Wells MF: *Patient care standards: Collaborative planning & nursing interventions,* St Louis, 2000, Mosby.

UTMB v Hohman, 6 SW 3d 767 (Tex App), 1999.

Walton M: *The Deming management method,* New York, 1986, Putnam.

Walton M: *Deming management at work,* New York, 1990, Putnam's Sons.

Watkins v Unemployment Compensation Board of Review, 689 A2d 1019 (Pa Commonwealth), 1997.

Weidman v Ketcham, 15, NW 2d 426 (NY), 1938.

Wheatley M: *Understanding just in time,* Hauppauge, NY, 1997, Barron's.

White House Domestic Policy Council: *Health security: The president's report to the American people,* Washington, DC, 1993, The Council.

Yoder-Wise PS: *Leading and managing in nursing,* ed 3, St Louis, 2003, Mosby.

Yount L: *Patients' rights in the age of managed care,* New York, 2001, Facts On File, Inc.

Index

Page numbers followed by f indicate figures; t, tables; b, boxes.

Notes

Notes

Notes

Notes

Notes

Notes

Notes